THE CARDIOLOGY COMPANION
A Socratic Approach to Clinical Insights

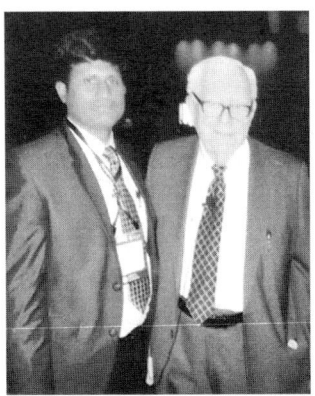

Prabir Kumar Das with Eugene Braunwald in Washington DC, USA during the 63rd Annual Scientific Conference of American College of Cardiology and Convocation for Fellow of American College of Cardiology (FACC) in 2013.

THE CARDIOLOGY COMPANION
A Socratic Approach to Clinical Insights

Third Edition

Prabir Kumar Das
MBBS FCPS (Int Med) MD (Cardio) FACC (USA) FCSI
Professor and Former Head
Department of Cardiology
Chittagong Medical College
Bangladesh

Foreword
Abdul Malik

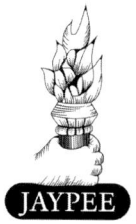

JAYPEE BROTHERS MEDICAL PUBLISHERS
The Health Sciences Publisher
New Delhi | London

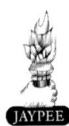 **Jaypee Brothers Medical Publishers (P) Ltd**

Headquarters
EMCA House, 23/23-B
Ansari Road, Daryaganj
New Delhi 110 002, India
Landline: +91-11-23272143, +91-11-23272703
+91-11-23282021, +91-11-23245672
e-mail: jaypee@jaypeebrothers.com

Corporate Office
4838/24, Ansari Road, Daryaganj
New Delhi 110 002, India
Phone: +91-11-43574357
Fax: +91-11-43574314
e-mail: jaypee@jaypeebrothers.com

Overseas Office
JP Medical Ltd
83 Victoria Street, London
SW1H 0HW (UK)
Phone: +44-20 3170 8910
e-mail: info@jpmedpub.com

EU GPSR Authorised Representative
Logos Europe, 9 rue Nicolas Poussin
17000, La Rochelle, France
Phone: +33 (0) 6 67 93 73 78
e-mail: contact@logoseurope.eu

Website: www.jaypeebrothers.com
Website: www.jaypeedigital.com

© 2026, Jaypee Brothers Medical Publishers

The views and opinions expressed in this book are solely those of the original contributor(s)/author(s) and do not necessarily represent those of editor(s) or publisher of the book.

All rights reserved. No part of this publication may be reproduced, stored or transmitted in any form or by any means, electronic, mechanical, photocopying, recording or otherwise, without the prior permission in writing of the publishers.

All brand names and product names used in this book are trade names, service marks, trademarks or registered trademarks of their respective owners. The publisher is not associated with any product or vendor mentioned in this book.

Medical knowledge and practice change constantly. This book is designed to provide accurate, authoritative information about the subject matter in question. However, readers are advised to check the most current information available on procedures included and check information from the manufacturer of each product to be administered, to verify the recommended dose, formula, method and duration of administration, adverse effects and contraindications. It is the responsibility of the practitioner to take all appropriate safety precautions. Neither the publisher nor the author(s)/editor(s) assume any liability for any injury and/or damage to persons or property arising from or related to use of material in this book.

This book is sold on the understanding that the publisher is not engaged in providing professional medical services. If such advice or services are required, the services of a competent medical professional should be sought.

Every effort has been made where necessary to contact holders of copyright to obtain permission to reproduce copyright material. If any have been inadvertently overlooked, the publisher will be pleased to make the necessary arrangements at the first opportunity.

Inquiries for bulk sales may be solicited at: jaypee@jaypeebrothers.com

The Cardiology Companion: A Socratic Approach to Clinical Insights

Third Edition: **2026**

ISBN: 978-93-6616-007-8

Printed at: Samrat Offset Pvt. Ltd.

Dedicated to
*My father (late) Chitta Ranjan Das,
mother (late) Chaya Rani Das*

Foreword

Cardiovascular diseases are the leading cause of morbidity and mortality in Bangladesh. With economic development, increasing urbanization, and population aging, heart diseases are increasing alarmingly here. Last few decades witnessed a tremendous development in the field of management of heart diseases in our country. Management of heart diseases needs a holistic approach including proper clinical assessment, investigation before offering drug treatment, intervention, surgery, etc. Also, appropriate preventive measures are important to handle heart diseases in the community. Heart diseases in our country have some unique features which, to some extent, differ from that in western countries. These features are described in question-and-answer format in this book. I feel delighted to see Prabir Kumar Das, one of my students of MD (Cardiology) of late 1980s in the National Institute of Cardiovascular Diseases, Dhaka the time while I was its Director, is going to publish the remarkable book *Cardiology Query*. In this book, the author has done a masterful job of finding out the queries on various aspects of cardiology and providing up-to-date solution of these queries. All current issues of cardiology have been covered, including queries related to ongoing COVID-19 and the heart. A separate chapter on Heart Diseases in South Asians presents the unique attributes of heart diseases among peoples in this geographical teritory. Keeping pace with the rapid development in the field of cardiology new chapters with interest on current issues have been included. I believe this edition will be of immense help to students of various postgraduate courses including MD (Cardiology), Diploma in Cardiology, FCPS (Cardiology), FCPS (Internal Medicine), MRCP, and others. Also, undergraduate medical students interested in cardiology will be benefited. This will contribute to enrich the bulk of published book in the field of cardiology in our country. The book has been presented in question-answer format, a Socretian method of learning, i.e., learning by recognizing one's own ignorance.

I congratulate the author and strongly recommend it, which will be interesting and valuable resource to cardiology residents, clinicians, specialists, generalists, trainees at all levels, and also teachers and apply the information in the care of patients with heart diseases.

Abdul Malik
MBBS (Dhaka) MRCP (UK) FCCP (USA) FCPS (BD)
FRCP (Glasgow) FRCP (Edin) FACC (USA)
National Professor Brig (Retd)
President, National Heart Foundation
and Research Institute, Bangladesh

Preface to the Third Edition

After wide acceptance of the second edition of the book by students of cardiology of Bangladesh at both postgraduate and undergraduate level, the third edition is made available within a short span of time by M/s Jaypee Brothers Medical Publishers (P) Ltd, New Delhi, India. This new edition is intended to reach the readers of various countries of the world. With the aim to make it more appealing and self-explanatory, the new title of the book is coined. *The Cardiology Companion: A Socratic Approach to Clinical Insights* is expected to generate global interest of the readers of cardiology and stimulate their clinical insight. Heart diseases being a rapidly increasing health problem with having some special attributes here, a separate chapter is dedicated on these aspects. The book is written on Socretian method of learning, i.e., learning by identifying one's own ignorance. The book has been designed making a comprehensive overview of all aspects of cardiology starting with the age-old clinical to modern interventional and preventive aspects. A new chapter on Application of Artificial Intelligence in the field of cardiology has been added with a step toward recent advancement in cardiology. Other chapters are also rewritten keeping pace with the latest advancement in the field of cardiology.

I am thankful to M/s Jaypee Brothers Medical Publishers (P) Ltd, New Delhi, for publishing the third edition of the book and their sincere effort in making it available globally. I strongly believe that this will go a long way to disseminate the message of the book to large groups of readers in various countries of the world.

Prabir Kumar Das

Preface to the First Edition

"Question and Answer" is the way whereby wisdom could be learned by recognizing one's own ignorance. Socrete's own particular style of teaching was by question and answers. He is still recognized as the master of those who know.

Cardiology being a fast-growing area in Medicine queries on various issues in cardiology and their solution may make its learning exciting, enjoyable, and easy. It may also help in self-assessment. About 900 queries on different aspects of cardiology in 31 chapters have been met that include 130 summary tables and 100 figures. Each chapter starts with an introductory comment and a quotation relevant to the topic. *Cardiology Query* will be a basic review for the students of cardiology, as well as cardiologists. Queries regarding basic aspects of cardiology, clinical, interventional, and preventive cardiology have been given in a comparative format. Efforts are made to incorporate all current issues with a list of further reading and references at the end of each chapter, which may help the readers in getting extended information on relevant topics. A separate chapter on Heart Diseases in South Asians is included to highlight the unique features of heart diseases among this populations.

I hope this book will stimulate the thinking process of the readers and they will be encouraged to learn more.

Prabir Kumar Das

Contents

1. Anatomy and Physiology of Cardiovascular System 1
2. Symptoms and Signs of Cardiovascular Disease 4
3. Investigations and Procedures 22
4. Coronary Artery Disease 82
5. Acute Rheumatic Fever and Chronic Rheumatic Heart Disease 136
6. Valvular Heart Diseases 144
7. Congenital Heart Diseases 188
8. Infective Endocarditis 223
9. Diseases of Myocardium 233
10. Pericardial Diseases 248
11. Hypertension 259
12. Heart Failure and Cardiogenic Shock 272
13. Cardiac Arrhythmias 295
14. Cardiac Arrest and Sudden Cardiac Death 320
15. Syncope and Hypotension 332
16. Cardiac Pacing (Including Implantable Cardioverter Defibrillator, Cardiac Resynchronization Therapy and EP Study) 337
17. Cardiac Pharmacology 359
18. Interventional Cardiology 394
19. Diseases of the Aorta 415
20. Pulmonary Heart Diseases (Pulmonary Embolism, Cor Pulmonale, and Sleep Disordered Breathing) 421
21. Peripheral Vascular Diseases 432
22. Diabetes and Heart Diseases 438
23. Pregnancy and Heart Disease 444
24. Renal Diseases and the Heart 450
25. Cerebrovascular Diseases and the Heart 454

26. Anesthesia, Surgery, and Heart Diseases 461
27. Neoplastic Heart Disease and Cardio-oncology 464
28. Air Pollution, Toxins, and the Heart 468
29. Traumatic Heart Disease 472
30. Genetics and Heart Diseases 474
31. Heart Diseases in the Elderly: Geriatric Cardiology 478
32. Heart Diseases in Women 483
33. Systemic Diseases Involving the Heart 489
34. Heart Diseases in South Asia 495
35. Artificial Intelligence in Cardiology 501
36. Preventive Cardiology 509

Index 515

Abbreviations

A_2	:	Aortic Component of Second Heart Sound
ABP	:	Ambulatory Blood Pressure
ACC	:	American College of Cardiology
ACEI	:	Angiotensin Converting Enzyme Inhibitor
ACS	:	Acute Coronary Syndrome
ADA	:	American Diabetic Association
AF	:	Atrial Fibrillation
AHA	:	American Heart Association
AICD	:	Automatic Implantable Cardioverter Defibrillator
AKI	:	Acute Kidney Injury
ALCAPA	:	Anomalous Left Coronary Artery from Pulmonary Artery
ALS	:	Advanced Life Support
AMI	:	Acute Myocardial Infarction
AML	:	Anterior Mitral Leaflet
AMP	:	Adenosine Monophosphate
Ao	:	Aorta/Aortic
AoV	:	Aortic Valve
A-P	:	Antero-posterior
AP	:	Aorto-pulmonary
APTT	:	Activated Partial Thromboplastin Time
AR	:	Aortic Regurgitation
ARF	:	Acute Rheumatic Fever
AS	:	Aortic Stenosis
ASCVD	:	Atherosclerotic Cardiovascular Disease
ASD	:	Atrial Septal Defect
ASO	:	Antistreptolysin-O Titer
AT	:	Angiotensinogen
ATP	:	Adult Treatment Panel
A-V	:	Arteriovenous
AV	:	Atrioventricular
AVD	:	Aortic Valve Disease
AVNRT	:	Atrioventricular Nodal Re-entrant Tachycardia
AVR	:	Aortic Valve Replacement
AVRT	:	Atrioventricular Re-entrant Tachycardia
BB	:	Beta(b)-blocker
BLS	:	Basic Life Support
BMI	:	Body Mass Index
BMS	:	Bare Metal Stent
BMV	:	Balloon Mitral Valvuloplasty
BP	:	Blood Pressure
BPM	:	Beats Per Minute

CABG	:	Coronary Artery Bypass Grafting
CABS	:	Coronary Artery Bypass Surgery
CAD	:	Coronary Artery Disease
CADI	:	Coronary Artery Disease in Indians
CAG	:	Coronary Angiography
CCB	:	Calcium Channel Blocker
CCF	:	Congestive Heart Failure
CCR	:	Cardiocerebral Resuscitation
CCU	:	Coronary Care Unit
CeVD	:	Cerebrovascular Disease
CFI	:	Color Flow Imaging
CHB	:	Complete Heart Block
CHD	:	Congenital Heart Disease
CHF	:	Chronic Heart Failure
CKD	:	Chronic Kidney Disease
CK-MB	:	Creatine Phosphokinase (MB Isoform)
CM	:	Cardiomyopathy
CMC	:	Closed Mitral Commissurotomy
CMV	:	Closed mitral valvuloplasty
CNS	:	Central Nervous System
CO_2	:	Carbon Dioxide
COP	:	Cardiac Output
COPD	:	Chronic Obstructive Pulmonary Disease
CPAP	:	Continuous Positive Airway Pressure
CPB	:	Cardiopulmonary Bypass
CPR	:	Cardiopulmonary Resuscitation
CRP	:	C-reactive Protein
CRT	:	Cardiac Resynchronization Therapy
CS	:	Coronary Sinus
CSC	:	Canadian Cardiovascular Society (Functional Class)
CSM	:	Carotid Sinus Massage
CT	:	Computed Tomography
CVD	:	Cardiovascular Disease
CVP	:	Central Venous Pressure
CVS	:	Cardiovascular System
CWD	:	Continuous Wave Doppler
CXR	:	Chest X-ray
D1, D2	:	First and Second Diagonal Branches (of LAD)
DBP	:	Diastolic Blood Pressure
DC shock	:	Direct Current Shock
DCA	:	Directional Coronary Atherectomy
DCM	:	Dilated Cardiomyopathy
DE	:	Dimensional Echo (2-DE)
DES	:	Drug Eluted Stent

DFG	: Deoxy-fluro Glucose
DIC	: Disseminated Intravascular Coagulation
DM	: Diabetes Mellitus
DORV	: Double Outlet Right Ventricle
DPPI	: Dipeptidyl Peptidase Inhibitor
DTA	: Descending Throcic Aorta
DVD	: Double Vessel Disease
DVR	: Double Valve Replacement
DVT	: Deep Vein Thrombosis
ECG	: Electrocardiogram
Echo	: Echocardiography
ED	: Emergency Department
EDM	: Early Diastolic Murmur
EDP	: End Diastolic Pressure
EDRF	: Endothelium Dependent Relaxation Factor
EDV	: End Diastolic Volume
EEG	: Electroencephalogram
EF	: Ejection Fraction
EJV	: External Jugular Vein
ELISA	: Enzyme-linked Immunosorbent Assay
EMD	: Electomechanical Dissociation
EPS	: Electrophysiological Study
ERC	: European Resuscitation Council
ESC	: European Society of Cardiology
ESM	: Ejection Systolic Murmur
ESR	: Erythrocyte Sedimentation Rate
ETT	: Exercise Treadmill Test/Exercise Tolerance Test
F	: French (Diameter of Catheter)
FBG	: Fasting Blood Glucose
FDG	: Fluro Deoxy-Glucose
FDP	: Fibrin Degradation Product
FFA	: Free Fatty Acid
FFR	: Fractional Flow Reserve
FH	: Familial Hypercholesterolemia
FMC	: First Medical Contact
FPG	: Fasting Plasma Glucose
GAS	: Group A *Streptococcus*
GFR	: Glomerular Filtration Rate
GLP	: Glucagon like Peptide
GP	: Glycoprotein
GTN	: Glyceryl Trinitrate
H(O)CM	: Hypertrophic (Obstructive) Cardiomyopathy
Hb	: Hemoglobin
HB	: His Bundle

HDL	:	High Density Lipoprotein
HIT	:	Heparin-induced Thrombocytopenia
HIV	:	Human Immunodeficiency Virus
HMG	:	4-hydroxy 3-methoxy Glutaryl CoA
HR	:	Heart Rate
HRT	:	Hormone Replacement Therapy
HTN	:	Hypertension
H-V	:	His-ventricular
IABP	:	Intra-aortic Balloon Pump
ICD	:	Implantable Cardioverter Defibrillator
ICH	:	Intracerebral Hemorrhage
ICM	:	Ischemic Cardiomyopathy
ICU	:	Intensive Care Unit
IE	:	Infective Endocarditis
IFG	:	Impaired Fasting Glucose
IGT	:	Impaired Glucose Tolerance
IHD	:	Ischemic Heart Disease
IJV	:	Internal Jugular Vein
IM	:	Intramuscular
INR	:	International Normalized Ratio
IPPV	:	Intermittent Positive Pressure Ventilation
ISA	:	Intrinsic Sympathomimetic Activity
ISI	:	International Sensitivity Index
IV	:	Intravenous
IVC	:	Inferior Vena Vava
IVS	:	Interventricular Septum
IVUS	:	Intravascular Ultrasound
JNC	:	Joint National Committee
JVP	:	Jugular Venous Pressure
K$^+$	:	Potassium
LA	:	Left Atrium
LAA	:	Left Atrial Appendage
LDL	:	Low Density Lipoprotein
LIMA	:	Left Internal Mammary Artery
LMC	:	Left Main Coronary Artery
LMWH	:	Low Molecular Weight Heparin
LP(a)	:	Lipoprotein(a)
LV	:	Left Ventricle
LVAD	:	Left Ventricular Assist Device
LVEDP	:	Left Ventricular End-diastolic Pressure
LVEF	:	Left Ventricular Ejection Fraction
LVF	:	Left Ventricular Failure
LVH	:	Left Ventricular Hypertrophy
LVIDd	:	Left Ventricular Internal Dimension at End Diastole

LVIDs	:	Left Ventricular Internal Dimension at End Systole
LVOT	:	Left Ventricular Outflow Tract
METs	:	Metabolic Equivalents
MetS	:	Metabolic Syndrome
MI	:	Myocardial Infarction
MPI	:	Myocardial Perfusion Imaging
MR	:	Mitral Regurgitation
MRA	:	Magnetic Resonance Angiogram
MRI	:	Magnetic Resonance Imaging
MS	:	Mitral Stenosis
MUGA	:	Multigated Acquisition
MVO	:	Mitral Valve Orifice
MVP	:	Mitral Valve Prolapse
MVR	:	Mitral Valve Replacement
NCEP	:	National Cholesterol Education Program
OCT	:	Optical Coherence Tomography
OGTT	:	Oral Glucose Tolerance Test
OMI	:	Old Myocardial Infarction
OMV	:	Open Mitral Valvuloplasty
PA	:	Pulmonary Artery
PAD	:	Peripheral Arterial Disease
PAPVC	:	Partial Anomalous Pulmonary Venous Connection
PCI	:	Percutaneous Coronary Intervention
PCWP	:	Pulmonary Capillary Wedge Pressure
PDA	:	Patent Ductus Arteriosus
PE	:	Pericardial Effusion
PEA	:	Pulseless Electrical Activity
PEm	:	Pulmonary Embolism
PET	:	Positron Emission Tomography
PFO	:	Patent Foramen Ovale
POBA	:	Percutaneous Old Balloon Angioplasty
PS	:	Pulmonary Stenosis
PSVT	:	Paroxysmal Supraventricular Tachycardia
PT	:	Prothrombin Time
PTCA	:	Percutaneous Transluminal Coronary Angioplasty
PV	:	Pulmonary Valve
PVC	:	Premature Ventricular Contraction
PVD	:	Peripheral Vascular Disease
PVR	:	Pulmonary Vascular Resistance
PWD	:	Pulse Wave Doppler
QWMI	:	Q Wave Myocardial Infarction
RA	:	Right Atrium
Rt-PA	:	Recombinant Tissue Plasminogen Activator
RVH	:	Right Ventricular Hypertrophy

RVI	:	Right Ventricular Infarction
RVOT	:	Right Ventricular Outflow Tract
SA	:	Sinoatrial
SK	:	Streptokinase
SV	:	Single Ventricle
SVC	:	Superior Vena Cava
SVD	:	Single Vessel Disease
SVG	:	Sephenous Vein Graft
TAPVC	:	Total Anomalous Pulmonary Venous Connection
TAVI	:	Transcatheter Aortic Valve Implantation
TAVR	:	Transcatheter Aortic Valve Replacement
TB	:	Tuberculosis
TG	:	Triglyceride
Tn I	:	Troponin I
TOD	:	Target Organ Damage
TR	:	Tricuspid Regurgitation
TV	:	Tricuspid Valve
TxA2	:	Thromboxane A2
UFH	:	Unfractionated Heparin

CHAPTER 1

Anatomy and Physiology of Cardiovascular System

"Blood by the beat of the ventricles flows through the lungs and heart and is pumped to the whole body."
—Willium Herbey (1578–1657)

■ INTRODUCTION

The heart is situated in the middle mediastinum, partially overlapped by the neighboring lungs. It is conical in shape. Its base is above and faces backward and to the right, and the apex is downward, facing forward and to the left. The heart has its own automaticity and rhythmicity.

Q1. What are the components of cardiovascular system (CVS)? Give its functions.

Ans. Components of CVS:
- The heart provides the driving force for the CVS.
- Arteries serve as distribution channels to the organs.
- Microcirculation capillaries serve as the exchange region.
- Veins serve as blood reservoirs and collect blood to return to the heart.

The primary function of CVS is convection, i.e., mass movement of fluid is caused by a difference in pressure between two points. It:
- Distributes substrates and O_2 to all body cells.
- Controls blood flow to the skin and extremities to enhance or retard heat transfer to the environment.
- Distributes hormones to distant sites.
- Aids in body defense mechanisms by delivering antibodies, leukocytes, and platelets to different areas of the body.

Q2. What is the difference between the left and the right ventricles—structurally and functionally?

Ans. Left ventricle (LV) pumps blood through the systemic circulation. It is cylindrical in shape and has a three-times thicker wall than does the right ventricle (RV). It ejects blood, primarily by reducing the cross-sectional area of the cylinder (area = πr^2, i.e., change in volume area is function of change in the radius squired). The LV works much harder than the RV because of the higher pressure in the systemic circulation. Consequently, the LV is more commonly affected by disease process than the RV **(Fig. 1.1)**.

Right ventricle pumps relatively large volumes of blood at low pressure through the pulmonary circulation. The RV ejects blood by the concurrent

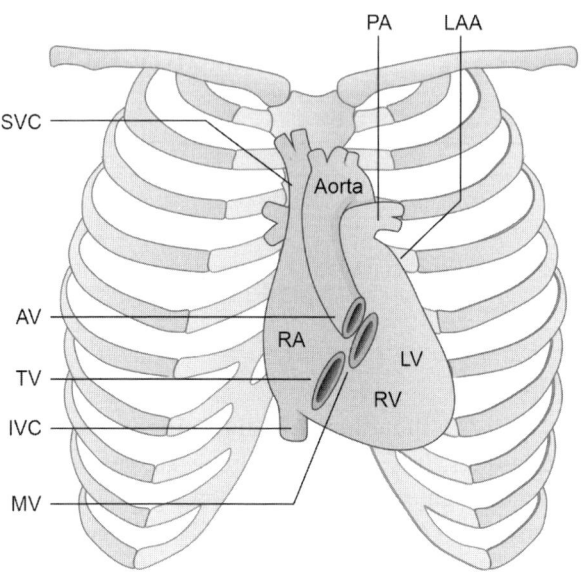

Fig. 1.1: The heart chambers, great vessels, and valve location. (AV: aortic valve; IVC: inferior vena cava; LAA: left atrial appendage; MV: mitral valve; PA: pulmonary artery; RA: right atrium; RV: right ventricle; LV: left ventricle; SVC: superior vena cava; TV: tricuspid valve)

shortening of the free wall and bulging of IVS into the RV (The bellow's function). The normal cross-sectional area of RV is crescent shaped. If the RV must eject blood against high pressure for prolonged periods (as seen in pulmonary hypertension), it assumes a much more cylindrical appearance, and there is thickening of RV free wall, i.e., in right ventricular hypertrophy (RVH).

Q3. What are the special features of coronary circulation?
Ans.
- The right and the left coronary arteries distribute blood in large part but not exclusively to their own half of the heart. Coronary arteries are compressed by the contracting myocardium during systole (a distinctive feature). Blood flow in the coronary artery is maximal during diastole and minimal during systole. During systole, no pressure difference does exist between the myocardium and LV, hence flow is not possible. During diastole, a pressure difference does exist, and the elasticity of the aorta propels blood through the coronary circulation.
- Normally, hemoglobin releases approximately 50% of its arterial O_2 content to the myocardium. This is in contrast to the remainder of the body at rest, where hemoglobin releases only approximately 25% of its O_2 content.
- As almost all O_2 is extracted during passage through capillaries in myocardium, coronary sinus blood is completely desaturated. Thus,

the heart cannot call upon a venous O_2 reserve when facing increased demands, e.g., during exercise and is largely dependent upon the ability of the coronary vasodilatation. Release of adenosine (from degradation of AMP by 5'-nucleotidase) produces an extremely strong vasodilator response.
- Coronary arteries are functional end arteries. Small anastomosis existing are of no functional importance, i.e., these are not enough to maintain blood supply when one is occluded (thus prevent infarction). In the face of chronic ischemia, these anastomoses enlarge and establish collateral supply to the affected area, which is often essential for its viability.
- Coronary arteries contain both α and β receptors. The α (vasoconstrictor) activity is rather weak, allowing the vasodilator (β) response to predominate. There is no sympathetic cholinergic vasodilator fiber in the myocardium.
- In a right dominant system, right coronary artery (RCA) supplies approximately 16% and left coronary artery (LCA) supplies 84% of the flow, of which 66% is from left anterior descending artery (LAD) and 33% is from the left circumflex artery (LCx).

SUGGESTED READING

1. Applied embryology, anatomy and physiology of the heart. In: Manchanda SC (Ed). Oram's Clinical Heart Disease, 3rd edition. New Delhi: CBS Publisher & Distributors; 1999. pp. 1-28.
2. Functional anatomy of the heart. In: Fuster V, Walsh R, Harrington RA (Eds). Hurst's the Heart, 13th edition. New York: Mc Graw-Hill; 2011. pp. 63-92.
3. O'Melley CD, Saunders JB (Eds). Lionardo da Vinci on the Human Body. Greenwich House; 1982. p. 233.

CHAPTER 2

Symptoms and Signs of Cardiovascular Disease

"There is a disorder of the breast, marked with strong and peculiar symptoms, considerable for the kind of danger belonging to it. The seat of it and sense of strangling and anxiety with which it is attended may make it not improperly be called angina pectoris."
—William Heberden (1768)

■ INTRODUCTION

Evaluation of symptom and signs of patients before going for laboratory investigations is both desirable and cost-effective. It guides downstream testing and establishes crucial bond between a patient and a doctor. This chapter deals with queries on cardiovascular history and physical examination.

Q1. What are the cardiovascular causes of cough?
Ans. Cough is a defense mechanism that helps to protect the airways from irritants and clear it of unwanted materials. Common cardiovascular causes are:
- Conditions causing raised left atrial (LA) pressure and pulmonary venous hypertension that result in interstitial or pulmonary edema: left ventricular failure (LVF), mitral stenosis (MS), and LA myxoma
- Pulmonary embolism
- Compression of recurrent laryngeal nerve by a greatly enlarged LA Ortner's syndrome patent ductus arteriosus (PDA), and aortic aneurysm
- Compression of tracheobronchial tree, e.g., aortic aneurysm
- Congenital cyanotic heart disease in particular Eisenmenger's syndrome

Q2. How patterns of cough give clues to underlying disease?
Ans.
- Pink frothy and voluminous sputum with shortness of breath—pulmonary edema
- Cough precipitated by exercise or sexual intercourse with associated hemoptysis—tight MS
- Nighttime cough with orthopnea or paroxysmal nocturnal dyspnea (PND) with or without wheeze—congestive heart failure (CHF)
- Paroxysmal "brassy" cough often with stridor—aortic aneurysm
- Intractable chronic nonproductive cough—medication like angiotensin-converting enzyme inhibitor (ACEI), amiodarone, and methotrexate.

Q3. What are the cardiac causes of dyspnea? How is it graded?

Ans. Dyspnea is an undue awareness of the effort of respiration. Dyspnea can occur on exertion. However, as the disease progresses, it occurs even at rest.

Cardiac cause of dyspnea are: Left ventricular failure, valvular disease, coronary artery disease, cardiomyopathy, congenital heart disease, and pericardial disease. Dyspnea can be an anginal equivalent due to stiff ventricle from ischemia.

The New York Heart Association (NYHA) functional and therapeutic classification of dyspnea:
- *Grade 1:* No dyspnea, but heart disease
- *Grade 2:* Dyspnea on severe exertion
- *Grade 3:* Dyspnea on mild exertion
- *Grade 4:* Dyspnea at rest

Patients who have dyspnea at rest that goes away with exertion usually have psychogenic etiology for their symptoms. Hyperventilation, in contrast to dyspnea, is an increase in rate and depth of respiration. The patient refer to feeling hunger for air, frequently caused by anxiety.

Q4. What is orthopnea and paroxysmal nocturnal dyspnea?

Ans. *Orthopnea:* It is the shortness of breathing that occurs within minutes of lying down and relieved within a few minutes of sitting upright. When reclining, blood returning from lower limb results in an increase in LA and pulmonary venous pressure causing increased pulmonary congestion and stiffness, which incite reflexes that trigger the sensation of shortness of breath. The diaphragm encroaches on the vital capacity of the lung in reclining position adding to the shortness of breathing. With assumption of upright posture venous return decrease, the diaphragm goes down and improves the situation within minutes.

Causes: Causes include severe LV dysfunction, subtle LV failure, increased pulmonary venous pressure, e.g., MS.

Paroxysmal nocturnal dyspnea: It is the shortness of breath (a suffocating feeling) that occurs after the patent has been lying in bed for several hours. The patient usually awakens several hours after retiring (typically between 1 and 3 AM) with severe shortness of breath. Relief is obtained only by getting out of bed, sitting in a chair, dangling the legs or standing. Unlike with orthopnea, sitting up does not cause relief in 1–2 minutes. Shortness of breath usually lasts from 10 to 30 minutes.

Paroxysmal nocturnal dyspnea is more common in patient with poor LV function who have peripheral edema. After the patient retires to bed at night, it takes 1–2 hours for edema fluid from the lower limbs to return to the heart. An extra volume of fluid precipitates LV failure, this causes an increase in LA pressure that results in pulmonary edema. Cough is often associated with the feeling of suffocation and with the production of frothy blood-stained sputum.

Q5. Enumerate the cardiovascular causes of edema. What are the features of cardiac edema?
Ans. Cardiovascular causes of edema are:
- CHF
- Constrictive pericarditis*
- Venous obstruction**
- Pregnancy
- Drugs—calcium antagonists, estrogen, nonsteroidal anti-inflammatory drugs (NSAIDs), and steroids

Features of cardiac edema:
- It is determined by gravity, occurs bilaterally—lower limbs in ambulant patient and sacral area, in bedridden patent.
- It is pitting, i.e., the tissue pits when pressed firmly for 10 seconds by the thumb.
- It is progressively worse during the day and often absent on initial rising (as fluid is redistributed on lying down).
- In severe heart failure, leg edema is followed by edema in trunk, face, ascites, and pleural effusion (anasarca).

Q6. What is palpitation? How it occurs?
Ans. Palpitation is an unpleasant awareness of the heartbeat. It may result from an increased awareness of the normal heartbeat, the sensing of slow or rapid heartbeat, or an irregular heart rhythm. The normal heart beat may be sensed when the patient is anxious, excited, exercising or lying on the left side. The most common arrhythmias to be felt as palpitation are premature ectopic beats and paroxysmal tachycardias. Ectopic beats frequently give rise to a sensation of missed beats or extra beat. Patients with supraventricular tachycardia are aware of the sudden onset of rapid beating, whereas those with atrial fibrillation may be conscious of its irregularity.

Q7. What are the cardiac causes of chest pain?
Ans. Chest pain is one of the common symptoms of heart disease. The causes are:
- Ischemic heart disease (IHD)—myocardial infarction, stable angina, and unstable angina
- Valvular diseases—aortic stenosis (AS), aortic regurgitation, and mitral valve prolapse
- Pulmonary embolism

---
*Occurs weeks after appearance of ascites.
**Commonly unilateral—one leg more than other. Left leg more than right.

- Pulmonary hypertension
- Pericarditis
- Aortic dissection
- Hypertrophic cardiomyopathy

Q8. How chest pain of angina pectoris differs from that in myocardial infarction?

Ans. Difference in chest pain of angina pectoris and myocardial infarction are shown in **Table 2.1**.

TABLE 2.1: Differentiating points: Anginal pain and pain of myocardial infarction.

Point	Angina pectoris	Myocardial infarction (MI)
Onset of pain	During or immediately after exercise	More common in morning
Duration	Usually 5–15 minutes	Constant for 30–60 minutes; may last intermittently for days
Precipitating factors	Exercise, anger, cold weather, heavy meals, sometimes smoking, and sexual activity	Thrombus and/or ruptured atheromatous plaque; extrinsic precipitating factors may be absent
Relieving factors	Rest or nitroglycerine	Morphine, beta blocker, completion of MI given relief
Association	Usually nil	Nausea, vomiting, diaphoresis, and dyspnea

Q9. How you differentiate anginal pain from pain due to anxiety state?

Ans. Anxiety state may produce chest pain where neurocirculatory asthenia and panic may be etiologic factor **(Table 2.2)**.

TABLE 2.2: Difference between angina and pain of anxiety state.

Points	Angina pectoris	Anxiety states
Prevalence	Usually in men over 40 years	Common in women and young men
Location	Retrosternal	Left inframammary region
Radiation	Arms, one or both neck or chin	Left scapula, left arm and left side of neck
Nature of pain	Pressure, tightness, sense of constriction	Dull ache, stabbing or shooting
Aggravating factor	Exercise or effort	Not exercise, may be provoked by anxiety state
Relieving factor	Rest or nitrates	Spontaneous or by tranquillizers
Duration of pain	5–15 minutes	Seconds, minutes to hours
Association	Nil	Chocking hyperventilation, palpitation, breathlessness pressure or hyperventilation

Q10. What is cyanosis? How cyanosis occurs in heart failure?
Ans. Cyanosis is a bluish discoloration of the skin and mucus membrane caused by an increased amount of deoxygenated hemoglobin in blood flowing through these regions. Cyanosis is not apparent if the blood hemoglobin is <5 g/L. Therefore, it may not be apparent in severely anemic patients.

Central cyanosis is seen in warm as well as cold areas. Peripheral cyanosis is seen only in cold areas such as nail beds, nose, cheeks, earlobes and outer surface of lips, where sluggish flow allows a marked reduction in oxygenated hemoglobin to occur in the capillaries. Central cyanosis occurs due to poor oxygenation in the lung or congenital right to left shunts. It is not usually recognized if arterial O_2 saturation is lowered to about 50%. In patients with congenital heart disease, cyanosis is usually observed when a R-L shunt is 25% of the left ventricular output. Cyanosis becomes worse during exercise, because R-L shunting increases. It does not improve by inhalation of 100% O_2.

Cyanosis in heart failure: Severe heart failure causes a low cardiac output and diminished circulation time and commonly cause peripheral cyanosis. Heart failure may add to central cyanosis when severe pulmonary edema results in decreased O_2 saturation in the lung. Conversely, cor-pulmonale causes central cyanosis, but if severe heart failure occurs, the peripheries become cold, and peripheral cyanosis is superadded. The combination of central cyanosis and peripheral cyanosis carries a poor prognosis.

Q11. What is differential cyanosis and reversed differential cyanosis?
Ans. Differential cyanosis means that the fingers are pink, but the toes are cyanotic (and usually clubbed). The situation is seen with PDA with a reversed right to left shunt due to pulmonary hypertension (Eisenmenger's syndrome). Deoxygenated blood flows from the pulmonary artery through the ductus into the aorta distal to the region of the carotid and subclavian arteries. Cyanosis spares the upper extremity.

Reversed differential cyanosis may be caused by transposition of the great vessels with coarctation of the aorta. Blood from the RV ejected into the aorta reaches the head and upper limbs but cannot reach the lower limb; hence upper segment is cyanosed, but blood from the LV ejected into the pulmonary artery flows through the PDA to the descending aorta and reaches the legs, which are therefore less cyanotic.

Q12. How the pulse helps in cardiac physical diagnosis?
Ans.
- Absent pulse—occlusion (thrombotic and embolic), arteritis, and anatomical aberration
- Delayed pulse—radio-femoral delay in coarctation of the aorta

- Low volume—in acute myocardial infarction (AMI), shock, MS, cardiac tamponade, and constrictive pericarditis
- High volume—in AR, hyperdynamic circulations (pregnancy, anemia, and thyrotoxicosis)
- Anacrotic—low volume pulse with slow, prolonged upstroke, as in severe AS
- Collapsing—high volume with rapid rise and fall; also called water hammer pulse
- Pulsus bisferiens—in combined AS and AR; a double peak can be felt.
- Pulsus paradoxus—a substantial inspiratory fall (>10 mm Hg); occurs in severe asthma and pericardial tamponade.
- Pulsus alternans—an alternative large and small volume pulse; found in severe LV dysfunction.
- Irregularly irregular pulse—irregular in rate, rhythm and volume; seen in atrial fibrillation. It is due to variable ventricular filling resulting from irregular atrial contraction.

Q13. How the appearance of a patient gives clues to cardiac illness?

Ans. Appearance may reveal important clues to underlying cardiac illness or associated conditions.

- *Apprehensive facies:* It is produced by pain and anxiety, and is a feature of acute MI, dissecting aneurysm of aorta, acute pulmonary edema, and pulmonary embolism.
- Head nodding movements secondary to the ballistic force of severe aortic regurgitation (AR) (de Musset's sign)
- *Malar flush:* A rosy malar prominence with dilated venules in the peripherally cyanosed skin of patients with long-standing MS
- *Down syndrome:* A flattened occiput, disproportionately small head, epicanthal folds that give the impression of slanted eyes, and a mouth held open by a large protruding tongue are the characteristics of Down syndrome. Here, various degree of endocardial cushion defect may produce combination of ASD, VSD, and valvular regurgitation.
- *Myxedema:* Puffy lids, scanty, dry hairs, coarse, dry skin, expressionless face, and enlarged tongue are the features. These patients have cardiomyopathies (due to increased interstitial fluid and fat infiltration) and pericardial effusion with high cholesterol content.
- *Williams syndrome:* A broad forehead, puffy cheeks, low ears, hypertelorism (eyes set widely apart) with strabismus, an upturned nose with a long philtrum, a wide protruding mouth, dental abnormalities, and a hypoplastic mandible. It is associated with supravalvular AS.

- *Hypertelorism:* It is associated with Pfeiffer syndrome, especially supravalvular AS and Hurler syndrome with MR. It also occurs in Down syndrome and Nonan's syndrome.
- *Xanthelasma:* Yellowish plaque of cholesterol deposits seen in patients with hypercholesterolemia **(Figs. 2.1A and B)**.

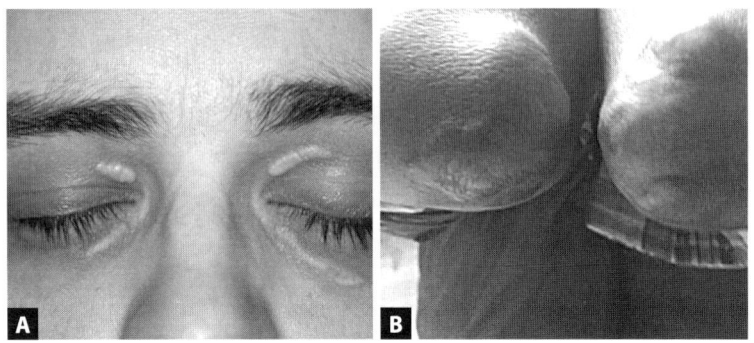

Figs. 2.1A and B: (A) Xanthelasma and (B) tendon xanthoma around both elbows.

- *Arcus lipidicus:* A thick band that begins inside the limbus allowing a rim of iris pigment to be seen between the arcus and the sclera. It is associated with hypercholesterolemia or coronary artery disease (CAD).

Q14. How extremities give clue to cardiac lesions?
Ans.
- *Turner syndrome:* Short stature and cubitus valgus are the features. Coarctation of the aorta is commonly associated. When web neck, cubitus valgus, short stature, and hypogonadism present in males, the condition is called Ullrich-Noonan syndrome. Pulmonary stenosis is the most common abnormally associated with it.
- *Holt-Oram syndrome:* Triphalangeal thumb, fingerized thumb lying in the same plane as the fingers, so that it is difficult to oppose thumb with fingers), and polydactyly are the signs of Holt-Oram syndrome. Distal radial and ulnar deformities cause difficulty in pronation and supination. Secundum type ASD is associated **(Fig. 2.2)**.
- *Marfan syndrome:* Increased height, long fingers (spider finger), elongated face, high arched palate, narrow palms, flat feat, kyphoscoliosis, subluxation of lens, mitral valve prolapse (MVP), mitral regurgitation (MR) (minimal or severe), and AR (due to dilated aortic root, prolapse of aortic cusp or aortic dissection) are the characteristics.
- *Ellis Van Crevel's syndrome:* Short extremities, polydactyly, dysplastic teeth and nail, and large VSD or single atrium are associated.

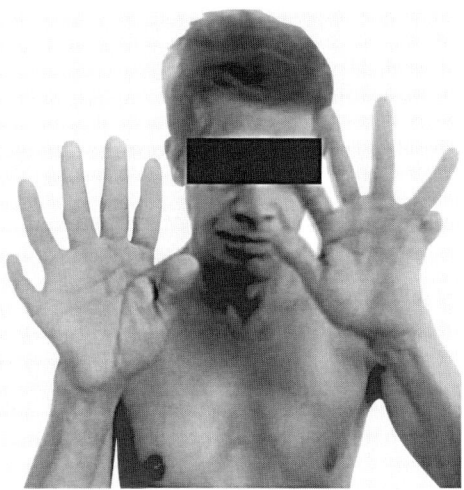

Fig. 2.2: Polydactyly in Holt-Oram syndrome.

Q15. What is jugular venous pressure (JVP)?
Ans. The mean level of JVP above right atrial level is a measure of the central venous pressure. Thus, bedside examination of JVP gives an estimate of right atrial pressure (i.e., central venous pressure). The normal right atrial pressure seldom exceeds 5 mm Hg, which is equivalent to a column of blood of roughly 7 cm height (1 mm Hg = 1.4 cmH$_2$O). This means that if a patient with normal right atrial pressure sits upright, the JVP should not be >7 cm above the mid right atrium (RA).

Q16. What is the importance of examination of neck vein?
Ans. A considerable amount of important data concerning the hemodynamics of the right and left side of the heart can be found by examination of jugular vein in the neck. Main objective is estimation of the central venous pressure and inspection of the waveform. In systole, the internal jugular veins (IJVs) are in continuity only with the RA. In diastole as the tricuspid valve (TV) is open, the jugulars are in continuity with the RA and the right ventricle (RV). Therefore, examination of the jugular vein may reveal the wave form and pressure in the RA and RV without the need for catheterization.

Q17. What are the causes of raised JVP?
Ans. The causes are:
- Right heart failure (isolated or secondary to left heart failure)
- Pulmonary hypertension (acute, e.g., pulmonary embolism or chronic)
- Tricuspid regurgitation (TR)
- Pulmonary stenosis
- Pericardial tamponade
- Constrictive pericarditis

- Others—tricuspid stenosis, canon waves [due to complete heart block ventricular ectopic etc.], fluid overload, superior vena cava (SVC) obstruction (nonpulsatile)

Q18. Why 45° inclination is done during examination of JVP?
Ans.
- Usually maximum pulsation of the IJV is observed when the trunk is inclined by less than 30° steeper and patients with cardiac disease are examined most effectively in the 45° position.
- At 45° inclination, in the normal individual, pulsation is not usually visible or just visible at the root of the neck. In this position, the perpendicular height of the venous pulsation from the sternal angle is 5 cm, as the distance from sternal angle to mid RA is 5 cm, indicating that the JVP is normal. Any filling or pulsation seen above this level indicates an elevated JVP. It is thus convenient to start the examination with the patient propped up at 45° angle.

Q19. Is it mandatory to put the patient at 45° inclination during measuring JVP?
Ans. No, the internal JVP expressed as centimeter of blood, is measured as the vertical distance between a horizontal plane passing through the sternal angle and another horizontal plane drawn through the highest point of visible internal jugular pulsation with the patient at any angle of inclination. The exact position is unimportant in measurement; rather the position should allow one to observe the top of the pulsation. Again, the distance between the mid RA and sternal angle is also the same (i.e., 5 cm) regardless of the patient's position. Hence, position does not influence the calculation of total venous pressure (as shown above), although influence the upper limit of the pulsation.

When the venous pressure is very high, the upper limit of the pulsation may not be visible until the patient sits upright. It may remain in intracranial cavity, i.e., in sigmoid sinus which continues as IJV outside cranial cavity. In this position, direct measurement from sternal angle to the upper limit of the pulsation is the measurement of internal jugular pressure. Conversely, in a patient with low venous pressure, venous waves may not be visible until the patient is placed in the supine position (sometimes with the leg elevated to increase venous return).

It must be realized that the venous pressure should be the same regardless of the inclinations of the patient. Assessment of the venous waveform requires the patient to be placed at a level of inclination at which pulsations are best seen. In patients with markedly elevated JVP, it may be necessary to elevate the trunk >45°, sometimes to as much as 90°.

Q20. What is the importance of sternal angle in the examination of JVP?

Ans.
- Sternal angle is a convenient reference point in the measurement of JVP. Central venous pressure is the perpendicular height above the mid RA (usually 6–8 cmH$_2$O). In healthy individual, this level is same as that of the sternal angle. In whatever position the patient may be sitting, standing, lying or intermediate postures, it represents the zero position in the venous system. Veins above this level are collapsed, veins below are filled to varying degree. Judgement as to whether venous pressure is raised will depend upon the height above the sternal angle at which the venous pulsation can be recognized.
- In the average patient, the mid RA lies approximately 5 cm below the sternal angle regardless of the body position.

The total measurement of the venous pressure is the vertical distance of the venous pulsation from the sternal angle + distance of mid RA to sternal angle, i.e., 5 cm.

Q21. How will you measure the venous pressure in the bedside?

Ans. The right IJV is utilized with the sternal angle as the reference point **(Fig. 2.3)**. It is desirable to use an examining table or bed that can be easily adjusted over a range, e.g., 0 to 45°. For examination of very high venous pressure, the sitting position (90°) is necessary.
- The neck should be relaxed, so that the sternomastoid muscle is relaxed.
- The patient is positioned with the trunk elevated between 30° and 45°, i.e., the optimum degree of elevation that allows one to observe the upper limit of the venous pulsation.
- Internal JVP is measured as the vertical distance between a horizontal plane, passing through the sternal angle and another horizontal plane drawn through the highest point of visible internal jugular pulsation **(Fig. 2.4)**. It is expressed as a centimeter of blood.

Venous pressure (i.e., RA pressure) is the distance of the venous pulsation from sternal angle + distance of mid RA to sternal angle, i.e., 5 cm.

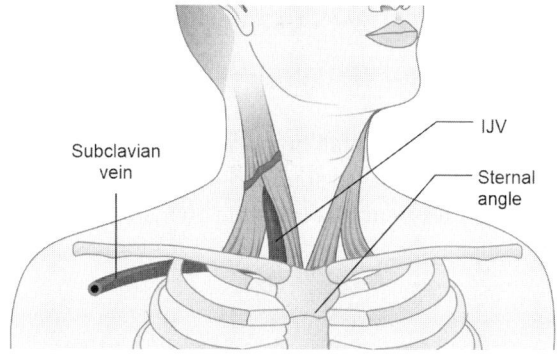

Fig. 2.3: Neck anatomy. (IJV: internal jugular vein)

14 Symptoms and Signs of Cardiovascular Disease

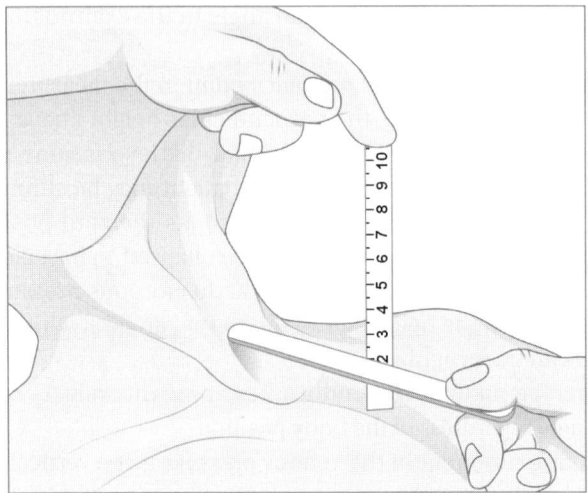

Fig. 2.4: Bedside measurement of venous pressure.

When the venous pressure is very high, the upper limit of the pulsation may not be visible until the patient sits upright. In this position, direct measurement from sternal angle to the upper limit of the pulsation is the measurement of internal jugular pressure.

Q22. What are the significance of waves in neck vein?
Ans. The normal JVP reflects phasic changes in the atrium and consists of two (sometimes three) positive waves and two negative troughs.

Waves of JVP are:
- *'a' wave:* It is produced by venous distension due to RA contraction. It precedes ventricular systole and thus the S_1 and carotid pulse (a-atrial systole).
- *'c' wave:* It is produced by the transmitted carotid impulse at onset of systole and the bulging of the TV in the RA (c-convergence of TV into RA).
- *'v' wave:* Rise in RA pressure by continuing venous filling while the TV is closed (v-venous filling).
- *'x' descent:* It is produced by RA relaxation followed by descent of tricuspid ring during early RV systole.
- *'y' descent:* It is produced by fall in RA pressure as TV opens and pent-up venous blood floods into RV at start of diastole. It is the deepest and most rapid collapsing movement that is visible on inspection **(Fig. 2.5)**.

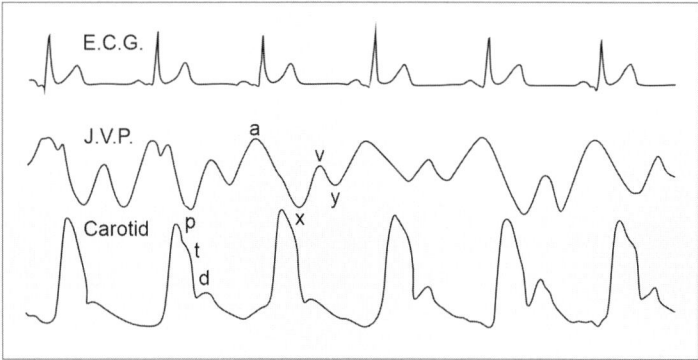

Fig. 2.5: Jugular venous waves, with corresponding arterial waves (below) and ECG (above).

Q23. What are the abnormalities of the waves in JVP?
Ans.

- *Giant 'a' wave:* This wave occurs when the right atrial workload increases, i.e., RA contracts against obstructed TV, e.g., tricuspid stenosis, atresia or increased resistance to RA emptying, e.g., pulmonary stenosis and hypertension.
- *Cannon wave:* This wave occurs when atrium contracts against a closed TV as in AV dissociation, e.g., CHB. In patient with CHB, atrium may contract at 72/min, ventricle at 30/min. At sometime, the atrium contracts against a closed TV. It may be necessary to observe the neck pulsations for more than 2 minutes to observe a cannon wave in CHB. Isolated cannon waves are sometimes seen with atrial, ventricular, and junctional beats.
- *Prominent 'v' waves:* This wave may be seen in TR, which may cause movement of ear lobes during systole. The v wave is visibly prominent because of rapid y descent consequent on the rapid fall of the very high atrial pressure. ASD causing right atrial diastolic overload may also produce prominent v wave.
- *Rapid 'y' descent:* It is seen in patient with very high atrial pressure with a normal TV opening. It is a typical feature of constrictive pericarditis (but not pericardial tamponade) and may be seen in severe RV failure.
- *Absent 'y' descent:* It is seen in cardiac tamponade (the high atrial pressure cannot empty into RV, because the major restriction in movement occurs during diastole).
- *Venous waves and arrhythmias:* Absent a wave in atrial fibrillation, because there is no atrial contraction (in atrial flutter multiple small a waves may be visible); irregular intermittent cannon a waves occur with CHB or ventricular ectopic beats.

Note: A very high venous pressure with the presence of large v waves and y descent is a valuable sign; because it signifies severe CHF and helps to exclude cardiac tamponade.

Q24. How to differentiate jugular venous pulsation from carotid?
Ans. Difference between jugular venous pulsation and carotid pulsation is shown in **Table 2.3**.

TABLE 2.3: Difference between jugular and carotid pulsation (**Fig. 2.5**).

Points	JVP	Carotid pulse
Postural variation	Present—high in supine, lowest during sitting up-right, and intermediate in between	No
Variation with respiration	Present; pressure falls during inspiration but waves more visible (as more blood go to right heart, contraction is more vigorous)	No
Upper limit of the pulsation	Yes (has definite upper limit)	No
Pattern of the pulse	Sinuous, prominent movement inward	Prominent movement out word
Waves per cardiac cycle	Two-a and v in sinus rhythm)	One
Finger pressure above clavicle	Often disappear	No effect
Palpation	Cannot be palpated; better seen	Easily palpable as a thrust
Hepatojugular reflux	Positive (more than 1 cm increase in JVP when right hypochondrial pressure applied for 30–60 second)	Negative

Q25. Which IJV is preferred—right or left?
Ans. Normally, the pressure in the right jugular is either slightly greater than, or the same as that in the left jugular vein. The right jugular is better than left for examination of JVP, as the communication to RA is direct here. In some atherosclerotic patients, left jugular pressure may be falsely raised by unfolded aortic arch posteriorly (compression on left innominate vein). A persistently left SVC that drains into the coronary sinus cause a slightly higher pressure in left jugular than right. It is especially likely in the presence of ASD. Nevertheless, if there is any difficulty in seeing a clearly pulsatile jugular vein on the right, both sides of neck should be carefully examined.

Q26. Which neck vein is preferable—internal or external jugular vein?
Ans.
- The internal jugular vein is preferable for examination; the external jugular vein (EJV) communicates with the SVC only after two near 90° angle turn (where EJV enters the subclavian and the subclavian enters SVC). It is difficult to communicate RA pressure accurately through two sharp turns.
- Being superficial, the EJV is subjected to external pressure by tight clothing, tie, etc.

- There is also a valve at the opening of EJV into subclavian.
- The EJV are occasionally either absent or too thready to be visible to necked eye. It may become narrow in CHF or shock and become invisible.

Q27. What is Kussmaul's sign?

Ans. It is the rise of JVP during inspiration. Normally, jugular pressure decreases during inspiration as more blood goes to RA. Kussmaul's sign is seen in patients with constrictive pericarditis. In this condition, the congested liver is compressed by the descending diaphragm and the right atrium and ventricles are prevented from distending by the rigid pericardium. This sign is also occasionally seen in severe right ventricular failure.

Q28. What are the conditions that produce low venous pressure?

Ans. A low JVP may result as a consequence of any condition causing a reduction in preload, e.g., hemorrhage and dehydration. An unexpectedly low venous pressure in patients with other signs of cardiac disease is commonly due to diuretic therapy.

Q29. Jugular venous pressure is raised but not visible? What are the possibilities?

Ans. The possibilities are:
- Jugular venous pressure is grossly elevated, and the upper limit of the pulsation is not visible. Pulsations may become apparent if the patient is placed in a more upright position. The upper level of pulsation may then be observed at the angle of the mandible, or the ear lobes may be observed to pulsate.
- Raised JVP is nonpulsatile, e.g., in SVC obstruction. Here, other features of SVC obstruction are apparent.

Q30. What are the characteristics of a good stethoscope?

Ans. For satisfactory cardiac auscultation, the following points are important:
- A shallow bell for low frequency sounds and low frequency murmurs. The bell accentuates the low frequency sounds and filters out the high-pitched tone. The stethoscope should be placed over skin with just enough pressure to seal the edge at the point of maximum impulse. With bell of stethoscope middiastolic murmur, third and fourth heart sounds, and all sounds outside the precordium are well heard. The stethoscope should be placed over skin with just enough pressure to seal the edge at the point of maximum impulse.
- A smooth, stiff, thin diaphragm for high frequency sounds. Diaphragm brings out the high frequencies and attenuates the low frequencies. When the diaphragm is used to attenuate high frequency sounds, it should be pressed very firmly against the skin. Heard well are soft high-frequency aortic and pulmonary blowing diastolic murmur and soft murmurs, splitting of S_1 or S_2.

- An internally smooth vinyl tubing is not over 12 inches (30 cm) long and 46 cm in internal diameter. Too long tubing attenuates heart sounds by room noise. A vinyl tube has been found to be more efficient for high frequency, because it allows less interference for reflected waves. Single tube is more flexible and portable.
- The largest ear tips, if possible, preferably of slightly soft rubbery material should be preferred. Head pieces are designed to point the eartips anteriorly. Metal headpieces are rotated to point the earpieces in the most comfortable direction.
- Pediatric-sized bell and diaphragm accessories are needed.

Q31. What are the areas of auscultation?
Ans. Four conventional areas are:
- *Mitral area (the cardiac apex):* Murmurs originating from the mitral valve are best heard in this area, but AS murmurs may be best heard at the apex, if RV occupies the apex.
- Aortic area (the second right intercostal space)—most murmurs arising from the AV are best heard in this position and radiates to the neck vessels.
- Aortic and pulmonary areas are clinical base of the heart, as these are located opposite to the apex, i.e., mitral area. This is in contrast to the anatomical base, which is formed by the left atrium.
- Pulmonary area (the upper left parasternal area; second interspace)
- Tricuspid area (the lower left sternal edge)

Other areas are:
- *Lower left parasternal area:* The murmur of AR is often best heard at the third or fourth intercostal space.
- *Left axilla:* For radiation of murmurs of MR
- *Over the carotids:* For radiation of murmurs caused by AS
- Below the left clavicle where the continuous murmur of PDA is best heard
- Just above the sternoclavicular joint for venous hum, upper epigastrium in patients with emphysema and with exacerbation of chronic obstructive pulmonary disease (COPD) (if the heart sounds are difficult to auscultate in other areas), the murmur of TR is best heard here.
- Posterior chest for bruits due to large bronchial collaterals in patients with coarctation of the aorta
- Over the spinous processes C_3 to L_2, in a flail MV.

It is to be noted that auscultatory areas do not indicate the location of the respective valves rather the sounds and murmurs originating from a particular valve. Thus, sounds heard in a particular area do not necessarily come from that particular valve, for example, murmurs originating at the aortic valve are frequently best heard in the mitral area.

Q32. How difference in intensity of S_1 occurs?

Ans. The first heart sound (S_1) is produced by the closure of the MV and TV. The intensity should be assessed with patient holding breath after a deep exhalation.

- Increased intensity of S_1 occur in tachycardia, MS, tricuspid stenosis, LA myxoma, short PR interval, and hyperthyroidism. In MS, S_1 has a typical slapping character. Here diastolic filling is prolonged, and the valves remain widely open up to the moment of ventricular contraction and thus close with great velocity.
- Diminished intensity of S_1 occur in heart failure, cardiogenic shock, MR (not due to prolapse), fibrosis and calcification of MV, prolonged PR interval, severe AR, and left bundle branch block (LBBB).
- Variation in intensity of S_1 occurs when there is varying relationship of atrial to ventricular contraction (or varying cycle length), e.g., atrial fibrillation, AV dissociation, complete AV block, and ventricular tachycardia.

Q33. What is a murmur? Classify it.

Ans. Murmurs are sounds resulting from vibrations set up by turbulent blood flow. Turbulence can be due to increased velocity of flow, obstruction, or regurgitation.

Etiologically murmur may be:
- *Innocent (or insignificant):* Murmurs without significant structural or physiologic abnormality in cardiovascular system (CVS). These are ejection systolic murmurs, usually faint in character, commonly found over the pulmonary area, and to a lesser extent over the cardiac apex; other signs of cardiac disease are completely absent. It may persist throughout childhood (due to enhanced cardiac contractility in children) and tend to attenuate or disappear with increasing age.
- *Physiologic:* Murmurs caused by disturbances in circulatory physiology, e.g., in anemia, pregnancy, high fever, thyrotoxicosis, and beriberi. These are also ejection systolic, best heard in pulmonary area.
- *Functional:* Murmurs caused by structural abnormality not involving the valves or murmurs of shunts. For example, MR due to LV dilatation (by IHD, hypertension, etc.), pulmonary ejection flow murmur in ASD, etc.
- *Organic:* Murmurs caused by valvular disease (stenosis and regurgitation), shunts, or vascular narrowing

Timing during cardiac cycle: Systolic, diastolic, and continuous.
- Systolic murmur begins after and ends at or before A_2 or P_2. It can be early systolic (e.g., acute severe MR and small muscular VSD), midsystolic (e.g., aortic and pulmonary stenosis, HCM, and innocent murmurs), late systolic (e.g. MVP), and holosystolic (e.g., MR, TR, and VSD).

- Diastolic murmurs can be early diastolic e.g., AR, PR, mid-diastolic (e.g., MS, atrial myxoma, tricuspid stenosis, and CHB), high diastolic (flow across AV valve in severe MR, large L-R shunt, and CHB), and late diastolic (e.g., MS in sinus rhythm, i.e., presystolic accentuation of MDM).
- Continuous murmurs begin in systole and continue throughout S_2 into part or all of diastole. These are loudest at the time of S_2, for example PDA, rupture of sinus of Valsalva, and aortopulmonary window.

Q34. How grading of intensity of murmur is done?
Ans. Murmurs are traditionally graded as:
- *Grade 1:* A very soft murmur that is (faintly) heard, the murmur may be missed during the initial examination.
- *Grade 2:* A soft murmur that is readily heard
- *Grade 3:* A loud murmur with no thrill
- *Grade 4:* A loud murmur with a thrill
- *Grade 5:* A very loud murmur heard when the edge of the stethoscope is applied to the area of maximal intensity.
- *Grade 6:* The loudest murmur audible with the stethoscope is removed from the chest wall.

Q35. How diagnosis of a murmur is done?
Ans. Following points are crucial for diagnosis:
- *Timing of the murmur:* It provides information regarding the cause of murmur. If the murmur is difficult to time, the observer should identify S_2 at the base, then slowly move the stethoscope down from the base to the apex, fixing the cardiac cycle with S_2 as the reference point.
- *Point of maximum intensity and radiation:* Murmurs due to pulmonary and TV lesions are generally well localized in the respective areas. Aortic and mitral murmurs however may radiate extensively. Aortic systolic murmur for instance may be best heard in the apical area. Systolic murmurs that radiate into the carotid arteries are usually aortic in origin. MR murmur usually radiates to axilla and left scapular area.
- *Quality and configuration of murmurs:* Rough murmurs are associated with obstructive lesions, e.g., AS, PS, etc. Blowing murmurs are typical of incompetent valve, e.g. MR. Murmur of MS is low pitched with a characteristic rumbling quality.
- *Behaviors with respiration:* Stroke output of the right heart increases during inspiration, while that of the left heart is reduced. A murmur originating on the right side will become louder during inspiration and that originating on the left side, during expiration.
- *Associated features:* These aid in diagnosis of a murmur, for example murmur of MS and aortic regurgitation may be missed unless heightened by clues. A wide pulse pressure and a loud S_1 are the clues for AR and MS, respectively.

SUGGESTED READING

1. Chamberlain EN, Ogilvie C (Eds). Chamberlain's Symptoms and Signs in Clinical Medicine, 10th edition. Butterworth-Heinemann: UK; 1980.
2. Constant J. Using internal jugular pulsations as a manometer for right atrial pressure measurements. Cardiology. 2000;93:26-30.
3. Glynn M, Drake WM, Hutchison's Clinical Methods an integrated approach to clinical practice. 23rd ed. Saunders Elsevier 2012.
4. Munro J, Edward C (Ed). Macleod's Clinical Examination, 8th edition. Churchill Livingstone: Edinburg; 1990.

Investigations and Procedures

"Findings of cardiovascular investigations and procedures make cardiology the most evidence-based medicine and allows interventions to be undertaken."
—Author of the book

▇ INTRODUCTION

Investigations aid in confirmation and exclusion of a clinical diagnosis done by history and physical examination. They also add independent information to clinical diagnosis. Investigations include bedside procedures such as electrocardiogram (ECG), chest X-ray (CxR), echocardiography (echo), and invasive procedures such cardiac catheterization and coronary angiography (CAG). Of these, CxR, echo, nuclear cardiology, cardiac computed tomography (CT), cardiovascular magnetic resonance (CMR), positron emission tomography (PET), cardiac catheterization, and CAG are cardiovascular imaging techniques.

▇ ELECTROCARDIOGRAM

Electrocardiogram is a fundamental tool to investigate various heart diseases. It is the gold standard for the diagnosis of cardiac arrhythmias and acute coronary syndromes. ECG is also very useful for the evaluation of palpitation, syncope, acute dyspnea, electrolyte disturbances, etc. Besides diagnosing various cardiac abnormalities, ECG has also been used in prognosis and risk stratification of many clinical conditions.

Q1. What is ECG?
Ans. Electrogram is any record produced by changes in electrical potential, e.g., ECG, electroencephalogram (EEG), etc. ECG is a graphical tracing of variations in electrical potential caused by excitation of the heart muscle and detected at body surface. The normal ECG is a graphical representation, showing positive and negative deflections resulting from change in voltage and polarity of atrial and ventricular electrical activity.

Electrocardiography is the making of a graphical record of variations in electrical potential caused by excitation of heart muscle that are detected at body surface.

Electrocardiograph is the instrument used for performing ECG.

Q2. What are the types of ECG recordings?
Ans.
- *12-lead ECG:* Routine ECG with 12 leads—3 bipolar limb leads (I, II, III), 3 technically augmented unipolar limb leads (avR, avL, avF), and 6 unipolar precordial leads (V_1-V_6)
- *Monitor ECG:* In CCU modified-bipolar chest lead is used with positive electrode at usual V_1 position, negative electrode near left shoulder, and a third electrode to a more remote area of chest (serves as ground). It is done to evaluate cardiac rhythm. For ischemia, detection positive electrode is to be placed in V_5 or V_6
- *Exercise ECG:* It is also a 12-lead ECG recorded every 90 seconds during exercise and every minute in recovery period. Since limb leads are applied to the torso in the exercising patient (rather than on the upper and lower extremities), some difference in QRS axis, morphology, and voltage from the usual is observed.
- *Ambulatory ECG monitoring:* Exploring electrode over V_1 and V_5, indifferent electrode over manubrium, and ground electrode over right lower ribs.
- *Intracardiac ECG:* It is done by attaching electrode catheter to V lead. His bundle electrocardiography and myocardial mapping (by electrical stimulation of various areas) are the examples of intracardiac ECG. It is also helpful in proper positioning of a pacing catheter "floated" into the heart without fluoroscopic guidance. Attachment of the V lead to the metallic hub of a pericardiocentesis needle permits ECG recording during the procedure. Touching the epicardium is indicated by ST elevation.

Q3. What are the causes of ST-segment elevation? How can they be differentiated?
Ans. Causes of ST-segment elevation include **(Table 3.1)**:
- Acute myocardial infarction (MI)
- Prinzmetal's variant angina
- Pericarditis
- Left ventricular (LV) aneurysm
- Early repolarization phenomena—normal variant

TABLE 3.1: ST-segment elevation—differentiating points.

Differentiating points	Acute MI	Variant angina	Pericarditis	LV aneurysm	Early repolarization
History	At risk for CAD	Migraines, Raynaud's syndrome	Pneumonia, recent UTI	History of MI	Young athletes, in blacks
Chest pain	Typical	Cyclic	Positional, pleuritic	None	None

Contd...

Contd...

Differentiating points	Acute MI	Variant angina	Pericarditis	LV aneurysm	Early repolarization
Duration	Less than hour (until Q appears)	Transient, (minutes) with pain	Hours to days	Months (after MI)	Constant (except with tachycardia)
Pattern of ST elevation	Convex up-ward	Convex	Concave	Convex	Concave notched J-point; fishhook appearance (at origin)
Location	Area supplied by occluded artery	Localized to spasm	Generalized	To wall-motion abnormality	Generalized
PR depression	None	None	Often generalized	None	Rare (inferior leads)
Pathologic Q waves	Enlarges as ST elevation decreases	May be present	None	Diagnostic	None

(CAD: coronary artery disease; MI: myocardial infarction; LV: left ventricular; UTI: urinary tract infection)

Q4. What are the patterns of T-wave inversions?
Ans. In general, T-wave changes are very nonspecific. T inversion may be seen in ischemia. It may also occur in many other conditions, e.g., hyperventilation, anxiety, stroke, and athletic heart syndrome. The following patterns of T-wave inversions are seen:
- Ischemic T inversion is symmetrical in shape and sharply pointed and deep, the peak being midway between the beginning and the end. ST segment hugs the baseline for a relatively long period of 0.24 seconds. Inverted T wave preceded by an isoelectric ST segment (with an upward convexity) is called 'coronary T', and when preceded by an elevated ST (with upward convexity) is called cave-plane T.
- Strain-pattern inverted T wave is blunt and asymmetrical; not particularly deep, ST segment is depressed and minimally concave upward. It is not isoelectric for any period (ST segment leaves QRS immediately). It is seen in ventricular hypertrophy.
- Secondary T inversion is an alteration of sequence of ventricular depolarization that produces secondary T-wave inversion in leads with

predominantly positive QRS, e.g., bundle branch block, ventricular pacing, ventricular ectopic beats, pre-excitation syndrome, etc.

Q5. What are the forms of ST-segment depression?
Ans. ST-segment usually has a mild-concave shape. It is taken from the QRS complex at junctional J-point, and curves imperceptivity into the early part of the T wave. In order of severity, the forms of ST-segment depression may be as follows:
- Horizontality of ST-segment: A horizontal ST-segment is usually abnormal.
- Upward slopping ST-segment depression—commonly seen with tachycardia.
- Plane ST-segment depression—seen in myocardial ischemia.
- Downward sloping ST-segment depression—seen in ischemia.

ST-segment depression may be associated with T-wave inversion. ST-segment depression >1 mm, horizontal (or plane), or downsloping is significant for ischemia.

Q6. What are the pitfalls in the ECG diagnosis of ischemia?
Ans.
- A single ECG is never diagnostic, since the transient reversible nature of the ischemic phenomena cannot be demonstrated in a single tracing.
- Separate ECGs recorded weeks, months, or years apart that show identical ST- and T-wave abnormality are unlikely to be reflecting myocardial ischemia. Ischemia is a dynamic process and is not expected to remain the same overtime.
- ST- and T-wave abnormalities mimicking ischemia can be produced by many other conditions including drugs, hypokalemia, pericarditis, myocarditis, left ventricular hypertrophy (LVH), etc.
- Minor ST-segment depression may be associated with T-wave inversion and is commonly reported as nonspecific ST-T-wave changes.

The diagnosis of myocardial ischemia, therefore, depends on the clinical evaluation of the patient and the ECG changes during and after spontaneous angina pectoris, whether it occurs at rest or during exertion.

Q7. How is ECG diagnosis of acute MI done?
Ans. Despite the advent of expensive and sophisticated cardiologic tests, such as troponin, creatine kinase-MB (CK-MB), ECG remains the most reliable and inexpensive tool for the confirmation of acute MI.

The conventional ECG features are as follows:
- ST-segment elevation—current of injury
- Q wave—necrosis (infarction)
- ST depression—ischemia

These terms are accurate but not appropriate for early diagnosis of acute infarction. Early ECG diagnosis is often made before the development of Q waves or at the stage of evolving Q waves.

In patients presenting with acute chest discomfort, diagnosis of acute MI is based on the following ECG findings:
- ST-segment elevation of ≥1 mm in two or more limb leads.
- ST-segment elevation of ≥2 mm in two or more precordial leads. Patients with diagnostic ST-segment elevation are classified as having probable Q-wave infarction.
- Abnormal Q waves, i.e., abnormally wide (0.04s) and deep (25% of the height of R wave) in a given lead. They may not be present on the initial tracing. They may manifest as early as 2 hours or as late as 12 hours from onset of symptoms, and therefore cannot be relied on for early diagnosis of MI.
- Evolutionary changes occur over the next 6–24 hours, i.e., ST-segment elevation recedes, Q waves become more apparent, and T-wave inversion occurs (T inversion occurs more rapidly with inferior infarction than with anterior infarction). In some patients evolutionary changes are delayed over 2–3 days.
- Reciprocal depression of ST-segment in leads opposite to those depicting ST elevation, provides important support to confirm the diagnosis (itself not diagnostic).
- ST-segment depression and positive CK-MB indicate probable non-Q wave infarction

If the initial ECG is nondiagnostic, the ECG should be repeated every 30 minutes for 2 hours to verify changes consistent with the diagnosis of infarction.

Q8. How does the left bundle branch block (LBBB) interfere with other ECG findings and their diagnosis?
Ans.
- *Myocardial infarction:* In most patients with LBBB, a diagnosis of acute or previous infarction cannot be made from the ECG findings. As the initial 0.04s vector (Q wave), the most diagnostic feature of MI, is abnormal in LBBB. The infarction pattern is obscured, and the expected abnormal Q wave will not be inscribed. However, in the presence of chest pain with LBBB (new or old), acute infarction is suggested by 3 ECG findings: Serial ECG changes (new LBBB), marked ST-segment elevation, and inscription of a new Q wave where it is not expected. Q waves in association with LBBB may signify anterior infarction with peri-infarction block.

  Ischemia: Myocardial ischemia cannot be diagnosed from ECG. ST-segment and T waves are directed opposite to the terminal QRS directions and hence, do not represent ischemia.
- *Left ventricular hypertrophy:* Since LBBB causes a derangement of normal vector forces, the diagnosis of LVH cannot be made. Voltage criteria for LVH are not valid here. However, extremely prominent voltage (SV_2+ RV_6

≥45 mm), together with a pattern of left atrial abnormality may indicate the presence of LVH.

Q9. What are the ECG findings of bundle branch block in acute MI? What is their significance?
Ans.
- *Right bundle branch block (RBBB):* In general, a RBBB pattern does not obscure the patterns of MI. The initial 0.04s QRS vector (the Q wave) remains normal in right-sided intraventricular conduction delay. In anterior wall MI as a result of the infarction, the initial r wave of the rsR complex in RBBB will disappear in right ventricular epicardial leads, resulting in a QR complex. Concomitant RBBB in anterior infarction indicates infarction of the interventricular septum (IVS), and this connotes an extensive degree of myocardial necrosis. In inferior wall MI, pattern is not obscured by the RBBB. This suggests that the proximal portion of the right bundle branch, which is supplied by the branches of the coronary artery is ischemic or infarcted.
- *Left bundle branch block:* The infarction pattern is obscured. Since the initial 0.04s vector is itself abnormal in LBBB, the expected abnormal Q wave will not be inscribed. A new LBBB in the setting of symptoms consistent with acute MI may be indicative of large anterior wall acute MI involving the proximal left anterior descending (LAD) coronary artery, and should be managed as ST elevation acute MI. In the presence of LBBB at baseline, the diagnosis of ST-segment elevation acute MI can be made from: Serial ECG changes, marked ST-segment elevation, and the inscription of a new q wave where it is not expected. Old infarction pattern, anterior or inferior, is lost with the development of LBBB.

Q10. What are the causes of Q wave other than MI?
Ans.
- *Pseudoinfarction:* Q wave may be observed is leads II, III, and aVF, when the arm leads are placed on the legs. Presence of, virtually, no ECG deflections (R or S wave) in lead I is the clue to this technical error. Due to incorrect lead placement, the interchange of right arm, left arm, and left leg electrodes results in market changes in the frontal plane leads mimicking MI. Lead misplacement will not alter the PQRS configuration in the precordial leads.
- *Transient Q:* Transient, reversible, severe myocardial ischemia may produce it. Conditions include coronary artery spasm and shock states such as pancreatitis, anaphylactic shock, adrenal insufficiency, and intracerebral hemorrhage.
- *Q in V_1 and V_2—other than MI:*
    - *Lead misplacement:* Placing the V_1 and V_2 electrode in a higher interspace than the fourth.

- *Change in anatomic position:* Patients with chronic obstructive pulmonary disease (COPD), with the heart assuming a vertical position and rotating clockwise.
- Abnormalities of interventricular conduction produce a Q pattern in leads V_1 and V_2. Of these, left anterior fascicular block, LBBB, and Wolff-Parkinson-White Syndrome (WPW) syndrome are most common.
- Altered direction of septal forces—septal activation may be directed inferiorly and perpendicular to the lead axis of V_1 and V_2.
- Hypertrophic cardiomyopathy (HCM)—if septum is hypertrophied, Q waves increase in depth and the resulting deep Q waves may mimic MI.
- Q waves may be found in leads III and aVL, and this can be up to 6 mm deep. Q wave of up to 0.04s wide, often occurs in normal individuals. If there is no Q wave in lead II or aVF, the Q wave in lead III should be ignored.
- Large Q waves or QS complexes are normally observed in lead aVR, because lead aVR looks into the cavity of the ventricle and faces the endocardial surface.
- In extreme clockwise rotation, lead V_1 faces the ventricular cavity, and the usual R wave may disappear resulting in a QS complex.
- In extreme counterclockwise rotation, all precordial leads may show q waves, thus qr complexes occur.

The above factors should be considered when the pretest likelihood for infarction is low and there is no supportive evidence for MI.

Q11. What are the minimum ECG criteria for LVH?

Ans. In LVH, the activating impulse must traverse the large muscle mass of the hypertrophied left ventricle and thus, the S wave in leads V_1 and V_2 is deep, and the R wave in leads V_5 and V_6 is tall **(Fig. 3.1)**.

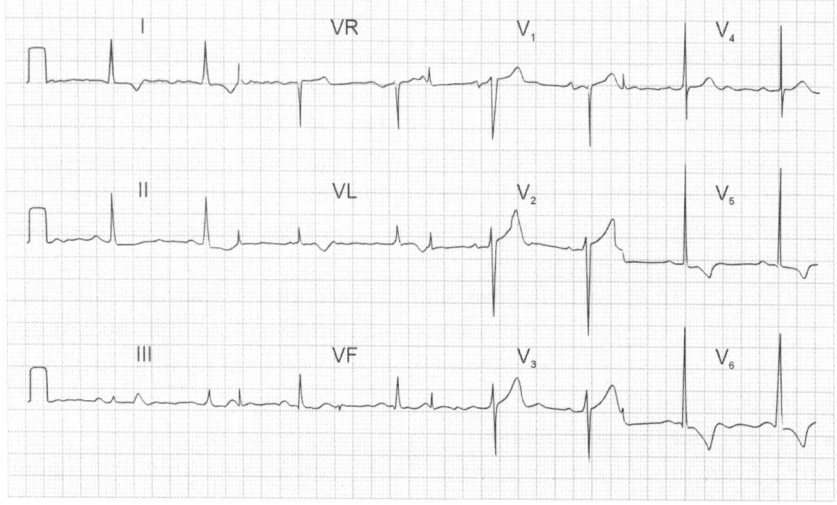

Fig. 3.1: Electrocardiogram (ECG) showing left ventricular hypertrophy (LVH).

- An S wave in lead V_1 or V_2 plus an R wave in lead V_5 or V_6 of >35 mm
- An R wave in V_5-V_6 >27 mm
- An R wave in aVL >11 mm

In LVH, the left atrium becomes enlarged to assist the decreased compliance of hypertrophied left ventricle. Thus, left atrial enlargement is an early ECG sign of LVH. The presence of left atrial enlargement and an ST-T-wave "strain pattern" in lead aVL, I, V_5, or V_6 increases the specificity and sensitivity, and indicates LVH if the voltage is borderline.

Left-axis deviation may be present in some cases, but it is not necessary for the diagnosis of LVH. The diagnosis of right ventricular hypertrophy (RVH), however, requires the presence of axis deviation. In presence of left anterior fascicular block, LVH is suggested when R wave in aVL >16 mm.

Q12. What are the common causes of LVH? What are the confirmatory investigations to detect LVH?
Ans. Common causes of LVH are: Hypertension, aortic stenosis (AS), HCM, aortic regurgitation (AR), mitral regurgitation (MR), coarctation of the aorta, patent ductus arteriosus (PDA), etc.

Echo [M-mode and two-dimensional echo (2-DE)] confirms the presence of LVH by measuring wall thickness and calculating LV mass.

Q13. What conditions could mimic LVH on ECG?
Ans. In absence of anatomic LVH, the following conditions may produce prominent LV voltage mimicking LVH on ECG:
- Left anterior fascicular block produces abnormally high voltage in leads I and aVL.
- Left bundle branch block—abnormal depolarization sequence produces abnormally high voltage.
- Wolff–Parkinson–White syndrome
- Acute myocardial ischemia—may be secondary to local intraventricular conduction delay.
- Others—young age (<25 years; R wave in V_5 or V_6 plus S wave in V_1 or V_2 should exceed 40 mm before the diagnosis of LVH can be made), thin-chest wall with closer proximity of the recording electrodes to the myocardial surface, black race (tend to have higher voltage than whites), left mastectomy (with close proximity of electrodes to myocardium).

Q14. What are the ECG features of RVH?
Ans. Electrocardiogram hallmarks of RVH include **(Fig. 3.2)**:
- Right-axis deviation of >110°
- A tall R wave in lead V_1 of ≥7 mm (in individuals more than 30 years of age)
- A deep S wave in lead V_6 or V_5 of ≥7 mm
- An R/S ratio in lead V_1 of ≥1

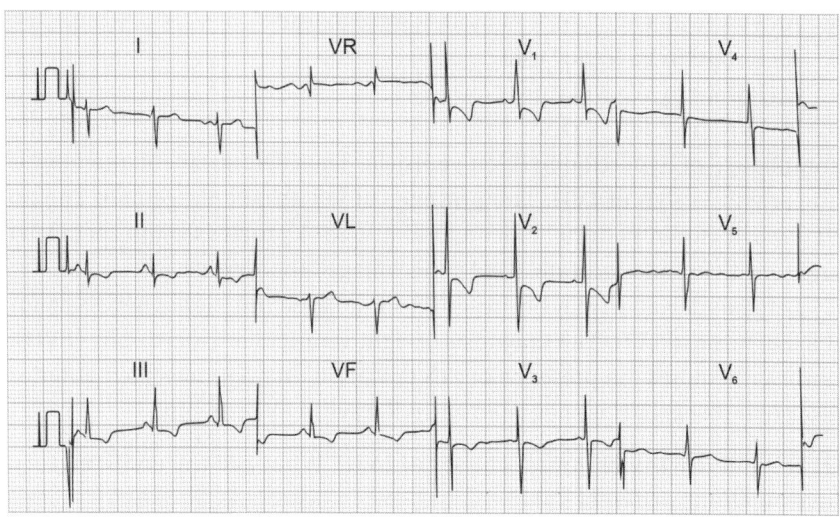

Fig. 3.2: ECG showing right ventricular hypertrophy (RVH).

- An R wave in V_1 plus an S wave in V_5 or V_6 of >9 mm

Any two of the above criteria indicate RVH.

Other findings that may be present are:
- A small q wave in lead V_1 (qR pattern) (since the normal location of the septum may be altered by the right ventricular mass, the initial force that depolarizes the septum may be directed from right to left and thus, q wave occurs in V_1). It is particularly seen in patients with congenital heart disease (CHD) and marked RVH.
- An ST-T-strain pattern in leads V_1-V_3 may be present and increases the specificity of the ECG criteria.
- Features of right atrial enlargement (P pulmonale) increase the probability of RVH.

Q15. What are the limitations in ECG diagnosis of RVH?
Ans.
- Right ventricular hypertrophy may be well advanced before ECG changes occur. Not infrequently, criteria for the diagnosis of RVH are not met in patients with clinical, echocardiographic, or hemodynamic evidence of this condition.
- Occasionally, a tall, pecked P wave in the inferior leads suggesting right atrial enlargement may be indirect evidence of RVH.
- A diagnosis of RVH should not be made in the presence of RBBB or WPW syndrome
- In patients with COPD and cor pulmonale, although right-axis deviation occurs, QRS axis may be directed posteriorly rather than anteriorly, resulting in normal, small, or even absent R wave in the right precordial

leads, thus anterior wall MI may be mimicked. As a general rule, when the diagnosis of COPD with cor pulmonale is known, the ECG diagnosis of MI should not be made without clinical correlation.
- The T-wave inversion in leads V_1-V_3 that may be seen in RVH can further mimic anterior wall myocardial ischemia or infarction.

In patients with COPD (predominant emphysema) with hyperinflation of the lung, ECG may show diffuse low voltage (with no QRS complex exceeding 5 mm in height in limb leads and 10 mm in height in chest leads). ECG criteria for diagnosis of RVH may not be valid. The QRS forces are directed superiorly, producing left-axis deviation. Hence, in the presence of pulmonary emphysema, left-axis deviation does not connote left anterior fascicular block.

The above factors should be considered when the pretest likelihood for infarction is low, and there is no supportive evidence for MI.

Q16. Besides RVH, what are the other causes of a tall R wave in lead V_1?
Ans.
- Right bundle branch block—if the QRS duration is ≥0.11 seconds, diagnosis of RBBB is considered; abnormal right-axis deviation is unexpected.
- Wolff-Parkinson-White syndrome—with an anterior oriented delta wave.
- True posterior infarction—T wave is upright in V_1-V_2.
- Hypertrophic cardiomyopathy
- A normal finding in children—adult configuration reaches by the age of 15 years.

Q17. What are the causes of RVH?
Ans.
- Rheumatic heart disease—mitral stenosis (MS), MR
- Congenital heart disease—tetralogy of Fallot (TOF), pulmonary stenosis, and Eisenmenger syndrome [in atrial septal defect (ASD), ventricular septal defect (VSD), and PDA]
- Chronic obstructive pulmonary disease
- Other causes of pulmonary hypertension (PH)—recurrent pulmonary embolism, primary PH

Q18. QRS duration greater than 0.12 seconds—what are the causes?
Ans. QRS durations is usually 0.04–0.10 seconds. QRS duration of more than 0.12 seconds may be due to:
- Complexes of ventricular origin—ventricular extrasystole (VES), ventricular tachycardia (VT), or ventricular-paced complex. The absence of associated preceding p waves and the presence of retrograde p waves are critical for confirming VES or VT, whereas identification of pacemaker spike recognizes a paced rhythm.
- Supraventricular tachycardia (SVT) with aberrancy.

- Bundle branch block: In RBBB—rabbit ear (rSR pattern) on the right-sided leads (V_1, V_2); wave complex looks normal if the terminal S wave on the left side (V_4, V_5, V_6) is disregarded. In LBBB—rabbit ears on the left-sided leads (V_5, V_6, and I) and Q waves in V_1-V_3.
- Wolff-Parkinson-White syndrome—short PR interval and delta wave present.
- Intraventricular conduction delay or peri-infarction block looks like a bundle branch block but cannot be identified as either RBBB or LBBB.

Q19. How is the differentiation of wide complex tachycardia made?
Ans. Wide complex tachycardia may be ventricular or supraventricular (with aberrant conduction) in origin. Points to consider in differentiating are:
- The clinical probability of a wide complex tachycardia being VT is 85%. The hemodynamic response to the tachycardia does not help differentiation (whether or not hypotension develops). If the patient is hemodynamically unstable, restore the normal cardiac rhythm with direct current (DC) cardioversion.
- When there is no time to carefully make a distinction, adenosine intravenous (IV) is acceptable for either SVT or VT, while IV verapamil is not an appropriate therapy for VT.

Q20. What are the atrial abnormalities on ECG?
Ans. The normal P wave results from the spread of electrical activity across the atrium. As the impulse spreads from right to left, the P wave is upright in leads I, III, and aVF, inverted in aVR, and may be upright, biphasic, or inverted in leads III, aVL, and V_1. It should not be higher than 2.5 mm in the unipolar leads and is usually <0.12 second in duration.
- P mitrale—broad, notched P wave in leads II and aVF (>2.5 mm wide). It is due to delayed depolarization of the left atrium. When the left atrium is enlarged, P wave is broad, biphasic in V_1.
- P pulmonale: Tall and peaked P wave (>2.5 mm high) is seen in leads II, III, and aVF. It is due to right atrial enlargement associated with lung disease, pulmonary embolism, or other causes of PH.
- Inversion of P wave (negative in leads in which it is positive): This usually occurs when there is abnormal propagation of the electrical impulse through the atria. Pacemaker not in the sinoatrial (SA) node but is in the atrioventricular (AV) node or below, as it occurs in junctional rhythm.
- Inversing of the P wave in leads and a positive P wave in aVR, with lead I being the mirror image of lead II. This may occur when the arm leads are reversed or in dextrocardia. In true dextrocardia there is a loss of R wave in leads V_4-V_6.
- P wave is absent or invisible due to presence of junctional rhythm or SA block.

- **P wave** is replaced by flutter wave with saw-tooth baseline in atrial flutter (**Fig. 3.3**) or fibrillatory wave in atrial fibrillation (AF).

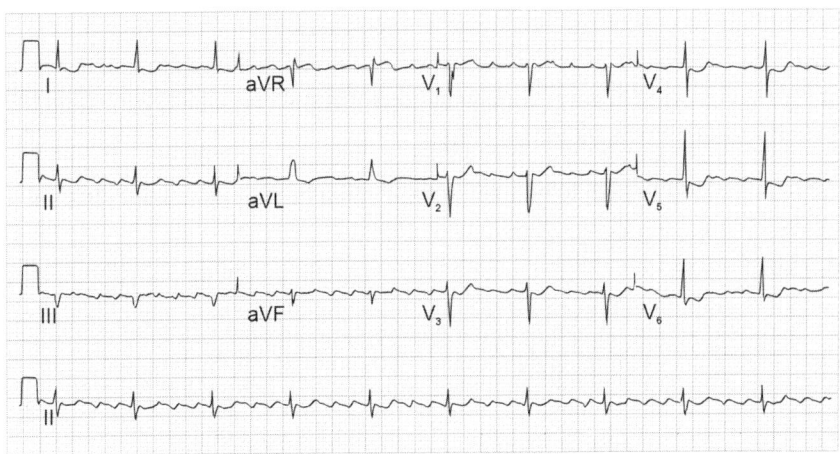

Fig. 3.3: Atrial flutter with 4:1 atrioventricular (AV) conduction.

Q21. What are the conditions mimicking acute MI on ECG?
Ans.
- Acute pericarditis—ST-segment elevation is concave as opposed to upward convexity with infarction. ST elevation is not confirmed to an anatomic coronary supply, it occurs in leads II, III, and aVF, and in the precordial leads.
- Left bundle branch block
- Chronic obstructive pulmonary disease
- Right ventricular pacing
- Wolff–Parkinson–White syndrome
- Left ventricular aneurysm and previous infarction
- Left ventricular hypertrophy—causing poor R wave progression in leads V_1-V_3 and ST elevation.
- Early repolarization changes—ST-segment is commonly elevated in leads V_2-V_5, or in leads II, III, aVF. ST-segment is usually concave, rather than convex; emergent Q waves and reciprocal depression are absent, T waves are often peaked and prominent.
- Prinzmetal angina in individuals with coronary artery spasm. ST elevation occurs during pain. It is rare; pain responds to nitroglycerin (NG), and the ST-segment returns to normal (in all patients presenting with atypical features of acute MI, NG should be administered before treating with thrombolytic agent).
- Acute myocarditis—usually causing nonspecific ST-T-wave changes. ST-segment elevation and Q waves may appear, simulating infarction.

- Acute cor pulmonale
- Tension pneumothorax

Q22. What do you mean by bundle branch block?

Ans. It is the impairment of conduction of impulse through one or more of the divisions of the intraventricular conduction system distal to (or within the lower portion of) the bundle of His.

The conduction fibers that participate in the depolarization of ventricular tissue are:
- The right bundle branch
- The common left bundle branch
- Anterior and posterior fascicles of the left bundle branch
- Also, there are septal fibers originating from the left bundle branch

Q23. How are the bundle branch block patterns classified?
Ans.
- *According to the degree of block:*
  - Incomplete—does not produce abnormal prolongation of the QRS interval (QRS interval <0.12 second and >0.10 second).
  - Complete—produce prolongation of the QRS interval (QRS interval >0.12s)
- *According to the bundle involved (right or left):*
  - Right bundle branch block
  - Left bundle branch block
  - Bilateral-bundle branch block-combinations:
    - RBBB and left anterior hemiblock (LAHB) or left posterior hemiblock (LPHB)—bifascicular block
    - RBBB and right and common LBBB
    - Right and both anterior and posterior divisions of LBBB
  - Fascicular block (hemiblock)—LAHB and LPHB

Q24. Compare and contrast between RBBB and LBBB.

Ans. Both RBBB and LBBB produce widening of QRS complex. Differences lie in wave pattern and their clinical significance **(Fig. 3.4 and Table 3.2)**.

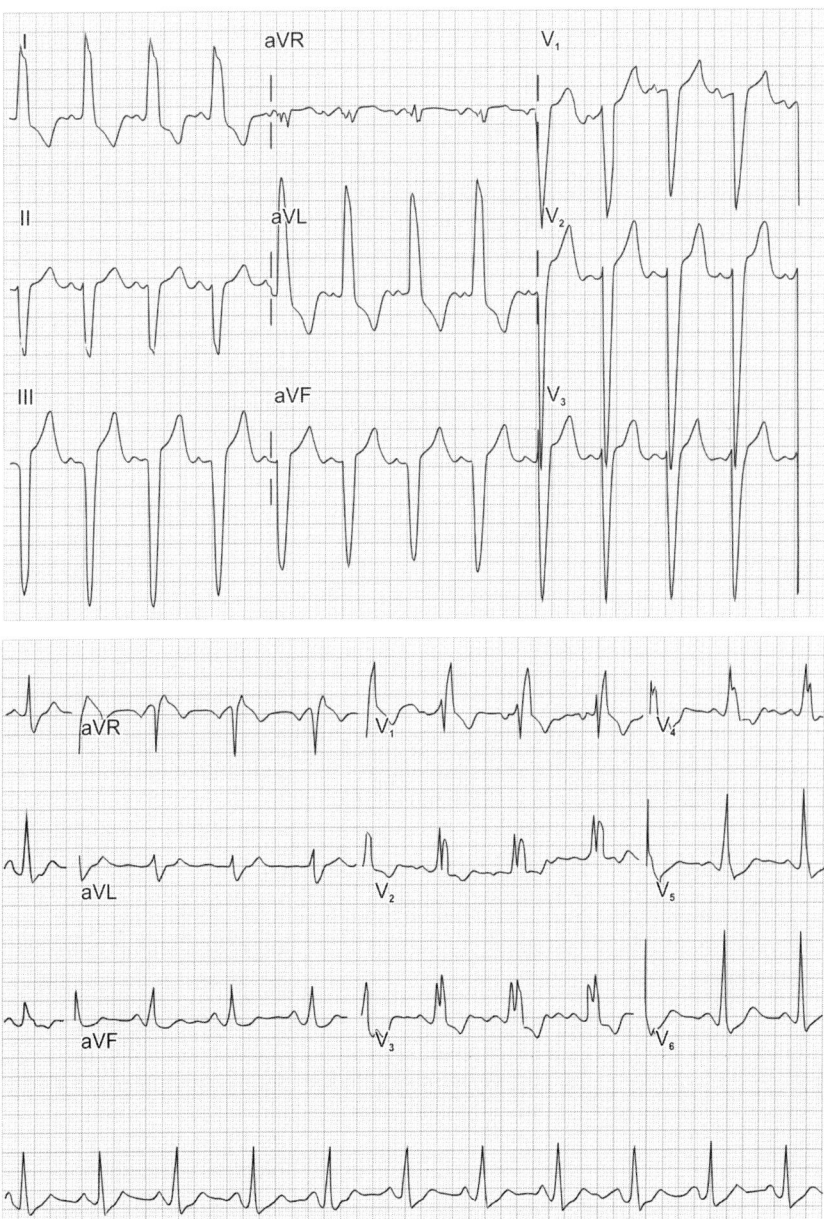

Fig. 3.4: Left bundle branch block (upper) and right bundle branch block (lower).

TABLE 3.2: Right bundle branch block (RBBB) and left bundle branch block (LBBB).

Points	RBBB	LBBB
Septal activation (from left to right)	Normal	Abnormal
QRS complex	M-shaped in V_1–V_2 (rsR', RSR', RSr'), Slurred S in V_5, V_6, I	M-shaped in V_5, V_6, I, QS in V_1
ST-segment	Usually normal	Elevated in V_1–V_4 (does not indicate MI)
Association with acute MI	More common with anteroseptal MI (IVS and right bundle has same blood supply from LAD artery)	Presence of new LBBB indicates ST-segment elevation acute MI
Association with acute MI	Presence of new RBBB itself does not qualify administration of thrombolytics	New LBBB itself qualifies thrombolysis in appropriate setting
Diagnosis of MI (acute or old)	Can be made (no effect on Q)	Cannot be made (initial QRS vector is abnormal)
Effect on LVH	No effect; diagnosis can be made on voltage criteria (if RBBB present on ECG)	Cannot be diagnosed (in presence of LBBB)
Rate-dependent conduction block	Yes (as RBBB has longest refractory period)	Nil
Association with heart disease	Less	More (permanent LBBB is almost always the result of organic heart disease)
Common causes	Rate dependency, cor pulmonale, myocarditis, cardiomyopathy, and pericarditis	Coronary heart disease, degenerative disease, LVH, cardiomyopathy, aortic stenosis, traumatic, and infective endocarditis

(ECG: electrocardiogram; IVS: interventricular septum; LAD: left anterior descending; LBBB: left bundle branch block; LVH: left ventricular hypertrophy; MI: myocardial infarction; RBBB: right bundle branch block)

Q25. What are the points to differentiate RBBB from RVH?

Ans. Both produce a tall R wave in right-sided precordial leads. Differentiating points are listed in **Table 3.3**.

TABLE 3.3: Difference between right bundle branch block (RBBB) and right ventricular hypertrophy (RVH).

Points	RBBB	RVH
Duration of QRS complex	≥0.12 second	<0.12 second
QRS configuration in V_1	rSR pattern	QR or pure R
QRS in leads V_5, V_6, I	Wide (with a wide S wave)	Normal
QRS axis	Normal	Rightward deviation (≥110°)
Ventricular activation time (time from beginning of QRS to the peak of R) in V_1	0.06–0.09s	0.04–0.05s

(RBBB: right bundle branch block; RVH: right ventricular hypertrophy)

Q26. What is bifascicular block? What is the significance?
Ans. Bifascicular block means the delay of conduction in right bundle branch along with one of the two fascicles of the left bundle branch, i.e., RBBB with LAHB or RBBB with LPHB **(Fig. 3.5)**.

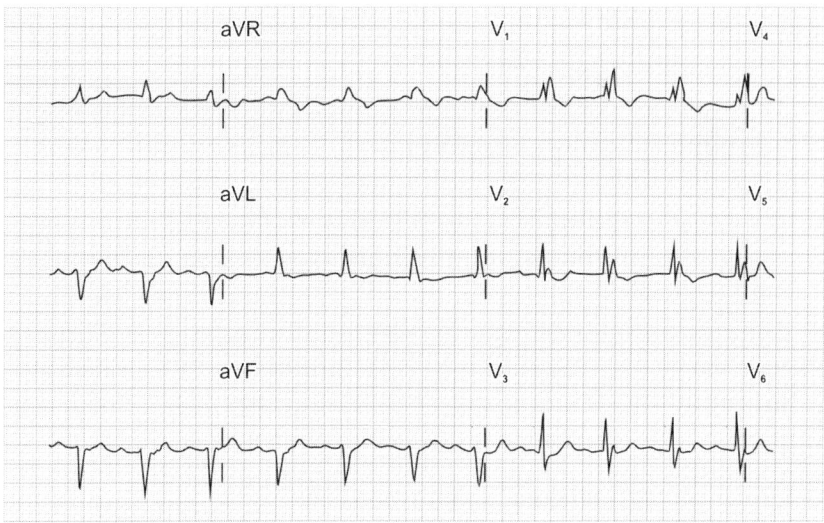

Fig. 3.5: Bifascicular block—RBBB and LAHB (QRS axis—90°).
(LAHB: left anterior hemiblock; RBBB: right bundle branch block)

- RBBB with LAHB most common type; presence of feature of RBBB and a left-axis deviation of 45–90°.
- RBBB with LPHB—combination of RBBB and a QRS axis of $+110^0$ or greater. Significance: In acute MI, the new development of bifascicular block implies extensive necrosis of the ventricular myocardium, including the

IVS. This condition needs the implantation of a temporary pacemaker (TPM). The degenerative process producing bifascicular block does not predict the development of complete heart block (CHB). If patient is asymptomatic, implantation of TPM is not needed. At times, bundle branch block is intermittent.
- Sometimes RBBB and LBBB may also alternate in the same tracing.
- The posterior fascicle is thick and short, has a double blood supply from LAD artery and right coronary artery (RCA), and is not commonly damaged.

■ HOLTER MONITORING

Prolonged electrocardiographic recording in patients engaged in normal daily activities is the most useful way of documenting and quantitating frequency and complexity of an arrhythmia, correlating it with patient's symptoms, and evaluating effect of antiarrhythmic therapy on arrhythmia. In addition, some recorders can document alteration of QRS, ST, and T contours.

Q1. What are the types of ambulatory ECG recordings available?
Ans. Major types of ambulatory ECG recordings include Holter monitors, event monitors, and implantable loop recorders (ILRs).
- *Holter monitor:* Continuous ECG recordings (e.g., 24- or 48-hours-cassette tape recorders, or digital loop recorders). 24-hours-Holter recorders are satisfactory if symptoms occur on an almost daily basis.
- *Event monitor:* Patient-activated device, especially useful when a patient can predict symptoms of arrhythmia and symptoms are infrequent (e.g., once a fortnight).
- *Implantable loop recorders:* An invasive monitoring device allowing long-term monitoring. These are sometimes indicated for investigating more infrequent episodes of syncope occurring greater than 1 month apart from each other, and noninvasive methods do not produce a diagnosis.

Q.2. What are the findings of Holter recordings?
Ans. Ambulatory recordings are usually read by an automated computer reader with subsequent eye verification. The following information are seen:
- *Heart-rate histogram:* Reveals heart-rate variability; flat tracing may indicate inactivity. A very flat trace may indicate a pacemaker. A decreased heart-rate variability, hence flat tracing may occur in diabetic patients and patients with MI (anterior > inferior). Here, a predominantly sympathetic control (and reduction in parasympathetic) decreases the fibrillation

threshold and predisposes to ventricular fibrillation (VF). A sudden jump in heart rate may signify episodes of arrhythmia.
- *Ectopic beat counter:* Narrow and broad-complex premature beats, couplets, triplets, VT and SVT episodes and pauses may be counted.
- *Rhythm strips:* Including main rhythm during recording, examples of arrhythmias recorded (including onset and offset), rhythm during episodes noted in patient's diary, and rhythm during maximum and minimum heart rate.
- *Ischemia episodes:* ST-segment depression ≥0.1 mV indicates silent or symptomatic ischemia.

Q.3. What information does Holter monitoring provide for patients with ischemic heart disease (IHD)?
Ans.
- *Silent ischemia:* It is the most important diagnostic tool. Nocturnal ST-segment changes may be an indicator of 2- or 3-vessel coronary artery disease (CAD) or left main stem stenosis.
- Detection of Prinzmetal angina.
- Post-MI evaluation—detection of frequency and complexity of ventricular ectopy, these are predictors of increased cardiovascular morbidity and mortality.
- Effectiveness of antiarrhythmic therapy

Q4. When are Holter monitoring findings considered to be positive?
Ans.
- *Arrhythmia:*
  - Bradyarrhythmias or tachyarrhythmias **(Fig. 3.6)** associated with symptoms.
  - Sinus pauses >3 seconds

  Second degree AV block type II

Ischemia: Indicated as ST-segment depression ≥0.1 mV. Several arrhythmias, such as sinus bradycardia (35–40 beats/min), sinus arrhythmias (with pause up to 3 seconds), SA-exit block; second degree AV block type 1, wandering pacemaker, junctional escape complexes, and premature atrial or ventricular contractions may not be abnormal. Again, early depolarization (i.e., normal ST elevations) which sinks to baseline with increasing heart rate, should not be misinterpreted as ischemia.

Correlation of the ECG information with patient's symptoms is an important component of complete interpretation.

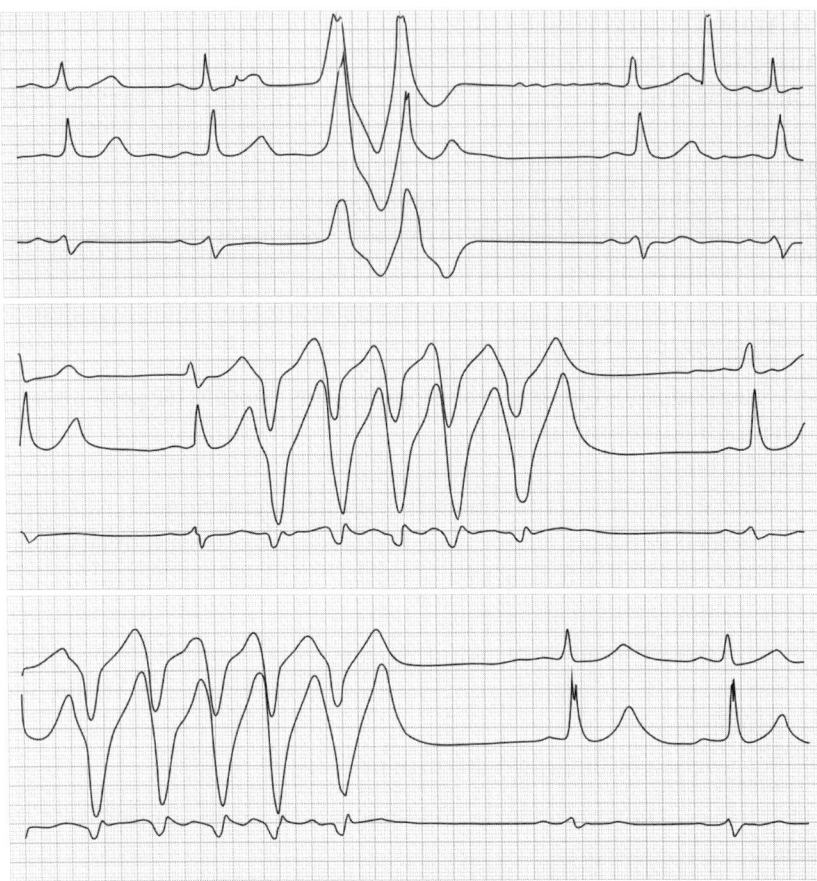

Fig. 3.6: Holter monitor showing multifocal ventricular ectopics, couplets, salvo, and nonsustained ventricular tachycardia (VT).

Q5. What is an ILR?
Ans. Implantable loop recorder (ILR) is used for patients with infrequent and transient symptoms, where neither Holter recorders nor 30-day-event recorders are helpful. Here, a small device is inserted under the skin at about the second rib on the left, anteriorly and is activated by passing a special magnet over it. The device can be configured to store patient-activated episodes, automatically activated recordings, or a combination of these.

■ EXERCISE TREADMILL TEST

Physiological stress of exercise places a major demand on the cardiopulmonary system. Hence, exercise is utilized to test cardiac performance and function. Thus, exercise ECG, that evaluates the response of cardiovascular system to exercise under carefully controlled conditions, can provide diagnostic, prognostic, and functional information.

Q1. What is Exercise Treadmill Test (ETT)?

Ans. Exercise treadmill test, also called exercise tolerance test, is the noninvasive evaluation of cardiovascular system's response to exercise under carefully controlled conditions using a treadmill. As the test is done in a treadmill, it is also designated as treadmill test (TMT).

Q2. What role does exercise ECG have in the diagnosis of CAD?

Ans.
- In patients with chest pain of uncertain etiology and a normal resting ECG, a standard exercise test is useful in the diagnosis of CAD. It is most valuable in confirming or excluding the diagnosis of CAD in patients with an intermediate pretest probability of CAD on the basis of age, sex, symptoms, and risk factors. Typically, these are adult male patients with some atypical anginal features and a normal ECG, who may or may not have risk factors for CAD. If typical anginal discomfort occurs during exercise and/or there is horizontal or downsloping ST-segment depression of ≥1 mm during test in these patients, it is virtually diagnostic of CAD.
- Exercise testing adds little to diagnosing CAD in patients with high pretest probability of CAD (i.e., adults with a history of typical angina with one or more risk factors), exercise test is positive usually. For these patients, invasive testing is preferred for a more definitive diagnosis, and possible intervention. A negative test may well be a false negative test in these patients.
- In patients with low pretest probability of CAD (i.e., young patients with a typical history of angina and normal resting ECG), a negative exercise test is highly reliable for excluding the diagnosis of significant CAD.

Thus, the main use of ETT is as a gateway to other imaging modalities and evaluation of prognosis.

Q3. What are the limitations of exercise ECG in the diagnosis of CAD?

Ans.
- Exercise ECG testing has a low specificity and sensitivity (65% sensitivity and 85% specificity). As a screening test for CAD in persons without symptoms, exercise ECG is not helpful. The ST-segment response to exercise in this group has a poor predictive accuracy. A positive test is often a false positive test in those patients with low pretest probability of CAD.
- ST depression is a representative of global subendocardial ischemia. It does not localize ischemia to an area of myocardium, or identify the coronary artery involved. ST depression in the inferior leads (II, aVF) is most often caused by the atrial repolarization wave (which begins in the PR segment and may extend to the beginning of ST-segment). Thus,

ST-segment changes, isolated to the inferior leads, are more likely to be a false positive response unless profound (i.e., >1 mm).
- ST depression during exercise may be obscured by baseline ECG abnormalities as in LBBB, LVH with repolarization abnormalities, WPW syndrome, digitalis therapy, ventricular paced rhythm, mitral valve prolapse (MVP). ST-depression is also not interpretable in previous coronary artery bypass graft and Q-wave MI.
- Ischemic ST depression normally occurs in the lateral leads (I, V_4-V_6). Isolated inferior or anterior changes are often false positive findings.
- Exercise testing is not useful for patients with claudication, severe lung problems, arthritis, poor physical fitness, or other conditions that limit the ability to exercise.
- The viability of myocardium cannot be determined with stress ECG.
- Rarely, severe cardiac diseases can cause an inadequate cardiac response to exercise—chronotropic incompetence.

Q4. What is the Bruce protocol?
Ans. Protocols have been developed by many investigators for exercise ECG testing. The one developed by Bruce and coworkers is the most popular, both because it is most extensively validated and because it can be performed relatively quickly. The Bruce protocol is used for diagnostic and prognostic evaluation of otherwise fit, stable patients with suspected CAD.

In this protocol, each stage lasts 3 minutes. During stage I, the patient walks at 1.7 mph up to a 10% grade. Energy expenditure for the average person is estimated to be 4.8 metabolic equivalents (METs) during this stage. Both speed and grade rise with each stage. It is unusual for patients to complete stage V (5.0 mph, 18% grade). An initial zero-and-one-half stage (1.7 mph at 0%, then 5% grade) is used for modified Bruce protocol. The modified Bruce protocol is useful for frail and elderly subjects, and as a limited protocol for risk assessment in patients stabilized after an episode of suspected unstable angina (UA).

Q5. What is an age-predicted maximum heart rate (APMHR)?
Ans. It is well known that maximum heart rate (MHR) decreases with age, thus most equations incorporate age. The most common formula is:
APMHR = 220 – Age

By convention, most clinicians accept a heart rate of 85% of the predicted maximum as reflective of near maximal exercise, a level of exercise that yields a sufficiently sensitive test.

Q6. What is a submaximal exercise test?
Ans. In a submaximal test, the goal for a patient is not to reach his or her maximum tolerated exercise capacity, but to stop at a level lower than that. The goal can be defined as a heart rate of 70% of maximum predicted, a heart

rate of 120 beats/min, or the completion of a certain stage of a protocol. A submaximal test is typically used for patients undergoing stress testing within 1 week after an acute MI.

Q7. How does exercise heart rate influence the test results?
Ans. Heart rate is considered as an index for the intensity of exercise. In general, the closer a patient gets to his or her predicted MHR, the more intense the exercise is, the more stress is placed on the cardiopulmonary system, and the more sensitive the test will be. Conventionally, a heart rate of 85% of predicted maximum is considered as reflective of a near maximal exercise to yield a sufficiently sensitive test. If maximal heart rate does not exceed 85% of APMHR during testing and there are no substantial ECG changes, the test is usually read as nondiagnostic. If there are substantial ECG changes, the test is read as abnormal regardless of the heart rate achieved.

A rapidly rising heart rate at low levels of exercise can indicate severe deconditioning.

Q8. What information to be included in an exercise ECG report?
Ans. Following points to be included:
- Protocol used
- Duration of exercise (time and stage)
- Peak treadmill speed and grade
- Peak workload in MET or VO_2 max
- Functional capacity
- Maximum heart rate achieved and percentage of APMHR
- Resting and peak blood pressure (BP)
- Symptoms—chest pain, dizziness, syncope, etc.
- Arrhythmias
- Electrocardiographic changes

Q9. What may be the exercise ECG test results?
Ans. It may be normal (negative), abnormal (positive), nondiagnostic, strongly positive, false positive.
- *Positive ETT-criteria:*
  - Horizontal or downsloping ST depression ≥1 mm, relative to PQ segment, 80 ms after the J-point (junction between QRS complex and ST-segment). It is the diagnostic hallmark.
  - ST elevation ≥1.0 mm in leads without Q waves, or not after a prior MI. In the presence of a normal resting ECG, ST elevation indicates severe ischemia (spasm or a critical lesion).
  - Typical anginal symptoms when associated with ST- or T-wave changes
  - Failure of BP to rise during exercise, or a decrease in systolic blood pressure (SBP) (ischemic LV dysfunction).

- Arrhythmias—sustained SVT, AFs, atrial flutter, junctional rhythm, nonsustained VT, second- or third- degree AV block.
- Increase in QRS voltage (ischemic LV dysfunction).

■ *Nondiagnostic ETT:* Those in which the subject does not achieve 85% of APMHR and has no abnormal ECG changes, or in which baseline ECG changes are present that obscure ST changes.

■ *False positive ETT (positive results with normal coronary artery):* These are particularly common in patients with a low pretest likelihood of CAD, e.g., asymptomatic young women, and patients with hyperkinetic heart syndrome (those with sympathetic overactivity, emotional lability, and resting tachycardia). Other associations are: Hyperventilation, hypertension [especially with LVH and strain pattern, prolapsing mitral valve (MV), hypertrophic cardiomyopathy (contraindicated in obstructive type)], dilated cardiomyopathy (DCM), AS, and resting ECG abnormalities (LBBB, WPW syndrome, digoxin, and tricyclic antidepressant therapy, coronary artery spasm, etc. (**Fig. 3.7**).

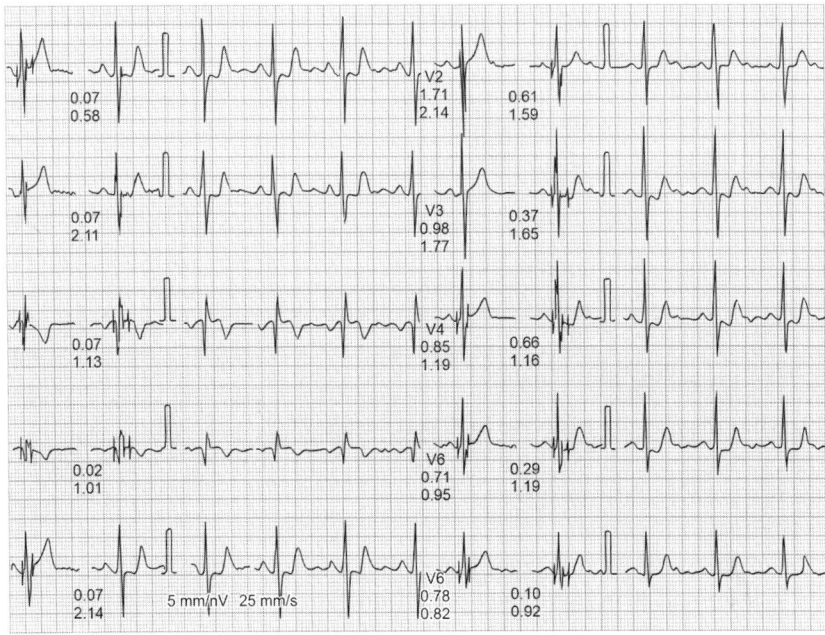

Fig. 3.7: Horizontal ST depression of >2 mm in a 40-years-old female, subsequently CAG was normal (thus, ETT result is false positive).

ST-segment changes in inferior leads alone (in absence of change in lateral leads especially V_5) are likely to be false positive result.

■ *Strongly positive ETT:* A test is strongly positive when ST depression appears at low workload <6 min in modified Bruce protocol, during first or second stage of the Bruce protocol, especially if exercise is terminated by the patient during one of those stages (**Fig. 3.8**). Abnormal BP response (failure to increase SBP ≥120 mm Hg, or a sustained decrease ≥10 mm Hg, or below resting level), ventricular arrhythmias—reproducible, sustained (>30 seconds), or symptomatic VT.

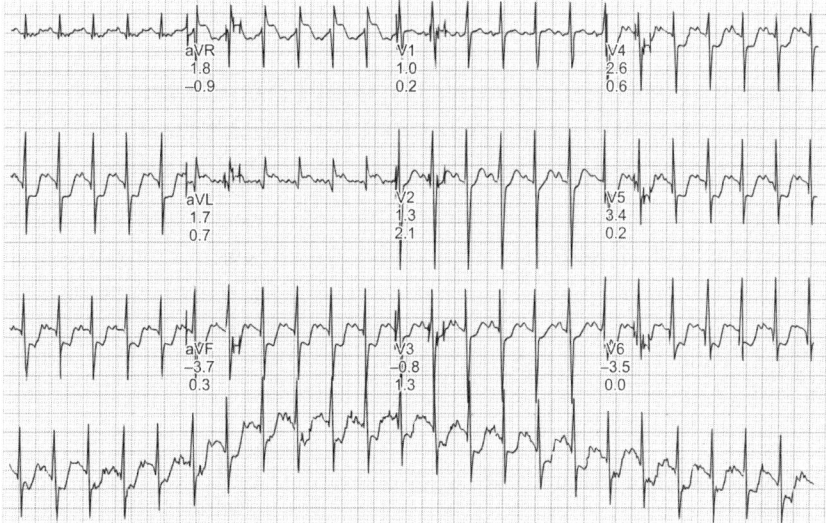

Fig. 3.8: Strongly positive ETT result (horizontal ST depression of >2 mm in stage I) in a 60-years-old male; subsequent CAG revealed multivessel CAD.

A strongly positive ETT indicates a relatively high likelihood (>70%) of severe CAD (multivessel disease or left main-stem disease) and is associated with adverse prognosis.

- *False negative ETT (negative result in the presence of CAD):* A rapidly rising heart rate at low levels of exercise may occur in severe deconditioning and/or severe cardiopulmonary disease. Heart rate may quickly reach to 85% of APMHR, but still insufficient load on the heart to produce a positive ETT result. Hence, the result may be false negative. Some baseline ECG abnormalities may obscure ST changes during exercise, e.g., LBBB, ventricular paced beats, WPW syndrome, ST abnormalities of SVT, or AF, etc. Thus, the result may be false negative.

If clinical impression is that the exercise ECG result is a false positive, or a false negative, or nondiagnostic, then one should apply the best-performed exercise add-on that is available. This could be CAG, but usually it will be nuclear perfusion.

CARDIOVASCULAR IMAGING TECHNIQUES

These include:
- *Nonionizing radiation techniques:*
  - Using ultrasounds—echo and Doppler

- Using radiowaves—CMR imaging
- Positron emission tomography scanning
- *Ionizing radiation techniques:*
  - X-ray
  - Nuclear cardiology—using gamma rays
  - Cardiac CT

CARDIAC RADIOLOGY (INCLUDING COMPUTED TOMOGRAPHY, CARDIOVASCULAR MAGNETIC RESONANCE, POSITRON EMISSION TOMOGRAPHY)

In various heart diseases, chest radiography may reveal changes in cardiac anatomy as well as pulmonary vasculature at a low cost. Clinical diagnosis done on the basis of physical signs can be ascertained by doing a simple CxR. A secundum ASD can be incorrectly diagnosed as MS because of similar physical signs, although the radiological signs of the two entities are quite different. Conversely, the radiological findings need to be correlated with clinical and other laboratory findings.

Q1. What are the patterns of cardiac chamber enlargement on chest X-ray?
Ans.
- *LV enlargement:* Left ventricle type cardiomegaly; left cardiophrenic angle is obtuse, and LV apex may be seen inside the diaphragm through the fundic gas.
- *RV enlargement:* Right ventricle type cardiomegaly; left cardiophrenic angle is acute, and the apex of the heart seems to be elevated above the diaphragm. Retrosternal space is obliterated on the left lateral view.
- *Left atrial enlargement:* Double contour of right border, straightening of the left border (contributed by enlarged left auricular appendage); esophagus is pushed back on barium swallow examination.
- *Right atrial enlargement:* Right border formed by the right atrium becomes more convex.
- *Aortic enlargement:* Aortic knuckle becomes prominent, sometimes unfolded. Ascending aorta becomes dilated in AS (due to poststenotic dilatation).
- *Pulmonary artery (PA) enlargement:* Pulmonary conus becomes full, sometimes convex (in PH or poststenotic dilatation).

Q2. Huge cardiomegaly without specific chamber dilatation—what are the possibilities?
Ans. Causes of huge cardiomegaly are:
- Multiple valvular disease
- Pericardial effusion

- Cardiomyopathy
- Ebstein anomaly (**Fig. 3.9**)

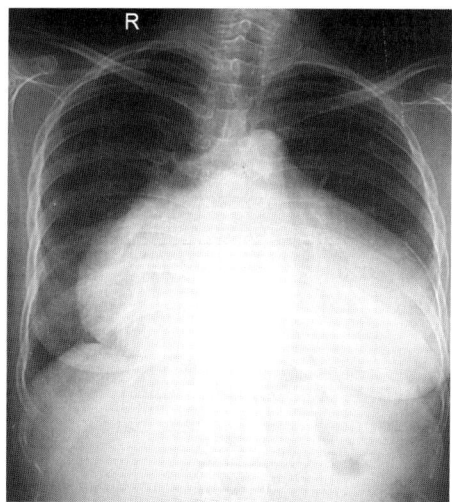

Fig. 3.9: Huge cardiomegaly in Ebstein anomaly.

Q3. What are the X-ray findings of pulmonary edema? What are the differential diagnoses?

Ans. Haziness in the lung, most prominent in the perihilar region in a bat-wing or butterfly pattern. This haziness has a ground-glass appearance. Opacity is due to edema fluid and lucency is due to air in the bronchial tree (*see* **Figs.12.2A and B**)

Differential diagnoses are:
- Noncardiac pulmonary edema, i.e., adult respiratory distress syndrome (ARDS)
- Bronchopneumonia

Q4. What are the radiologic features of PH?

Ans. Pulmonary hypertension may be:
- Pulmonary venous hypertension—upper-lobe diversion
- Pulmonary capillary hypertension—peribronchial cuffing, perihilar haze (bat-wing pattern), and Kerley B line
- Pulmonary arterial hypertension—full pulmonary conus

Q5. How do pulmonary vascular markings give clue to cardiac diseases?

Ans.
- *Pulmonary veins:* They become dilated when left atrial pressure increases. Dilated upper lobe veins in chronically elevated left atrial pressure as in MS is called upper lobe diversion.

- *Pulmonary artery:* Full pulmonary conus (instead of normal concavity) is a sign of pulmonary arterial hypertension. Pulmonary conus becomes bulged in shunt anomalies (due to large flow). Lower lobe PAs are more dilated in shunt anomalies due to the gravitational effect. In Eisenmenger syndrome, peripheral PAs are attenuated (called peripheral pruning).
- *Pulmonary capillaries:* Congested capillaries due to raised left atrial pressure cause peribronchial cuffing and pulmonary edema. Dilated lymphatics at lung base, in an attempt at draining the edema fluid produces Kerley B line. Pulmonary capillary hemorrhage, resulting from ruptured bronchopulmonary anastomotic sites, produces hemosiderosis (engulfment of iron particles by macrophage with secondary calcification).

Also, pleural effusion, especially right sided, may occur in chronic heart failure (CHF).

Q6. How to differentiate various shunt anomalies on chest X-ray?
Ans. Three commonly found shunt anomalies have characteristic radiological features **(Table 3.4 and Fig. 3.10).**

TABLE 3.4: Shunt anomalies on chest X-ray-differentiating points.

Point	ASD	VSD	PDA
Age	Usually adult	Younger	Usually adult
Cardiomegaly	RV type	LV type	LV type
Leftward shift	Yes	No	No
Pulmonary plethora	Marked	Less marked	Less marked
Inverted comma sign*	Yes	Nil	Nil
Pulmonary edema	Never	May occur	May occur

*Dilated right lower pulmonary artery.
(ASD: atrial septal defect; LV: left ventricle; PDA: patent ductus arteriosus; RV: right ventricle; VSD: ventricular septal defect)

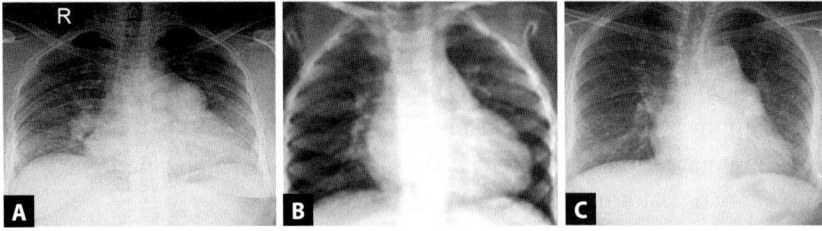

Figs. 3.10A to C: Chest radiograph of (A) ASD, (B) VSD (B), and (C) PDA.

Q7. What are the radiological findings of left atrial enlargement?
Ans. Left atrium is posteriorly situated (not to the left), hence not visible on posteroanterior view. However, if enlarged, it goes more posteriorly and produces a double contour on the right border (right and left border at different

levels with lung intervening). On the left border, it produces a bulge below the pulmonary conus due to an enlarged left auricular appendage contributing to the straightening of left border **(Fig. 3.11)**. Left atrial enlargement may also produce splaying of the left bronchus (upward displacement).

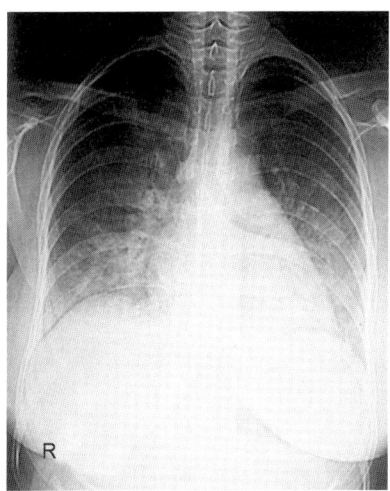

Fig. 3.11: Left atrial enlargement in mitral stenosis.

Q8. What are the differences between left ventricle and right ventricle type apex on CxR?
Ans. When left ventricle enlarges, it presses the diaphragm down, and the angle between the diaphragm and the apex is obtuse.

When right ventricle enlarges, it lifts the apex up from the diaphragm. As a result, the angle between the apex and the diaphragm becomes acute.

Q9. What is upper lobe diversion? What is the mechanism?
Ans. When left atrial pressure increases, there is raised pulmonary venous pressure (i.e., pulmonary venous hypertension). Pressure increases more in lower zone pulmonary veins due to hydrostatic reasons. Hence, there is a tendency to develop pulmonary edema. To prevent the development of pulmonary edema, the lower lobe pulmonary veins undergo active vasoconstriction. As a result, blood is diverted from lower lobe veins to upper lobe. This is called upper lobe diversion (or cephalization). It is evident on the chest radiograph as dilated linear radio-opaque lines. It is a protective phenomenon to prevent the development of pulmonary edema. It is most commonly seen in mitral valvular diseases (also may develop in other conditions producing raised left atrial pressure).

Q10. What are the cardiac conditions where calcification may be found on CxR?
Ans. These are:
- Aortic knuckle (eggshell calcification)—in old age due to atherosclerosis

- Pulmonary hemosiderosis—in MS **(Fig. 3.12A)**
- Pericardial calcification—in constrictive pericarditis and tubercular pericarditis **(Fig. 3.12B)**
- Aortic valve—senile or rheumatic AS
- Coronary arteries—atherosclerotic
- Others—calcification of LV thrombus, left atrial thrombus, etc.

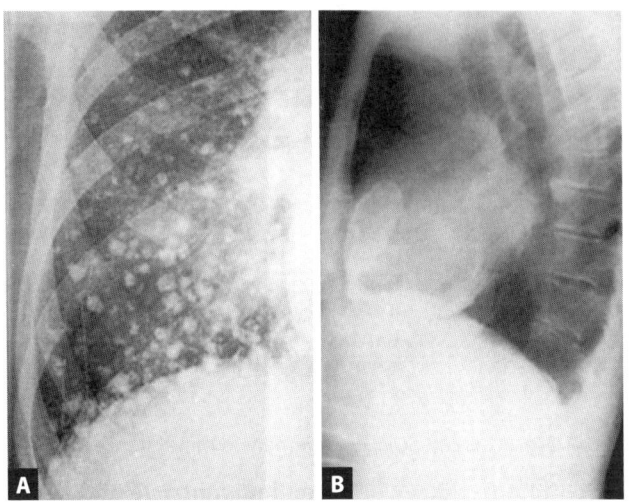

Figs. 3.12A and B: Pulmonary hemosiderosis in MS (A), and pericardial calcification on lateral view (B).

Q11. What are the various ways of imaging coronary arteries?
Ans.
- Coronary angiography—gold standard
- Computed tomography angiography
- Magnetic resonance angiography (MRA)

Q12. What are the ways of estimating ejection fraction (EF)?
Ans.
- Echocardiography—most commonly done
- Left ventriculography (LV graphy)—using contrast during catheterization.
- Radionuclide ventriculography—using radiotracers
- Cardiac magnetic resonance imaging (MRI)—most reliable

Q13. What is the principle of CMR?
Ans. Hydrogen of the human body behave like magnets and align to an exposed magnetic field. When a body region can be excited by a pulse of radiowaves in a 1.5 T magnetic field at a resonant frequency of 63 MHz, all excited hydrogen nuclei rotate away from the direction of main magnetic field axis (the flip angle) and process in a coordinated manner which causes net magnetization. After the excitation phase is finished, the net magnetization

decays to the former position (relaxation), and the energy is transmitted as a radiosignal. Typically, this signal is formed into a radiowave echo by the scanner, such that it can be used for an image by a receiver antenna.

Q14. How is CMR a safe procedure? What are its advantages?
Ans. Physical interaction required for CMR is at the level of atomic nucleus. The frequency of radiowave absorption depends on the external magnetic field. MR does not interfere with the electrons on the outer atomic shell that are responsible for chemical bindings. Thus, it is fundamentally safe unlike ionizing radiation, such as X-ray which may interact with electrons binding damaging molecules such as deoxyribonucleic acid (DNA).

The advantages of CMR are: It is neither operator-dependent nor limited by acoustic window (problem faced in echo). It can differentiate ischemic cardiomyopathy (ICM) from nonischemic cardiomyopathy.

Q15. What are the cardiac conditions where CMR is diagnostic?
Ans. Cardiovascular magnetic resonance is gold standard for assessment of regional and global LV systolic function, MI, and viability and assessment of CHDs.

Clinical applications of CMR are:
- Coronary artery disease—Coronary magnetic resonance angiogram for coronary anomalies, LV function, and myocardial perfusion study (by wall-motion abnormality induced by ischemia using adenosine/dipyridamole).
- Heart failure and cardiomyopathy—differentiating DCM from ICM, HCM, arrhythmogenic right ventricular cardiomyopathy, etc.
- Congenital heart diseases—complex CHD, adult CHD after surgical correction. 3-D configuration and less operator dependence make it suitable for the purpose. A combination of CMR and transesophageal echo (TEE) is best.
- Pericardial diseases—pericardial constriction (where echo provides incomplete information), detection of small effusion
- Tumors—its relation to adjacent structures
- Others—aortic dissection, post heart transplantation, etc.

Q16. What is viable myocardium? How to detect it?
Ans. It means myocardium with impaired contractile function that is potentially reversible. Characteristic features of a viable myocardium are:
- Impaired systolic wall motion at rest
- Normal or reduced but not absent blood flow
- Preservation of cellular homeostasis—cell-membrane integrity and production of high-energy phosphate.

Most widely applied approach, now, is the evaluation of relative distribution of blood flow and of exogenous glucose utilization with 18F-fluorodeoxyglucose (FDG) by PET.

Q17. What informations are obtained from PET imaging?
Ans.
- Myocardial perfusion imaging (MPI)—identification of CAD, assessment of its extent and severity, and risk stratification of patients. It is especially useful in patients with equivocal or nondiagnostic single photon emission computed tomography (SPECT) myocardial perfusion studies.
- Assessment of myocardial viability
- Characterization of potentially vulnerable plaque, identification of preclinical coronary atherosclerosis—by PET/CT hybrid device
- Investigational—expression of transfected gene, cell trafficking, or probe molecular processes.

Q18. How to differentiate ICM from idiopathic DCM?
Ans. In addition to heart failure symptoms, LV dilatation, global hypokinesia, and a low EF and MR are all found in ICM as in DCM. Conduction abnormalities may develop in ECG that may obscure the evidence of previous MI. The points that differentiate ICM from DCM are shown in **Table 3.5**.

TABLE 3.5: Differences between ischemic cardiomyopathy and idiopathic dilated cardiomyopathy.

Points	ICM	DCM
H/O IHD	Usually present	Absent
Biventricular enlargement	May develop lately	Characteristic
Uptake of 18 F-FDG on PET	Inhomogeneous	Homogeneous
Myocardial blood flow	Reduced in distinct areas	Homogeneous
Viable myocardium	May be present	Usually absent
CAG	Obstructive coronary lesion	Nil
CMR (gadolinium enhancement)	Yes	No

(CAG: coronary angiography; CMR: cardiovascular magnetic resonance; DCM: dilated cardiomyopathy; FDG: fluorodeoxyglucose; H/O: history of; IHD: ischemic heart disease; ICM: ischemic cardiomyopathy; PET: positron emission tomography)

ECHOCARDIOGRAPHY

Echo is the evaluation of cardiac structure and function by images produced by ultrasounds. It has become a fundamental component of cardiac evaluation and after ECG, is the second most frequently performed cardiac diagnostic procedure. Echo is the initial-cardiac imaging test to evaluate cardiovascular structural, functional, or hemodynamic abnormalities. Doppler and color flow imaging allow reliable assessment of cardiac hemodynamics and blood flow. An accurate delineation of cardiovascular structure by echo and a reliable hemodynamic evaluation by Doppler have markedly reduced the necessity for cardiac catheterization before undertaking valvular and congenital heart surgery and intervention.

Q1. Mention the echocardiographic modalities with their utility.
Ans. An echocardiographic examination begins with real time 2-DE, which produces high-resolution images of cardiac structures and their movements. The commonly done echocardiographic modalities are:
- *Motion-mode:* Derived from 2D-tomographic images and graphically represents the motion of cardiac structures. It is used primarily to measure cardiac chamber size, timing of cardiac events, and to display subtle abnormalities of cardiac motion.
- *Two-dimensional echo:* It allows visualization of cardiac structures in real time.
- *Doppler echo:* It is used to reliably assess cardiac hemodynamics and blood flow.
  - Pulsed-wave Doppler (PWD)—it is location-specific; location determined by placement of "sample volume". The same crystal sends and receives sound beams reflected from moving red cells from a specific location (determined by sample volume).
  - Continuous wave Doppler (CWD)—sends ultrasound waves and receives the reflected waves continuously with the use of two separate crystals. It records all the velocities along the beam path, hence used to detect and record the highest flow velocity available.
  - Color-flow imaging (CFI; color Doppler)—a form of PWD, displays blood flow in different colors (usually red, blue, green), or their combinations, depending on their velocity, direction, and turbulence. Flow toward the transducer is coded in shades of red, and that away from the transducer, in shades of blue. Turbulence is coded in a shade of green. Therefore, abnormal blood flow is easily recognized by combination of multiple colors according to direction, velocity, and degree of turbulence. The width and size of abnormal intracardiac flow are used to evaluate the degree of valvular regurgitation or cardiac shunt.

Other special modalities (done in selective cases) are:
- *Transesophageal echo:* It improves resolution of 2-DE images owing to proximity of major cardiovascular structures (heart, aorta, PAs) to esophagus. It is done to evaluate MV lesions, (left atrium, or left atrial appendage), intracardiac mass, aortic lesions, etc.
- *Contrast echo:* Encompasses two modalities: One using agitated saline to identify a intracardiac right-to-left (R-L) shunt and to improve the Doppler signal from right side of the heart, and the other using gas-filled microbubbles that can pass through the pulmonary circulation to improve

the delineation of LV endocardial border and to assess myocardial perfusion.
- *Stress echo:* Patients may have normal resting studies but will show wall-motion abnormalities with stress-induced ischemia. Treadmill testing, bicycle exercise, or pharmacologic agents, such as dobutamine, dipyridamole, or adenosine may be used as stressors. It is an excellent method for comparing wall motion, myocardial perfusion, pressure gradient, pulmonary pressure, valvular regurgitation before and after a stress to identify a pathological condition that is not apparent at rest. Stress myocardial perfusion echo can be used to identify ischemic myocardium. To induce a perfusion defect, adenosine, or dipyridamole are administered to create a *coronary steal*, so that myocardial segments, subtended by a stenotic coronary artery, show a decrease in myocardial perfusion.
- *Tissue-Doppler imaging (TDI):* Records motion of myocardial tissues. Tissue has velocity much lower than that of blood flow, but amplitude larger than those produced by blood. TDI has enhanced the ability to assess systolic and diastolic function.
- *Three-dimensional echo (3-DE):* Improvement in ultrasound-transducer technique created harmonic transducer allowing real time 3-DE.
- *Intraoperative echo*: For monitoring patients during cardiac surgery.
- *Digital echo*: Recording and displaying echocardiographic data in a digital form. Digital storage of images has many advantages compared with the traditional videotape system. It permits further offline digital measurement and analysis of images. The echocardiographic recordings can be viewed and manipulated by computers. Computer-generated images are ideal for quantitation as in stress echo. All modern echo machines have capabilities for digital image acquisition to review and analyze further.

Q2. How situs is determined on echo? How to identify right ventricle on echo?

Ans. A sequential approach to determine the cardiac situs is necessary to detect cardiac malposition and to diagnose complex CHD. The first step is to determine the atrial situs and to assess the venous inflow patterns to the atria. Then, AV connections are defined, and ventricular morphology and position are determined. Finally, ventriculoarterial relationships are evaluated.

Atrial situs is determined by using subcostal view. In atrial situs solitus (normal position), the morphologic right atrium is to the right and morphologic left atrium is to the left. Atrial and visceral situs are always concordant. Location and morphology of the atria are determined by 2-DE. The morphological right atrium contains eustachian valve, and its appendage is shorter and broader than that of left atrium. Left atrium lacks eustachian valve and has a more rounded shape than right atrium. Left atrial appendage is long and thin and has a narrower atrial junction compared to that of right. After that, the orientation and morphology of ventricles are determined from relative position of AV valves, and presence or absence of chordal attachments into septum is determined. Finally, identification of great arteries and their respective connections are determined. Normally, pulmonary valve lies slightly anterior and to the left of the aortic valve. PA then courses posteriorly and bifurcates. Course and bifurcation are most reliable signs to identify great arteries. Transposition occurs when great arteries arise from opposite ventricles. In D-transposition, ventricular relationship is normal. In L-transposition, AV discordant is present, so that the morphological right ventricle lies to the left of morphological left ventricle.

Echocardiographically, right ventricle is identified by the following features:
- Right ventricle has tricuspid AV valve; in comparison with mitral annulus, tricuspid annulus is positioned slightly closer to the cardiac apex.
- Right ventricle has a moderator band and a trabeculated endocardial surface (LV surface is smooth).
- It has a triangular cavity (left ventricle is ellipsoidal).
- Right ventricle has chordae inserted into ventricular septum.

Q3. What are the echocardiographic findings of myocardial ischemia and infarction?

Ans. Myocardial ischemia reveals following findings on echo:
- Segmental wall motion abnormalities on M-mode (due to high sampling rate, wall motion is recorded extremely well in M-mode)
- Absence of normal systolic thickening
- Systolic thinning—thickness of LV wall is more in diastole than in systole

In MI:
- Segmental wall-motion abnormalities on M-mode
- Thin, echogenic LV wall-segment—in old infarction.
- Change of wall thickness (as in ischemia)—it provides more accurate means than wall motion does. Recent MI tends to be overestimated, as a result stunning and old MI tends to be underestimated because of "tethering effect" on the normal muscle. The involved vessel can be predicted from the wall-motion abnormalities detected.

It is to be noted that the lack of wall-motion abnormality does not exclude possibility of an obstructed artery—obstruction may be partial, and ischemia may be absent in resting state. Also, collaterals may preserve myocardial function despite severe, or even total obstruction.

Q4. How to measure LV function on echo? What are the limitations?

Ans. Calculation of LV systolic function on echo is done by measuring EF, which is done by dividing stroke volume (SV) by end-diastolic volume (EDV):

$$EF = SV\,(EDV - ESV)/EDV$$

Normally, ventricle ejects more than half of its EDV. Average EF (as determined by M-mode or 2-DE) is 63–69%.

On 2-DE, EF is measured by modified Simsons method. Here, left ventricle is visualized in apical 4- or 2-chamber view and endocardial borders outlined in end-diastole, and endsystole is equidistant along the left ventricle—usually at the tips of MV and at the level of papillary muscles along with determination of LV length.

With M-mode echo, LV internal diameter is measured in left parasternal long-axis view at MV tips. LV internal diameter at the end of diastole (LVIDd), interventricular septal (IVS) and left ventricular posterior wall (LVPW) are measured at the end of diastole, coincident with the R-wave ECG. The end-systolic dimension, LV internal diameter at end-systole (LVIDs) is measured at the peak of contraction.

Grading of LV dysfunction:
- Mild dysfunction: 36–45%
- Moderate dysfunction: 28–35%
- Severe dysfunction: <28%

Limitations of M-mode measurement: LV shape may vary. CAD affects different myocardial segments varyingly, and produces regional wall-motion abnormality. Thus, linear measurement across different segments may vary.

Q5. How is the assessment of wall motion abnormalities done in IHD?
Ans. Left ventricle is divided into 16 regional segments by 3 longitudinal axis views (parasternal long-axis, apical 4-chamber, and apical 2-chamber) at 3 levels—basal, mid, and apical, and by parasternal short-axis views at same 3 levels—basal, mid, and apical. These 16 segments can be recorded from either 3 longitudinal views or three short-axis views.

These 16 segments are:
- *6 segments at basal level:* Anterior, lateral, posterior, inferior, septal, and anteroseptal
- *6 segments at mid-level:* Anterior, lateral, posterior, inferior, septal, and anteroseptal
- *4 segments at apical level:* Anterior, lateral, septal, inferior (derived from apical 4- and 2-chamber views, not parasternal long-axis view, as apex is not visualized). A given segment can be evaluated in more than one view.

Wall-motion abnormalities may be: Hypokinesia, akinesia, dyskinesia, etc.

Q6. What are the segmental wall motion abnormalities on echo?
Ans.
- *Normal:* Wall thickness increases in systole; left ventricle contracts concentrically toward its center.
- *Hypokinesia:* Decreased wall motion; occurs in ischemia, myocarditis, MI

- *Akinesia:* Absence of contraction and relaxation; occurs with myocardial scarring in old MI.
- *Dyskinesia:* Paradoxical wall motion, i.e., outward contraction in systole and inward contraction in diastole. It occurs in LV aneurysm.
- *Hyperkinesia:* Increased wall motion seen with acute ischemia or with stress testing.

Q7. What is the relationship between abnormalities of LV motion and thickness with coronary supply?
Ans. Presence of regional wall motion abnormality in 2-DE can predict the involved vessel.
- *Parasternal long-axis view:* Visualize anterior IVS and posterior LV free wall, LVPW. This IVS is supplied by LAD artery of left coronary artery (LCA). The basal 1–2 cm is supplied by S_1 (1st septal perforator). LVPW (as seen in this view) is usually supplied by the left circumflex artery (LCx) (not routinely involved with infective MI with obstruction to PDA).
- *Apical 4-chamber view:* All three coronary arterial territories are seen. The apex and distal half to two-thirds of IVS are supplied by LAD artery. The proximal third of IVS is usually supplied by PDA, and the lateral free wall by the branches of LCx.
- *Apical 2-chamber view:* Basal half or two-thirds of posterior wall is supplied by PDA. The rest of left ventricle is supplied by LAD artery.
- *Parasternal short-axis view:* LAD artery supplies anterior portion of LV free wall and posterior half of IVS. PDA supplies the posterior-medial portion of LV free wall as well as posterior half of IVS. LCx supplies posterolateral portion (in this view). Also, PDA may arise from LCx in left dominant system.

Q8. How is diastolic LV dysfunction assessed?
Ans. The MV PWD signal can indicate LV diastolic function by determining E/A ratio. An E/A ratio <1.0 indicates diastolic dysfunction in patients up to 50 years of age. In those >50 years of age, a ratio of <0.5 is taken as an indicator of diastolic dysfunction.

Q9. How is pulmonary arterial pressure measured on Doppler?
Ans.
- From the transtricuspid pressure difference calculated from the tricuspid regurgitation (TR) jet added to an estimate of right atrial pressure (10 mm Hg).
- Assessment of diameter of inferior vena cava (IVC) and its degree of collapse during inspiration.

Q10. What are the conditions that lead to right ventricular volume overload on echo?
Ans. These are:
- Atrial septal defect
- Pulmonary regurgitation

- Tricuspid regurgitation
- Anomalous venous connection—partial anomalous pulmonary venous connection (PAPVC), total anomalous pulmonary venous connection (TAPVC), etc.

Q11. How does stress echo help in diagnosis?

Ans. Stress echo has two main utilities—assessment of myocardial ischemia and detection of myocardial viability.

- During stress, reduction of wall motion (in a segment which contracts in resting state) indicates that the segment is subtended by flow-limiting stenotic coronary artery.
- Improved function of an impaired segment during low-dose pharmacological stress indicates that the segment is viable-stunned or hibernating.

Q12. What are the intracardiac masses diagnosed on echo?

Ans. Common intracardiac masses diagnosed on echo are:
- *Thrombus*: It becomes echogenic as it becomes organized.

Thrombus may be formed in left atrial appendage (in AF), left ventricle (after anterior transmural MI, in DCM), in right ventricle [in deep vein thrombosis (DVT)]. Mural thrombus is common at LV apex or overlying large akinetic, dyskinetic, or aneurismal segments **(Figs. 3.13A and B)**.

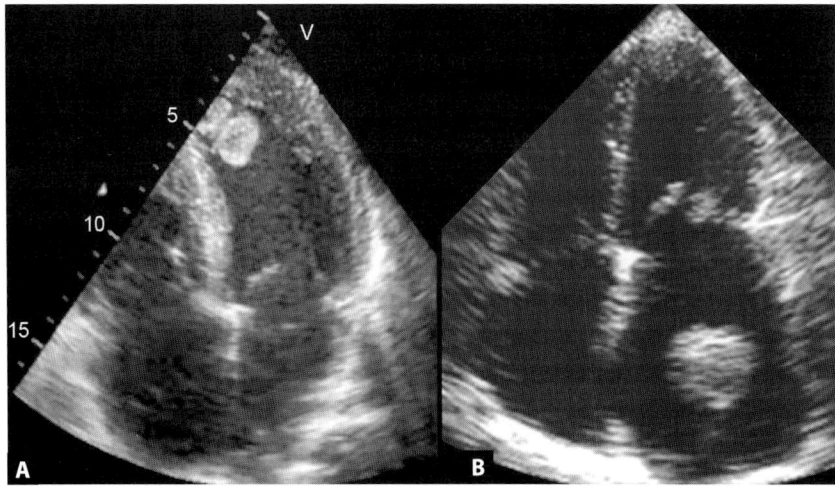

Figs. 3.13A and B: LV thrombus in anterior (MI) (A), and LA thrombus in MS (B). (LA: left atrial; LV: left ventricular; MI: myocardial infarction; MS: mitral stenosis)

- *Cardiac myxoma:* It is commonly in left atrium. It has a characteristic bright, gelatinous loculated appearance. It is usually attached by a pedicle to interatrial septum and may prolapse through the MV.
- *Foreign bodies:* Catheter tips, tips of pacemaker lead, etc.

Q13. What are the echo appearance of vegetations?

Ans. These are echogenic structures attached to cardiac valves, having the following features:
- Site attached to low pressure side of valve or defect, e.g., atrial side in MR, ventricular side in AR, right ventricular side in VSD, etc.
- Lower echogenicity compared to the valve to which it is attached
- Mobile
- Lesions are multiple.
- Borders are ill-defined, friable, and have a flimsy appearance.

Q14. How does echo aid in invasive procedures?

Ans. Echo can be used to monitor various invasive procedures, such as pericardiocentesis, intra-aortic balloon catheter placement, performing an atrial balloon septostomy in transposition of the great arteries (TGA), doing a balloon mitral valvotomy in MS, TEE during catheter ablation and cardiac surgery. Occasionally, echo may be used instead of fluoroscopy to monitor an invasive examination, as in pregnant patients to minimize ionizing radiation.

Q15. What is the utility of echo in critically ill patients?

Ans.
- Assessment of LV function
- Pericardial effusion/tamponade
- Volume status
- Others—valvular pathology, R-L shunt, etc.

Q16. What is IVUS? Give its application.

Ans. It is the invasive method for the detection of structure and composition of diseased coronary arteries, dynamic changes before, after, and late after percutaneous coronary intervention (PCI) by applying ultrasound intravascularly. It permits 360° characterization of arterial lumen dimensions in regions that are difficult to assess by using conventional CAG, such as left main coronary artery (LMCA), ostium of LAD artery, LCx, and RCA. Three-dimensional reconstruction of the arterial wall may be performed when a mechanical pull back of IVUS catheter is done at a fixed rate **(Figs. 3.14A to C)**.

Utilities in PCI:
- Characterization of baseline plaque composition, vessel size, and lesion accessibility to select best single device, combination of devices in PCI.
- Confirm (or refute) angiographic estimation of stenosis severity, particularly in regions that are difficult to visualize by CAG.
- Assess anatomical results and detect complications (e.g., dissections) and residual stenosis following PCI.

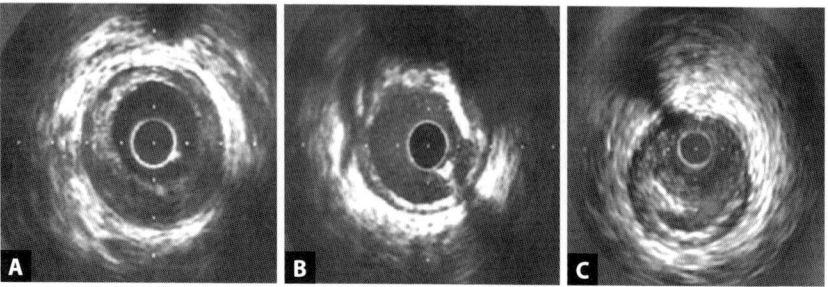

Figs. 3.14A to C: IVUS showing concentric soft plaque (A), calcified plaque (B), and intimal dissection (C).

Q17. What is optical coherence tomography (OCT)?

Ans. It is the novel, noninvasive real-time, tomographic catheter-based imaging technique that uses light and fiberoptic technology to obtain unique details of the coronary arteries on a microscopic scale. It delivers near-infrared light to the wall of the coronary artery through small-diameter optical fibers. The light that illuminates the vessel is absorbed and reflected by the vascular tissues to different degrees. Different tissue types have different optical characteristics. Thus, lipid-rich tissue can be differentiated from fibrous and calcified tissue. It provides cross-sectional imaging of coronary arteries at a high resolution (4-10 microns), permitting plaque characterization and identification of the thickness of fibrous cap. OCT can also be used to assess early and late results in patients undergoing PCI.

NUCLEAR CARDIOLOGY

It is the noninvasive radionuclide cardiac imaging with stress–nuclear cardiology procedures done for diagnosis and risk assessment of patients with suspected or known CAD. Gated SPECT imaging of myocardial perfusion is the most commonly performed imaging procedure. Although echo, CT, and CMR may increasingly be used, the ability of SPECT MPI to provide objective, quantitative assessment of myocardial perfusion and function may continue to offer standardized procedures at moderate expense that are not highly technology-dependent.

Q1. What is nuclear cardiology?

Ans. It is the noninvasive radionuclide imaging of the heart including myocardial blood flow, metabolism, and function. The most commonly performed imaging procedure in nuclear cardiology is SPECT MPI of myocardial perfusion.

Q2. What is MPI?

Ans. Single photon emission computed tomography is the most commonly performed MPI technique. Here, after injection of a chosen radiotracer (technetium or thallium), the isotope is extracted from blood by viable myocardium and retained for some period. Photons are emitted from the myocardium in proportion to the magnitude of tracer uptake, in turn related to perfusion. Gamma camera captures the gamma-ray photons and converts the information into digital data representing the magnitude of uptake and location of emission **(Flowchart 1)**.

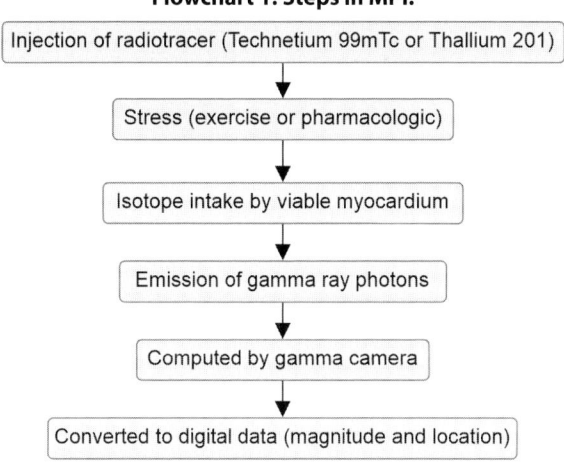

Flowchart 1: Steps in MPI.

Q3. What are the indications of MPI?
Ans.
- Diagnosis of CAD—chest pain evaluation, e.g., negative ETT with high suspicion of CAD, positive ETT with low probability of CAD, nondiagnostic ETT, and when ETT is uninterpretable, e.g., LBBB.
- Evaluation of physiological importance of known CAD, e.g., borderline CAD (lesion 40–70%), small vessel stenosis, evaluation before PCI and heart transplantation, identification of hibernating myocardium.
- Assessment after therapeutic intervention, e.g., PCI, coronary artery bypass grafting (CABG), or symptomatic improvement after medical treatment.
- Risk stratification—UA, stable angina, post MI, those undergoing noncardiac surgery.
- Identification of MI with angiographically normal coronary artery.

Q4. What are the types of perfusion defects in MPI?
Ans.
- *Fixed:* Absent tracer uptake (photon-deficient areas) that remains unchanged on both rest and stress. It may be due to scar or viable myocardium (hibernating). Metabolic scan or PET differentiates.

- *Reversible:* Defect present on initial stress images but resolves on rest, or delayed images indicating ischemic myocardium **(Figs. 3.15A and B)**.

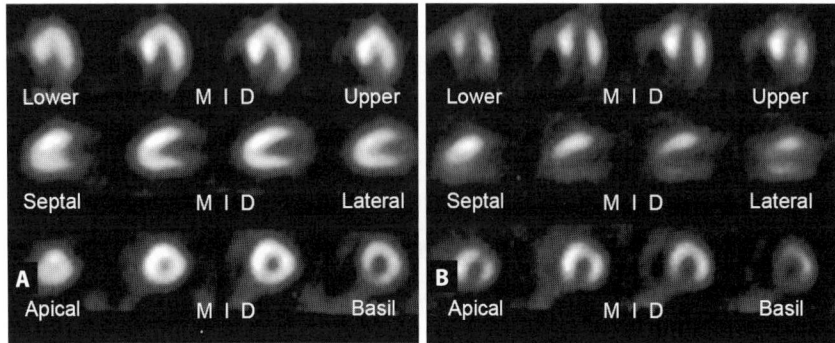

Figs. 3.15A and B: MPI showing normal perfusion at rest (A); reversible perfusion defect with impaired perfusion in inferior segment during exercise (B). (MPI: myocardial perfusion imaging)

- *Partially reversible:* Defect present on stress images and partially resolves on rest, i.e., do not fill completely. It indicates a mixture of scar and ischemic myocardium.
- *Redistribution:* Defect large on rest and absent on stress testing. It is seen after revascularization, e.g., acute MI with thrombolysis, PCI, or autolysis after MI.

Q5. What is myocardial viability? How is it detected?
Ans. Viable myocardium means myocytes with sufficient blood flow and preserved metabolic activity. If blood flow is severely reduced, metabolic pathways are inhibited and cell membrane is disrupted. Thus, with severe flow reduction, MPI provides information regarding viability. However, in regions in which reduction in blood flow is less severe, metabolic scan using FDG is needed to identify clinically relevant viability. Tracers reflecting cation flux-thallium-201 or electrochemical gradient, e.g., sestamibi or tetrofosmin are also suitable.

Q6. What are stunned and hibernating myocardium?
Ans. These are adaptive mechanisms of myocardium to a temporary or sustained reduction in coronary blood flow. Myocardial function is depressed at rest, but myocytes remain viable.

In stunned myocardium, LV function is depressed at rest, but perfusion is preserved as it is observed after a transient period of ischemia followed by reperfusion.

In hibernating myocardium, LV function and perfusion both are depressed at rest as an adaptive response to chronic and repetitive episodes of ischemia.

CARDIAC CATHETERIZATION AND CORONARY ANGIOGRAPHY

Cardiac catheterization is the insertion and passage of small plastic catheters into arteries, veins, and the heart and other vascular structures. It has become a standard laboratory procedure to measure cardiovascular hemodynamics (i.e., pressure, cardiac output, oximetry data, etc.), acquire radiologic image of coronary arteries (i.e., CAG) and cardiac chambers, and visualize aorta, PA, and peripheral vessels. Now, cardiac catheterization has evolved from diagnostic modality to therapeutic modality through numerous catheter-based interventions, e.g., angioplasty, stenting, closure of congenital defects like ASD and PDA.

Q1. What are the routes of cardiac catheterization?
Ans.
- *Arterial (for left heart catheterization):*
  - Brachial route (Sones technique)—by cut-down or percutaneous puncture. It is often used for:
- Patients on anticoagulants
- Aortic coarctation (prevents effective steering of catheters from leg)
- Patients with intermittent claudication (severe aortoiliac disease) or aortoiliac surgery
- Uncontrolled hypertension (hemostasis easier from brachial route)
- Occasionally, when aortic valve stenosis is severe and a dominant feature.
  - Femoral route—by percutaneous puncture of right femoral artery (Judkins technique). It is most often used, because it is easier, associated with less complication, and does not get in the way of the X-ray camera.

Situations where femoral route is used are:
- Several (two or more) previous brachial catheterizations
- Patients with a right subclavian bruit
- Patients with Raynaud's phenomenon
- Young women with atypical chest pain (who may have small brachial arteries and a tendency to arterial spasm)
  - Radial route—used for quick ambulation after CAG
- *Venous (for right heart catheterization):*
  - Femoral route—usually preferred for ASD and most CHD, temporary pacing-lead insertion (who had thrombolysis for acute MI).
  - Brachial route is usually preferred for:
- Patients on anticoagulation
- Temporary pacemaker lead insertion (who need to travel via air)
  - Subclavian—for lead insertion in permanent pacemaker.
  - Internal jugular—for PA catheterization (Swan-Ganz) and central venous pressure (CVP) monitoring.

Q2. What are the commonly used catheters?

- *Right heart catheters:*
  - Cournand catheter: It is an end-hole catheter, used for measurement of right atrial, right ventricular, PA, and pulmonary capillary wedge pressure.
  - NIH catheter has closed end with multiple side holes in close proximity to the tip. It can record pressure in different chambers. It is used for visualization of right ventricle (right ventriculography), right atrium, and PA by hand injection of dye.
  - Swan–Ganz balloon-tipped flow-directed catheter: The ballon allows the catheter to float with the flow of blood from the great veins, through the right heart chambers, and into the PA.
- *Left heart catheters* (**Fig. 3.16**):
  - Judkins catheters: It is used for CAG via femoral approach. These are end-hole catheters of 7 or 8 Fr size that taper to 5 Fr near the tip, polyethylene or polyurethane catheters containing either steel braid or nylon within the wall that provide excellent torque control needed for coronary cannulation.

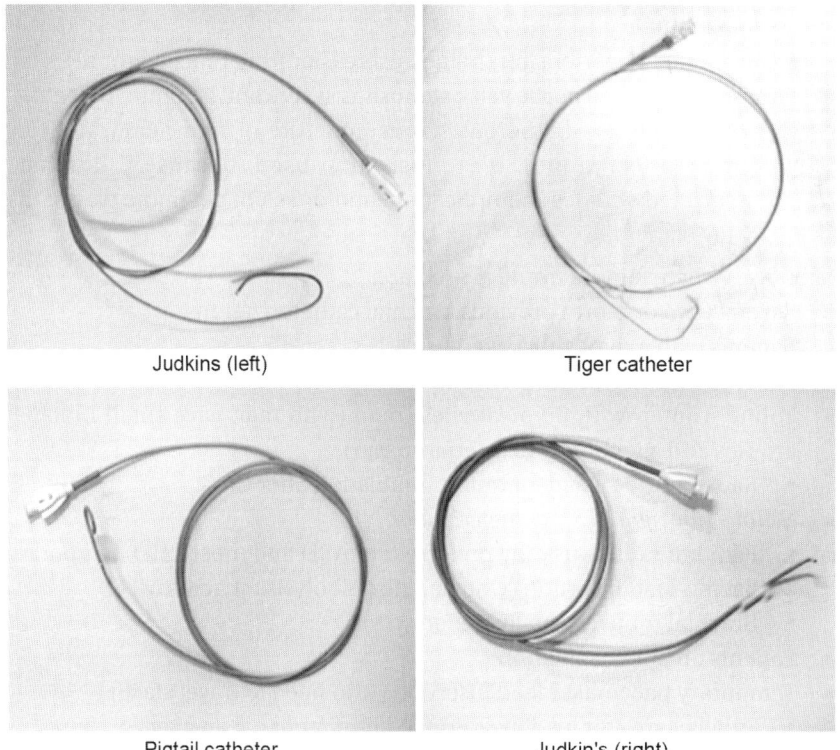

Fig. 3.16: Left heart catheters.

- Left Judkins catheter: It has two angled segments, a curve near the tip, and is designed to engage the left coronary ostium while bracing against the opposite aortic wall. A left Judkins catheter with a 4 cm curve is commonly referred to as JL4. In 95% cases, JL4 is adequate for catheterization of left coronary. In patients with a widened aortic root (due to disease or hypertension), JL4 may be too short to allow successful engagement, and a JL5 or JL6 may be needed.
- The right Judkins catheter is straight other than at the tip. It is designed to be torqued into the right coronary ostium.
  - Tiger catheter: It is used for angiography of both coronaries through transradial route.
  - Amplatz catheter: It is used for CAG and PCI.
  - Extra backup (EBU) catheter: It is used for transradial PCI and CAG.
  - Pigtail catheter: A closed-end catheter with multiple side holes near its tip (having a configuration of a pigtail at its distal end) is used for left ventriculography and aortography). LV injection and aortic injection of contrast are done by power injector. Pigtail configuration prevents myocardial staining during the procedure.
  - Sones catheter: It has an end hole and four side holes within 7 mm of the tip. It has a variety of curves; 7 and 8 Fr. size taper to a 5 Fr. external diameter near the tip. Sones catheter can be used for CAG and left ventriculography by the branchial approach. It is often helpful in navigation through a tortuous subclavian artery into the ascending aorta. It is most helpful in crossing a tight aortic valve when other catheters have failed.

Q3. Why is cardiac catheterization done under local anesthesia?
Ans. Cardiac catheterization is performed on a fully conscious patient under local anesthesia. General anesthesia is not usually used as:
- It interferes with hemodynamics and O_2 saturations.
- Patients under general anesthesia cannot indicate if they develop angina or other symptoms.
- Patients are required to perform respiratory maneuvers, coughing, etc.
- Patients are sometimes required to perform exercise during the test. General anesthesia may be required in pediatric cases.

Q4. What is Seldinger technique?
Ans. It is the method of introducing cardiac catheter by percutaneous approach, usually through femoral vessels (artery or vein).

The steps in Seldinger technique are:
- Percutaneous puncture of the vessel through and through by a Seldinger needle (with its solid obturator in place).
- Obturator is removed and a syringe is attached to the needle cannula.

- Slow withdrawal of the cannula that brings the tip of the cannula back into the vessel lumen. This is recognized by the sudden ability to withdraw venous blood freely into the syringe (femoral venous route), or a brisk spill into the syringe (in femoral arterial route).
- Syringe is removed from the cannula and a soft tipped J-guide wire is advanced down the lumen of the needle.
- The needle is withdrawn over the stationary wire (after the guide wire has been advanced safely into the vessel). A small (1 cm) skin incision is made with a scalpel and the track is dilated.
- The sheath with the dilator is introduced trough the guide wire.
- The inner dilator is removed to permit catheter introduction.

Q5. What is a guide wire?
Ans. Guide wire is the means that serves as the rail over which different catheters and other devices travel during catheterization and intervention.

The characteristics of a guide wire are:
- Length (in cm), e.g., 150 cm—may be short or long
- Diameter (in inch), e.g., 0.035–0.038 inches
- Tip configuration, e.g., J-tipped, straight, etc.

Uses of a guide wire are:
- Diagnostic—during catheter introduction by Seldinger technique, and exchange of catheters subsequently. Although some catheters may be inserted directly over the guide wire, this is now common practice to place an introducing sheath over the guide wire and then advance the catheter through the sheath.
- Therapeutic—guide wires are essential components for cardiac interventions like percutaneous transluminal coronary angioplasty (PTCA) and ballon valvuloplasty.

Guide wires vary in configuration (e.g., J- shaped in CAG), floppy (very soft), intermediate stiff to extra stiff, and in length (short and exchange length). A key principle of wire deployment is to avoid endothelial disruption. Therefore, soft-tipped wires should be used, which can also negotiate tortuous vessels. Stiffer wires are useful in PTCA for difficult lesions or total occlusions and provide a good rail over which to advance balloon and stents. During CAG, J-configuration and flexibility of the guide wire allow it to pass safely through most iliac arteries, even with considerable tortuosity and arteriosclerotic irregularities. Guide wires used in interventional procedures are specially designed that combine tip stiffness, radiographic visibilit y, and precise torque control so that it can be steered.

Q6. What is the use of vascular sheath?
Ans. Vascular sheath (the commonly used one is Cordis sheath) is a device that allows catheter introduction and exchange of catheter during catheterization

and intervention. Cordis sheath has an inner dilator. It is equipped with a back-bleed valve (to control bleeding around the catheter) and a side arm to provide a means of administering fluid and pressure monitoring, with the catheter in place. The sheath-and-dilator assembly is inserted over the guide wire as a unit, following which the dilator is removed to permit catheter introduction. The sheath and dilator are rotated as they are advanced progressively through the soft tissues. If excessive resistance is encountered, it may be necessary to remove the dilator from the sheath and to introduce the dilator alone before attempting to introduce the combination. The dilator (and wire) being removed, the sheath is flushed by withdrawing blood and administering heparinized saline solution. Again, the sheath should be flushed immediately after each catheter is introduced or withdrawn every 5 minutes during the catheterization to avoid encroachment of blood and potential thromboembolism from within the sheath **(Fig. 3.17)**.

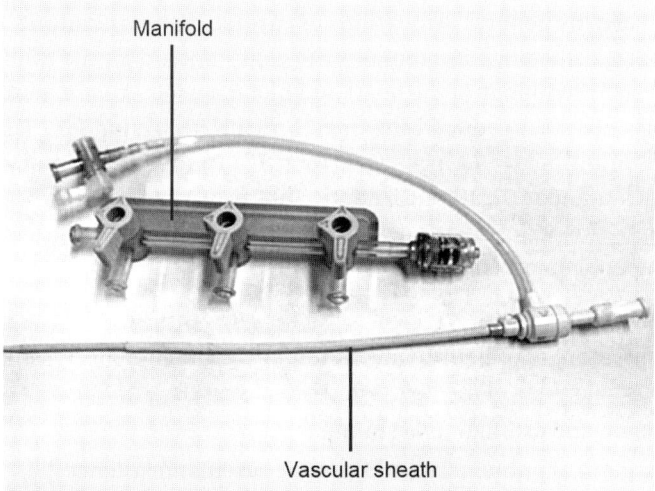

Fig. 3.17: Vascular sheath and manifold.

Q7. What is a manifold system?
Ans. It is a specially designed device used in left heart catheterization, commonly during CAG (hence, called coronary manifold). It consists of a syringe, connecting tubing, a series of three-way taps, which connect the catheter to a pressure transducer, a saline-flash circuit, and a contrast-agent reservoir **(Fig. 3.17)**. Manifold provides a closed system with which blood can be withdrawn from the catheter and discarded, all under the control of a series of stop corks. Sometimes a fourth port is connected to an empty plastic bag and is used as a discard port for blood and air bubbles, so that the syringe need not be disconnected from the manifold at any time during the procedure.

Precautions:
- Before starting any series of contrast injections, blood should always be aspirated from the catheter, so that there is no air bubble in the catheter and tubing.
- While flushing with saline, catheter should be connected to manifold tubing.

Q8. What are the sizes of a catheter and introducer sheath?
Ans.
- Size of a catheter is its outer diameter expressed in French units:
  1 Fr = 0.33 mm
- Size of an introducer is the French number of the largest catheter that passes freely through it:
  A 7 Fr introducer accepts 7 Fr catheter, but has an outer diameter >7 Fr.

Q9. What are the general indications of cardiac catheterization?
Ans. Cardiac catheterization remains the gold standard for the evaluation of anatomy and physiology of the heart and blood vessels. Although the advent of Doppler echo has reduced the need for catheterization for diagnosis of CHD and adult heart disease, rapid increase in the use of interventional techniques mandates catheterization. Today, cardiac catheterization and angiography are performed as a combined procedure for diagnostic purpose and therapeutic intervention.

The main indications are:
- Measurement of pressure, waveforms, and estimation of O_2 saturation in various chambers of the hearts and blood vessels.
- Detection and estimation of shunts
- Assessment of pulmonary and systemic vascular resistance
- Estimation of cardiac output and ventricular function
- Coronary angiography, including selective angiocardiography
- Detection and estimation of valve stenosis and regurgitation
- Various interventional procedures and implantation of pacemakers
- Electrophysiological studies and endomyocardial biopsy

Q10. What are the special catheterization techniques?
Ans. Some special catheterization techniques are:
- Trans-septal heart catheterization, e.g., in mitral balloon valvuloplasty
- Intra-aortic balloon counterpulsation
- Catheterization in adult CHDs, and heart transplant patients
- Endomyocardial biopsy
- Pericardiocentesis (under catheterization)

Q11. What are the contraindications to cardiac catheterization?
Ans.
- Absolute—refusal of a mentally competent patient to consent to the procedure
- Relative—uncontrolled ventricular irritability; the risk of VT/fibrillation during catheterization increases
- Uncorrected hypokalemia or digitalis toxicity
- Uncontrolled hypertension that predisposes to myocardial ischemia and/or heart failure during angiography
- Decompensated heart failure
- Severe allergy to radiographic contrast agents
- Anticoagulated state (prothrombin time: 18 second)
- Severe renal failure
- Intercurrent febrile illness

Q12. List some potential complications of cardiac catheterization. What are the factors predisposing to increased mortality?
Ans.
- Local vascular (at access site) hematoma, delayed hemorrhage, pseudoaneurysm, arteriovenous (A-V) fistula, arterial thrombosis and embolism, local cellulitis, phlebitis, arteritis, injury to nerve, etc.
- Vasovagal reactions
- Allergic reactions (to contrast agent)
- Arrhythmias—VT, VF, asystole, marked bradycardia, CHB, SVT.
- Myocardial infarction—in UA.
- Cerebrovascular accidents—by thromboembolism.
- Death
- Others—cardiac perforation, renal failure, infections, knotting of catheters.

Factors predisposing to increased mortality are:
- Age: Infants (<1 year), elderly (>60 years)
- New York Heart Association (NYHA) class IV
- Left main-stem disease
- Combined valvular disease and CAD
- LV dysfunction: Left ventricular ejection fraction (LVEF) <30%
- Severe noncardiac disease—renal failure, advanced cerebrovascular, peripheral vascular, and pulmonary disease
- Interventional procedures involving cardiac catheterization

Q13. What are the normal pressure in cardiac chambers?
Ans.
- Right atrial (central venous) pressure: 5 mm Hg (range: 0–8 mm Hg)
- Right ventricular systolic pressure: 25 mm Hg (range: 15–50 mm Hg)

- Right ventricular end-diastolic pressure: 5 mm Hg (range: 0–8 mm Hg)
- Left atrial (pulmonary capillary wedge) pressure: 10 mm Hg (5–15 mm Hg)
- Left ventricular systolic pressure: 125 mm Hg (90–140 mm Hg)
- Left ventricular end-diastolic pressure: 10 mm Hg (5–15 mm Hg)
- Aortic systolic pressure: 125 mm Hg (90–140 mm Hg)
- Aortic diastolic pressure: 75 mm Hg (60–90 mm Hg)

All pressures are estimated as multiples of five—*Rules of five* of pressure values.

Q14. What is a shunt? Classify it.

Ans. A central circulatory shunt may be defined as abnormal communication between pulmonary and systemic circulation connecting either of the two parts of cardiac chambers, or the great vessels. Shunts are classified as listed in **Box 3.1**.

> **BOX 3.1:** Classification of shunt.
>
> - Direction of flow:
>   - Left-to-right, e.g., ASD, VSD, and PDA
>   - Right-to-left, e.g., TOF and Eisenmenger syndrome
>   - Bi-directional
> - Level of shunt:
>   - At atrial level, e.g., ASD patent foramen ovale
>   - At ventricular level, e.g., VSD rupture sinus into right ventricle, coronary A-V fistula (into right ventricle), PDA with PR
>   - At pulmonary artery level, e.g., PDA: PDA, aortopulmonary window, anomalous LCA from PA (ALCAPA)
>
> (ASD: atrial septal defect; VSD: ventricular septal defect; PDA: patent ductus arteriosus; TOF: tetralogy of Fallot; PR: pulmonary regurgitation; PA: pulmonary artery)

Q15. How is shunt detected on catheterization?

Ans. Shunt detection is done by:

- Oximetry method: Percent saturation of O_2 is measured in blood samples drawn sequentially from PA, superior vena cava (SVC), and IVC. A left-to-right shunt is detected and localized if a significant "step up" in O_2 saturation is found in one of the right heart chambers. A significant step-up is defined as an increase in O_2 saturation that exceeds the normal variability, that might be observed if multiple samples were drawn from that cardiac chamber **(Table 3.6)**.

The simplest way to screen for a left-to-right shunt is to sample SVC and PA blood and see the difference of O_2 saturation. If there is a O_2 step up of 8%, a left-to-right shunt may be present at atrial, ventricular, or great vessel level, and a full oximetry run should be done.

Criteria for significant step-up:

TABLE 3.6: Significant oxygen (O_2) step up in different chambers.

Level	% O_2 saturation
Atrial (SVC to RA)	11
Ventricular (RA to RV)	10
Great vessel (RV to PA)	5

(O_2: oxygen; PA: pulmonary artery; RA: right atrium; RV: right ventricle; SVC: superior vena cava)

Arterial desaturation (i.e., O_2 saturation: 95%) persisting after 100% O_2 administration by face mask, suggests presence of a R-L shunt. For detection of R-L shunt, oximetry is done from pulmonary vein, left atrium, left ventricle, and aorta. Pulmonary venous blood is fully saturated. Therefore, the site of R-L shunt may be localized by noting which left heart chamber is the first to show desaturation, i.e., a stepdown in O_2 saturation. If left atrial saturation is normal, but desaturation is present in left ventricle and in the systemic circulation, the R-L shunt is across a VSD.

- Catheter trajectory—may show the location of the shunt.

Q16. What are the indications of selective angiocardiography?
Ans. Angiocardiography is an effective way of visualizing and localizing the site of the shunt. Complicated lesions commonly require angiographic delineation before surgical intervention. It also helps to assess all other cases more completely.
- Right atrial injection is done for detecting:
  - Ebstein anomaly
  - Tricuspid atresia
  - Right atrial tumors
- Right ventricular injection done to detect:
  - Fallot's tetrad: Confirm the diagnosis with regard to the site of obstruction, degree of aortic overriding, and site of VSD.
  - Pulmonary stenosis: Site of obstruction (valvular or infundibular)
  - TGA and double outlet right ventricle (DORV) to outline the origin of great vessels
  - Miscellaneous: To visualize pulmonary arterial tree in pulmonary embolism, detect TR, right-sided cardiomyopathy
- LV injections (usually made in a retrograde fashion) are done to assess:
  - Mitral regurgitation—its presence and severity.
  - LV function and aneurysm, particularly during CAG
  - Left ventricular outflow tract (LVOT) obstruction—aortic, subaortic, supra-aortic, and the degree of obstruction.

- Ventricular septal defect—location of defect or Gerbode defect.
- TGA, DORV—to diagnose the origin of great arteries.
- Miscellaneous—diagnosis of hypertrophic obstructive cardiomyopathy (HOCM), detection of ostium primum ASD, and endocardial cushion defects.
- Left atrial injection—is rarely done as pulmonary arteriography is easier and usually delineates the left atrium satisfactorily on levophase. It is done by trans-septal puncture.

An ASD is best defined bt selective injection of right upper lobe pulmonary vein by hand injection. It frequently opacifies the pulmonary arterial tree. The technique is also undertaken in cases of pulmonary atresia.

Aortic injection done retrogradely (like LV graphy). It is done for:
- Detection of AR and its severity
- Detection of coarctation of aorta, aortic arch syndrome, aneurysm (dissecting, syphilitic), rupture sinus of Valsalva, etc.
- Diagnosis of aorto- pulmonary septal detect
- Pulmonary artery injection—it is done for:
  - Visualization of PA and its branches, e.g., in PA stenosis
  - Detection of pulmonary A-V fistula
  - Determination of anomalous pulmonary venous drainage.
  - Detection of left atrial tumors, e.g., left atrial myxoma (in levophase).

CORONARY ANGIOGRAPHY

It includes performing and recording angiographic images of coronary arteries, storing digital image data, and displaying it for analysis and review. CAG is the primary method of defining coronary anatomy that provides the anatomic map to define site, severity, shape, and distribution of stenosis. Also, the presence of any intracoronary thrombus, mass of myocardium served, coronary flow index, presence of collateral, coronary spasm (by provocative test), myocardial bridge can be ascertained by CAG. Functional significance of coronary stenosis is assessed by doing fractional flow reserve (FFR). Left ventriculography is included in CAG, enabling visual analysis of wall motion, EF, presence of viable myocardium, and presence of MR.

Q1. Name the coronary arteries and their main branches as they are commonly identified by CAG.
Ans. Although there are two coronary arteries, angiographically there are three—LAD artery, LCx, and RCA **(Fig. 3.18)**.

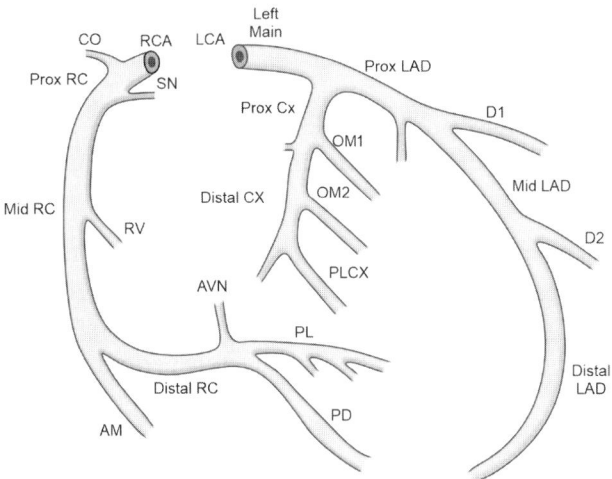

Fig. 3.18: Coronary arteries and their branches. (AM: acute marginal; AVN: atrioventricular node; Cx: circumflex artery; LAD: left anterior descending; LCA: left coronary artery; LCx: left circumflex artery; OM1,2: obtuse marginal1,2; PL: posterior left ventricular; PD: posterior descending; RC: right coronary; RCA: right coronary artery; RV: right ventricle; SN: sinoatrial node)

Q2. What is the information derived from CAG?
Ans. Information:
- Anatomic map of coronary artery—size, severity, shape of stenosis, location of CAD determined as an aid to planning PCI and CABG
- Characteristics of distal vessels—size, presence of atherosclerotic disease, mass of myocardium served
- Identification of collateral vessels and their functional importance
- Coronary spasm—ascertained by provocative maneuver
- Index of differential coronary flow—functional significance of stenosis done by measuring coronary flow at rest and during intense coronary-dilator stimuli. Difference is the flow reserve capacity.

Q3. What are the views for CAG?
Ans.
- *Left coronary artery:* Six standard radiographic views are: anteroposterior (AP), lateral, left anterior oblique (LAO) cranial, LAO caudal, right anterior oblique (RAO), and RAO caudal. Cranial and caudal views use approximately 20° angulation.
  A steep RAO cranial view helps separate the LAD artery from overlapping diagonal vessels.
  The AP caudal view opens out the left main stem.

- *Right coronary artery:* Two standard radiographic views are: LAO and RAO. The distal RCA is opened out using the LAO cranial view during examination.
- *Nonselective CAG:* Contrast injection in the sinus of Valsalva is done to evaluate ostial lesions and anomalous coronary ostium or coronary bypass graft.

Q4. What are the indications for CAG?
Ans. The American College of Cardiology (ACC)/American Heart Association (AHA) class I indication is when there is a consensus that CAG is indicated, and class II indication is when CAG is frequently performed but there is no consensus).

- *Limiting angina pectoris:*
  - Chronic stable angina poorly controlled by medicines, or intolerant to medications—class I indication
  - Unstable angina—high-risk cases, and those refractory to medical therapy—class I indication.
- *Acute MI:*

  Patients with persistent pain or unresolved ECG changes after thrombolytic therapy.
  - Patients with postinfarction complications, such as recurrent ischemia or mechanical complications, e.g., VSD
  - Patients with significant angina after MI or with a positive stress test
  - Patients with post-MI complications—CHF, cardiogenic shock

  Following non-ST elevation MI
  - Those requiring primary angioplasty for acute ST elevation MI
- *Abnormal stress test result:*
  - High-risk stress test predictive of left main and/or multivessel CAD—class I indication
  - Positive stress test without high-risk features—class II indication.
- Ventricular arrhythmias and dysfunction:
  - A history of sustained VT or sudden cardiac death (without any obvious metabolic cause)—class I indication.
  - LV dysfunction of unknown etiology with EF < 40% (to rule out CAD)—class I indication.
- *Valvular heart disease*—patients requiring valve surgery who have angina and an abnormal ECG—class I indication. CAG is done before valve surgery for men >40 years, and women >50 years of age to rule out clinically silent CAD (younger patients may require CAG if cardiac risk factors are present).

- *Preoperative:*
  - Patients with angina or a positive stress test who are to undergo major vascular surgery—class I indication
  - Planned major nonvascular surgery—class II indication.
  - Patients with CHD—to rule out concomitant coronary anomalies or atherosclerotic disease (if symptomatic).
  - Miscellaneous: Asymptomatic patients are at risk for CAD (whose safety is important for occupational purpose, e.g., pilot), abnormal resting ECG that requires a confirmatory diagnosis of CAD (may be important to remove anxiety for CAD)—class II indication.

Q5. What are the limitations of CAG?
Ans.
- There may be inter- and intraobserver variability in grading stenosis severity in CAG. Sometimes the severity of a lesion may be difficult to gauge on the basis of visual estimation alone.
- Angiography only provides an outline of the lumen (the so-called luminogram). The morphology of plaque cannot be assessed.
- Angiogram can underestimate the presence of atheroma because of outward remodeling of the arterial wall, i.e. adaptove enlargement of coronary artery in response to plaque formation, maintaining a relatively consistent inner lumen (the "Glagov phenomenon").
- Angiography can only visualize arteries >200 µm in diameter.
- Dynamic phenomena that are not active at time of CAG, such as "hit-and-run" events resulting from coronary embolization or thrombosis and subsequent resolution, coronary artery spasm may have LV scar but does not result in coronary angiographic findings.

Q6. What is coronary dominance?
Ans. Coronary dominance identifies the coronary artery, which crosses the crux of the heart (the junction of the posterior AV groove with the posterior interventricular groove) and therefore, generally supplies the basal posterior IVS of the left ventricle. The same artery commonly gives rise to the AV nodal artery in the region of, or just beyond, and the crux. In approximately 85%. of humans, the RCA is dominant. In the remainder 15%, the LCx is dominant, however, codominance does occur.

Note: The term may seem misleading; it is not simply the degree of importance. As LCA is more important as it supplies bulk of the myocardium.

Q7. What is damping and ventricularization?
Ans. Damping means fall in overall catheter-tip pressure, and ventricularization means fall in diastolic pressure only. These indicate restriction of coronary inflow because of insertion of the catheter tip into a

proximal coronary stenosis, or due to an adverse catheter lying against the coronary wall. Vigorous injection may predispose to dissection of proximal coronary artery. Hypotension and arrhythmia may follow. The catheter should be withdrawn gently to restore flow. Damping and ventricularization are more common with RCA—small caliber, ostial spasm around catheter tip, subselective engagement of conus branch, and true ostial stenosis are reasons for it.

Q8. What are the pitfalls of CAG?
Ans. Pitfalls may lead the inexperienced coronary angiographer to a mistaken conclusion. These are:
- Superselective injection—LAD artery, LCx, especially when LMCA is short and its bifurcation is early.
- Total occlusion—absence of vascularity in a portion of heart may indicate total occlusion; usually collateral channels permit visualization of distal occluded artery.
- Myocardial bridges—LAD artery, diagonal and marginal branches dip intramyocardially; overlying myocardium acts to compress artery in systole.
- Coronary spasm—commonly at the catheter tip in RCA.
- Anomalous coronary artery—origin from ectopic site or single coronary artery.
- Ostial lesion—may be overlooked.

Q9. How to assess the degree of coronary lesion on a CAG?
Ans. For routine clinical evaluation, one quantitatively estimates the degree of stenosis visually. Multiple views of the regions of interest are obtained over a range of projection angles to best define the three-dimensional geometry of the lesions. Severity of a lesion is based on percent diameter stenosis compared to a "normal" reference segment (e.g., a 75% stenosis is a lesion that narrows the lumen diameter by approximately 75%). Formal quantitative CAG, or the use of calipers can improve the measurement of coronary lesions.

Q10. How to categorize the severity of coronary stenosis?
Ans. The visual grading system to assess the degree of stenosis is qualitative. Severity of coronary stenosis is usually assessed as the estimated amount of luminal loss and is graded as mild (70–80% reduction in cross-sectional area), moderate (80–90%), and severe (90–99%).

There is a squared relationship between cross-sectional area and diameter. Location within the coronary artery tree, morphology of lesion (concentric vs. eccentric), and presence of an ulcerated plaque are also important and should be mentioned **(Fig. 3.19)**.

Diameter reduction: Mild: ≤40% stenosis, intermediate: 40–70%, and significant: ≥70%.

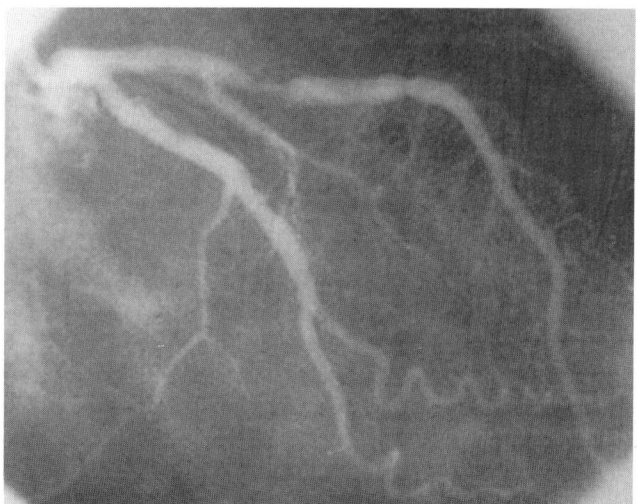

Fig. 3.19: CAG showing severe eccentric 95% LAD stenosis.

Q11. What are the advantages of transradial catheterization?
Ans. Transradial approach is associated with: Fewer vascular complications, more patient comfort, rapid ambulation, lower procedural cost, and reduced hospital stay.

Q12. What are the situations where transradial approach is the most suitable?
Ans. It is most suitable in:
- Patients with high risk of bleeding—elderly, obese, women, those with renal impairment, and those on multiple antithrombotic therapy, especially glycoprotein (GP) II_b/III_a inhibitor.
- Those with severe peripheral arterial disease, patients with bilateral aortoiliac bypass graft and aortic aneurysm, patients with previous femoral complications after catheterization.
- Primary PCI—in patients treated by aggressive antithrombotic agents; life-threatening access-site bleeding complications can be avoided.

Q13. What are the situations where transradial approach is contraindicated?
Ans. It is not indicated in:
- Presence of forearm A-V fistula
- Proven absent ulnar collateral circulation—determined by modified Allen test.
- Small, heavily calcified radial artery
- Intra-aortic balloon pump (IABP), and all other devices or procedures needing access that is larger than 8 Fr catheter.

Q14. What is a modified Allen test?

Ans. It is done before performing any transradial approach to confirm presence of ulnar collateral, in absence of which transradial approach is contraindicated.

The following steps are undertaken in the test:
- Simultaneous compression of radial and ulnar artery followed by several flexion—extension movement of fingers (leading to blenching of palm).
- Ulnar compression ceased
- Time of restoration of color noted: <5 seconds: Normal, 5–10 seconds: intermediate, and ≥10 seconds: abnormal.

In the same manner, a reverse Allen test may be undertaken for transulnar approach.

Q15. What are the complications of transradial approach?

Ans.
- Radial artery spasm—females, patients with small body mass index (BMI), smokers, persons with small radial artery are more prone.
- Radial occlusion—more prone are those with low difference between sheath and artery, diabetics, repeated procedure and low dose of anticoagulation use.
- Asymptomatic loss of radial pulse
- Symptomatic finger or hand ischemia
- Others—bleeding at puncture site, radial false aneurysm, A-V fistula.

Q16. What is SYNTAX scoring system?

Ans. It is an angiographic tool for grading the complexity and extent of CAD. This scoring system was developed during the *SYNTAX* (*Syn*ergy between PCI with *Tax*us and Cardiac Surgery) trial. It is an important prognostic tool for risk stratification of patients with multivessel disease who are being considered for coronary revascularization, and selecting the most appropriate modality. It is also validated for predicting clinical outcomes in patients undergoing primary PCI in ST-segment elevation MI (STEMI) and non-ST-segment elevation MI (NSTEMI). In this scoring system, a lesion is defined to be significant when it causes >50% luminal diameter reduction by visual assessment in a vessel >1.5 mm in diameter using a multiplication factor 2 for nonocclusive, and 5 for occlusive lesions. Up to 12 lesions are identified within the coronary tree, and each lesion is assessed for its severity, including total occlusion and side branches, and their size. Calculation is done automatically by using an online algorithm. A SYNTAX score of II is also developed on the basis of anatomic score, age, creatinine clearance, LVEF, unprotected LM disease, and side branches and their size.

Q17. What information is obtained by LV graphy?

Ans. Quantitative LV graphy calculates LV volumes. SV is determined by subtracting the endsystolic LV volume from the end-diastolic LV volume. EF is the SV divided by the end-diastolic LV volume. EF provides a measurement of global LV systolic function. Regional systolic wall motion is assessed by grading each segment of the left ventricle as hyperkinetic, normal, hypokinetic, akinetic, or dyskinetic. Space-occupying lesions within the LV chamber, e.g., thrombus, may be identified. Finally, assessment of MV competence is made. MR is graded as mild (1+), moderate (2+), moderately severe (3+), or severe (4+).

Q18. What are FFR and instant wave-free ratio (iFR)?

Ans. Fractional flow reserve is the guide wire-based physiological assessment of severity of coronary lesions during PCI. FFR allows determination of coronary stenosis severity, independent of baseline hemodynamics, BP, and heart rate. It is done by measuring distal coronary and aortic pressure during maximum hyperemia. An FFR of <0.75 predicts ischemia, and if it is ≥0.75, PCI may be deferred.

Fractional flow reserve allows determining culprit stenosis in patients with multivessel disease, and evaluation of ostial lesions, LM lesions, serial lesions, and side branch stenosis that may be ambiguous on CAG.

In the era of expensive drug-eluting stents (DES), FFR can be used to limit intervention only to flow-limiting lesions.

Instant wave-free ratio is the updated version of FFR that reduces adenosine cost, used to induce hyperemia during the procedure. It is also a physiological assessment determining whether a stenosis is causing limitation in flow in coronary arteries with subsequent ischemia. Like FFR, it is performed with high-fidelity pressure wires that are passed distal to coronary stenosis.

Q19. What are the indications of renal angiography during CAG?

Ans.

- Hypertensive patients with the onset of hypertension before 30 years, or after 55 years of age
- Malignant, accelerated, or resistant hypertension
- Unexplained renal dysfunction, development of azotemia with an angiotensin-converting enzyme inhibitors (ACEI)/angiotensin II receptor blockers (ARB)

Q20. What is the difference between CAG and CT angiography?

Ans. Invasive CAG is the gold standard technique for anatomical delineation of coronary artery, allowing intervention when needed. Noninvasive evaluation of coronary arteries by CT angiography has some advantages and applicability as listed in **Table 3.7**.

TABLE 3.7: Cardiac computed tomography (CT) angiography and coronary angiography (CAG).

Points	Cardiac CT angio	CAG
Invasiveness	Noninvasive	Invasive
Temporal resolution*	Lower (8 ms)	Higher (60–220 ms)
Spatial resolution**	Low (0.2 mm)	Excellent (0.4–0.5 mm)
Plaque characterization	Possible—soft, calcified, mixed	Not possible
Regular and slow HR during test	Needed	Not needed
Ionizing radiation	More	Less
Indication	Rule out CAD, coronary anomaly	Gold standard for diagnosing CAD
Intervention	Not possible	Possible, where indicated

*Time taken to acquire an image
**The narrowest distance between two objects that can be distinguished by the detector.

SUGGESTED READING

1. American College of Sports Medicine. ACSM's Guidelines for Exercise Testing and Prescription, 6th edition. Baltimore, USA: Lippincott-Williams and Wilkins; 2000.
2. Cheitlin MD, Alpert JS, Armstrong WF, Aurigemma GP, Beller GA, Bierman FZ, et al. ACC/AHA Guidelines for the Clinical Application of Echocardiography: Executive Summary. A report of the American College of Cardiology/American Heart Association Task force on Practice Guidelines (Committee on Clinical Application of Echocardiography). Developed in collaboration with the American Society of Echocardiography. J Am Coll Cardiol. 1997;29(4):862-79.
3. Goldschlager N, Goldman MJ. Principles of Clinical Electrocardiography, 13th edition. East Norwalk, Connecticut: Lange Medical Publications; 1989.
4. Grossman W. In: Baim DS (Ed). Grossman's Cardiac Catheterization, Angiography, and Intervention, 7th edition. Philadelphia: Lipincott-Williams and Wilkins; 2006.
5. Hendel RC, Berman DS, Di Carli MF, Heidenreich PA, Henkin RE, Pellikka PA, et al. ACCF/ASNC/ACR/AHA/ASE/SCCT/SCMR/SNM 2009 Appropriate Use Criteria for Cardiac Radionuclide Imaging: A Report of the American College of Cardiology Foundation Appropriate Use Criteria Task Force, The American Society of Nuclear Cardiology, the American College of Radiology, the American Heart Association, the American Society of Echocardiography, the Society of Cardiovascular Computed Tomography, the Society for Cardiovascular Magnetic Resonance, and the Society of Nuclear Medicine. J Am Coll Cardiol. 2009;53(23):2201-29.
6. Jefferson K, Rees S. In: Rees S (Ed). Clinical Cardiac Radiology, 2nd edition. London, UK: Butterworth-Heinemann Ltd; 1980.
7. Kennedy HL. Use of long-term (Holter) electrocardiographic recordings. In: Zipes DP, Jalife J (Eds). Cardiac Electrophysiology: From Cell To Bedside, 4th edition. Philadelphia: WB Saunders Co Ltd; 2004.

8. Kim HW, Afshin F, Klem I, Rehwald W, Kim RJ. Magnetic resonance imaging of the heart. In: Fuster V, Walsh RA, Harrington RA (Eds). Hurst's The Heart, 13th edition. USA: Mc Graw-Hill; 2011.
9. Klocke FJ, Baird MG, Lorell BH, Bateman TM, Messer JV, Berman DS, et al. ACC/AHA/ASNC guidelines for the clinical use of cardiac radionuclide imaging-executive summary: a report of the American College of Cardiology/American Heart Association Task Force on Practice Guidelines (ACC/AHA/ASNC Committee to Revise the 1995 Guidelines for the Clinical Use of Cardiac Radionuclide Imaging). Circulation. 2003;108(11):1404-18.
10. Schlant RC, Adolph RJ, DiMarco JP, Dreifus LS, Dunn MI, Fisch C, et al. Guidelines for electrocardiography. A report of the American College of Cardiology/American Heart Association Task Force on Assessment of Diagnostic and Therapeutic Cardiovascular Procedures (Committee on Electrocardiography). J Am Coll Cardiol. 1992;19(3):473-81.
11. Schlant RC, Friesinger GC 2nd, Leonard JJ. Clinical competence in exercise testing. A statement for physicians and the ACP/ACC/AHA Task Force on Clinical Privileges in Cardiology. J Am Coll Cardiol. 1990;16(5):1061-5.

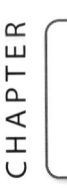

Coronary Artery Disease

"Vessels in the elderly, through the thickening of the tunics, restrict the transit of blood."
—Leonardo da Vinci

■ INTRODUCTION

Coronary artery disease (CAD) is the leading cause of death worldwide. The incidence of CAD is increasing in low- and middle-income countries (LMICs) due to high prevalence of CAD risk factors related to environmental and lifestyle changes. CAD results from atherosclerotic involvement of coronary arteries and their complications. It is a slowly progressive disease with long incubation period that produces few symptoms until late into its course or complicated by thrombus formation. Thus, CAD is manifested either as chronic CAD, where coronary flow and myocardial oxygen (O_2) supply is inadequate in relation to the demand, or where coronary atheroma is complicated with superimposed thrombus, resulting in acute coronary syndrome (ACS). CAD is a disease with high mortality, but it is also highly predictable, treatable, and preventable with existing knowledge.

■ CORONARY RISK FACTORS

Q1. What are CAD and ischemic heart disease (IHD)?

Ans. These are diseases of coronary arteries, resulting from development of atheromatous plaque in coronary arteries and its complications. Obstructive coronary lesions lead to ischemia in myocardium, the entity known as *ischemic heart disease*. But IHD may also manifest in patients with no apparent CAD, such as in coronary embolism, and conditions leading to a demand–supply mismatch. Also, myocardial infarction with nonobstructive coronary arteries (MINOCA), and ischemia with nonobstructive coronary arteries (INOCA) manifest as IHD without CAD. Hence, all CAD may produce IHD, but all IHD may not be CAD.

Q2. What are manifestations of IHD?

Ans. Ischemic heart disease clinically manifests as either stable IHD (SIHD), i.e., chronic stable angina, or as ACS. The spectrum of ACS includes ST-segment elevation myocardial infarction (STEMI), and non-ST-segment elevation ACS (NSTE-ACS), which consists of non-ST-segment elevation myocardial infarction (NSTEMI) and unstable angina (UA). Patients with typical symptoms without persistent (>20 minutes continuously) ST-segment elevation in at least two contiguous electrocardiogram (ECG) leads, but with elevation of myocardial biomarkers >99% percentile of normal are classified as having NSTEMI.

Other manifestations are: Silent ischemia, angina equivalent, heart failure (HF), cardiac arrhythmia, and sudden cardiac death (SCD).

ST-segment elevation myocardial infarction represents the most malignant presentation of CAD resulting from acute thrombus—mediated closure of a coronary artery with the exception of inaugural SCD.

Q3. What is SIHD?
Ans. Here, atheromatous plaque in coronary arteries is stable, and there is no thrombus formation. Besides plaque other factors contributing are endothelial dysfunction, microvascular disease, vasospasm, etc.

This entity comprises patients with:
- Chronic stable angina
- Asymptomatic ischemia
- Prior MI
- Prior coronary revascularization
- Patients with nonobstructive coronary atherosclerosis.

Q4. What is atherosclerosis?
Ans. It is a chronic, systemic immunoinflammatory, fibroproliferative disease of intima of medium and large vessels fueled by lipids.

Inflammation is particularly frequent and intense in ruptured plaques beneath the thrombus. Low-density lipoprotein (LDL) is proinflammatory. Endothelial cell function disrupts with the loss of nitric oxide (NO) production by oxidized LDL. LDL lowering stabilizes coronary lesion by modifying its structure and composition. Thus, the likelihood of coronary plaque rupture and thrombosis is reduced by lowering the LDL level. It is a heterogenous disease having both chronic and acute manifestations with long incubation period, with prolonged period of inactivity, followed by sudden manifestation of deadly complications of atheroma—MI, UA, and stroke often without warning.

It produces stenosis of some vessels, e.g., coronary, cerebral, and peripheral arteries, but aneurysm in some, as in the aorta. Also, ectasia may coexist with stenosis in same arteries.

Q5. What is a risk factor? How to classify CAD risk factors?
Ans. Risk factor is a characteristic or feature of an individual or population that is present early in life and is associated with an increased risk of developing future diseases.

Risk factors of CAD may be:
- *Conventional:*
  - Major risk factor:
- Inherited (unmodifiable)—increasing age, male sex, race, positive family history (F/H) of premature CAD (before the age of 55 years in male, before 65 years in female), menopause (in female).
    - Acquired (modifiable)—smoking, diabetes mellitus (DM), dyslipidemias, hypertension
  - Minor risk factors: Obesity, sedentary lifestyle, type A personality (stressful, competitive living)
- *Emerging:* Newer and novel factors are now incriminated against CAD. These include—lipid factors, e.g., lipoprotein (a) [LP(a)], high triglyceride (TG), small LDL particles and non-lipid factors, e.g., C-reactive protein (CRP), homocysteine, fibrinogen, and plasminogen activator inhibitor-1 (PAI-1).

Q6. How to classify lipoprotein profile?

Ans. Fasting lipid profile is done (after 9–12 hours fast). Adult Treatment Panel (ATP)-III classification of lipoprotein levels is shown in **Table 4.1**.

TABLE 4.1: Lipoprotein profile—classification.

Total cholesterol	
Desirable	<200 mg/dL
Borderline high	200–239 mg/dL
High	≥240 mg/dL
LDL-cholesterol	
Optimal	<100 mg/dL
Above optimal	100–129 mg/dL
Borderline high	130–159 mg/dL
High	160–189 mg/dL
Very high	≥190 mg/dL
HDL-cholesterol	
Low	<40 mg/dL
High	≥60 mg/dL
Serum triglycerides	
Normal	<150 mg/dL
Borderline high	150–199 mg/dL
High	200–499 mg/dL
Very High	≥500 mg/dL

Q7. How to calculate LDL-cholesterol (C) from total cholesterol (TC), TG, and high-density lipoprotein (HDL)-cholesterol (C)?

Ans. LDL-C is calculated by using the following equations:

$$\text{LDL-C (mg/dL)} = \text{TC} - \left(\frac{\text{TG}}{5} + \text{HDL-C}\right)$$

Q8. What is the role of HDL-C?

Ans. High-density lipoprotein-cholesterol protects against atherosclerosis by removing excess cholesterol from peripheral tissue such as blood vessels and moving it back to the liver where it can be excreted in bile. It also prevents oxidation of LDL-C.

Low HDL-C levels are an independent risk factor for CAD. In Framingham Heart Study, there was a 10% increase in CAD for each 4 mg/dL decrease in HDL-C. A low level of HDL is particularly common among South Asians and considered to contribute to the increasing CAD incidence here.

Adult treatment panel III report of National Cholesterol Education Program (NCEP) classifies HDL-C level of <40 mg/dL as low and a level of 60 mg/dL or more as high.

Q9. How is LDL linked to CAD?

Ans. Low-density lipoprotein is proinflammatory. Oxidized LDL produces loss of NO production that leads to disruption of endothelial cell function with increase in its permeability. Lipoproteins enter subendothelially and engulfed by macrophage to form foam cells, thus initiating atheroma formation. Lowering LDL modifies lesion structure and composition of atheroma. Thus, it reduces the likelihood of coronary plaque rupture and thrombosis.

Q10. How is TG related to risk of CAD?

Ans. Triglycerides bring about changes in LDL particle size, density, and composition producing smaller, denser, and more atherogenic particles. Higher intake of carbohydrate (high glycemic load) coupled with higher prevalence of insulin resistance generally results in higher serum levels of TG that significantly lower LDL-C giving a false sense of security. The true risk of CAD in people with high TG is represented by the non-HDL cholesterol level (non-HDL-C = TG-HDL), which can be calculated even in a nonfasting state.

Q11. What are a good, bad, ugly, and deadly cholesterols?

Ans. High-density lipoprotein brings cholesterol to liver from peripheral sites and reduces the risk of atherosclerosis. Thus, it is good cholesterol. LDL produces atherosclerosis by being engulfed by LDL receptors of macrophage at site of atheroma. So, it is bad cholesterol. TG, by itself, does not cause atherosclerosis but brings about changes in LDL that leads to formation of atheroma. Thus, it acts as ugly cholesterol. LP(a) is not only atherogenic but it is also thrombogenic and antifibrinolytic. Hence, it is called deadly cholesterol.

Q12. Why is LP(a) called deadly cholesterol?
Ans. Lipoprotein (a) is often the link between atherosclerosis and thrombosis. The atherogenicity of LP(a) is 10-times higher than LDL. LP(a) is also highly thrombogenic and antifibrinolytic by virtue of its homology to plasminogen. Hence, it is called deadly cholesterol. It is a strong independent-risk factor for CAD in many populations, including South Asians.

Q13. What are the ATP-IV guidelines on treatment of blood cholesterol in reducing atherosclerotic cardiovascular (ASCVD) risk in adults?
Ans. Adult Treatment Panel-IV focuses on treatment proven to reduce ASCVD events. It is not a comprehensive approach to lipid management. These guidelines are not a replacement for clinical judgement.

It is an evidence-based treatment guideline for blood cholesterol to reduce ASCVD risk, based on randomized controlled trials (RCTs). ATP-IV, unlike ATP-III, does not offer a comprehensive approach to detection, evaluation, and treatment of lipid disorders. Here, fixed doses of cholesterol-lowering drugs to reduce ASCVD risk are used. It has the following aspects:

- Four statin-benefit groups—for primary and secondary prevention of ASCVD events (with the exception of no ASCVD event reduction in those with New York Heart Association (NYHA) class II–IV HF, or receiving maintenance hemodialysis).
  - Those with clinical atherosclerotic CVD
  - Those with LDL-C ≥190 mg/dL
  - Diabetics aged 40–75 years with LDL-C: 70–189 mg/dL and without clinical ASCVD
  - Those with LDL-C: 70–189 mg/dL, and estimated 10-year ASCVD risk ≥7.5%, and without clinical ASCVD or diabetes
- Identifies high-intensity (to maximally lower LDL-C) and moderate-intensity statin therapy for secondary and primary prevention. It does not support the use of LDL-C target. No data shows that adding a nonstatin drug to high-intensity statin therapy will provide incremental ASCVD risk reduction benefit with an acceptable margin of safety. High-intensity daily dose lowers LDL-C by approximately ≥50%, moderate-intensity approximately 30–50%, and low-intensity <30%.
- Appropriate intensity of statin therapy should be used to reduce ASCVD risk; no RCT evidence to support continued use of specific LDL-C and/or non-HDL-C treatment targets.
- New—the Pooled Cohort Equations (PCE) to estimate 10-year ASCVD risk.
- More accurately identifies higher risk individuals for statin therapy and focuses statin therapy on those most likely to benefit, also indicates those high-risk groups that may not benefit (based on RCT data).

Q14. What is the treatment approach for lowering cholesterol? What are the criticisms of treat-to-target approach?
Ans. These are:
- "Treat-to-target"
- Lower cholesterol is better
- Risk-based treatment approach
- Treating to LDL-C goal may mean that a suboptimal dose of statin is used (because goal is achieved).
- What the target should be, any additional ASCVD risk reduction with lower target, adverse effect of multidrug therapy that might be needed to achieve a specific goal.
- Many clinicians use the target as LDL-C <70 mg/dL, and LDL-C <100 mg/dL for secondary and primary prevention (non-HDL-C target is 30 mg/dL or higher).
- RCT shows ASCVD events reduced by using maximum tolerated statin in those groups shown to be benefited.
- Primary prevention with statins reduces total mortality as well as nonfatal ASCVD events.
- In many cases, individuals with familial hypercholesterolemia (FH) are unable to achieve an LDL-C goal <100 mg/dL. These patients are not treatment failure, as observational data has shown significant reduction in ASCVD events with high-intensity statin use without achieving specific LDL-C goal.
- In age ≥70 years, if estimated 10-year risk is ≥7.5%, statin therapy reduces ASCVD. Advancing age is the strongest risk factor as it represents cumulative-risk factor exposure.

Risk Assessment Work Group (RAWG) provides guidelines on selected individuals not included in the four statin benefit group.

Q15. What are the utilities of nonstatin therapy?
Ans. Nonstatin therapies do not provide acceptable ASCVD risk reduction benefit compared to their adverse effects in routine prevention of ASCVD. Also, RCT data is not available on treatment of hypertriglyceridemia, optimal age for initiating statin therapy to reduce lifetime risk of ASCVD, and use of non-HDL-C in treatment decision making.

Q16. What is the common pattern of dyslipidemia in South Asians? How does it differ from that of Americans?
Ans. South Asians have borderline elevation of LDL, low levels of HDL, high levels of TG, and high levels of LP(a). The most common patterns of dyslipidemia seen in South Asians compared with that in Americans are shown in **Table 4.2**.

TABLE 4.2: Dyslipidemia in Asian Indians—comparison with Americans.

Lipids	Relative serum concentrations
Total cholesterol	Similar
LDL (bad cholesterol)	Similar
Small, dense LDL	Higher
Triglyceride (ugly cholesterol)	Higher
HDL (good cholesterol)	Lower
LP(a)	Higher

Q17. How does hyperinsulinemia act as a CAD risk factor?

Ans. Insulin resistance and hyperinsulinemia lead to endothelial inflammation, thus hyperinsulinemia promotes atherosclerosis and acts as a CAD risk factor. It is also accompanied by hypertriglyceridemia, low HDL, hypofibrinolysis, hypertension, central obesity, and predominance of small, dense LDL. These are the components of metabolic syndrome (MetS).

Q18. What is MetS? How is it diagnosed?

Ans. Metabolic syndrome is a cluster of multiple cardiometabolic risk factors in the same individual. People with MetS are at high risk for the development of cardiovascular diseases (CVD), chronic kidney diseases (CKD), and cerebrovascular diseases (CeVD). The excessive presence of MetS in South Asians is likely the cause for the twofold rise in type 2 DM (T2DM) and an alarming increase in incidence of CVD. The American Heart Association (AHA) defines level of various components of MetS as shown in **Table 4.3**.

TABLE 4.3: The American Heart Association (AHA) criteria for diagnosis of metabolic syndrome (MetS).

Risk factor	Defining level
Abdominal obesity (inches): WC	
Men	>40 (>35 in South Asians)
Women	>35 (>32 in South Asians)
Triglycerides (mg/dL)	>150
HDL-C (mg/dL)	
Men	<40
Women	<50
BP (mm Hg)	>130/>85
Fasting glucose (mg/dL)	>110 (ADA >100)
Presence of any three of the above five major criteria constitutes MetS.	

(ADA: American Diabetes Association; BP: blood pressure; HDL-C: high-density lipoprotein-cholesterol; WC: waist circumference)

Q19. When should hypercholesterolemia be treated?

Ans. A positive association between elevated serum TC levels and CAD is primarily due to the high level of LDL-C. The ATP-III guideline provides LDL-C cutpoint for initiating dietary and drug therapy, and also a target LDL-C level after therapy. Here, dietary therapy is generally recommended for 3-6 months before initiation of drug treatment.

- As a primary prevention for persons without CAD, treatment and target cutpoints vary according to the presence of other risk factors for CAD (risk factors are age <45 years for men and <55 years for women, F/H of MI or sudden death of first degree relative before 55 years for male or 65 years for female, smoking, hypertension, and DM).
  - For patients with less than two risk factors, lipid-lowering drug therapy is given if LDL-C is >190 mg/dL, target is to reduce it <160 mg/dL.
  - Those with more than two risk factors, drug therapy is given if LDL-C is more than 160 mg/dL, goal is to reduce it to <130 mg/dL.
- As a secondary prevention, i.e., for patients with definite coronary heart disease (CHD) or other atherosclerotic diseases, drug therapy is recommended if LDL-C is >130 mg/dL with a goal of bringing it to <100 mg/dL.

Q20. How is cigarette smoking a CAD risk factor?

Ans. Cigarette and tobacco materials have more than 5,000 toxic chemicals and 10^5-10^{17} free radicals. These are the number one CAD risk factors among Bangladeshis that are related to their oxidative stress. CAD risks due to smoking are:

- Hemodynamic changes—due to nicotine and its sympathomimetic activation and resulting increased cardiac contractility, heart rate, and systolic blood pressure (SBP). Increased O_2 demand, coronary vasoconstriction, and decreased O_2-carrying capacity due to formation of carboxyhemoglobin lead to ischemia.
- Endothelial dysfunction—endothelium releases NO, tissue plasminogen activator (tPA), prostacyclin, and PAI-1. Endothelium-dependent vasodilatation is decreased in smoking.
- Prothrombotic state—by altered platelet activity, alteration in antithrombotic and prothrombotic factors. Coronary plaque becomes vulnerable with higher extracellular content and tendency to rupture.
- Proinflammatory effect—by chronic vascular inflammation.
- Lipid metabolism—lower HDL, increased TG, TC, and LDL, increased oxidized LDL; increased hepatic lipase activity leads to production of small, dense LDL and small, dense HDL-C (no protective effect).
- Glucose metabolism—increases the risk of T2DM; nicotine stimulates catecholamine release from adrenal medulla, thus increasing insulin resistance.

- Cardiac remodeling—nicotine increases expression of angiotensin-converting enzyme (ACE) and production of angiotensin-II, thus producing left ventricular hypertrophy (LVH) and left atrial (LA) enlargement.

Q21. How does CRP act as a risk factor for CAD?
Ans. C-reactive protein, a part of innate immunity, is now a major cardiovascular (CV) risk factor (as atherosclerosis is a chronic inflammatory condition). Absolute vascular risk is higher in individuals with raised high-sensitivity CRP (hs-CRP) and low LDL than in those with a raised LDL but low hs-CRP. The risk is linear across the full range of its serum level, but a level >3 mg/dL is considered high risk.

Q22. What are the characteristic features of obesity in Asian Indians?
Ans. South Asians have a higher prevalence of abdominal obesity, fatty infiltration of liver, ectopic fat deposition, and a higher percentage of body fat compared with other races. This increased adiposity manifests as MetS. Abdominal obesity is increased, especially when associated with a body mass index (BMI) >25 kg/m^2. Hence, the National Obesity and MetS Summit has revised the diagnostic cutoffs for BMI and waist circumference for South Asians as listed in **Table 4.4**.

TABLE 4.4: Recommended body mass index (BMI) for South Asians.

Categories	BMI
Normal	18–22.9 kg/m^2
Overweight	23–24.9 kg/m^2
Obesity	>25 kg/m^2
Abdominal waist circumference	Men >35 in (90 cm), women >32 in (80 cm)

Q23. What are vulnerable plaque and vulnerable myocardium?
Ans. Vulnerable plaques are plaques that are prone to rupture and put patients at risk for ACS and SCD following rupture. These have a large lipid core and a thin fibrous cap. These plaques may be angiographically unimpressive and hemodynamically insignificant. Thus, the majority of acute MI (AMI) occur due to sudden total occlusion at sites of mild to moderate stenosis with a vulnerable plaque. On the other hand, angiographically severe stenosis results in severe angina, but rarely results in MI. Thus, there is a paradigm change in CAD pathogenesis.

Vulnerable myocardium may be ischemic and nonischemic. Ischemic includes patients with old MI, UA, myocardial scarring, etc. Nonischemic includes cardiomyopathies [dilated cardiomyopathy (DCM), hypertrophic cardiomyopathy (HCM), right ventricular cardiomyopathy], aortic stenosis, long QT syndrome (LQTS), Brugada syndrome (BrS), Wolff–Parkinson–White (WPW) syndrome, sick sinus syndrome, atrioventricular (AV) block, etc.

Vulnerable blood is a serological marker, which predicts patient's risk of CV complications. These are: Abnormal lipid profile [high LDL, low HDL, high LP(a)], high inflammatory marker, e.g., hs-CRP, markers of MetS, e.g., DM, hyper TG, increased D-dimer, PAI-1, reduced tPA, smoking, cocaine abuse, etc. Vulnerable patients are subjects who are susceptible to ACS or SCD based on the triad of plaque, blood, and myocardial viability.

Q24. What are the techniques to characterize plaque composition?
Ans. These are: Intravascular ultrasound (IVUS), intravascular optical coherence tomography (OCT), virtual histology, and near-infrared spectroscopy (NIRS). IVUS can detect remodeling, plaque burden, calcium; OCT detects necrotic core, fibrous cap thickness, macrophages. IVUS with virtual histology can detect necrotic core, calcium, and collagen. NIRS can detect the necrotic core.

- IVUS allows visualization of the disease in vessel wall and provides cross-sectional and longitudinal images of atherosclerotic plaques. It is based on transmitting and receiving high-frequency sound waves through a low-profile catheter. IVUS allows identification of hemodynamically significant lesions that may be underestimated by angiography, particularly in nonocclusive plaques with positive remodeling. It delineates the degree of calcification, plaque burden, and arterial remodeling. It differentiates highly echogenic components such as calcium and dense fibrous tissue from echolucent tissue, such as lipid and necrotic core. However, it cannot clearly differentiate between fibrous and fatty plaques. Also, it cannot detect thin core fibroatheromas (TCFAs). IVUS is an excellent tool for detecting remodeling, a major feature of advanced atherosclerotic plaques. Here, large plaques can appear to be nonobstructive on coronary angiography (CAG) and ruptured plaques may be realized as larger than the nonruptured one. No other imaging modality can show remodeling better than IVUS.
- *OCT:* It is the highest resolution (5–20 μm) intravascular imaging technique that identifies plaque rupture, fibrous cap erosion, intracoronary thrombus, and TCFA location. OCT can identify several high-risk plaque characteristics, including eccentric plaque distribution, intimal laceration, ruptured plaque, large high-attenuation lipid pool covered with thin fibrous cap, calcium deposition (low attenuation), lumen thrombus (including differentiation between high-attenuation red and low-attenuation white thrombus), microchannels, etc. OCT is the only imaging tool with enough resolution to identify fibrous cap thickness of 65 μm or less, which is lowest in patients with AMI, intermediate in UA, and highest in chronic stable angina. It can predict no-flow phenomenon

with large lipid cores which undergo percutaneous coronary intervention (PCI) for ACS. It is the gold standard for identifying neovascularization.
- Virtual histology, and NIRS—noninvasive technique using optical device, i.e., light to measure tissue oxygenation and perfusion

Q25. What is vascular remodeling?
Ans. Vascular remodeling is the phenomenon of harboring large atheroma without luminal obstruction. It takes place in high-risk atherosclerosis. It promotes higher stress at the level of fibrous cap and makes the plaque vulnerable to rupture. Remodeling may be positive or negative. Positive remodeling is more common in ACS, and negative remodeling more in chronic stable angina cases.

Q26. What is the AHA classification of atherosclerotic lesions?
Ans.
- *Type I:* Microscopic
- *Type II:* Fatty streak
- *Type III:* Preatheroma lesions
- *Type IV:* Atheroma
- *Type V:* Lesion with positive remodeling (increase of vessel-external boundary without luminal narrowing)—may be the following:
  - Type Va—lesion (fibroatheroma with prominent fibrous connective tissue around lipid core).
  - Type Vb—calcified core
  - Type Vc—fibrotic with no or minimal lipid core.
- *Type VI:* Lesion—complex disease, including plaque rupture, erosion, or intraplaque hemorrhage).

Type I–III are clinically silent.

Q27. How does DM act as a CAD risk factor?
Ans. Diabetes accelerates the natural process of atherosclerosis. Accelerated atherosclerosis in a person with diabetes may be attributed to coexistent hypertension, hyperlipidemia, obesity, and insulin resistance. Diabetes carries a greater burden of additional known major CV risk. DM is a risk factor of CAD, but the risk starts to increase long before the onset of clinical diabetes. This is due to the hyperinsulinemic state that promotes atherosclerosis and CAD. By the time the patient develops diabetes, atherosclerosis is far advanced and equivalent to having CAD. Hence, diabetes is called a CAD equivalent and the target of LDL-C in diabetics is similar to that in patients with CAD.

Q28. Does atherosclerotic CAD differ in diabetic patients compared to nondiabetics?
Ans. It has been found that people with diabetes have a greater number of affected coronary vessels (multivessel CAD), more diffuse distribution

of lesions, and greater narrowing of the left main (LM) coronary artery than people without diabetes. Patients with diabetes undergoing cardiac catheterization for MI, percutaneous transluminal coronary angioplasty (PTCA), or planned coronary artery bypass grafting (CABG) have significantly more severe CAD and a decreased coronary collateral.

Q29. What is syndrome X?
Ans. There are two types of syndrome X—metabolic and cardiac. MetS X is MetS.

In contrast to MetS X, a cardiac syndrome X (microvascular angina) exists in those patients who have anginal symptoms, normal coronary arteries on catheterization, but small, more distal occlusive disease. Both syndromes may coexist inside the same patient.

Q30. What are the implications of concurrent diabetes in ACS?
Ans. Overall, individuals with diabetes do significantly worse than nondiabetics in the setting of AMI. In hospitals, the mortality rate among people with diabetes with MI remains twice that of people without diabetes. This is due to an increased propensity to develop myocardial rupture, reinfarction, shock, and congestive HF (CHF) among diabetic patients.

Blood glucose level may rise due to increased catecholamine surge associated with AMI. In MI setting, blood glucose should be controlled with insulin.

Delayed complications of MI are also more common among diabetics. Survival and recurrent CV events among patients with diabetes after MI are closely related to post-MI ejection fraction (EF), the presence of multivessel CAD, and the prothrombotic state associated with diabetes.

Although β-blockers are relatively contraindicated in diabetes, they are of benefit after MI and should be given, especially in anterior MI. Hypoglycemia developing in patients on insulin or on oral agents may be masked and requires frequent monitoring.

Q31. How reliable is angina as an indicator of ischemia in diabetic patients?
Ans. Diabetic individuals have increased incidence of silent ischemia and MI due to the development of autonomic neuropathy. Hence, angina is not a reliable marker of ischemia in this situation. Because of this, it is important to do a thorough evaluation of nonspecific symptoms, symptoms of angina equivalents [e.g., shortness of breath (SOB) and tiredness], or symptoms of early CHF in individuals with long-standing diabetes.

Q32. How is hyperinsulinemia related to CAD?
Ans. An increased prevalence and severity of CAD have been reported in patients with hyperinsulinism. Hyperinsulinemia is associated with dyslipidemia, enhanced proliferation of cells composing atherosclerotic

plaque, and increased production of PAI. The physiologic response to hyperinsulinism and insulin resistance is glucose intolerance and the development of frank DM.

Q33. Regarding CAD risk, which hypertension is more important?
Ans. An increase in SBP indicates that the heart has to pump more vigorously.

The workload falling on the heart is more. As a result of increased workload,

myocardial hypertrophy occurs. LVH is a risk factor for future cardiac events.

An increase in diastolic pressure means that the heart cannot relax adequately. Diastolic compliance decreases and coronary flow, which occurs mainly in the diastole, is hampered. Diastolic dysfunction and HF results. Recent studies reveal SBP to be a stronger predictor of events from CAD than diastolic blood pressure (BP). Isolated systolic hypertension is highly correlated with CV risk and is important to control. The relationship is shown to be stronger for SBP than diastolic BP; the risk for CAD progressively increases for an increase in SBP.

Q34. How is obesity related to CAD?
Ans. Obesity is associated with several CV risk factors—hypercholesterolemia, hypertension, and glucose intolerance. Central obesity with increased waist-to-hip ratio is viewed as a more accurate predictor of CAD. This android pattern of fat distribution is more metabolically active and highly associated with dyslipidemia. Obesity among adults is associated with increased left ventricular (LV) mass, and rarely cardiomyopathy, which independently increases CV morbidity and mortality. Central obesity is part of insulin resistance syndrome or syndrome X, which appears to increase the risk for CAD in both sexes.

Q35. Is sedentary lifestyle a predictor of CAD?
Ans. There is nearly a twofold increase in the risk for development of CAD and death among sedentary persons compared to active persons. A sedentary lifestyle is also associated with obesity, hypertension, NIDDM, and hypercholesterolemia. On the contrary, regular physical activity prevents obesity, may allow weight loss, and promote control of BP and dyslipidemias. Among patients who had MI, controlled cardiac rehabilitation programs with early ambulation significantly reduce CV mortality.

Q36. How does exercise improve CV health?
Ans. Exercise improves glucose tolerance and insulin sensitivity, thus helps in the control of diabetes. It aids in the control of hypertension. Exercise improves O_2 uptake in the heart, increases fibrinolysis, and increases coronary artery diameter. Exercise reduces sensitivity of the myocardium to the effect of catecholamines and thus reduces risk for ventricular arrhythmias and

SCD. Exercise lowers LDL-C, and vigorous exercise is believed to increase HDL-C and as such reduce cardiac events. Exercise training may increase regression and reduce the progression of coronary lesions in CAD.

ANGINA PECTORIS AND CHRONIC CORONARY ARTERY DISEASE

Q1. What is angina pectoris?
Ans. Angina pectoris is a syndrome characterized by discomfort in the chest or an adjacent area that is associated with myocardial ischemia due to an imbalance between myocardial O_2 supply and demand.

Q2. What are the types of angina?
Ans. Two basic types are stable angina and UA. Anginal symptoms are defined as stable if there is no substantial deterioration in symptoms over several weeks. Angina is said to be unstable when the symptom pattern worsens abruptly (increase in severity, frequency, and duration) without an obvious cause of increased myocardial O_2 consumption. In stable angina, a stable (fixed) coronary artery obstruction is present, which limits O_2 delivery during the time of increased metabolic demands. The severity of the obstruction determines the threshold for cardiac ischemia. In UA, coronary lesion becomes unstable and nonocclusive intracoronary thrombi develop on the ruptured coronary artery plaque. Local vasoconstriction also occurs.

Other less common presentations of angina are:
- *Atypical angina:* The presenting symptoms do not include all the classic features of angina, for instance, pain or discomfort other than substernal in location (neck, jaw, epigastrium, etc.).
- *Variant angina:* It is a relatively rare syndrome related to coronary artery spasm. Chest pain usually occurs at rest; they are often cyclic, occurring at the same time of day. The angina is frequently marked by ST-segment elevation (or depression) and dysrhythmias including heart block and even ventricular tachycardia (VT). The spasm can occur in normal coronary vessels or in proximity to fixed lesions.
- *Decubitus angina:* This angina occurs with change in posture, on lying position and is believed to be caused by a shift in blood volume.
- *Nocturnal angina:* It occurs at night and is frequently associated with nightmares.
- *Angina equivalents:* In this atypical presentation, patients do not perceive angina as pain. They have dyspnea, profound fatigue, weakness, lightheadedness, nausea, diaphoresis, presyncope, or syncope.

Q3. What is stable angina?
Ans. It is the condition resulting from transient myocardial ischemia due to an imbalance between myocardial O_2 supply and demand. It is caused by a fixed or stable atheroma in the coronary artery.

Q4. How is stable angina graded?
Ans. The Canadian Society of Cardiology (CSC) classification of stable angina:
- *Class I:* Angina on extraordinary exertion, no angina with ordinary activity
- *Class II:* Slight limitation of ordinary activity; pain on climbing >1 flight of stairs
- *Class III:* Marked limitation of ordinary physical activity; pain on climbing 1 flight of stairs
- *Class IV:* Inability to carry on any activity; angina at rest or with normal activity.

Q5. What factors make chest pain more likely to be ischemic in origin?
Ans. Most patients describe angina as vague chest discomfort. The presence of risk factors for CAD such as hypertension, DM, smoking, hypercholesterolemia, F/H of IHD, and advanced age increase the likelihood that the chest discomfort is being caused by myocardial ischemia.

Q6. What is the characteristic of a typical anginal attack?
Ans. The chest pain or pressure, heaviness or weight-like sensation located in the substernal area, brought on by exertion that often radiates across the midthorax into the left arm (ulnar aspect), neck, or jaw, lasting constantly for 2–15 minutes, and relieved by rest or nitroglycerin (NG). It is often associated with SOB. Angina is aggravated by cigarette smoking, heavy meals, anger, cold weather.

Q7. Who are the patient subsets in whom ACS is most likely to be missed?
Ans.
- *Young:* Incidence of AMI is increasing in the youth (age <40 years). High index of suspicion is needed in youth who develop typical or atypical anginal symptoms, particularly if there is a history of tobacco abuse or a F/H of premature CAD.
- *Elderly:* More prone to atypical presentations with dyspnea (as angina equivalent).
- *Women:* Tend to present with longer delay from symptom onset, tend to be older, have more comorbid diseases (e.g., diabetes), and have more atypical presentation. Postmenopausal women assume the same risk as their male counterparts for CAD.
- *Diabetics:* Presentations are more frequently silent or atypical.
- *Drug abusers and alcoholics:* Etiology of their chest pain may not be evaluated objectively.
- *Frequent flyers:* With repeated visit to the emergency department (ED), a tendency to dismiss complaints from these groups of patients accumulates.

Atypical presentation: 10% of AMI and UA are missed because of atypical presentation.

- *Comorbid psychiatric and somatoform diseases:* Psychiatric diagnosis in a patient who complains of chest pain should always be a diagnosis of exclusion.
- *Pre-existing gastrointestinal (GI) disease:* Epigastric or chest pain in these patients may be misleading and may be attributed to their underlying chronic diagnosis rather than ACS.

Q8. What are the varieties of acute chest pain that are unlikely to be due to ACS?
Ans. These are:
- Pain localized to skin or chest wall that can be reproduced by local pressure
- Pain localized to a small area of chest (<3 cm in diameter) or pain that radiates to right lower chest
- Sharp, stabbing pain aggravated by deep breathing or rotating the chest
- Pain worse in supine position and relieved by sitting or leaning forward (suggesting pericarditis).
- Pain lasting <15 seconds is rarely ischemic in origin

Q9. What are typical and atypical ischemic chest pain?
Ans. Heberden provided the first description of typical ischemic chest pain in 1768: A painful sensation in the breast accompanied by a strangling sensation, anxiety, and occasional radiation of pain to the left arm and is associated with exertion and relieved with rest.

Typical anginal pain is a discomfort in chest and adjacent areas, usually brought on by exertion, beginning gradually and reaching its maximum intensity over a period of minutes, and relieved by rest or by nitrates within minutes. A delay of more than 5–10 minutes before relief of the pain, or pain lasting >20 minutes suggest AMI. Pain >10 minutes, or pain occurring at rest indicates UA.

Q10. What is the location and radiation of anginal pain?
Ans. Anginal pain may be felt anywhere between the diaphragm and mandible, but it is most often substernal, or on the left side of the chest. It tends to be diffuse. It commonly radiates to the arm (usually the inner aspect of the arm and more commonly the left), but it may radiate to neck, throat, mandible, and shoulder.

Q11. How long does an episode of angina last?
Ans. Anginal symptoms typically last 3–5 minutes. If symptoms last longer than 20 minutes, they are usually due to myocardial necrosis (infarction) or are noncardiac in origin. Also brief, fleeting pains (lasting less than 1 minute) are rarely cardiac.

Q12. What are the CV causes of acute chest pain?
Ans. These are:
- Acute coronary syndrome:
  - Unstable angina
  - Acute MI
- Pulmonary embolism
- Acute aortic dissection
- Acute pericarditis

Q13. How does ECG guide therapy in acute chest pain?
Ans.
- ST-segment elevation >1 cm in two or more leads—STEMI. Urgent coronary reperfusion by PCI or thrombolytic therapy is warranted.
- Flat or downsloping ST depression or T-wave inversion—UA or NSTEMI. Antithrombotic agents (heparin) to prevent STEMI along with antiplatelet and other anti-ischemic agents advocated.
- No ECG changes—observation with repeat ECG, cardiac markers, and exercise ECG (in some).

Q14. What changes on ECG may be seen with angina?
Ans. The classic ECG changes of myocardial ischemia are horizontal ST-segment depression in leads corresponding to the anatomic regions of the heart. Besides, there may be transient changes in T wave or conduction abnormalities.

Symptoms with associated ECG changes that resolve strongly suggest myocardial ischemia. A normal ECG does not exclude ischemia as being the cause of chest pain.

There is fairly close correlation between ischemic ECG abnormalities and the anatomic site of coronary obstruction. Ischemic changes in the inferior leads (II, III, aVF) indicate right coronary or circumflex artery disease. Abnormal changes in the anterior precordial leads suggest left anterior descending (LAD) artery disease and change in the left lateral (V_5-V_6) or high lateral leads (I, aVL) implies either diagonal or circumflex artery disease.

The presence of Q wave is usually a specific indicator of MI.

The presence of left bundle branch block (LBBB) in patients with angina is associated with significant LV dysfunction and may reflect multivessel CAD.

Q15. What may be the causes of angina in patients with normal CAG findings?
Ans. Causes of angina without flow-limiting CAD may be: Vasospastic angina, misinterpreting CAG, misdiagnosis of flash (or stump) coronary occlusion at site of major bifurcation, increased subendocardial pressure leading to coronary compression, hyperdynamic ventricular contraction with elevated

wall tension. Also, concealed diffuse coronary atherosclerosis [revealed by fractional flow reserve (FFR) or IVUS], endothelial dysfunction, coronary spasm, and myocardial bridges may be causes of myocardial ischemia without critical stenosis.

Q16. What is meant by syndromic presentation of CAD?
Ans. Coronary artery disease being a dynamic process, structural alteration, i.e., atherosclerotic plaque and functional alteration of coronary circulation is involved. It can be modified by lifestyle, pharmacotherapy, and revascularization, which results in stabilization and regression of disease process. A stable plaque may turn into a vulnerable one by an increase in its lipid core with thin fibrous cap. Also, vulnerable blood with an abnormal lipid profile, high inflammatory markers, and coexistent vulnerable myocardium make a patient vulnerable and susceptible to ACS. Thus, it is a syndrome, i.e., chronic coronary syndrome (CCS) where a vulnerable patient may develop ACS. In this way, CAD is a continuum that may present as either ACS or as CCS. European Society of Cardiology used the term CCS in their 2019 and 2024 guidelines to describe the clinical presentation of CAD during stable periods, particularly those preceding or following ACS. Here, CCS is defined as a range of clinical presentations or syndromes that arises due to structural and/or functional alterations related to chronic diseases of the coronary arteries and/or microcirculation. It may be symptomatic or asymptomatic. Although stable for a long time, it is frequently progressive and may destabilize at any time leading to ACS.

Q17. What are the clinical presentations of CCS?
Ans.
- Stress-induced angina or equivalent with obstructive CAD
- Angina or equivalent with no obstructive CAD, i.e., angina with non-obstructive coronary arteries (ANOCA), INOCA
- Stabilized phase after ACS, PCI, or CABG
- LV dysfunction or HF of ischemic origin
- Asymptomatic with abnormal coronary anatomical or functional test

Q18. What is the stepwise approach for a suspected case of CCS?
Ans.
- *Step 1:* Clinical evaluation—including ruling out noncardiac causes of chest pain and ACS, with 12-lead ECG, basic blood tests, and few other selective tests.
- *Step 2:* Cardiac examination—echocardiography (echo) to rule out LV dysfunction and valvular heart disease, estimating clinical likelihood of obstructive CAD to guide further noninvasive and invasive testing.
- *Step 3:* Diagnostic testing to establish diagnosis and determine the patient's future risk.

- *Step 4*: Lifestyle and risk factor modification combined with a combination of antianginal medications. Coronary revascularization is considered if symptoms are refractory to medical treatment, or if high-risk CAD is present. If symptoms persist after ruling out obstructive CAD, coronary microvascular disease and vasospastic angina should be considered.

Q19. Who are the high-risk patients with adverse CV event?
Ans. High-risk categories for adverse CV event are patients with:
- *Exercise tolerance test (ETT):* Duke Treadmill Score ≤10
- *Stress single photon emission computed tomography (SPECT) or positron emission tomography (PET) perfusion imaging:* Area of ischemia ≥10% of LV myocardium
- *Stress echo:* ≥3 of 16 segments with stress-induced hypokinesia or akinesia
- *Stress cardiovascular magnetic resonance (CMR):* ≥2 of 16 segments with stress perfusion defects, or ≥3 dobutamine-induced dysfunctional segments
- *Coronary computed tomography (CT) angiography:* LM disease with ≥50% stenosis, 2-vessel disease with ≥70% stenosis, including the proximal LAD artery, or small vessel disease of proximal LAD artery with ≥70% stenosis with FFR-CT ≥0.8.

Q20. What are the indications of invasive CAG in case of suspected CAD?
Ans. Coronary angiography is recommended to diagnose CAD in individuals with a very high (>85%) clinical likelihood of disease, severe symptoms refractory to guideline-directed medical therapy (GDMT), angina at low level of exercise, and/or high event risk. In individuals with de novo symptoms highly suggestive of obstructive CAD that occur at low level of exercise, CAG with a view towards revascularization is recommended. Radial route is the preferred access site with pressure assessment [FFR/instantaneous wave-free ratio (iFR)] to evaluate the functional severity of intermediate nonleft main stenosis prior to revascularization. It is also recommended to confirm or exclude the diagnosis of obstructive CAD or ANOCA/INOCA in individuals with an uncertain diagnosis on noninvasive testing.

To rule out obstructive CAD in individuals with low to moderate pretest likelihood, coronary CT angiography is recommended as the preferred diagnostic modality.

Q21. What is the role of exercise ECG in the diagnosis of CAD?
Ans. The concept of exercise ECG testing arose from the observations of ST-segment depression caused by exercise-induced ischemia. In patients with chest pain of uncertain etiology and a normal ECG, a standard exercise test is useful in the diagnosis of CAD. Exercise ECG provides useful information about patients with normal baseline ECGs who are at high risk for CAD. It is less useful when the pretest probability of CAD is low. Exercise ECG is

best used in the evaluation of a patient at intermediate risk with an atypical history, or a patient at low risk with a typical history.

Q22. What is the importance of exercise ECG in patients with CAD?
Ans.
- Exercise ECG helps to ascertain whether a patient is at high risk for future adverse events—prognosis of patients with stable angina largely depends on the exercise capacity and the stage at which ischemia is induced.
- It is used to identify a safe limit for exercise in patients with stable angina.
- For some patients, exercise testing is used to evaluate the response to antianginal therapy. Here, a maximum capacity stress test is performed to determine the functional benefit of the therapy.

Q23. How to stratify risk in stable angina?
Ans.
- High risk—postinfarction angina, poor effort tolerance, ischemia at low workload, LM disease, triple vessel disease on CAG, and poor LV function
- Low risk—predictable exertional angina, good effort tolerance, ischemia only at high workload, single vessel disease or minor double vessel disease on CAG, and good LV function.

Q24. How is stress testing utilized for risk stratification of patients with CAD?
Ans. Stress testing with exercise or pharmacologic agents identifies patient with low, intermediate, or high risk for subsequent cardiac events.
- *High risk (>3% annual mortality):*
  - Severe LV dysfunction (EF <35%)—resting and on exercise.
  - High-risk treadmill score ≥11
  - Stress-induced perfusion defect—large (particularly, if any), multiple moderate-sized defect, defect with LV dilatation, or increased lung uptake (thallium-201).
  - Large, fixed perfusion defect with LV dilatation or increased lung uptake (thallium-201).
  - Stress-echocardiographic evidence of extensive ischemia, or echocardiographic wall-motion abnormalities (involving more than two segments) developing at low dose of dobutamine (≤10 mg/kg/min) or at a low heart rate (<120 beats/min).
- *Intermediate risk (1–3% annual mortality rate):*
  - Mild/moderate LV dysfunction [left ventricular ejection fraction (LVEF): 35–49%]
  - Intermediate-risk treadmill score ≥8
  - Stress-induced moderate perfusion defect without LV dilatation or increased lung uptake (thallium-201).

- Stress-echocardiographic evidence of limited ischemia with a wall-motion abnormality only at higher dose of dobutamine involving ≤2 segments.
- *Low risk (<1% annual mortality risk):*
  - Low-risk treadmill score ≥5
  - Normal or small myocardial perfusion defect at rest or with stress
  - Normal stress-echocardiographic wall motion, or no change of wall motion during stress

Patients identified as high risk are generally referred to as CAG independent of their symptomatic status.

Q25. When to do CAG in chronic stable angina?
Ans. In chronic stable angina, CAG with a view to consider revascularization is done in patients with refractory symptoms of ischemia despite optimal therapy; those with high risk, noninvasive test results. It is also considered in those with occupation or lifestyle that require a more aggressive approach, e.g., pilot and fireman.

Q26. Outline treatment of stable angina.
Ans.
- Identification and treatment of precipitating factors—anemia, hypertension, tachycardia, CHF, and valvular disease
- Control of risk factors—DM, hypertension, and dyslipidemia
- General and nonpharmacological measures—lifestyle modification
- Pharmacological—aspirin, β-blockers, NG (sublingual or long-acting oral), ACE inhibitors (ACEI), calcium-channel blockers, and lipid-lowering agents. ACEI and β-blockers decrease morbidity and mortality in LV dysfunction following MI. Again, aspirin, ACEI, and lipid-lowering agents decrease morbidity and mortality in chronic stable angina with preserved LV function. All these three are indicated in CAD patients with or without angina.
- Revascularization—when an unacceptable level of angina persists despite medical management, patient has troublesome side effects from anti-ischemic drugs, and/or exhibits a high-risk result in noninvasive testing, coronary anatomy should be defined to allow selection of appropriate technique for revascularization. Type of revascularization is selected on the basis of coronary anatomy, LV function, and other comorbidities. PCI (PTCA, stenting, atherectomy) done in single and double vessel disease. CABG done in triple vessel and LM disease.

Q27. What are the uses of antianginal drugs?
Ans. Nitrates, β-blockers, and calcium-channel blockers are three drugs used as initial therapy to control anginal attack as shown in **Table 4.5**.

TABLE 4.5: Antianginal drugs—uses.

Drugs	Uses
Nitrates	• Acute anginal episode; sublingually—drug of choice • Short-term prophylaxis (up to 30 mm)—nitroglycerin tablet used sublingually before activities known to precipitate angina • IV nitroglycerin (10–20 µg/min) in unstable angina (and acute MI with ongoing chest pain) • Long-acting oral nitrate—often used as secondary therapy to alleviate anginal symptoms and increase exercise tolerance
β-blockers	• Effort-induced angina—primary therapy • After MI—reduced incidence of reinfarction, sudden death, and improved survival • Patients with hypertension and angina • Use of IV β-blockers in unstable angina and acute MI, in patients with ongoing chest pain (or persistent hypertension)
Calcium-channel blockers	(As effective as β-blockers in relieving angina and improving exercise tolerance) • Used in combination with β-blockers when initial treatment with β-blockers is not successful • Preferred agents in patients with history of asthma, copd, or severe peripheral vascular disease • In variant (vasospastic) angina—drug of choice • Unstable angina—when β-blockers and nitrates fail to relieve symptoms of ischemia • In patients undergoing PCI—to prevent coronary artery spasm • In non-ST segment elevation MI—may prevent reinfarction

(COPD: chronic obstructive pulmonary disease; IV: intravenous; MI: myocardial infarction; PCI: percutaneous coronary intervention)

Q28. What are the limitations of aspirin as an antiplatelet agent for secondary prevention of CHD?

Ans.

- Aspirin is associated with GI side effects that may prompt patients to discontinue its use, as well as bleeding side effects that may be life-threatening.
- There appears to be a population of patients that is "aspirin resistant".
- Patients taking aspirin may have recurrent ischemic episodes attributable to the relatively weak platelet inhibition provoked by aspirin.
- Aspirin may interact adversely with other medications, such as ACEI.

Unlike aspirin, clopidogrel acts by interfering with platelet adenosine diphosphate (ADP) receptor activation. Blockade of this single pathway may be more potent than thromboxane A_2 inhibition.

It is because it acts independently of the arachidonic acid pathway, the antiplatelet activities of aspirin and clopidogrel are synergistic.

Q29. What are the types of CABG? What are the patient subsets for which CABG is offered?

Ans. Types of CABG:
- Conventional CABG—under cardiopulmonary bypass (CPB)
- Minimal invasive CABG—four categories (based on approach and use of CPB):

Port-access CABG, off-pump approach, including minimally invasive direct CABG (MIDCAB), and off-pump CAB (OPCAB). Hybrid procedure includes minimally invasive coronary bypass surgical procedure on the LAD coronary artery with PCI on remaining vessels.

CABG provides more complete revascularization. It has more survival benefits; in patients with LV dysfunction and multivessel disease, LV function improves after CABG. CABG is done more on older (more on female), sicker patients with more proportion of UA, triple vessel disease, previous CABG or PCI, LV dysfunction, and with more comorbid conditions such as hypertension, DM, and peripheral vascular disease.

Q30. Compare between venous and arterial graft.

Ans. Both arterial and venous grafts are used for coronary artery bypass.

They differ in respect of indication, outcome, and long-term patency as listed in **Table 4.6**.

TABLE 4.6: Grafts for coronary artery bypass.

Venous graft	Arterial graft
Diameter matching with coronary—not closer	Closer
Vasodilatory property—not maintained	Maintained (endothelin-dependent)
Intimal hyperplasia occurs	Nil
Perioperative spasm—less	More
Venous graft atherosclerosis (VGA*) occurs	Nil
Late graft patency—less	More
Late attenuation—more	Extremely low
Grafting time—less	More
In cardiogenic shock—more preferred	Less
Indication—distal RCA, OM artery, diagonals	LAD (routinely done)
Subsequent PCI—may be needed	Not needed

*VGA: Different from native coronary atherosclerosis—circumferential, not encapsulated, and extremely friable (embolization may occur).
(LAD: left anterior descending; OM: obtuse marginal; PCI: percutaneous coronary intervention; RCA: right coronary artery)

Q31. How to prevent CAD?
Ans.
- *Primordial:* Prevent development of risk factors of CAD (population-based strategy)—lifestyle modification.
- *Primary:* Control of risk factors (high-risk, individual-based strategy)—LSM and drugs.
- *Secondary:* Prevent progression of CAD by aggressive drug therapy—antiplatelet, β-blocker, statin, ACEI/angiotensin-II receptor blockers (ARB), etc.

Q32. What are the prognostic factors in CAD patients?
Ans.
- LV function—strongest predictor of long-term survival; EF is the measure of degree of LV dysfunction. Resting LVEF or exercise LVEF: <35% indicate high risk (>3% annual mortality), and LVEF: 35–49% indicates intermediate risk (annual mortality: 1–3%).
- Number of stenosed coronary arteries, and severity of atherosclerotic involvement
- Evidence of a recent coronary plaque rupture—higher risk for cardiac death or nonfatal MI
- General health and noncoronary comorbidity

Q33. What are the determinants of risk in CAD?
Ans. Four main determinants of risk in CAD are:
- Extent of ischemia
- Number of diseased vessels
- LV function
- Electrical substrate

Points to ponder:
- In patients with angina who are not considered to be at high risk, survival is similar for surgery, PCI, and medical management.
- Aspirin, ACEI, lipid-lowering agents–indicated in patients with or without angina; they decrease morbidity and mortality in chronic stable angina with preserved LV function. ACEI is specially indicated in patients with low EF, CKD, DM, and hypertension.
- Coronary revascularization (PCI and CABG) is highly efficient in relieving symptoms, and may be considered for patients with moderate to severe ischemic symptoms who are not controlled by and/or are dissatisfied with medical therapy even if they are not in a high-risk subset.
- PCI—good outcome unlikely in complex lesion, long, eccentric, calcified lesion, lesion in a bend or within a tortuous vessel, lesion that involves a branch or contains active thrombus. In single vessel disease—objective is to relieve symptom by PCI.

ACUTE CORONARY SYNDROME (UNSTABLE ANGINA AND ACUTE MYOCARDIAL INFARCTION)

Q1. What is ACS?

Ans. Acute coronary syndrome refers to any constellation of clinical symptoms resulting from an acute alteration in coronary plaque, leading to a temporary or permanent occlusion by formation of thrombus. Ruptured atherosclerotic plaque leading to thrombus formation is the basic mechanism in ACS. ACS includes UA, NSTEMI, and STEMI.

It represents a continuum that shares a common initiation when an atheromatous plaque is ruptured or fissured. Plaque rupture causes platelet deposition at the site of injury followed by thrombus formation. Once intracoronary thrombus in a patient with UA becomes transiently or persistently occlusive, myocardial necrosis and non-ST-segment elevation or STEMI occurs.

Q2. What is the spectrum of ischemic syndrome?

Ans. Ischemic syndrome is a spectrum as shown in the **Flowchart 4.1**.

Flowchart 4.1: Ischemic syndrome-spectrum.

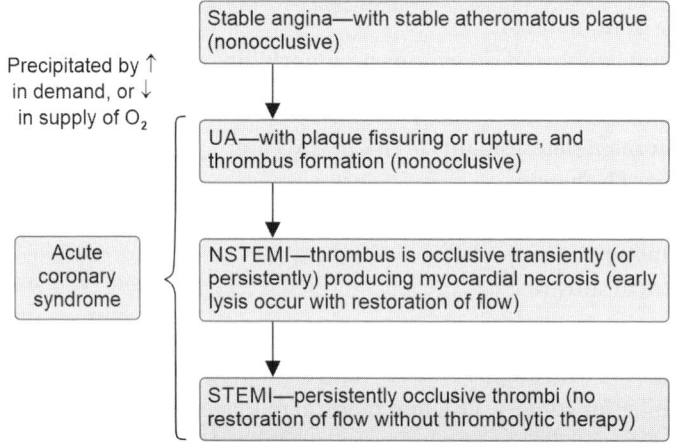

(NSTEMI: non-ST-segment elevation myocardial infarction; STEMI: ST-segment elevation myocardial infarction; UA: unstable angina)

Q3. Define UA?

Ans. Unstable angina is a syndrome resulting from an increased coronary arterial obstruction due to plaque rupture and thrombus formation. It includes patients with either:
- Crescendo angina (more severe and frequent) superimposed on chronic stable angina
- Angina at rest
- New-onset angina (within 1 month) which is brought on by minimal exertion.

Unstable angina includes a heterogenous population with single or multivessel disease, with or without prior MI and an uncertain outcome.

Q4. In patients with UA, what is unstable?
Ans. The intracoronary plaque responsible for angina is unstable or "ruptured"; platelet aggregation occurs and thrombus develops on the unstable lesion. Local vasoconstriction also occurs. This causes acute impairment of O_2 delivery and angina.

The clinical picture is also unstable—the patient may develop chronic stable angina, the condition may progress to MI in the ensuing days or weeks (10-20% of patients), or UA symptom may be unresponsive to full medical treatment and may continue as such.

Q5. What is the implication of angina developing in patients with PTCA and CABG?
Ans. Recurrent angina after PTCA is encountered in 20-30% patients within first 6 months and is associated with angiographic restenosis. MI is unusual because stenosis reflects vascular smooth-muscle proliferation rather than thrombus formation or unstable lesion. When UA occurs 6 months or more after PTCA, a new active lesion is likely to be present.

Unstable angina in patients with previous CABG carries a worse long-term prognosis. It occurs more with venous graft, due to more rapid progression of the disease. Reduced possibility of a new revascularization procedure is also a major problem.

Q6. How useful is ECG in evaluating patients with UA?
Ans. Common ECG findings include ST-segment depression and T-wave inversion. Transient ST elevation may also occur. These changes are usually resolved with relief of pain. Approximately 20% of patients with UA who have NSTEMI confirmed with cardiac enzyme elevation have no ischemic ECG changes. ECG can be used for risk stratification of patients with UA. Patients with ST-segment deviation (ST depression or transient ST elevation) ≥0.5 mm or new LBBB are at increased risk for death or MI after 1 year. The new persistent symmetric T-wave inversion in the anterior precordial leads is a marker for high-grade LAD or LM coronary artery disease. These patients are at an increased risk of infarction. Persistence of ST-T changes may also suggest NSTEMI.

Q7. Define AMI.
Ans. Acute MI is ACS resulting from transiently or permanently occlusive coronary thrombus, leading to myocardial necrosis. Permanent occlusion of coronary arteries produces STEMI or transmural MI. Transient occlusion (i.e., occlusion followed by reopening) produces NSTEMI (subendocardial infarction).

Q8. How are infarcts classified?
Ans.
- *Pathologic classification (by size):*
  - Microscopic (or focal)
  - Small: <10% of the left ventricle
  - Medium: 10–30% of the left ventricle
  - Large: >30% of the left ventricle
- *By location*: Anterior, lateral, inferior, posterior, septal, or a combination
- *According to the morphologic appearance:*
  - Acute: 6 hours–7 days
  - Healing: 7–28 days
  - Healed: 29 days or more

Note: The clinical and ECG timing of MI may not be the same as the pathologic timing of an acute infarct.

Q9. What are the forms of AMI?
Ans.
- *On gross inspection—transmural and subendocardial:* In transmural infarction, myocardial necrosis occurs in full thickness of ventricle. In subendocardial (nontransmural), infarction necrosis occurs in subendocardium, the intramural myocardium, or both without extending all the way through the ventricular wall to the epicardium. In transmural infarction, myonecrosis occurs in a wavefront manner, starting in the subendocardium, then extends across full thickness to subepicardium. To start with, all MI are subendocardial in location. The LV myocardium contracts in a centripetal manner, contractile force being maximal in subendocardial region. Thus, subendocardium is the area that bears the brunt of coronary occlusion despite the presence of adjacent intraventricular blood.

   An occlusive coronary thrombus produces transmural infarction of myocardium supplied by the artery **(Fig. 4.1)**. Nontransmural infarction occurs in the presence of severely narrowed, but still patent coronary artery. The patchy nontransmural infarct may arise from fibrinolysis or PCI of an originally occlusive thrombus with restoration of blood flow.

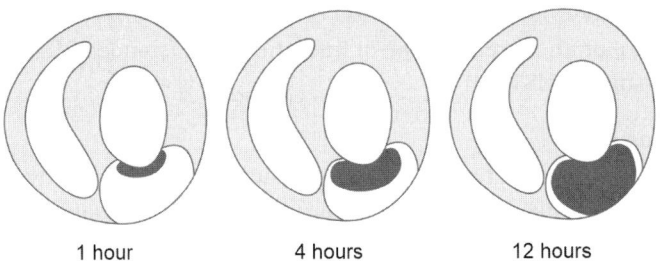

1 hour   4 hours   12 hours

Fig. 4.1: Time course of MI—myonecrosis starts subendocardially and extends subepicardially (completed in 12 hours).

- *On ECG changes—Q-wave and non-Q-wave infarction:*
  On the basis of evolution of ECG pattern over several days, MI was divided into Q-wave and non-Q-wave infarct during the prefibrinolytic era. Q-wave MI (QWMI) was synonymous with transmural infarct, and non-QWMI was referred to as subendocardial infarct.
- *STEMI and NSTEMI—transmural infarcts produce ST elevation in ECG:*
  STEMI and subendocardial infarction produce NSTEMI. Majority of patients presenting with STEMI develop Q wave in leads overlying the infarct zone, i.e., QWMI if reperfusion therapy (thrombolytic or PCI) is not undertaken. With greater use of reperfusion therapy, the majority of STEMI do not go to QWMI. Hence, all STEMI are not QWMI, although all QWMI were STEMI to start with. So, the current terminology is STEMI and NSTEMI (in place of QWMI and non-QWMI).

Q10. What is the difference between STEMI and NSTEMI?
Ans. STEMI and NSTEMI are two entities in myocardial infarction. Their differences are shown in **Table 4.7**.

TABLE 4.7: Difference between NSTEMI and STEMI.

Parameter	NSTEMI	STEMI
Coronary occlusion	Subtotal	Total
Extend of infarct	Subendocardial	Transmural
Residual myocardium	More	Less
Early ischemia and reinfarction	More	Less
ECG	ST depression, T inversion, No Q	ST elevation, Q dev.
Cardiac enzymes	Low	High
Thrombolytics	Not recommended	Recommended
Heparin	Indicated	Only when rtPA used (class IIa)
CAG and intervention	Indicated more	Indicated as pr. PCI
Mortality	Less	More

(CAG: coronary angiography; ECG: electrocardiogram; NSTEMI: non-ST-segment elevation myocardial infarction; PCI: percutaneous coronary intervention; rtPA: recombinant tissue plasminogen activator; STEMI: ST-segment elevation myocardial infarction)

Q11. What is NSTEMI?
Ans. In NSTEMI (non-QWMI, in older classification), myocardial necrosis occurs without ECG evidence of transmural injury, i.e., ST elevation **(Fig. 4.2A)**. As ST elevation does not occur, it is not followed by development of Q wave **(Fig. 4.2B)** (hence, the old term non-QWMI).

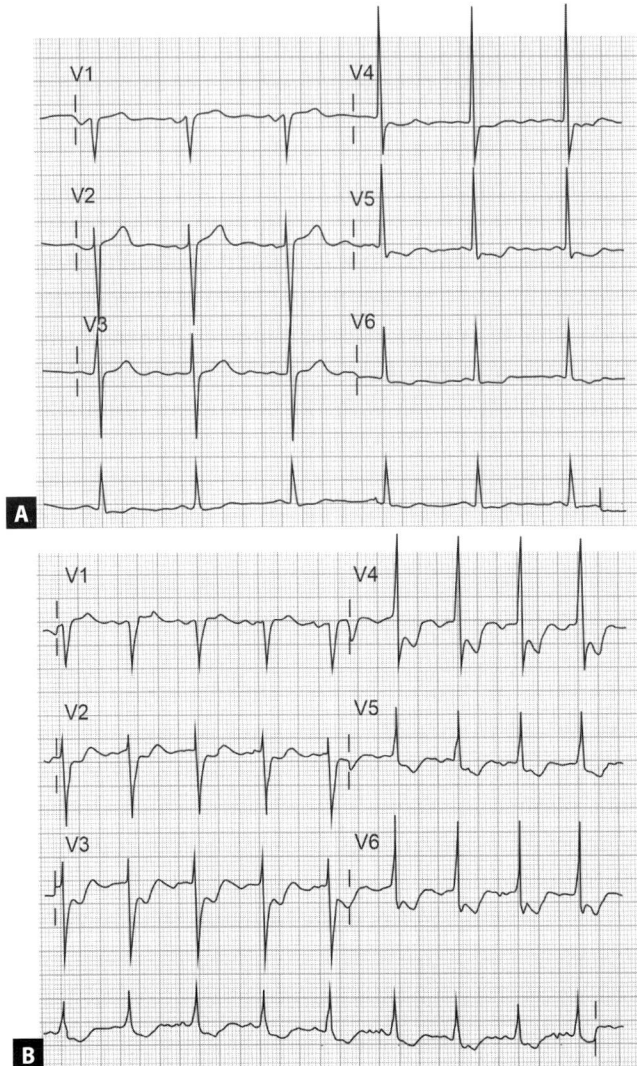

Figs. 4.2A and B: NSTEMI. (A) ST depression in V_5–V_6; (B) Widespread ST depression with no Q wave (after 18 hours). (NSTEMI: non-ST-segment elevation myocardial infarction)

Patients with ongoing chest pain without ST-segment elevation on ECG have either UA or NSTEMI. The distinction is made by cardiac enzyme analysis. NSTEMI and UA are together leveled as NSTE-ACS.

Q12. What are the pitfalls in ECG diagnosis of NSTE-ACS?
Ans. More than 50% of NSTE-ACS may have normal or nondiagnostic ECGs. Ischemia occurring in a territory not well represented in conventional 12-lead ECG such as circumflex artery or acute marginal branch of right coronary artery, or the patient may have episode of ischemia that is missed on

initial ECG. Hence, tracing is repeated every 20–30 minutes until symptoms resolve, or the diagnosis of MI is established or refuted.

Q13. How is risk scoring done in NSTE-ACS?
Ans. Risk assessment for patients with NSTE-ACS:
- Thrombolysis in Myocardial Infarction (TIMI) risk score identifies seven independent risk factors. Some of these correlate directly with death or recurrent ischemic events. These are: Age ≥65 years, ≥3 CAD risk factors, known CAD (>50% stenosis), prior aspirin, ≥2 anginal episodes in prior 24 hours, ST elevation ≥0.5 mm of initial ECG, and increased cardiac enzymes. This rapid assessment at initial evaluation identifies high-risk patients who can derive benefit from an early invasive strategy and more intensive antithrombotic therapy.
- Global Registry of Acute Coronary Events (GRACE) scoring is more complex than TIMI risk score that uses a larger number of weighted risk factors.

Q14. What are the clinical predictors of high risk in NSTE-ACS?
Ans. Nine clinical predictors for high risk NSTE-ACS patients are: CHF, hypertension, age: ≥75 years, DM, prior stroke, prior CABG, peripheral artery disease, estimated glomerular filtration rate (eGFR): <60, and current smoking.

Q15. How is MI redefined?
Ans. The European Society of Cardiology (ESC)/American College of Cardiology (ACC) in 1999 redefined MI as follows:
- *Criteria for acute, evolving, or recent MI:* Typical rise and gradual fall (troponin), or more rapid rise and fall creatine phosphokinase MB (CK-MB) of biochemical markers of myocardial necrosis with at least one of the following:
  - Ischemic symptoms
  - Development of pathologic Q waves on the ECG
  - ECG changes indicative of ischemia (ST-segment elevation or depression)
  - Coronary artery intervention (e.g., of coronary angioplasty)
  - Pathologic findings of AMI
- *Criteria for established MI:* Any of the following criteria:
  - Development of new pathologic Q wave on serial ECGs. The patient may or may not remember previous symptoms. Biochemical markers of myocardial necrosis may have been normalized depending on the length of time that has passed since the infarct developed.
  - Pathologic finding of a healed or healing MI.

Q16. What are the implications of the new definition of MI?
Ans.
- Detection of minimal quantities of myocardial necrosis. Any amount of myocardial necrosis should be leveled as infarction. Measurement of cardiac troponin allows this detection, it is very sensitive as well as specific.
- It will result in more cases identified, thereby allowing appropriate secondary prevention. Increased sensitivity of the defining criteria for MI would mean more cases are identified.
- It will identify more infarcts and more episodes of reinfarction in patients with progressive CAD.
- Patients who undergo coronary revascularization (coronary angioplasty or bypass surgery) are at high risk for myocardial damage or rather MI according to the new definition. This has been highlighted by the new, more sensitive cardiac marker.
- Increasing the specificity of diagnostic criteria will result in elimination of noncases, thereby leading to reduced costs for hospital stay and secondary prevention.
- An increase in sensitivity of the criteria for AMI might entail negative consequences for some patients who are not currently labeled as having had an MI.

Q17. What is the World Health Organization (WHO) definition of MI?
Ans. In studies of disease prevalence by WHO, MI was defined as a combination of two of the three characteristics:
- Typical symptoms, i.e., chest discomfort
- Typical ECG pattern involving development of Q waves
- Enzyme rise

Q18. Justify use of thrombolytics in ACS?
Ans. Thrombolytic therapy is clearly indicated in STEMI, but not in NSTE-ACS (UA or NSTEMI). It has been shown to decrease mortality and to preserve LV function in patients with STEMI. But it is associated with worse overall outcome among patients with UA and NSTEMI.

In UA, the coronary lesion is nonocclusive and platelet rich. Partial lysis induced by thrombolytics may expose clot bound thrombin, platelets are activated, and the condition may be worse. Hence, thrombolytic therapy in UA cannot be generally recommended at present. It would appear that these patients need an agent to prevent thrombus from progression, so antithrombotic agent (heparin) and antiplatelets (aspirin, clopidogrel, etc.) are most appropriate. Moreover, as thrombin in UA is nonocclusive, thrombolytic agents would not be expected to dramatically improve coronary blood flow as they do in STEMI.

In NSTEMI, only partially occluding thrombus is present. Early lysis of thrombus occurs with spontaneous restoration of coronary flow in these patients. Here also, antiplatelets and antithrombotic agents are most appropriate to prevent development of STEMI in these patients. Thrombolytic agents would not be expected to improve coronary blood flow anymore, rather they may expose the patient to risk of bleeding.

However, patients with UA or NSTEMI should be followed with serial ECG. If there is persistent ST elevation of more than 1 mm in two or more contiguous leads, or new LBBB indicating acute transmural injury, then this mandates prompt administration of thrombolytic therapy.

Q19. What is the importance of estimation of cardiac troponins (cTn) in patients with ACS?

Ans. Serologic analysis for cardiac contractile proteins called troponins [troponin I (TnI) and troponin T (TnT)] is increasingly utilized in ACS.

- An elevated troponin is diagnostic of NSTEMI (UA and NSTEMI are closely related conditions in the spectrum of ACS).
- Risk stratification in UA—elevations of either TnT or TnI have been shown to be independent predictors of adverse outcomes such as recurrent angina, nonfatal MI, or death. Whereas normal troponin levels are associated with low risk for cardiac death.

Q20. What is the goal of treatment of UA?

Ans.

- Relieving symptoms—NG, β-blockers, and to a less extent calcium-channel blockers reduce the risk of recurrent ischemia.
- Reducing risk of MI—by antiplatelets (aspirin, clopidogrel) and antithrombotic agents (heparin).
- Revascularization—PTCA in patients with favorable anatomy, and CABG in some selected cases eliminates ischemia.

Q21. What is the advantage of low molecular-weight heparin (LMWH) over unfractionated heparin in patients with UA?

Ans. These include:

- Predictable anticoagulant effect caused by increased bioavailability
- Fixed dosing by means of subcutaneous (SC) injection
- More effective thrombin inhibition because of increased antifactor II_a and antifactor X_a activity
- Lower rate of thrombocytopenia
- Cost saving—because partial thromboplastin time (PTT) levels do not have to be followed to monitor anticoagulant activity.

Q22. What are the markers that predict adverse outcomes in patients with UA?

Ans. Although LV function and extent of CAD ultimately determine long-term prognosis, markers that predict adverse outcomes such as MI and death are:

- Age: >75 years
- Prolonged ongoing rest pain (>20 minutes)
- Recurrence of chest pain within 48 hours after admission
- Pulmonary edema is caused by ischemia, angina with new or worsening rales, S_3 or mitral regurgitation (MR), and angina with hypotension
- ECG findings—rest angina with dynamic ST changes ≥1 mm or T-wave inversion, new bundle branch block.
- Cardiac markers—elevated cTn (TnT or TnI, >0.1 ng/mL: High risk; 0.06–0.1 ng/mL: Medium risk, and <0.06 ng/mL: Low risk).

Q23. Compare and contrast between inferior and anterior wall MI.

Ans. Comparison of inferior and anterior wall MI and their contrasting features are shown in **Table 4.8**.

TABLE 4.8: Inferior and anterior wall infarction—difference.

Points	Inferior MI	Anterior MI
Size of infarct	Smaller	Larger
Artery involved	RCA, LCx artery (if dominant)	LAD, LCx arteries
RV infarction	May occur	Nil
Symptoms	Vomiting more (parasympathetic)	Sweating more (sympathetic)
Sign	Bradycardia more	Tachycardia more
Arrhythmias	Heart block—more, CHB reverts	PVC, VT, VF—more, CHB—if develops need pacing
Cardiogenic shock	Less, only if RV infarction	More
Investigations		
LV function	Usually normal	May be reduced
Cardiac enzymes	Less elevated	More elevated
Therapy		
Analgesic	Pethidine may precipitate bradycardia	Morphine, pethidine ±
SK	Less beneficial	Benefit more
ACEI	Benefit ±	Definitely beneficial
Beta-blocker	Benefit ±	Benefit definite
Prognosis	Better	Depends on LV function

(ACEI: angiotensin-converting enzyme inhibitors; CHB: complete heart block; LAD: left anterior descending; LCx: left circumflex; LV: left ventricular; MI: myocardial infarction; PVC: premature ventricular contraction; RCA: right coronary artery; RV: right ventricular; SK: streptokinase; VF: ventricular fibrillation; VT: ventricular tachycardia)

Q24. What are the unique features of right ventricular (RV) infarction?

Ans. Right ventricular infarction develops in association with infarction of adjacent interventricular septum and inferior LV walls. Classic presentations are hypotension, clear lungs, and elevated jugular venous pressure (JVP). Kussmaul's sign in the setting of inferior STEMI is highly predictive of RV involvement. Judicious volume replacement, early revascularization, pacing (if needed), and in refractory cases, mechanical circulatory support are modalities of treatment. In contrast to left ventricle, right ventricle can sustain long periods of ischemia but still demonstrate excellent recovery of contractile function after reperfusion.

Q25. How does atrial infarction occur?

Ans. Atrial infarction often occurs in conjunction with ventricular infarction; appendage is involved more frequently and associated with atrial fibrillation (AF) and thrombus formation.

Q26. What is an "infarction at a distance"?

Ans. STEMI may occur at a distance from a coronary occlusion when collateral vessels perfuse an area of the ventricle and viability depends on that collateral circulation. An occlusion of coronary artery providing the collateral leads to STEMI at a distance. For example, with gradual occlusion of RCA, collateral developing from LAD artery can keep viability of inferior wall intact. An occlusion of LAD artery at a latter period may cause infarction of distal inferior wall.

Q27. What is ischemic cardiomyopathy?

Ans. Ischemic cardiomyopathy is symptomatic HF due to ischemic myocardial dysfunction, diffuse fibrosis, multiple MI, and hibernation, alone or in combination. Ischemic symptoms may disappear as HF symptoms dominate. Some patients may not have any angina symptoms or MI. Those with extensive multivessel disease and viable myocardium may derive benefit from CABG.

Q28. What are the new paradigms of development of MI?

Ans. According to the old paradigm, high-grade coronary stenosis frequently leads to STEMI than do less obstructive lesions. But new paradigm is that STEMI can result from sudden thrombotic occlusion at the sites of noncritical stenosis that are strategically located, whereas more severe lesions lead to chronic CAD. Thus, there is a paradigm shift in the causation of MI.

Q29. What are thrombolytic agents?

Ans. Currently, four thrombolytic agents are approved for use worldwide: streptokinase (SK), alteplase, reteplase, and tenecteplase (TNK). The last three agents were developed via recombinant deoxyribonucleic acid (DNA) technology to improve fibrin specificity, and to increase the duration of activity to enhance bolus dosing.

Q30. What are the indications in the use of thrombolytics?

Ans. In-hospital thrombolytic therapy should be administered to those patients who present to a non-PCI-capable hospital within 12 hours of symptom onset, if transfer for primary PCI (PPCI) (the preferred reperfusion strategy) cannot be completed in a timely fashion [door-in to door-out time (DIDO) ≤30 minutes, or time of arrival to non-PCI-capable hospital to leaving for the PCI-capable hospital], or anticipated first medical contact to device time is of 120 minutes, and there is no evidence of HF or cardiogenic shock. It is recommended that because of increased bleeding risk very early (within 2-3 hours), with intend to perform, revascularization after thrombolytic administration should be limited to rescue PCI (should be attempted in those patients who fail thrombolysis and have significant myocardium in jeopardy).

Q31. Why are fibrinolytic agents not used in NSTE-ACS?

Ans. Fibrinolytic agents simultaneously exert clot-dissolving and procoagulant actions, a partially occlusive thrombus may be converted into a completely occlusive one in NSTEMI and UA. Hence, fibrinolytic agents must not be used in NSTE-ACS. The risk of bleeding will be increased besides the risk of total thrombotic coronary occlusion.

Q32. Justify the long-term use of NG in STEMI.

Ans. In the absence of angina or HF, routine long-term use of NG in STEMI patients provides no clear benefit. Hence, its use beyond the first 48 hours in patients without angina or left ventricular failure is not beneficial.

Q33. What factors determine myocardial viability following MI?

Ans. Viability of myocardium following STEMI depends on: Rate of development of occlusion, quantity of myocardium supplied by obstructed vessel, presence of collaterals, level of myocardial metabolism, presence and location of stenosis in other coronary arteries, etc.

Q34. How does RV infarction differ from LV infarction?

Ans. As left ventricle has to pump blood into systemic circulation with high pressure and its wall thickness is three times more than right ventricle, left ventricle is more prone to infarction, and for all practical purpose infarction means LV infarction unless categorically mentioned. Isolated RV infarction seldom happens. It is usually associated with inferior wall infarction of left ventricle. Differentiating features of LV and RV infarction are shown in **Table 4.9**.

TABLE 4.9: Left ventricular and right ventricular infarction—differences.

Points	LV infarction	RV infarction
Incidence	Common	Uncommon
Artery involved	LAD, LCx arteries	RCA, LCx artery (if dominant)
LVF	Common	Rare
Size of infarct	Bigger	Smaller
Cardiogenic shock	Due to severe pump failure	Due to inadequate filling of left ventricle
Fluid	Contraindicated	Indicated
Prognosis	Less favorable	Better

Q35. What is the importance of estimation of cTn in the diagnosis of MI?

Ans. Cardiac troponin (TnI or TnT) is the preferred biomarker for myocardial damage. It has nearly absolute myocardial tissue specificity as well as high sensitivity, thereby reflecting even microscopic zone of myocardial necrosis. Troponins are released into plasma, so that reliable diagnostic sensitivity (≥90%) is reached by 12–16 hours, and maximal activity is reached by 24–36 hours. Both TnI and TnT remain elevated for 10–14 days. Hence, in patients admitted 48–72 hours after onset of symptoms, particularly when associated with minimal myocardial damage, TnI or TnT are preferred diagnostic markers (CK-MB returns to normal after 48–72 hours). Blood levels of troponin at presentation predict risk in patients with AMI.

Q36. How is ECG helpful in patients with MI?
Ans.

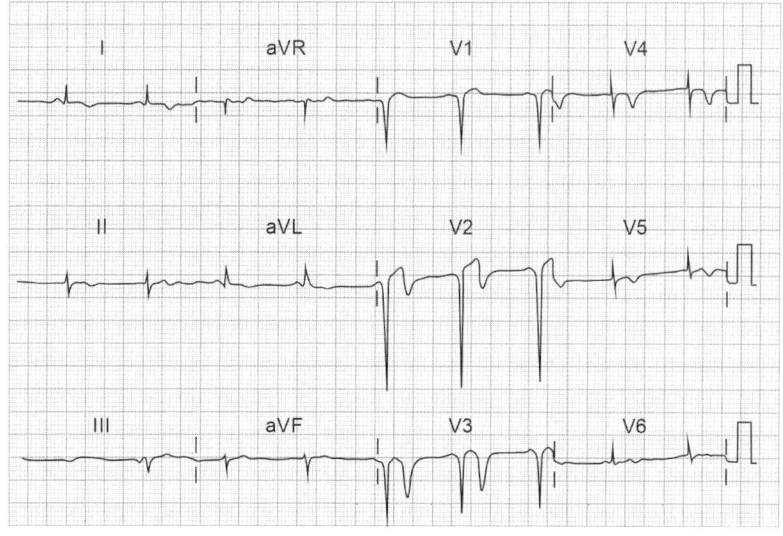

Fig. 4.3: Anteroseptal MI (ST segment elevated) with Q-wave and T-wave inversion after 24 hours of chest pain onset.

- *Diagnostic:* Presence of any one of the following in the setting of chest pain diagnoses AMI **(Fig. 4.3)**:
  - New or presumably new Q waves (at least 30 ms wide and 0.20 mV deep) in at least two leads from any of the following:
    - Leads II, III, aVF
    - Leads V_1-V_6
    - Lead 1 and aVL
  - New or presumably new ST-T segment elevation or depression (≥0.10 mV measured 0.02 s after J-point in two contiguous leads of the above-mentioned lead combinations).
  - New, complete LBBB in the appropriate clinical setting.
  Size of infarction:
    - Involvement of 2–3 leads indicates small infarct
    - Involvement of 4–5 leads indicates a moderate infarct
    - Involvement of 6–7 leads indicates a large infarct
    - Involvement of 8 or more leads indicate an extensive infarct **(Fig. 4.4)**

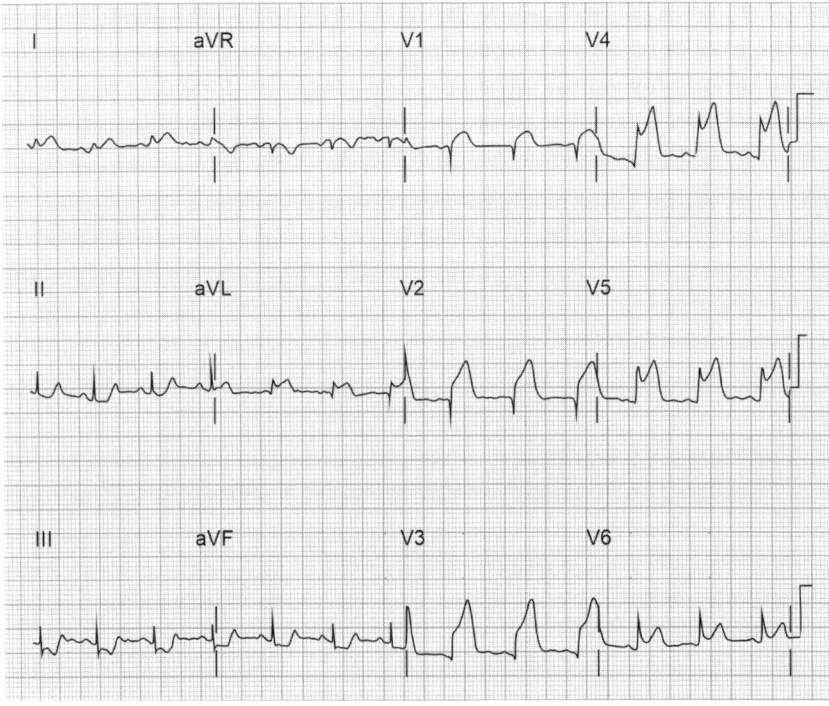

Fig. 4.4: Extensive infarction (ST elevation in 8 leads).

- *Therapeutic:* ECG results dictate rapid treatment with thrombolytic agents. Patients with ST-segment elevation in two or more contiguous leads or a bundle branch block masking ST-segment changes occurring

within 12 hours of onset of symptoms are candidates for thrombolytic therapy.
- *Prognostic:* ST elevation can be divided into subgroups that are correlated with the infarct-related artery, and prognosis of the patient as shown in **Table 4.10**.

TABLE 4.10: ST-elevation in electrocardiogram (ECG)—prognosis.

Infarct site		ECG findings	Anatomy of occlusion	Prognosis
Anterior	Extensive anterior	V_1–V_6, I, aVL and fascicular or BBB	Proximal LAD artery (proximal to first septal)	Usually more extensive
	Anterior	V_1–V_6	Mid-LAD artery (proximal to D_1 but distal to S_1)	LV function impaired; mortality and morbidity more
	Anteroseptal	V_1-V_4	Distal LAD (distal to D_1), or diagonal itself	LVF, cardiogenic shock may occur
	Anterolateral	V_4–V_6, I, aVL		
Inferior	Small inferior	II, III, aVF	Distal RCA or LCx artery (if left dominance)	Good (AV block, usually temporary)
	Moderate or large inferior associated	II, III, aVF associated		Intermediate (cardiogenic shock may occur in RV infarction)
	RV infarction	V_1, V_3R, V_4R	Proximal RCA or LCx artery (if left dominance)	
	Posterior infarction	R > S in V_1, V_2		
	Lateral	V_5, V_6		

(AV: atrioventricular; BBB: bundle branch block; ECG: electrocardiogram; LAD: left anterior descending; LCx: left circumflex; LV: left ventricular; LVF: left ventricular failure; RCA: right coronary artery; RV: right ventricular)

Q37. What are the limitations of ECG in the diagnosis of AMI?
Ans.
- ECG changes may be absent in some patients with AMI. Absence of changes during pain provides evidence but no proof that pain is not ischemic in nature.
- In patients with pre-existing LBBB, ST elevation for diagnosis of AMI is not applicable.
- If reperfusion occurs very early (within an hour of onset of symptoms), the ECG may be normalized, signifying an aborted MI.

Q38. What is the importance of ECG in thrombolytic therapy?

Ans. ECG findings of a patient with appropriate history (i.e., typical chest pain over 15 minutes) indicate need for thrombolysis. Patients with ST-segment elevation of 1 mm in two or more adjacent limb leads, or 2 mm in two or more adjacent chest leads, or new LBBB are candidates for thrombolytic therapy. Patients with typical history suggesting MI but initial ECGs are nondiagnostic should be repeatedly evaluated by 12-lead ECG as frequently as every 10–15 minutes during first 4–6 hours in order to identify ST elevation as soon as possible **(Fig. 4.5A)**. Conversely, ST-segment elevation in the absence of suggestive symptoms should raise such possibilities as early repolarization, pericarditis, and previous infarction with aneurysm formation.

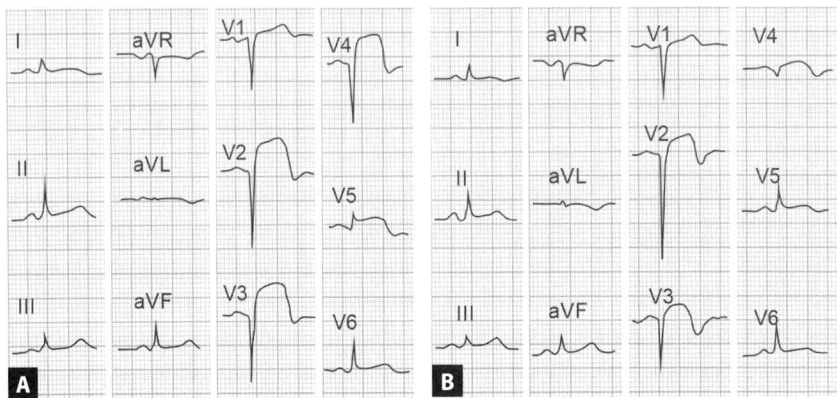

Figs. 4.5A and B: STEMI (A) before and (B) after thrombolysis.

Resolution of ST-segment elevation on serial ECG predicts reperfusion (often occurs about 1 hour after starting thrombolytics) **(Fig. 4.5B)**. PVC and runs of VT often occur as result of reperfusion injury and may serve as a marker of the time of reperfusion.

Q39. What is the benefit of thrombolytic therapy?

Ans. The benefit of thrombolysis has been well documented in the management of AMI, regardless of age, sex, and most baseline characteristics.

However, the patients who derive the most benefit are those treated earliest and those at highest risk, such as the elderly and those with anterior MI. Elderly patients (aged 75 years or older) should not be excluded primarily because of their age or the perceived increased risk of bleeding. The beneficial effects of thrombolysis, as demonstrated in numerous studies, are decrease in mortality, improvement in LV function, fewer arrhythmias, and improved long-term survival.

In addition to prevention of infarction or decrease of infarct size, and probable improved electrical stability of the heart with decreased arrhythmia, benefit of a patent artery may include a favorable effect on ventricular remodeling, improved diastolic function, low incidence of cardiac rupture, provision of collateral flow, and later improvement in systolic LV function. There is improvement in overall long-term survival.

Q40. When is thrombolytic therapy favored over PCI in STEMI?
Ans. According to ACC/AHA guidelines, thrombolytics are favored over PCI in the following cases:
- Patients not in shock
- No contraindication to thrombolysis
- Who present early—<3 hours of pain onset
- Who have no invasive option, e.g., catheterization laboratory unavailable
- Delay in performing PCI

Q41. What is TIMI flow grade?
Ans.
- *Grade 0:* Complete occlusion of infarct-related artery
- *Grade 1:* Some penetration of contrast material beyond the point of obstruction, but without perfusion of distal coronary bed
- *Grade 2:* Perfusion of the entire infarct vessel into the distal bed but with delayed flow compared with a normal artery
- *Grade 3:* Full perfusion of the infarct vessel with normal flow

Q42. What are the contraindications of thrombolytic therapy?
Ans.
- *Absolute:* Prior intracranial hemorrhage, ischemic stroke <3 months, known cerebral arteriovenous malformations or malignancy, aortic dissection, head injury <3 months, and any active bleeding
- *Relative:* BP >180/120 mm Hg, ischemic stroke >3 months, prolonged traumatic cardiopulmonary resuscitation (CPR), recurrent internal bleeding <2–4 weeks, active peptic ulcer disease, noncompressible puncture, warfarin use, pregnancy, prior exposure, or allergy to SK

Q43. What are the indications of PCI in ACS?
Ans.
- *UA and NSTEMI:* High-risk cases with:
  - Prolonged rest pain >20 minutes
  - Dynamic ST changes >1 mm
  - Hemodynamic—third heart sound (S_3) gallop, new MR, pulmonary edema, or severe LV dysfunction
  - Electrical instability
  - Raised biomarker (>0.1 µg/L)
  - Prior PCI, CABG in 6 months
- *STEMI:*
  - Primary PCI **(Figs. 4.6A and B)**—experienced operator, door-to-balloon (DTB) time <90 minutes, patient not eligible for thrombolytics, high-risk for stroke, those in shock

- Rescue PCI—persistent chest pain or ST elevation after lytic therapy
- Delayed PCI (secondary)—post-MI pain, CHF, sustained VT, and positive predischarge stress test result.

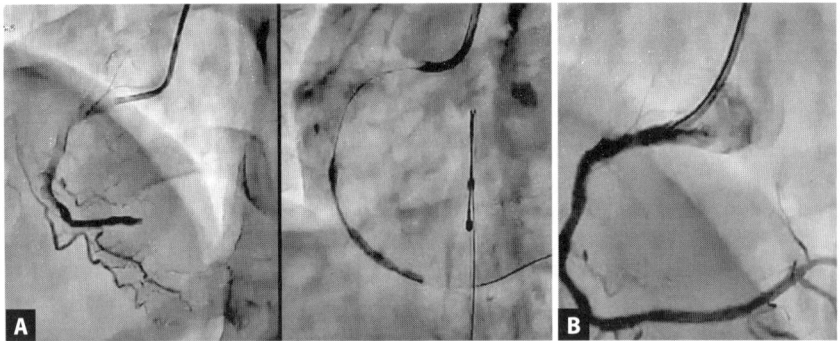

Figs. 4.6A and B: Primary PCI in complete occlusion of RCA (A) before and (B) after stenting. (PCI: percutaneous coronary intervention; RCA: right coronary artery)

Q44. When is PCI preferred over fibrinolysis in STEMI?
Ans. In STEMI, PCI provides better short- and long-term prognosis compared to fibrinolysis. It should be the preferred treatment strategy for patients presenting with STEMI to a facility experienced with and capable of performing PCI.

In general, PCI is preferred over thrombolytics in the following situations:
- In all patients, if facilities for immediate CAG and PCI are available within 90 minutes of first medical contact (i.e., DTB time), PCI is the preferred therapy with better reperfusion as well as short and long-term benefits. It is also associated with a reduction in the incidence of intracranial hemorrhage compared to fibrinolytic therapy when PCI is possible within 90 minutes.
- Cardiogenic shock—the more the mortality risk from STEMI, the more is the benefit; Because of the relative lack of efficacy of lytic therapy in patients with cardiogenic shock or prior CABG, PCI should be undertaken for such cases.
- When there is an increased risk of bleeding and there are other contraindications to fibrinolytics.
- When diagnosis of STEMI is in doubt (CAG will confirm it).

However, if facilities for immediate CAG and PCI are not available, or if the DTB time is more than 90 minutes, thrombolytic therapy, unless contraindicated, should be instituted within 30 minutes of first medical contact (i.e., door-to-needle time). Also, if a long delay (>3 hours) is anticipated, therapy may still be considered while arrangements for PCI are made (facilitated PCI).

Q45. How is pain in AMI alleviated? Why is it important?
Ans. Pain relief is provided in two ways:
1. Attacking pain directly with narcotics, i.e., morphine
2. Anti-ischemic therapy—reperfusion (with thrombolytics or mechanical, in selected cases), β-blockers (if appropriate), nitrates, and O_2 administration.

It is necessary to relieve pain promptly, because pain precipitates autonomic disturbances that may trigger malignant arrhythmias and hypotension and may increase infarct size.

Q46. What are infarct expansion and infarct extension?
Ans. An increase in size of infarcted segment by acute dilatation and thinning of the area is called infarct expansion **(Fig. 4.7)**. LV apex, the thinnest region of left ventricle, is particularly vulnerable to infarct expansion. It results in higher incidence of ventricular aneurysm, HF, and higher mortality.

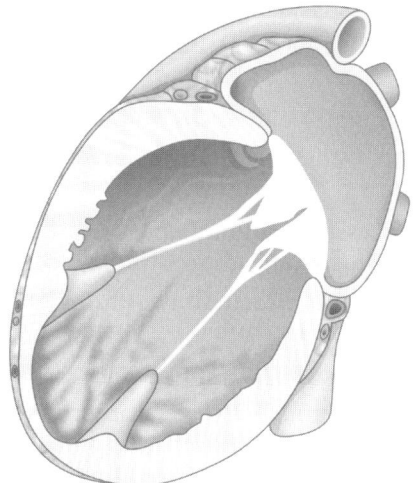

Fig. 4.7: Infarct expansion and ventricular remodeling.
(following an anterior wall infarction)

Q47. What is ventricular remodeling?
Ans. It is the change in size, shape, and thickness of left ventricle following MI **(Fig. 4.7)**, involving both the infarcted and noninfarcted segments. A combination of infarct expansion (dilatation and thinning) and hypertrophy of residual noninfarcted myocardium causes remodeling. It influences ventricular function and prognosis and hence needs to be prevented pharmacologically. Acute full-thickness MI is often followed by thinning and stressing of the infarcted segment with progressive dilatation and hypertrophy of the remaining ventricle, producing ventricular remodeling. If it continues, HF may supervene. ACEI, by reducing ventricular afterload, can counteract ventricular remodeling.

Infarct extension is the appearance of an infarct at a new location in left ventricle.

Q48. What are the atypical features of STEMI?
Ans. These are: Classic angina pectoris (without severe, prolonged episodes of pain), HF (dyspnea), atypical location of pain, e.g., epigastric etc., central nervous system (CNS) manifestations such as stroke [reduction of cardiac output (COP) in a patient with cerebral atherosclerosis], syncope, extreme weakness, nervousness, acute indigestion, peripheral embolization, psychosis, etc.

Q49. What are the causes of raised TnI other than AMI?
Ans.
- Cardiac—myocarditis, pericarditis, takotsubo cardiomyopathy, tachyarrhythmia, CHF, hypertensive emergencies, aortic stenosis, aortic dissection, coronary spasm, cardiac procedures (like endomyocardial biopsy, ablation, CABG, and PCI), infiltrative diseases, e.g., amyloidosis, etc.
- Noncardiac—pulmonary embolism, pulmonary hypertension (PH), trauma, hypothyroidism, hyperthyroidism, renal failure, sepsis, shock, and toxicity

Two negative cTn assays, 6 hours apart, are needed to exclude MI. Although with newer high-sensitivity troponin (hsTn) assays, a single measurement of <5 ng/L can exclude two thirds of "high-risk" cases at presentation.

Multimarker approach such as simultaneous assessment of cTn, hs-CRP, and B-type natriuretic peptide (BNP) can improve risk stratification of patients with NSTE-ACS.

Q50. How are antianginal drugs selected?
Ans. Things to consider are:
- History of asthma or chronic obstructive pulmonary disease (COPD) with wheeze-calcium antagonists or nitrates preferred; β-blockers may not be tolerated.
- Chronic stable angina with symptomatic conduction disease—long-acting nifedipine, amlodipine, and nicardipine preferred. Nitrates and ranolazine are alternatives.
- Suspected Prinzmetal angina—calcium antagonists and long-acting nitrates; β-blockers may aggravate the condition.
- Symptomatic PAD—calcium antagonists are preferred
- Significant depressive illness, sexual dysfunction, sleep disturbance, nightmares, and fatigue—β-blockers are avoided.

- Patients with LV dysfunction after MI, with or without symptoms of HF; amlodipine can be given if angina persists despite β-blockers after using nitrates.
- Hypertensive patients with angina pectoris—β-blockers or calcium antagonists along with an ACEI. Among the β-blockers, carvedilol is preferred for its more robust effect on BP.

Q51. Compare between PPCI and thrombolytic therapy in AMI.
Ans. Primary PCI and thrombolytic therapy are reperfusion strategies for AMI. Comparison between the two are shown in **Table 4.11**.

TABLE 4.11: Primary PCI versus thrombolytic therapy in AMI.

Points	Thrombolytic	Primary PCI
Indication	STEMI	STEMI, NSTEMI
Benefit	Confined to first 12 hours	Beyond 12 hours
Reperfusion	Less	More complete
Bleeding	Cerebral hemorrhage may occur	Risk less
Early reocclusion	Less	More
Cardiogenic shock	Beneficial	Benefit doubtful
Mortality benefit	More	Less

Q52. What is the present position of pharmacoinvasive (PI) therapy as reperfusion strategy in STEMI?
Ans.
- Timely thrombolysis followed by PCI is a reasonable alternative of PPCI in STEMI.
- Tenecteplase is given in bolus, it is fibrin-specific and causes minimal depletion of fibrinogen.
- TNK administered early followed by PCI within 3–24 hours after initiation of thrombolytic therapy regardless of success of thrombolysis.
- Current data supports the strategy of early routine PCI after fibrinolysis rather than the conservative approach of fibrinolytic therapy only, i.e., PI strategy.
  The STREAM (Strategic Reperfusion Early After Myocardial Infarction) trial proved that a strategy involving early fibrinolysis with bolus TNK, and adjunctive pharmacotherapy followed by PCI offer similar efficacy as PPCI in patients with STEMI who present within 3 hours of symptom onset, and who cannot undergo PPCI within 1 hour of first medical contact.
- PI strategy is safe with lower thrombus burden, better TIMI-3 flow at the time of procedure.

Q53. What are the types of PCI done in STEMI?
Ans. These are:
- Primary PCI—reperfusion therapy of choice, DTB time <90 minutes, patient not eligible for fibrinolytics, high risk for stroke, and those in cardiogenic shock.
- Rescue PCI—within 12 hours, and 2 hours after lytic therapy—where fibrinolytics fails to reperfusion, or a severe stenosis present in the infarct-related artery with persistent chest pain or ST elevation.
- Facilitated PCI—fibrinolytics immediately before planned PCI in selected high-risk patients when PPCI is not immediately available and bleeding risk is low.
- Pharmacoinvasive—reasonable alternative to PPCI.
- Delayed (secondary) PCI—post-MI pain, CHF, sustained VT, and positive predischarge stress test. When spontaneous or exercise-induced ischemia occur (whether or not fibrinolytics is received).

Q54. What is the current status of thrombolytic therapy as a reperfusion strategy?
Ans. Thrombolytic therapy remains the preferred reperfusion strategy in patients with STEMI who present within 12 hours of symptom onset when timely PPCI is not available, and no contraindication to thrombolysis is present. Although PPCI has superseded thrombolysis as the preferred reperfusion strategy, in most patients presenting with STEMI, the most recent American College of Cardiology Foundation (ACCF)/AHA STEMI guideline continues to favor thrombolytic therapy over PPCI as the primary reperfusion strategy in patients who:
- Present within 12 hours of symptom onset
- Have no invasive option (catheterization laboratory unavailable, timely vascular access not possible), or face a delay of >120 minutes from first medical contact to PCI
- Are not in cardiogenic shock
- Have no contraindication to thrombolytic therapy. However, because of concerns about bleeding complications, incomplete patency, and early reocclusion rates with thrombolytic therapy for STEMI, which is associated with better clinical outcome, PPCI is reperfusion strategy of choice. Moreover, PPCI is now safely and successfully performed at centers without onsite cardiac surgery backup.

Despite the growing availability of PPCI, thrombolytic therapy will remain as the most common and important reperfusion strategy for STEMI, taking into account the growing burden of CVD worldwide, particularly in developing countries including Bangladesh.

Q55. What are the reperfusion strategies for STEMI patients?

Ans. These are:
- Thrombolytic intervention
- PPCI
- Combined—PI strategy, rescue PCI, and facilitated PCI

Q56. Compare and contrast different combined reperfusion therapies undertaken in STEMI.

Ans. Pharmacoinvasive therapy, rescue PCI, and facilitated PCI are three combined reperfusion therapies undertaken in STEMI cases. Their difference from each other are shown in **Table 4.12**.

TABLE 4.12: Combined reperfusion strategies in STEMI.

Points	Pharmacoinvasive	Rescue	Facilitated
Indication	Routinely-all cases	*Failed thrombolysis	As a bridge to PCI
Thrombolytic used	In usual dose	In usual dose	At reduced dose
Time of PCI	3–24 hours of thrombolytic	After 2 hours	As primary PCI
Use of thrombolytic	Primary	Primary	Secondary
PCI done in	All cases	Some	All cases
Outcome	Comparable to PPCI	Satisfactory	Doubtful
Present status	Widely practiced	In some	Not practiced

*Less than 70% ST-segment resolution at 90 minutes or ongoing chest pain.
(PPCI: primary percutaneous coronary intervention)

Q57. How is time related to myocardial reperfusion in AMI?

Ans. "Time is myocardium"—degree of myocardial salvage following AMI is related to timely reperfusion, with the 2–3 hours' time point representing the critical window to minimize mortality and morbidity. There is a golden first hour and an ominous twelfth hour after symptom onset (no survival benefit beyond 12 hours). Serious bleeding and latent myocardial rupture occur with late therapy.

If PPCI is undertaken, DTB time should be <90 minutes. Every 30 minutes of delay in PPCI results in a 7.5% increase in 1-year mortality. The net benefit of PPCI over thrombolysis may be neutralized if door-to-stent time for PCI is 60 minutes longer than door-to-needle time for thrombolysis.

Also, timely use of thrombolytic therapy is the most important factor in predicting benefit of thrombolysis. Thrombolytics can only effectively "dissolve" an intracoronary thrombus if they are used rapidly after the onset of thrombosis. By opening up the thrombosed coronary artery, "borderline" areas of ischemic myocardium may be saved. After a few hours, the clot undergoes a hardening process, which makes it resistant to breakdown by plasmin. Thus, delay in administering thrombolytics can reduce their effectiveness. The use of thrombolytic agents within 6 hours of presentation confers the most survival benefit, although effectiveness has been shown up to 12 hours, especially in high-risk infarctions.

Q58. What is the utility of PI therapy?
Ans. In PI therapy, routine early CAG and provisional PCI in 3–24 hours are done to avoid recurrent ischemia related to incomplete recanalization and propagation of platelet-rich thrombus following fibrinolysis. Prothrombotic effect of plasminogen activators and showering of platelet-rich thrombi into microcirculation occur when full dose of thrombolytics is used before PCI for STEMI. PI therapy should be undertaken for all high-risk STEMI patients, and should be considered in all patients following successful thrombolysis. It is appealing as many patients do not have access to PPCI within 120 minutes of their first medical contact and may be important for those who live some distance from PCI capable centers.

Q59. What is the principle of pharmacological therapy in STEMI?
Ans. After administration of aspirin and initiation of reperfusion strategies, and administration of appropriate beta-blockers, all patients with STEMI should be considered for renin–angiotensin–aldosterone system (RAAS) blockers, particularly high-risk patients (elderly, anterior infarction, previous infarction, Killip class II or greater, and asymptomatic patients with LV dysfunction on imaging).

In the absence of angina or HF, routine long-term use of NG in STEMI patients provides no clear benefit. Hence, its use beyond the first 48 hours in patients without angina or LVF is not beneficial.

Q60. What are the principles of use of antiplatelet agents in STEMI?
Ans. All patients with STEMI should receive dual antiplatelet therapy (aspirin and others) for 12 months according to the following regimen:
- Clopidogrel 75 mg/day in patients with STEMI treated with medical therapy alone, lytic therapy, or PCI
- Prasugrel 10 mg/day in patients treated with PCI
- Ticagrelor 90 mg twice daily in patients treated with medical therapy alone or PCI
- Cangrelor intravenous (IV), a potent fast-acting P2Y12 inhibitor in subjects requiring PCI.

Q61. Which patients should receive ACEI in MI and how long to continue it?
Ans. Although ACEI may benefit most patients with AMI, it is generally recommended for patients with:
- Heart failure

- Large anterior MI (with ST elevation in anterior leads or LBBB)
- LVEF <40% or large wall-motion defects on echo

Angiotensin-converting enzyme inhibitors can be given within 24 hours of onset of AMI unless there is hypotension (SBP <100 mm Hg). If there is no evidence of LV dysfunction in 4–6 weeks, therapy can be stopped. With significant LV dysfunction, therapy should be continued indefinitely.

Q62. What is the role of β-blockers in ACS?
Ans.
- Acute MI—by antagonizing the hyperadrenergic state that often accompanies MI, β-blockers reduce heart rate and BP. This reduces myocardial O_2 demand, limits infarct size, and relieves ischemic pain. The incidence of free-wall rupture is also reduced. β-blocking agents should be administered orally to patients with normal or mildly impaired LV function within the first 24 hours of AMI unless complicated by hypotension, bradycardia or symptoms of CHF, or otherwise contraindicated, e.g., bronchial asthma. Patients with sinus tachycardia, AF with rapid ventricular rate, hypertension (BP >140/90 mm Hg), or continuing or recurrent ischemic pain are suitable for early IV β-blocker therapy.
- Use of β-blockers is also recommended in non-ST-segment elevation AMI.
- In UA, β-blockers are the most useful drugs to reduce myocardial O_2 demand. It is started with IV bolus, titrated to reduce heart rate to 50–60 beats/min at rest, to achieve beta blockade within hours. In low-risk patients, oral therapy is appropriate. Cardioselective agents such as metoprolol or atenolol are used to prevent side effects.

Q63. How to interfere with intracoronary thrombus in AMI?
Ans. Intracoronary thrombus developing on fissured or ruptured atheromatous plaque has two major components—platelet and fibrin.
- Platelet adhesion and aggregation are inhibited by aspirin and clopidogrel.
- Thrombolytic agents, e.g., SK, recombinant tissue plasminogen activator (rtPA) promote the breakdown of fibrin through conversion of the endogenous proteolytic enzyme plasminogen into active plasmin. Fibrin is cleaved into fibrin degradation product (FDP).
- Heparin prevents the progression or recurrence of thrombosis in the coronary arteries. Heparin is essential in the first 24 hours to maintain patency rates with rtPA, although it is not necessary to achieve reperfusion. In contrast to fibrin selective agents (rtPA), SK or anisoylated plasminogen SK activator complex (APSAC) attacks clot-bound as well as circulating fibrinogen, which leads to high levels of FDP that inhibit platelet aggregation. Hence, it is recommended that heparin is not to be started immediately, but an activated partial thromboplastin time (APTT)

be drawn 4 hours, and heparin be stated when APTT returns to less than twice control (about 70 seconds).

Acute myocardial infarction patients with ST elevation who are not treated with thrombolytic agents, LMWH is a class-IIa indication as an alternative to unfractionated heparin.

Q64. What is the role of heparin in ACS?
Ans.
- *In AMI:*
  - Heparin with thrombolytics—as an adjunct to therapy with tPA, IV heparin has been shown to improve late patency, otherwise there is a high risk of reocclusion. There is no data to advocate the routine use of IV heparin with SK unless the patient has another indication for heparin therapy.
  - Heparin with direct angioplasty—heparin IV is recommended for patients undergoing percutaneous interventions (class I indication).
  - Heparin without thrombolysis:
- To prevent or treat thromboembolism from left heart—IV heparin is used in AMI patients with AF, with large and especially anterior infarction, and those with history of previous stroke.
- To prevent or treat deep vein thrombosis and pulmonary embolism—SC heparin is used.
- *In UA:* Heparin is recommended for all UA patients except those at low risk. It reduces the risk of development of MI. Unfractionated or LMWH SC are used. Anticoagulant response with LMWH is more predictable and is superior in preventing development of MI.
- *In NSTEMI:* LMWH SC or IV unfractionated heparin is recommended (class-IIa recommendation). LMWH has been shown to be superior to unfractionated heparin in reducing cardiac events.

Q65. When is tPA preferred over SK as thrombolytic agent?
Ans. Both have been shown to limit infarct size, preserve ventricular function, and improve survival rates. SK is the most frequently used thrombolytic agent worldwide. It is less expensive compared with rtPA and anistreplase, which are more expensive. The tPA is preferred in:
- Patients with extensive infarction—ST-segment ↑ in ≥8 leads
- Patients <75 years with large anterior infarction. In patients >75 years, SK carries less risk of cerebral bleeding than rtPA.
- Patients who are allergic to SK, or if SK was used in the prior 12 months (as neutralizing antibodies are still present)
- Patients with second infarction, in particular, if it is complicated by pulmonary edema, indicating very high risk
- Recent streptococcal infection
- Hypotension SBP <100 mm Hg

Q66. What is "door-to-needle" time?

Ans. It is the time interval between the arrival of the patient with AMI in the emergency room and the administration of thrombolytic therapy. The shortest possible door-to-needle time is needed to allow quick administration of thrombolytics after onset of chest pain (i.e., pain-to-needle time). A door-to-needle time of less than 30 minutes should be the goal.

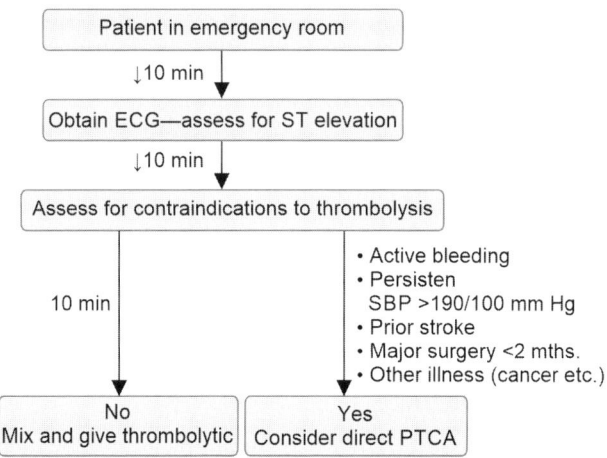

Flowchart 4.2: Time frame for thrombolytic administration.

(ECG: electrocardiogram; PTCA: percutaneous transluminal coronary angioplasty; SBP: systolic blood pressure)

SK: 1.5 million units/1 h, or tPA: 15 mg bolus (also in parts with cardiogenic shock and stroke).

Then, 50 mg/30 min and 35 mg in 1 hour.

Regarding administration of thrombolytic agent in acute MI- the sooner is the better. Every effort should be made to bring the patient to the emergency room within 1–2 hours of onset of chest pain. Thrombolysis should be started in the emergency room if there is any delay in transferring to CCU. Investigations like blood and chest X-ray should not delay thrombolysis. Administration of thrombolytics in the emergency room by the ED physician is now the standard care for MI.

Q67. When is MI itself an absolute contraindication for thrombolysis?

Ans. One situation in which a patient with documented MI should never be given thrombolytics is aortic dissection. The infarction is due to mechanical compression of the coronary artery openings near the aortic valve, rather than thrombosis. Thrombolytics would likely prove rapidly fatal. About 75% of aortic dissection victims will have an abnormal ECG, which may show signs of regional infarction.

Q68. If bleeding complication occurs, how to reverse thrombolytic therapy?

Ans. Bleeding complications occur in 5% of patients receiving thrombolytics.

It mostly occurs at the site of invasive procedure (i.e., puncture site). Intracranial bleeding is the most dangerous (occurs in about 0.5% of cases).

In the initial evaluation of the bleeding patient, all vascular sites should be inspected, and pressure should be applied if needed. Blood should be sent for crossmatching. Aspirin and heparin therapies should be discontinued. If necessary, protamine sulfate (1 mg per 100 U of heparin, not to exceed 50 mg in 10 minutes) is given to reverse heparin effect.

For severe bleeding, cryoprecipitate and fresh-frozen plasma should be given (especially if fibrinogen level is <100 mg/dL). Platelets can be given when bleeding time is prolonged. If life-threatening bleeding continues, antifibrinolytic drugs may be considered.

Q69. Should diuretics be used in HF due to AMI?

Ans. Diuretics should not be used initially as treatment of pulmonary congestion in AMI, because intravascular pressure is initially normal (unless there was existing CHF). Pulmonary edema with transudation of fluid into the lungs may induce hypovolemia. Administration of diuretics may reduce preload. These may lead to a progressive decline in systemic BP and coronary perfusion pressure. Their use should be guided by hemodynamic measurements from a Swan–Ganz catheter [pulmonary capillary wedge pressure (PCWP) >18 mm Hg and cardiac index (CI) >2.2 L/min/m^2, i.e., Forrester class II]. Also, if high filling pressure, i.e., PCWP >18 mm Hg, persists after achieving adequate output with positive inotropic agents and/or vasodilators, diuretics may be added with caution. Their use may become appropriate later if salt and water retention occur and LV filling pressure becomes excessively high.

Q70. What are the hemodynamic features of cardiogenic shock in MI?

Ans. Hemodynamic features of cardiogenic shock are similar to that of LVF without cardiogenic shock, except that arterial pressure is lower and CI is reduced.

These are:
- *Low CI:* <1.8 L/min/m^2
- *Persistent hypotension:* SBP <90 mm Hg for >30 minutes
- *Elevated LV filling pressure:* PCWP >18 mm Hg

Shocks may also occur in AMI when PCWP is low, e.g., overdiuresis, dehydration, GI bleeding after thrombolysis, and reduced LV filling as in RV infarction.

Q71. What is invasive monitoring in patients with AMI?

Ans. Invasive monitoring is done in certain patients with complicated MI, especially when vasodilator and inotropic agents are needed. The objective is to maintain an adequate COP and BP without inducing tachycardia, and while maintaining a filling pressure that is normal or minimally increased.

Invasive monitoring consists of:
- Inserting an arterial line for continuous measurement of arterial pressure for all hypotensive patients, especially those in shock and receiving vasopressor agents. Radial artery is the preferred site, although brachial and femoral arteries can be used.
- Insertion of Swan-Ganz balloon flotation catheter—measurement of pulmonary artery (PA), PCWP [equivalent to left ventricular end-diastolic pressure (LVEDP)], right atrial (RA) pressure, and COP (by thermodilution). It permits, in setting of low COP, to distinguish between inadequate ventricular filling pressure and inadequate systolic function. The former is treated by volume expansion, and the latter by inotropic support and afterload reduction.
- Foley catheter for the measurement of urine output.

Q72. What are the indications of invasive monitoring in AMI?
Ans. The goal of invasive monitoring is to maintain ventricular performance, support BP, and protect jeopardized myocardium. It is indicated in:
- Severe or progressive CHF and RV failure from suspected RV infarction
- Persistent hypotension—cardiogenic shock or hypovolemic (occasionally)
- Suspected mechanical complications—ventricular septal defect (VSD), papillary muscle rupture, and cardiac tamponade
- Monitoring response to vasodilator with SBP <100 mm Hg
- Monitoring response—COP and ventricular filling pressure to inotropic therapy
- Hemodynamic compromise severe enough requiring intra-aortic balloon pump (IABP)
- Arterial monitoring—BP cuffs are likely to be underestimated in hypotension with peripheral vasoconstriction.

Q73. Is invasive monitoring needed for all patients with AMI?
Ans. The patients with clinically uncomplicated MI, circulatory status can be assessed by careful clinical evaluation—heart rate, rhythm, BP, auscultation of lung fields for pulmonary congestion, examination of skin and mucus membrane for evidence of adequacy of perfusion, measurement of urine output, chest radiographs for pulmonary congestion, and arterial sampling for partial pressure of oxygen (PO_2), partial pressure of carbon dioxide (PCO_2), and PH (when hypoxia, metabolic are acidosis suspected).

The catheter used for invasive monitoring (Swan–Ganz and arterial), even when used correctly, are not totally complication free.

Q74. What is the role of vasodilators in cardiogenic shock and LVF in patients with AMI?
Ans. Vasodilators play an important role in the management of post-MI HF by means of afterload reduction. They reduce wall stress and decrease O_2

requirement. Vasodilators also improve COP by decreasing afterload and systemic vascular resistance. It is preferable that hemodynamic monitoring with Swan-Ganz catheter is done when one gives a vasodilator to reduce the ventricular filling pressure to <18 mm Hg.

- Nitroglycerin IV—drug of choice; it is anti-ischemic and less likely to produce coronary steal. In patients with pulmonary edema with adequate SBP (≥100 mm Hg), it is the preferred drug. NG is titrated to achieve a mean arterial pressure of approximately 70 mm Hg.
- Nitroprusside IV—may be added if afterload reduction is warranted. In severe pulmonary edema, nitroprusside may be essential.

If SBP is <100 mm Hg, treatment should be initiated with a positive inotropic agent, with the subsequent addition of a vasodilator if adequate BP is achieved.

Q75. What is the optimum LV filling pressure? How is it achieved in AMI?
Ans. Optimum LV filling pressure or end-diastolic pressure (assessed by PCWP) is the highest pressure that may be achieved without causing pulmonary edema—usually 16-20 mm Hg, while maintaining adequate COP and coronary perfusion.

- In raised LV filling pressure—a vasodilator may reduce it, but an IV inotropic agent such as dobutamine may be needed.
- A low LV filling pressure (low PCWP)—accompanies RV infarction and reduced blood volume (e.g., in vomiting). It is corrected by volume loading with IV normal saline. Large volume may be needed. The target central venous pressure (CVP) for fluid administration is approximately 15 mm Hg.

Q76. What is the role of inotropes in patients with HF post MI?
Ans.
- In cardiogenic shock—if the systolic BP is <80-90 mm Hg, dopamine 2-7 µg/kg/min is given and is associated with increase in stroke volume, COP, renal blood flow, and peripheral resistance to a modest degree. Some patients may need norepinephrine to maintain arterial pressure.
- In patients with extensive pulmonary edema who are normotensive, an IV inotropic agent, usually dobutamine is added along with NG. The infusion should be initiated at 2.5 µg/kg/min and should be increased to maintain adequate systemic pressure and at the same time, does not increase heart rate by more than 10-15%. Hemodynamic monitoring should be done. Ventricular filling pressure should be reduced to <18 mm Hg while maintaining adequate BP.
- In patients with SBP <100 mm Hg with evidence of peripheral hypoperfusion, and in patients with pulmonary edema, therapy should be initiated with an inotrope (dopamine), not a vasodilator, which may be subsequently added if adequate BP is achieved.

Q77. Compare dopamine and dobutamine as inotropes in HF after AMI.
Ans. Dobutamine, in dose 2.5–15 µg/kg/min, has a combined inotropic and vasodilator effect, which reduces afterload. It increases COP and decreases filling pressure and increases coronary flow. It is less prone to cause tachycardia than dopamine. If used alone, it may produce immediate hypotension. Dopamine, in dose 2.5–5.0 µg/kg/min, improves COP and increases renal blood flow. It increases the heart rate more than dobutamine. With higher dose, it produces renal and peripheral vasoconstriction and increases filling pressure, offsetting some of the positive inotropic effect. Low-dose dopamine can be used in conjunction with dobutamine.

Q78. Does use of positive inotropes increase infarct size?
Ans. Inotropic agents, by increasing heart rate and myocardial contractility, are likely to increase infarct size. But, as long as the heart rate does not increase more than 10% above baseline, there is no increase in infarct size or incidence of reinfarction or arrhythmia. In this regard, dobutamine increases the heart rate less than dopamine, and it may increase coronary flow (acting as vasodilator).

SUGGESTED READING

1. 2012 ACCF/AHA/ACP/AATS/PCNA/SCAI/STS guideline for the diagnosis and management of patients with stable ischemic heart disease: executive summary: a report of the American College of Cardiology Foundation/ American Heart Association Task Force on Practice Guidelines, and the American College of Physicians, American Association for Thoracic Surgery, Preventive Cardiovascular Nurses Association, Society for Cardiovascular Angiography and interventions, and Society of Thoracic Surgeons. Circulation. 2012;126(25):3097-137.
2. Antman EM, Aneb DT, Armstrong PW, Bates ER, Green LA, Hand M, et al. ACC/AHA guidelines for the management of patients with ST-elevation myocardial infarction; A report of the American College of Cardiology/American Heart Association Task Force on Practice Guidelines (Committee to Revise the 1999 Guidelines for the Management of patients with acute myocardial infarction). J Am Coll Cardiol. 2004:44(3):E1-211.
3. National Cholesterol Education Program, National Heart Lung, and Blood Institute, National Institutes of Health. Third Report of the National Cholesterol Education Program (NCEP) Expert Panel on Detection, Evaluation, and Treatment of High Blood Cholesterol in Adults (Adult Treatment Panel III) Final Report. Bethesda, MD: NIH Publication No.02-5215; 2002.
4. O'Gara P, Kushner FG, Ascheim DD, Casey Jr DE, Chung MK, de Lemos JA, et al. 2013 ACCF/AHA Guideline for the Management of ST-Elevation Myocardial Infarction: A report of the American college of Cardiology foundation/American Heart Association Task Force on Practice Guidelines. Circulation. 2013;127(4).
5. Vrints C, Andreotti F, Koskinas KC, Rossello X, Adamo M, Ainslie J, et al. 2024 ESC guidelines for the management of chronic coronary syndromes. Eur Heart J. 2024;00:1-123.

CHAPTER 5
Acute Rheumatic Fever and Chronic Rheumatic Heart Disease

"Rheumatic fever does not deform the joints but kills the patient due to involvement of heart."
—William Charles Wells (1812)

■ INTRODUCTION

Although prevalence of rheumatic fever has decreased in the past few decades, chronic rheumatic heart diseases (CRHDs) are still the most commonly acquired heart disease in children and young people in Bangladesh. Rheumatic fever (RF) is an enigma with several unique features in its pathogenesis, clinical manifestations, treatment, and prevention.

Q1. What is RF?
Ans. Rheumatic fever is an acute, systemic inflammatory disease that occurs as a reaction to sore throat by group A beta hemolytic streptococcus bacteria.

Rheumatic fever with resulting rheumatic heart disease (RHD) is the most frequent cardiac disease in Bangladesh.

Q2. Why is the prevalence of RF and RHD high in low- and middle-income countries (LMICs)?
Ans. Higher prevalence of streptococcal throat infection resulting from overcrowding, poor living standard, and malnutrition is responsible for this high prevalence of RF and RHD in LMICs.

Q3. Why RF is the most common between the age of 5 and 15 years?
Ans. As the higher incidence of group A streptococcal (GAS) sore throat occurs in children between the age of 5 and 15 years, the peak age for attack of acute rheumatic fever (ARF) is in the same age range.

Q4. How frequently does valvular heart disease follow sore throat?
Ans. Valvular heart diseases are frequently sequale of streptococcal sore throat in a manner shown in **Flowchart 5.1**.

Flowchart 5.1 shows only 3% individuals with true streptococcal sore throat develop ARF after 3 weeks (on average). Pancarditis develops in about 50% of patients with the first attack of RF. Pericarditis and myocarditis usually resolve without residue, whereas 50% of patients with endocarditis develop CRHD after 10–20 years in temperate countries, and as early as 2 years in

Bangladesh and other developing countries. In 50% of CRHD patients, mitral valve (MV) is involved.

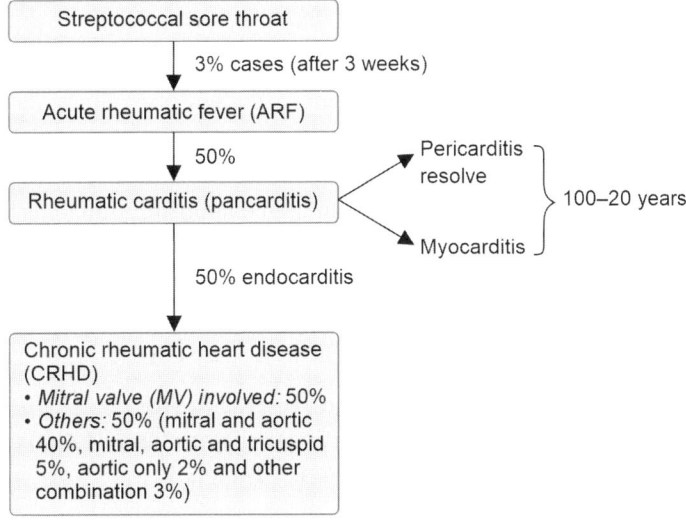

Q5. How is ARF diagnosed?
Ans. There is no definite diagnostic test. The *Jones criteria*, updated in 1992, were designed to aid in the diagnosis of the first episode of RF. RF can be diagnosed when an evidence of previous GAS sore throat is detected in conjunction with either two major manifestations, or one major and two minor manifestations. Major manifestations include arthritis, carditis, chorea, erythema marginatum, and subcutaneous nodules. Minor manifestations include fever, arthralgia, high erythrocyte sedimentation rate (ESR) or C-reactive protein (CRP), prolonged PR interval on electrocardiogram (ECG); if arthritis is used as a major criterion for the diagnosis, arthralgia cannot be used as a minor criterion. In some circumstances, the diagnosis of RF can be made without strict adherence to Jones criteria, as in cases of insidious onset carditis, or isolated cases of chorea when other causes have been excluded. The requirement of additional evidence of preceding streptococcal infection may be waived in this case. Streptococcal antibody may have already returned to normal level since the patient was first seen.

Q6. What are the unique features of RF?
Ans.
- Rheumatic fever is an enigma; its etiology, pathogenesis, diagnosis, and treatment are incompletely characterized.
- It licks the joints and bites the heart.

- Children <5 years are not commonly affected; recurrence is rare beyond 34 years. The earlier the heart is affected in life, more serious is the prognosis.
- One attack predisposes further attack and each recurrence increases risk of valvular damage.
- No diagnostic test is available—diagnosis depends on criteria developed by expert opinion (not controlled trial).
- Diagnostic criteria are frequently updated. Some countries like New Zealand and Australia have their own diagnostic guidelines [carditis diagnosed by echocardiography (echo)].
- Clinical evaluation is central to diagnosis of ARF. Echo is an excellent tool that may prevent overdiagnosis of ARF by excluding physiologic flow murmurs and undetected coronary heart disease (CHD).

Q7. Compare and contrast carditis and arthritis of ARF.
Ans. Carditis and migratory polyarthritis are major manifestations of ARF. They have some contrasting features listed in **Table 5.1**.

TABLE 5.1: Rheumatic carditis and arthritis comparison.

Carditis	Arthritis
Incidence: 40–60%	75%
Initial attack does not resolve	Resolve in ≤1 month
Attack always recurrent	Recurrenceless
Usual complication; RHD	Nil to rare
More severe with less arthritis	More severe with less carditis
Steroid therapy is mandatory	Aspirin is enough, or steroid rarely needed

Q8. What are the evolutionary changes in the diagnosis of RF?
Ans. Jones criteria developed for diagnosis of RF have undergone major modifications for four times in six decades **(Box 5.1)**.

BOX 5.1: Diagnostic criteria of rheumatic fever—evolutionary changes.
- *1944–5:* Major criteria suggested
- *1956:* Criteria modified, minor criteria added such as arthralgia, fever, and elevated phase reactant
- *1965:* Evidence of prior GAS infection (+ve throat culture), raised antistreptolysin O (ASO) titer incorporated as essential criteria for diagnosis
- *1992:* Revised criteria, they are guidelines for diagnosis of initial attack of RF, eliminated various elements of minor criteria-prolonged PR interval, leukocytosis, also abdominal pain, epistaxis, pulmonary findings, anemia, etc. It listed two exceptions that do not need evidence of antecedent GAS infection—chorea and insidious onset carditis
- *2004:* World Health Organization (WHO) algorithm for diagnosis of ARF and recurrent RHD:

Category	Criteria
– Primary episode of RF	– Two major or one major, and two minor manifestations plus evidence of GAS infection
– Recurrent RF without RHD	– Same
– Recurrent RF with established RHD	– Two minor manifestations plus evidence of GAS infection
– Rheumatic chorea and insidious onset carditis	– Other major manifestations or evidence of GAS infection not needed
– Chronic valvular lesions of RHD	– No need of any other criteria

- *2015:* American Heart Association (AHA) revised Jones criteria for diagnosis of RF.

(RF: rheumatic fever; ARF: acute rheumatic fever; RHD: rheumatic heart disease; GAS: group A streptococcal)

Q9. What are the Jones criteria?
Ans.
- *Major manifestations:* Carditis, polyarthritis, chorea, erythema marginatum, and subcutaneous nodule
- *Minor manifestations:* Clinical fever, polyarthralgia, laboratory-prolonged PR interval, elevated acute phase reactant (ESR, CRP, and leukocytosis)
- *Supportive evidences of GAS infection (within last 45 days):* Elevated or rising ASO, or other streptococcal antibody, or a positive throat culture, or rapid antigen test for GAS, or recent scarlet fever.

Q10. What is insidious onset carditis?
Ans. It is an unusual presentation of RF. Patients have no history of prior rheumatic symptom, but give history of malaise, lethargy, and poor appetite for past several months. On examination, a sign of carditis is unmistakable—children have murmurs, enlarged heart, sign of features of heart failure. Such

patients may have only one major manifestation—carditis, or atmost one major and one minor manifestation, such as low-grade fever or raised ESR. They do not fulfill the revised Jones criteria.

Q11. How long to continue therapy for secondary prevention of RF?
Ans. Secondary prophylaxis with penicillin for long period to prevent recurrence **(Box 5.2)**.

> **BOX 5.2:** Secondary prophylaxis in rheumatic fever.
> - For patients with rheumatic fever (RF) without carditis, prophylaxis should be continued for 5 years after the first attack of RF or up to age 21 years, depending on whichever is longer
> - For patients with RF and carditis but no residual valvular disease [or rheumatic heart disease (RHD)], prophylaxis should be extended for a period of 10 years or beyond adulthood, depending on whichever is longer
> - For patients with RF and carditis with residual valvular disease [chronic rheumatic heart disease (CRHD)], prophylaxis is recommended for the lifetime of the patients

When in some patients the diagnosis of RF is probable rather than definite, the duration of prophylaxis can be shortened in proportion to the double of what the physician has on the diagnosis.

Q12. Why is penicillin chosen for RF prophylaxis?
Ans. Penicillin has been proven to be the most efficacious antibiotic against GABHS, which is responsible for RF. Resistance of this organism against penicillin is virtually unknown, even after long-term use. These, along with its low cost, make penicillin the prophylactic agent of choice in this condition.

Q13. Antistreptolysin O titer is raised—what does it really mean?
Ans. Raised ASO titer (antibody against streptolysin O) provides solid evidence for recent GAS infection. A greater than twofold rise in ASO titer compared with convalescent titer is diagnosed. The probability of detecting a previous streptococcal infection can be increased by obtaining repeated ASO titer. A raised ASO titer, per se, is not indicative of RF unless present along with other manifestations (Jones criteria). On the contrary, a raised ASO titer can be found in conditions other than RF, such as rheumatoid arthritis, Takayasu's arthritis, systemic lupus erythematosus, and infective endocarditis. These conditions may mimic RF and even fulfill the Jones criteria, unless very carefully applied. ASO titer may also be raised in healthy children.

Again, in unusual presentations like insidious onset carditis and Sydenham's chorea—diagnosis of RF is made in absence of raised ASO titer. They appear after few months of sore throat when ASO titer is usually normalized.

Q14. Rheumatic fever licks the joints and bites the heart—what does it mean?

Ans. Polyarthritis and carditis are two major manifestations of RF. Arthritis produces swollen, hot, painful joints within a few hours. Salicylates and corticosteroids relieve arthritic features promptly. Even in absence of treatment, arthritis usually disappears within 3 weeks, and leaves no residual abnormalities. Hence, it is licking the joints (effusion only, no damage or biting). On the contrary, endocarditis of RF often produces signs of residual valvular damage, hence the biting, i.e., damage.

Q15. What are the Doppler echocardiographic criteria for the diagnosis of carditis?

Ans. World Heart Federation criteria for carditis causing valvular regurgitation [mitral regurgitation (MR) and aortic regurgitation (AR)] are:

Four criteria must be met:
- Seen in at least two views
- Seen in at least one view with jet length ≥2 cm in MR and ≥1 cm in AR
- Peak velocity ≥3 m/sec
- Pansystolic jet in at least one envelop

Q16. What is the current update on Jones criteria?

Ans. American Heart Association revised Jones criteria for diagnosis of RF in 2015, which is the most recent update. In this, to avoid overdiagnosis in low-incidence populations and underdiagnosis in high-incidence populations, variable diagnostic criteria were introduced (in line with Australian guidelines).

- *Major criteria for low-risk populations:* Carditis (clinical or subclinical), arthritis (polyarthritis only), chorea, erythema marginatum, and subcutaneous nodule
- *Major criteria for moderate to high-risk populations:* Carditis (clinical or subclinical), arthritis (including polyarthritis, monoarthritis, or polyarthralgia), chorea, erythema marginatum, and subcutaneous nodule
- *Minor criteria for low-risk populations:* Polyarthralgia (unless arthritis is major), fever ≥38°, raised ESR (≥50 mm) or CRP (≥3.0 mg/dL), and prolonged PR interval (unless carditis is major)
- *Minor criteria for moderate- and high-risk populations:* Monoarthralgia, fever ≥38°, raised ESR or CRP, and prolonged PR
- The American Heart Association suggests that clinical judgement has to be applied for "possible" RF in areas where RF remains common, and where it is not possible to fulfill the Jones criteria because of lack of laboratory facilities. It is reasonable to offer 12 months of secondary prophylaxis

followed by reassessment based on history, physical examination, and repeated echocardiography.

Point to ponder: During recurrence in pre-existing RHD, carditis may precipitate heart failure (HF), but it may not be possible to diagnose. ARF is diagnosed on the basis of minor manifestations and evidence of recent streptococcal infection (WHO criteria).

Q17. How RF leads to mitral valve disease—mitral stenosis (MS), MR, combined MS and MR?

- Chronic rheumatic heart disease, producing symmetric fusion of the commissures results in small, central, oval orifice in diastole (fish mouth in pathological specimens), leads to MS.
- CRHD leading to exclusive or predominant contraction and fusion of the chordate tendineae with little fusion of the commissures, leads to dominant MR results.
- With end-stage disease, thickened leaflets are so adherent and rigid that they cannot open or close, leading to combined MS and MR.

Q18. What are the common combined valvular lesions in CRHDs?
Ans.
- Mitral stenosis and MR are the most common. If left ventricle (LV) is dilated, MR is the dominant lesion, and if LV is not dilated, MS is the dominant lesion.
- *MS with AR:* MS reduces cardiac output, many of the peripheral signs as well as echocardiographic features of AR may be missing.
- MS with tricuspid regurgitation (functional)

Q19. How is bed rest advised to patients with RF?
Ans. Patients need and want bed rest in acute phase. Gradual mobilization is done when temperature, pulse and ESR return to normal, and evidence of acute arthritis and carditis disappears **(Table 5.2)**.

TABLE 5.2: Suggested bed rest in rheumatic fever.

Cardiac status	Management
No carditis	Bed rest for 2 weeks and gradual ambulation for 2 weeks (even if on salicylate)
Carditis but no cardiomegaly	Bed rest for 4 weeks and gradual ambulation for 4 weeks
Carditis with cardiomegaly	Bed rest for 6 weeks and gradual ambulation for 6 weeks
Carditis with heart failure	Bed rest till failure controlled and gradual ambulation

Q20. How does ARF lead to both morbidity and mortality?
Ans. Failure to put patients with ARF on antibiotic prophylaxis to prevent future attacks, leads to repeated episodes of ARF, scarring of valves, chronic valvular heart diseases, HF, and death, usually before middle age.

SUGGESTED READING

1. Gerber MA, Baltimore RS, Eaton CB, Gewitz M, Rowley AH, Shulman ST, et al. AHA guidelines on prevention of rheumatic fever and treatment of acute streptococcal pharyngitis: a scientific statement from the American Heart Association Rheumatic Fever, Endocarditis, and Kawasaki Disease Committee of the Council on Cardiovascular Disease in the Young, the Interdisciplinary Council on Functional Genomics and Translational Biology, and the Interdisciplinary Council on Quality of Care and Outcomes Research: endorsed by the American Academy of Pediatrics. Circulation. 2009;119(11):1541-51.
2. Gewitz MH, Baltimore RS, Tani LY, Sable CA, Shulman ST, Carapetis J, et al. Revision of the Jones criteria for the diagnosis of acute rheumatic fever in the era of Doppler echocardiography a scientific statement from the American Heart association. Circulation 2015;113:1806-18.
3. National Heart Foundation of Australia and the Cardiac Society of Australia and New Zealand. Diagnosis and Management of Acute Rheumatic Fever and Rheumatic Heart Disease in Australia: An evidence-based review. Melbourne, Australia; 2006.
4. Sika-Paotonu D, Beaton A, Raghu A, Steer A, Carapetis J. Acute rheumatic fever and rheumatic heart disease. In: Ferretti JJ, Stevens DL, Fischetti VA (Eds). *Streptococcus Pyogenes:* Basic Biology to Clinical Manifestations. Oklahoma City: University of Oklahoma Health Sciences Center; 2016.
5. World Health Organization. (2004). Rheumatic Fever and Rheumatic Heart Disease: Report of a WHO Expert Consultation, WHO Technical Report Series No. 923. [online]Available from https://iris.who.int/bitstream/handle/10665/42898/WHO_TRS_923.pdf. [Last accessed May, 2025].

CHAPTER 6

Valvular Heart Diseases

"No diagnostic procedure can visualize the heart valves as well as echocardiography. It has become the examination of choice for evaluating valvular heart disease."
—Harvey Feigenbaum

■ INTRODUCTION

A diseased valve may be stenotic (failing to open normally) or regurgitant (failing to close normally). In Bangladesh, valvular heart diseases (VHDs) are mostly rheumatic in origin. Age-related degeneration, e.g., calcific aortic stenosis (AS) and congenital lesions, such as congenital AS and pulmonary stenosis (PS) are also found. Percutaneous valvular interventions include mitral balloon valvuloplasty (MBV) for rheumatic mitral stenosis (MS) and pulmonary balloon valvuloplasty (PBV) for congenital PS. Valve surgery includes prosthetic mitral valve replacement (MVR) and aortic valve replacement (AVR). Prosthetic valve disease develops in some of the MVR and AVR patients.

Q1. How to classify VHDs?
Ans. Depending on their cause, type of valve involved, and the pathological process involved, VHDs are classified as shown in **Box 6.1**.

> **BOX 6.1:** Valvular heart disease (VHD)—classification.
>
> - *Etiologically:*
>   - Rheumatic—acute rheumatic fever (RF) and chronic rheumatic heart disease (RHD)
>   - Infective, i.e., infective endocarditis—acute (healthy valve) and subacute (diseased valve)
>   - Traumatic, e.g., mitral regurgitation following mitral balloon valvuloplasty
>   - Degenerative, e.g., CAVD (calcific aortic valve disease) and mitral valve prolapse (MVP)
>   - Miscellaneous—connective tissue disease, e.g., aortic regurgitation in Marfan syndrome and pulmonary stenosis in carcinoid syndrome
> - *Type of valve involved:*
>   - Native valve disease
>   - Prosthetic valve disease—metallic and bioprosthesis
> - *Pathologically:*
>   - Organic, i.e., valve itself is involved
>   - Functional, i.e., valvular involvement is secondary to right ventricular (RV) or left ventricular (LV) dilatation, e.g., tricuspid regurgitation (TR), MR

Q2. How are VHD patients staged?

Ans. Valvular heart disease patients are now classified by disease stages as follows:
- *Stage A:* Patients at risk of development of VHD
- *Stage B:* Asymptomatic patients with progressive VHD (mild to moderate severity)
- *Stage C:* Asymptomatic patients with severe VHD, with either normal RV or LV systolic function (*stage C1*), or decompensated ventricular function (*stage C2*).
- *Stage D:* Symptomatic patients with severe VHD.

Q3. How does clinical presentation vary in different VHDs?

Ans. Morphologically, the two categories of VHD, i.e., stenotic and regurgitant lesions vary in their clinical presentation as listed in **Box 6.2**.

> **BOX 6.2:** Clinical presentation of valvular diseases.
> - *Dyspnea:* Early in mitral valvular diseases (MVDs) as left atrial (LA) pressure increases early and pulmonary congestion develops. In aortic valvular disease, pulmonary congestion occurs late [until patients develop left ventricular (LV) dysfunction]
> - *Hemoptysis:* Develops early in MVD, more with mitral stenosis (MS) as pulmonary hypertension is more with overload of LA pressure than LA volume overload, as in mitral regurgitation (MR)
> - *Palpitation:* More in regurgitant lesions, such as aortic regurgitation (AR), MR. It may occur in MS when atrial fibrillation (AF) develops
> - *Chest pain:* Develops when pulmonary hypertension (stressing of pulmonary artery). It may also occur in obstructive lesions, e.g., MS, aortic stenosis (AS), pulmonary stenosis (PS)
> - *Thromboembolic phenomena:* When AF develops in MVD (more in MS due to overload of LA pressure, although LA size is more with MR)

Q4. What is the utility of echocardiography (echo) in the assessment of VHD?

Ans. Echocardiography is recommended in the following:
- Any murmur associated with cardiac symptoms
- A murmur of grade 3 or louder
- Any diastolic murmur. Wide availability of echo ensures that a correct diagnosis of valve anatomy and function is possible in every patient.

Q5. When is coronary angiography (CAG) done in VHD?

Ans. Coronary angiography is recommended to exclude concomitant coronary artery disease (CAD) in the following:
- Patients with CAD, angina, objective evidence of ischemia, or CAD-risk factors
- Chronic severe secondary mitral regurgitation (MR)
- Patients undergoing elective valve surgery.

Q6. Outline the general strategies for the management of rheumatic valvular diseases?

Ans. General strategies for drugs, intervention, and surgery for the management of rheumatic valvular diseases are as shown in **Box 6.3**.

BOX 6.3: Management of rheumatic valvular disease—general strategies.

- *Drug treatment:*
  - Prophylaxis for rheumatic fever—lifelong; all cases
  - Prophylaxis for infective endocarditis—in aortic regurgitation (AR), mitral regurgitation (MR), aortic stenosis (AS)
  - Digoxin—in atrial fibrillation (AF)
  - Betablocker—in mitral stenosis (MS), AS
  - Angiotensin-converting enzyme inhibitor (ACEI)—in MR and AR
  - Anticoagulants—in AF
- *Interventional:*
  - Mitral balloon valvuloplasty (MBV)—in MS
  - Transcutaneous aortic valve replacement (TAVR)—in AS
- *Surgical:*
  - Valvotomy [closed mitral valvotomy (CMV) and open mitral valvotomy (OMV)]—in MS
  - Valvuloplasty [mitral valve (MV) repair]—in MR
  - Valve replacement—mitral valve replacement (MVR), aortic valve replacement (AVR)

Q7. What are different interventional and surgical procedures available for VHDs?

Ans.
- *Interventional:*
  - Balloon mitral valvuloplasty (BMV) in symptomatic severe MS with mitral valve area (MVA) <1.5 cm² (type I indication), asymptomatic severe MS with new atrial fibrillation (AF) and suitable anatomy [no MR, no left atrial (LA) thrombus, mobile and noncalcified leaflets, no subvalvular changes], symptomatic with moderate MS with MVA >1.5 cm², severely symptomatic, severe MS with MVA <1.5 cm² with suboptimal anatomy (type IIb indication), in case of isolated MS.
- MitraClip system for MR > Grade III
  - PBV in PS
  - Aortic balloon valvuloplasty (ABV) in congenital AS
  - Transcatheter aortic valve replacement (TAVR) in AS
- *Surgical:*
  - Valvotomy—closed mitral valvotomy (CMV), open mitral valvotomy (OMV) in MS
  - Valvuloplasty—repair of mitral valve (MV) in MR, MitraClip in MR
  - Valve replacement—MVR and AVR (metallic, bioprosthetic). In chronic MR and aortic regurgitation (AR) with worsening symptoms, progressive radiological cardiac enlargement and deteriorating LV function on echo are indications for valve replacement. In acute AR,

immediate surgery is needed. In severe AS with classic symptoms, AVR is done. It is also done in asymptomatic AS with left ventricular dysfunction—in worsening symptoms, progressive radiological cardiac enlargement, deteriorating left ventricular function on echo.

▪ MITRAL STENOSIS

Q1. What are the causes of MS?
Ans.
- *Rheumatic fever:* 99% cases
- *Others:* Congenital, following radiotherapy (for chest or breast cancer), functional MS (extensive mitral annular calcification restricting annular motion).

Q2. What are the stages of MS?
Ans. The American College of Cardiology (ACC)/American Heart Association (AHA) guidelines (2014) for the management of VHD stages of MS are as follows:
- *Stage A (at risk of MS):* Asymptomatic; mild diastolic doming and normal transmitral flow velocity
- *Stage B (progressive MS):* Asymptomatic; diastolic doming, commissural fusion and increased transmitral velocity; MVA >1.5 cm^2, pressure half ($P_{1/2}$) time <150 ms, and mild to moderate LA enlargement
- *Stage C (asymptomatic severe MS):* Asymptomatic; all above plus $P_{1/2}$ time ≥150 ms (≥220 in very severe), MVA ≤1.5 cm^2 (≤1.0 cm^2 in very severe), severe LA enlargement, and pulmonary artery systolic pressure (PASP) >30 mm Hg
- *Stage D (symptomatic severe MS):* Symptomatic; exertional dyspnea, decreased exercise tolerance; MVA ≤1.5 cm^2 (≤1.0 cm^2 in very severe), $P_{1/2}$ time ≥150 ms (≥220 ms in very severe), severe LA enlargement, and PASP >30 mm Hg.

Q3. What are the grades of severity of MS?
Ans. Severity of MS as per ACC/AHA guidelines (2006) are as follows:
- *Mild MS:* MVA >1.5 cm^2, mean pressure gradient (MPG) <5 mm Hg, and PASP <30 mm Hg
- *Moderate MS:* MVA 1–1.5 cm^2, MPG 5–10 mm Hg, and PASP 30–50 mm Hg
- *Severe MS:* MVA <1.0 cm^2, MPG >10 mm Hg, and PASP >50 mm Hg.

Q4. What are the conditions other than MS that produce LV inflow obstruction?
Ans. The conditions other than MS that produce LV inflow obstruction are:
- LA myxoma

Ball valve thrombus in left atrium (usually associated with MS)
- Cor triatriatum (congenital membrane in left atrium)
- Infective endocarditis (IE) with large vegetation.

Q5. What are the other conditions producing a mid-diastolic murmur in the mitral area besides MS?
Ans. These are as follows:
- LA myxoma
- Ball valve thrombus
- Austin Flint murmur of AR
- Increased flow in ventricular septal defect (VSD)
- Severe MR
- Hypertrophic cardiomyopathy (HCM) (early diastolic flow into nondistensible left ventricle).

Q6. What are the changes in heart sounds in MS?
Ans.
- First heart sound (S_1) is loud when leaflets are flexible, due to sudden closure of widely apart mitral leaflets. It becomes variable in intensity after development of AF. Marked calcification and/or thickening of mitral leaflets reduce amplitude of S_1 due to diminished motion of leaflets. With end-stage disease, anterior and posterior mitral leaflets may be so adherent and rigid that they cannot open or shut. S_1 diminishes in intensity, or rarely even abolishes.
- P_2 becomes accentuated when pulmonary arterial pressure (PAP) rises, splitting of S_2 narrows and lastly becomes single.
- Others—pulmonic ejection sound of severe pulmonary hypertension (PH) and dilatation of PA, S_4 originating from RV (S_3 gallop originating from LV absent).

Q7. How does AF develop in MS?
Ans. Development of AF correlates directly with severity of MS, degree of LA dilatation, and age of the patient. It is episodic at first but then becomes more persistent. AF causes diffuse atrophy of atrial muscle, further atrial enlargement, and further inhomogeneity of refractoriness and conduction leading to irreversible, chronic AF. Thus, AF begets further AF.

Q8. How does AF alter the natural course of MS?
Ans. Atrial fibrillation may precipitate or worsen symptoms caused by loss of atrial contribution of LV filling and a short diastolic filling period when ventricular rate is not well controlled. Also, AF predisposes to LA thrombus formation and systemic embolism. Development of AF carries a worse overall prognosis in MS patients.

Q9. What are the LA changes in mitral valvular diseases (MVDs)?
Ans. The combination of MVD and atrial inflammation secondary to rheumatic carditis causes LA dilatation, fibrosis of atrial wall, and disorganization of atrial muscle bundle. These lead to disparate conduction velocities and inhomogeneous refractory periods. Premature atrial activation

caused by increased automaticity or re-entry may precipitate AF. In MS, there is pressure overload, and in MR there is volume overload of left atrium. AF is more frequent with MS than MR.

Q10. What causes hemoptysis in MS? How is it managed?
Ans. Causes of hemoptysis are as follows:
- Sudden, profuse hemoptysis occurs from rupture of thin-walled dilated bronchial veins, usually as a consequence of sudden rise in LA pressure, which act as collaterals draining from the distended pulmonary veins.
- Blood-stained sputum with attack of paroxysmal nocturnal dyspnea
- Pink, frothy sputum is a characteristic of acute pulmonary edema, with rupture of alveolar capillary
- Pulmonary infarction associated with heart failure (HF)
- Blood-stained sputum complicating chronic bronchitis
- Recurrent pneumonia in congested lung.

Treatment includes:
- Sedation with morphine
- Assumption of upright posture
- Aggressive diuresis—intravenous (IV) furosemide: 40–80 mg

These measures reduce pulmonary venous pressure and control hemoptysis.

Q11. What is the difference between three categories of MS?
Ans. Mitral stenosis is not symptomatic unless it is of severe degree. Besides severity, the three degrees of MS have some characteristic features listed in **Table 6.1**:

TABLE 6.1: Features of mitral stenosis (MS) of differing severity.

	Mild	Moderate	Severe
Mitral valve area (MVA) (cm^2)	1.5–2.0	1.0–1.4	<1.0
Mean LA pressure (mm Hg)	<12 mm Hg	12–20 mm Hg	>25 mm Hg
Symptoms	Asymptomatic	Usually asymptomatic (symptomatic with exertion and during pregnancy)	Symptomatic
Sign	Mid-diastolic murmur—short	Mid-diastolic murmur—shorter	Mid-diastolic murmur longer in duration
Complications	AF may occur	AF occurs	AF more common
	Infective endocarditis more	Infective endocarditis may occur	Rare

Contd...

Contd...

Intervention	Not usually needed	Needed before pregnancy	Always needed
Prophylaxis for RF	Always needed	Needed	Needed
Prophylaxis for IE	Needed	Needed	Needed

(LA: left atrial; AF: atrial fibrillation; RF: rheumatic fever; IE: infective endocarditis)

Q12. What is silent MS?
Ans. When mid-diastolic murmur of MS is inaudible due to marked enlargement of right ventricle that occupies the apex and reduced cardiac output (COP), the condition is called silent MS. The murmur may be audible in mid or posterior axillary line. These patients have extremely high PAP, with loud P_2, pulmonary ejection click, RV heave and sometimes tricuspid systolic murmur and Graham Steell murmur of pulmonary regurgitation (PR). These patients may be remarkably free from symptoms for a long time yet need valvotomy urgently (as MS is critical here).

Q13. Why is first heart sound loud in MS?
Ans. Sudden closure of the widely apart pliable MV leaflets produces loud S_1. The leaflets remain open at the onset of isovolumetric contraction because of the elevated LA pressure. Marked thickening and calcification of the MV reduce the loudness.

Q14. What are the auscultatory signs of pliable mitral leaflets?
Ans.
- Loud S_1
- *Opening snap (OS):* It is usually accompanied by loud S_1; it occurs when the movement of pliable mitral dome into the left ventricle suddenly stops.

Q15. What are the clinical indicators of severe MS?
Ans.
- *Symptomatology:* Patients with severe MS are usually symptomatic, often even at rest. AF often develops, which may precipitate pulmonary oedema and systemic thromboembolism. Development of pulmonary hypertension is a frequent feature, which may progress to right HF.
- *Semiology:* Palpable P_2, RV heave, features of right HF [edema, raised jugular venous pressure (JVP), and enlarged tender liver], loud P_2 on auscultation, mid-diastolic murmur of longer duration with short A_2–OS interval.

Q16. What is juvenile MS?
Ans. In the Indian subcontinent, MS tends to progress rapidly and frequently causing serious symptoms before the age of 20 years—the entity called juvenile mitral stenosis. The latent period between the initial attack of

rheumatic carditis and development of symptomatic MS may be as low as 2 years, whereas it is generally two decades in Western countries. In Bangladesh, about 30% of patients with MS belong to this entity. Development of severe degrees of PH is also faster in juvenile MS.

Q17. What are the radiologic findings of MS?

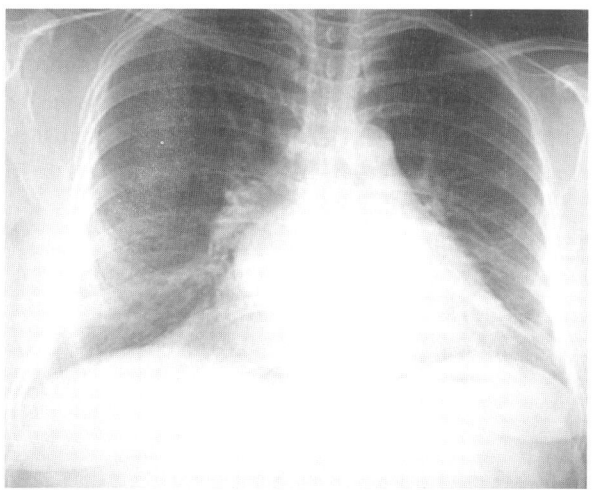

Fig. 6.1: Chest X-ray P/A view in mitral stenosis. (double contour right border; straightened left border)

Ans. The radiologic findings of MS are as follows:
- *Sign of LA enlargement:* Double contour right border (due to different levels of right atrium (RA) and dilated left atrium with intervening lung in between) **(Fig. 6.1)**.
- *Straightening of left border (mitralization):* Due to small aortic knuckle, full pulmonary conus, dilated left auricular appendage—all coming at same level.
- *Sign of pulmonary venous hypertension:* Upper lobe diversion
- *Sign of pulmonary capillary hypertension:* Pulmonary edema, Kerley B lines, and occasionally pulmonary hemosiderosis
- *Sign of pulmonary arterial hypertension:* Full pulmonary conus, feature of right ventricular hypertrophy (RVH) (reduction of retrosternal space in lateral view).

Q18. What are the M-mode echo and two-dimensional echo (2DE) findings of MS?
Ans.
- *M-mode:* E-F slope (mid-diastolic closing velocity) is reduced as mid-diastolic closure occurs at a slower rate due to the slow emptying of left atrium through narrowed mitral orifice and the valve is held open by a

persistent pressure gradient between left atrium and left ventricle. It may be used to quantitate severity of MS. Anterior motion of the posterior mitral leaflet (normally downwards in diastole)—due to thickening and commissural fusion, LA dilatation, and presence of PH loss of a dip of pulmonary valve on M-mode echocardioghaphy.

- *Two-dimensional echo:* Doming of AML (in rheumatic MS with pliable leaflets), thickening and relative immobility of PML, calcification (of tip of leaflet) or commissures, thickening and shortening of chordae (if marked, produce both stenosis and regurgitation), LA dilatation, usually the more the dilatation, the more severe the stenosis. LA thrombus (homogenous, more echogenic than underlying myocardium) with a thin lucent border between it and myocardium. Left ventricle assumes a D-shape (with development of severe PH and dilatation of RA and right ventricle). In parasternal short axis, MVA is planimetered, and stenosis is quantitated as mild, moderate, and severe. In mild MS, it is 1.6–2 cm^2, in moderate MS, it is 1–1.5 cm^2, and in severe MS, it is <1.0 cm^2 (**Figs. 6.2A and B**).

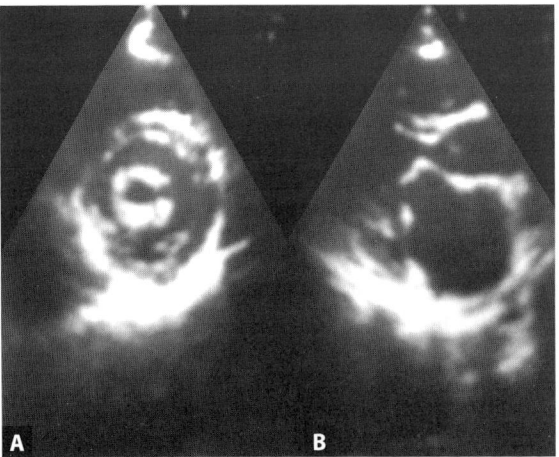

Figs. 6.2A and B: Two-dimensional echocardiography (2DE) in left parasternal short axis (A) and long axis (B) in severe mitral stenosis (MS).

Q19. What is the utility of Doppler echo in patients with MS?
Ans. Doppler echo provides anatomical as well as functional information of patients with MS.
- Severity of MS is assessed by measuring the transvalvular gradient and the stenotic MVA (by $P_{1/2}$ time method).
- *Hemodynamic consequences:* PH can be identified and quantified.
- Color Doppler study excludes any associated regurgitation.
- Beneficial effect of valvotomy can be assessed—reduction of transvalvular gradient, decrease of PAP, increase of MVA in postcommisurotomy

patients Doppler echo is superior to 2DE in calculating MVA (as orifice is irregular, planimetry is difficult). Any procedure induced MRs can be detected by color Doppler.

Q20. How does Doppler echo help in the assessment of MS?
Ans. Doppler echo [continuous wave Doppler (CWD), pulsed-wave Doppler (PWD), and color-flow imaging (CFI)] assesses hemodynamic aspects of MS—transmitral gradient, estimation of MVA (by $P_{1/2}$ time or continuity equation), and its severity, estimation of pulmonary artery pressure, etc. PWD (done in apical 4-chamber view with sample volume at tip of mitral leaflet in LV inflow) records high diastolic velocity (>1.5 m/s), spectral broadening in diastole, biphasic-Doppler recording, and an increased A-wave (absent in AF). CWD recording is similar to PWD, but it is better for recording high velocities. It can record MPG and peak pressure gradients across MV, measures MVA by using $P_{1/2}$ time, and estimates pulmonary artery pressure to assess PH. In mild MS, mean transmitral gradient is <5 mm Hg, in moderate MS it is 5–10 mm Hg, and in severe MS it is >10 mm Hg.

Color-flow imaging helps in qualitative diagnosis of MS—gives clue to location and direction of stenotic jet, thus helps in positioning Doppler sample volume and aligning Doppler cursor. It also helps in the identification of concomitant MR, AR, and tricuspid regurgitation (TR). CFI can also determine MVA (by proximal isovelocity surface area technique and color flow area method).

Q21. What is $P_{1/2}$ time? How does it determine MVA and its severity?
Ans. It is the time (in millisecond) needed for initial peak diastolic pressure gradient to decline by 50%. In MS, $P_{1/2}$ time range is from 100–400 ms, depending on severity (normal: 20–60 ms). In mild MS, $P_{1/2}$ time is 100–149 ms, in moderate MS, it is 150–220 ms, and in severe cases, it is >220 ms.

It has been found that a $P_{1/2}$ time of 220 ms correlates with an MVA of 1.0 cm². Thus, MVA can be derived by dividing 220 by the measured $P_{1/2}$ time. As $P_{1/2}$ time is a hemodynamic measurement, not dependent on MV orifice morphology, it is a more accurate measure of MVA, especially if the orifice is grossly irregular (difficult to planimeter), and after balloon mitral commissurotomy with irregular opening of the orifice. $P_{1/2}$ time is also much less influenced by heart rate and COP, although it may not be accurate in patients with coexistent MR and AR.

Q22. How is the assessment of severity of MS done on Doppler study?
Ans. It is done by measuring $P_{1/2}$ time, MPG, and valve area **(Fig. 6.3)**.

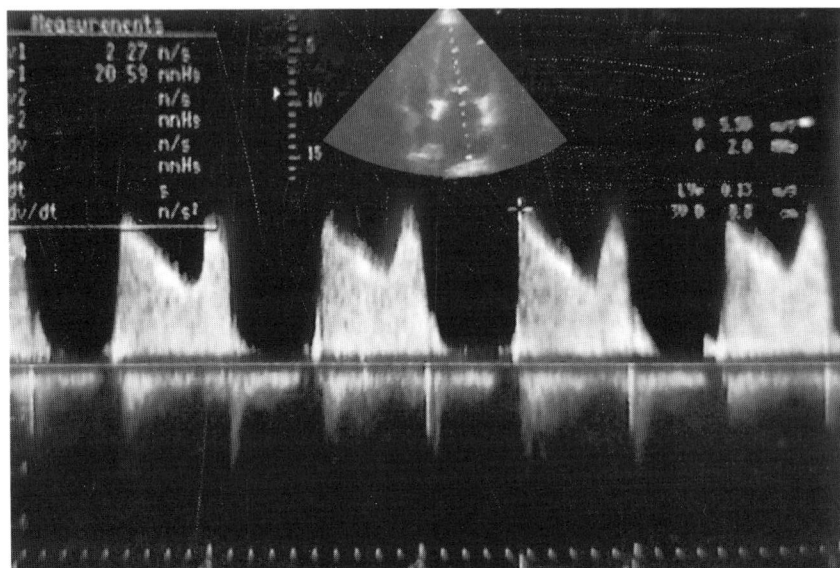

Fig. 6.3: Continuous wave Doppler (CWD) in patient with severe mitral stenosis (MS).

$P_{1/2}$ time, MPG, and MVA measurement with CWD categorizes severity of MS as shown in **Table 6.2**.

TABLE 6.2: Grading severity of mitral stenosis (MS).

Severity	Pressure half time (ms)	MPG (mm Hg)	Valve area (cm²)
Mild	100–149	<5	2.2–1.6
Moderate	150–220	5–10	1.5–1.0
Severe	>220	>10	<1.0

(MPG: mean pressure gradient)

Q23. What are the echocardiographic findings of severe MS?
Ans.
- *M-mode echo, 2DE findings:*
  - EF slop <10 mm/sec (persistently high LA pressure throughout diastole keeps leaflets open)
  - Anterior diastolic motion of PML (by large and more mobile AML)
  - Dilated RA and right ventricle; RVH
  - Severe sclerosis of AML and PML
  - PH (loss of 'a-dip' on M-mode)
  - Inferior vena cava (IVC) plethora
  - MVA less than 1 cm² (on planimetry)
- *Doppler echo findings:*
  - Transvalvular MPG >12 mm Hg
  - MVA <1 cm² (by $P_{1/2}$ time method)
  - At least mild TR
  - Raised PASP (measured from TR gradient).

Q24. How does echo guide suitability of balloon valvotomy in MS?

Ans. In general, a valve is suitable for valvotomy if there is significant MS with the following:
- Mobile and pliant anterior leaflet base
- No severe thickening of chordae
- No commissural calcium
- No more than mild MR
- No visible LA thrombus.

Q25. Does a patient with MS need catheterization?

Ans. With availability of Doppler echo, cardiac catheterization is rarely needed. The hemodynamic parameters, such as transvalvular gradient and pulmonary artery pressure correlate well with Doppler-estimated parameters. It may be indicated in elderly patients (>40 years.) to exclude CAD (by CAG). Catheterization may subject the patient to the risk of complications. It also places a heavy economic burden on patients and hospital resources.

Q26. What are the principles of drug therapy in MS?

Ans.
- Prevention of recurrent rheumatic fever by penicillin prophylaxis for beta-hemolytic streptococci
- Prevention and treatment of complications of MS, such as AF, congestive heart failure (CHF)
- Intervention at optimal time after monitoring the progression.

Q27. What is the treatment of MS with AF?

Ans.

Drugs: Digoxin, to slow ventricular rate, small dose of betablocker may be added when digoxin fails to control ventricular rate. Maintenance of sinus rhythm can be tried with quinidine (in new onset of AF). Anticoagulation with warfarin is imperative to prevent thromboembolism. International normalized ratio (INR) to be maintained between 2.0 and 3.0. It has to continue till sinus rhythm returns or valvotomy is done. If thromboembolic phenomenon occurs, warfarin is used even if the patient is in sinus rhythm and continued up to the time of valvotomy and 3-4 weeks thereafter.

- *Direct current (DC) cardioversion:* It can be effective in young patients if AF is of relatively recent onset (i.e., less than ½ year) and LA size is less than 5 cm. It is preceded by 3-4 weeks of anticoagulation to reduce risk of arterial embolism. Duration should be twice as long if echo reveals thrombus. If sinus rhythm is restored, anticoagulation is continued for another 3-4 weeks or until atrial activity returns. Digoxin must be stopped for 4 weeks before giving DC shock, otherwise lignocaine pretreatment is done. In patients who cannot be converted to or maintained in sinus rhythm, resting ventricular rate is maintained at 60-65 per minute with digoxin. If it is not possible, then a small dose of atenolol (25 mg/day) is added.

- *Interventional:* Some suggest that occurrence of AF is an indication for valvotomy (surgical or percutaneous). If thromboembolism occurs, MBV or closed mitral commissurotomy (CMC) should be withheld for 3-6 months. Open mitral commissurotomy (OMC) can be undertaken which allows removal of any atrial thrombi during the procedure. It is recommended that intervention should be done if recurrent thromboembolism occurs, even if the patient is asymptomatic.

Q28. How is mechanical relief achieved in MS?
Ans.
- *Closed mitral valvotomy:* Simple, inexpensive, good long-term outcome in suitable cases; general anesthesia is needed.
- *Open mitral valvotomy:* Valvotomy under direct visualization; concurrent annuloplasty for MR feasible; general anesthesia is needed.
- *Mitral valve replacement:* Feasible in all patients regardless of calcification or severity of MR; chronic anticoagulation with prosthetic valve. Annular-papillary muscle continuity is lost.
- *Balloon mitral valvuloplasty:* Percutaneous procedure under local anesthesia; no direct visualization of valve; good long-term outcome in selected cases; contraindicated in MR grade >2+.

Q29. When is MVR indicated?
Ans. Mitral valve replacement is recommended for symptomatic patients with severe MS [MVA <1.5 cm^2 in the New York Heart Association (NYHA) Class III or IV] whose valve are not suitable for valvotomy (BMV or surgical repair). Usually MVR is required for patients with combined MS and moderate to severe MR, those with extensive commissural calcification, severe fibrosis, and subvalvular fusion, and those who have undergone previous valvotomy. Generally, a mechanical valve is preferred when MVR for MS is necessary, and AF is present because of the need for chronic anticoagulation.

Q30. Recurrence of symptoms following mitral valvotomy—what are the possibilities?
Ans. Mitral valvotomy, whether percutaneous or operative and open or closed, is palliative rather than curative and even when successful, some degree of valve dysfunction remains. Recurrence of symptoms is often not caused by restenosis but may be caused by one or more of the following:
- An inadequate first procedure with residual stenosis
- Increased severity of MR (either at operation or developing subsequently)
- Progression of aortic or tricuspid valve (TV) disease
- Development of CAD.

Restenosis is due to turbulent flow in paravalvular region with leaflet calcification and stiffness and is not usually the result of recurrent rheumatic fever. These are like the changes occurring on a bicuspid aortic valve (BAV).

Q31. What is the role of digoxin in MS?
Ans. Digoxin is necessary in the following:
- *Atrial fibrillation:* To slow ventricular rate by its vagal effect.
- *Right HF:* To reduce symptoms by its positive inotropic effect.

It usually does not alter the hemodynamics and usually does not benefit patients with pure stenosis and sinus rhythm.

Q32. What are the ways of mechanical relief in MS?
Ans.
- Mitral balloon valvuloplasty
- Closed mitral valvotomy
- Open mitral valvotomy
- Mitral valve replacement

Q33. What are indications of valvotomy (CMV or BMV)?
Ans.
- Patients with significant symptoms (NYHA class II or greater).
- History of systemic embolism, even if patients are asymptomatic now (to prevent recurrent thromboembolism).
- Pregnancy with MS, midtrimester valvotomy (preferably MBV) done even if patient is not significantly symptomatic, it is done to avoid development of pulmonary edema in late pregnancy or after delivery.
- Patients with features of PH.
- *Echocardiographic parameters:*
  - Isolated MS no (or trivial) MR
  - MVA <1 cm^2 (even if patient is mildly symptomatic)
  - Mobile, noncalcified valve without significant subvalvular changes
  - Left atrium free of thrombus.

Q34. Compare between CMV and BMV?
Ans. Balloon mitral valvuloplasty is a structural intervention with balloon on stenosed MV, commonly done with Inoue balloon technique. It is the procedure of choice. Surgical CMV with metallic dilator is also practiced occasionally. The differences between the two are listed in **Table 6.3**.

TABLE 6.3: Comparison between closed mitral commissurotomy (CMC) and mitral balloon valvuloplasty (MBV).

Points	CMV	MBV
Route	Done through thoracotomy and atriotomy	Done percutaneously, through femoral vein
Dilatation done by	Metallic Tubb's dilator	Balloon inflation by contrast material
Cost	Less costly	More, especially if balloon is not reused
Efficacy	Good	Good with disposable balloon; may deteriorate if reused

Contd...

Contd...

Surgical and anesthetic hazard	Present	Absent
Hospital stay	7–10 days	1–2 days
Subsequent risk of thromboembolism	Reduced by removal of the left atrial appendage	Remains
Indication	Wider	Symptomatic patients with favorable valve morphology, patients with severe PH (even asymptomatic) who are high-risk candidates for surgery. Pregnant women (midtrimester), and old patients with serious extracardiac diseases (poor operative candidates)

(CMV: closed mitral valvotomy)

Q34. Differentiate between CMV and OMV.
Ans. Closed mitral valvotomy is a blind procedure done on beating heart through a side hole made on lateral chest wall. OMV is an open surgical procedure done under cardiopulmonary bypass that allows direct visualization of MV apparatus and adjacent structures. Thus, these two procedures have their unique features listed in **Table 6.4**.

TABLE 6.4: Difference between closed and open mitral commissurotomy.

CMV	OMV
Done on beating heart through a thoracotomy; blind procedure, dilatation done with metallic dilator. Risk of embolism from LA remains (hence, TEE should exclude thrombus in left atrium)	Done under cardiopulmonary bypass. Direct visualization of valves with debridement of calcium and splitting of fused commissures and chordae done; thrombus (if any) removed preoperative
Cost low	Cost very high
Hospital stay short	Longer
May be undertaken only in pure MS	May be undertaken in patients with coexistent lesions in other valves, which can be treated simultaneously

■ MITRAL REGURGITATION

Mitral valve apparatus anatomically includes MV leaflets, chordae tendineae, papillary muscles, and mitral annulus. Abnormalities of any of these structures may cause MR.

Q1. How do we classify MR?
Ans.
- *Clinically (depending on duration):* Acute (left atrium, left ventricle not dilated), and chronic (left atrium, left ventricle dilated)

- *Etiologically:* Primary (organic) and secondary (functional)—ischemic (maybe acute or chronic) and nonischemic
- *Type of leaflet motion:* Type I (normal motion), type II (increased motion), type IIIa (restricted opening), and type IIIb (restricted closure). In general, type II and type IIIa are usually caused by primary disorder of the leaflets, whereas type I and IIb have relatively normal leaflets, which are distorted by left ventricle and annular remodeling causing secondary MR.

Q2. How is the staging of chronic primary MR done?
Ans. The 2014 AHA/American College of Cardiology Foundation (ACCF) guidelines are as follows:
- *Stage A (at risk of MR):* Asymptomatic; mild MVP, mild MV thickening; no or small central MR jet <20% left atrium
- *Stage B (progressive MR):* Asymptomatic; severe MVP (with normal coaptation), rheumatic valve changes, and noncoaptation. Previous IE; central jet MR: 20–40% left atrium, angiographic grade 1–2+, mild LAE, no LVE, normal PAP
- *Stage C (asymptomatic severe MR):* Severe MVP (with noncoaptation), rheumatic valve changes and noncoaptation. Previous IE; central jet MR >40% left atrium, angiographic grade 3–4+, moderate or severe LAE, LVE, PH±
  - *Stage C1:* Left ventricular ejection fraction (LVEF) >60% and left ventricular end-systolic diameter (LVESD) <40 mm
  - *Stage C2:* LVEF ≤60% and left ventricular end-systolic volume (LVESV) ≥40 mm
- *Stage D (symptomatic severe MR):* Severe MVP (with normal coaptation), rheumatic valve changes and noncoaptation. Previous IE; central jet MR >40% left atrium or holosystolic eccentric jet MR; angiographic grade 3–4+, moderate to severe LAE, LVE, and PH with exertional dyspnea and poor exercise tolerance.

Q3. What are the stages of ischemic MR?
Ans. Ischemic MR is a subset of secondary MR caused by regional ventricular dysfunction from prior myocardial infarction (MI).
- *Stage A:* Following acute myocardial infarction (AMI); at risk stage
- *Stage B:* Symptomatic; progressive
- *Stage C:* Asymptomatic severe stage (prior to onset of HF symptoms)
- *Stage D:* Following onset of HF; symptomatic severe stage.

Q4. How does MR develop in rheumatic fever?
Ans. Acute rheumatic fever is a frequent cause of isolated severe MR among adolescents in developing countries including Bangladesh, that has a rapidly progressive course.

Here, chronic rheumatic heart disease (RHD) remains a common cause of MR. It results from shortening, rigidity, deformity, and retraction of one or both mitral cusps with associated shortening and fusion of the chordae tendineae and papillary muscles.

Q5. How does primary MR differ from secondary MR?

Ans. Primary and secondary MR are two distinctly different disease conditions with different pathophysiology, management strategies, and outcomes. Primary MR results from pathological process affecting the MV leaflets. Secondary MR develops as a result of annular dilatation and tethering of leaflets from geographic displacement of papillary muscles leading to restricted leaflet closure and incomplete coaptation during systole. It is a marker of significant regional or global LV dysfunction.

Primary MR, in the long run, may lead to secondary MR with development of significant LV dysfunction. Thus, MR begets MR.

Q6. What are the hemodynamic changes in acute MR?

Ans. In acute MR, there is marked elevation of pressure in the pulmonary vasculature, thus right-sided HF results. Here, murmur is not holosystolic (ends before A_2), loud P_2, paradoxical splitting of A_2 may be found. In severe acute MR secondary to AMI, Frank cardiogenic shock may develop. Afterload reduction with IV nitroprusside may be lifesaving.

Q7. How does acute MR differ from chronic MR?

Ans.

- In acute MR, the sudden burden of the regurgitant volume on normal chambers does not allow compensatory dilation of the left atrium and left ventricle. Consequently, marked elevations of left atrium and pulmonary venous pressure are produced, which may lead to acute pulmonary edema.
- In chronic MR, long-standing volume overload produces dilatation of left atrium and left ventricle. The major burden and threat of acute MR is to the pulmonary venous circulation and lung, whereas in chronic MR, the major burden is carried by left ventricle. The two conditions differ in the following aspects listed in **Table 6.5**.

TABLE 6.5: Difference between acute and chronic mitral regurgitation (MR).

	Acute	Chronic
Left atrium	Small, noncompliant	Large, compliant
Left ventricular	Not dilated; no dysfunction	Dilated; dysfunction occurs at a later stage
Symptoms	Sudden onset of dyspnea and pulmonary edema	Occur lately; fatigue and dyspnea
Sign	No left atrial pulsation in precordium, murmur is early or midsystolic	Precordial pulsation due to enlarged left atrium usual, murmur is pansystolic
	Patients usually in sinus rhythm	Atrial fibrillation may develop
	Large V-wave in wedge tracing	Lower V-wave in wedge tracing, except on effort

Valvular Heart Diseases

Q8. How does ischemic heart disease (IHD) produce MR?
Ans. Ischemic heart disease may produce acute as well as chronic MR.
- *Acute MR:* Rupture of papillary muscle by infarction, or papillary muscle dysfunction due to ischemia. MR is organic in origin.
- *Chronic MR:* Dilatation of left ventricle by long-standing ischemia, i.e., ischemic cardiomyopathy. Here MR is functional.

Q9. How is the degree of MR assessed clinically?
Ans.
- The greater the shifting of apex beat on palpation
- The greater and later the left parasternal movement (LA expansion)
- The louder and longer the apical systolic murmur
- The louder the S_3 and wider the splitting of S_2.
The greater the degree of MR.

Q10. Compare and contrast between MS and MR.
Ans. Mitral stenosis and MR are two opposite types of lesions with different clinical features, but have some overlapping features as discussed below in **Table 6.6**:

TABLE 6.6: Comparison between mitral stenosis (MS) and mitral regurgitation (MR).

Points	MS	MR
Sex	Female > Male	Male > Female
Cause	Mostly rheumatic (rarely congenital)	Varied cause
Symptoms	• Hemoptysis and systemic embolism are more common • Infective endocarditis uncommon • PH and RHF more	• Less common • More common • PH and RHF less common
Sign	• S_1 loud (unless calcified), S_2 not split, loud P_2 more common, S_3 never present. • Left parasternal lift is sustained (due to RVH) • Apex tapping, not shifted • OS present, if valve pliable. MDM longer, presystolic murmur present in sinus rhythm. • Apical pansystolic murmur usually absent (occ. heard due to transmitted TR)	• Never loud • S_2 usually split, loud P_2 less often S_3 commonly present and loud • Lift is less sustained and late (due to LA enlargement) • Apex hyperdynamic (forceful and ill-sustained) and shifted • OS rarely present • MDM if present, short; presystolic absent • Present
Investigation: CXR,	Cardiac shadow normal in TD	Enlarged, left ventricle type

Contd...

Contd...

ECG	RVH (if PH present) usual	LVH (RVH rare)
Echocardiography	Left atrium enlarged, left ventricle normal, E-F slope reduced, MV domed, MVO reduced; PH more	Left atrium hugely enlarged, LV volume overload with increased septal- and post- wall motion, E-F slope increased; AV closes early, MV leaflets noncoapted. MVO normal; PH less. Doppler signal in left atrium during systole
Hemodynamic data	LA pressure is usually greatly raised; gradient across valve in diastole; PVR may be severely raised	LA pressure raised less severely; no gradient usually. PVR is less often raised
Treatment	Vasodilators are contraindicated	Vasodilators are indicated (particularly helpful in acute MR)

Q11. How do we differentiate MS from MR on chest X-ray?
Ans. Both conditions cause LA enlargement, but MR also causes LV enlargement. Thus, MR causes cardiomegaly, but MS does not **(Fig. 6.4)**. Other radiological differences also exist as listed in **Table 6.7**.

TABLE 6.7: Radiological differences between mitral stenosis (MS) and mitral regurgitation (MR).

Points	MS	MR
Cardiomegaly	Nil	Yes
LAE	Less marked (pressure overload)	More (volume overload)
PH	Develops early	Late (capacious LV decompression into left atrium)
Pulmonary edema	More, early	Late, LV dysfunction in chronic MR; early in acute MR

(MR: mitral regurgitation; MS: mitral stenosis; LAE: left atrial enlargement; PH: pulmonary hypertension; LV: left ventricular)

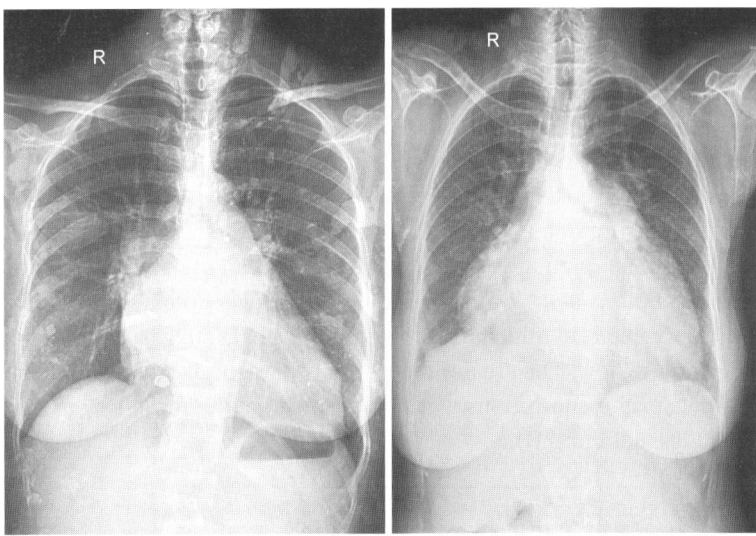

Figs. 6.4: MS (right) and MR (left) on chest X-ray P/A view.

Q12. What is the role of Doppler echo in evaluating patients with MR?

Ans. Doppler study is useful in diagnosing MR, determining its severity and cause.

- *Color-flow imaging* allows detection and visualization of regurgitant jet, including its direction and orientation within left atrium. It can determine the severity and cause of MR **(Fig. 6.5)**.
  - *Assessment of severity of MR:* It can be made semiquantitatively from the color-flow jet-length mapping:
    - *1+ (trivial):* Regurgitant jet is seen behind leaflets
    - *2+ (mild):* Jet extends one-third way back into left atrium
    - *3+ (moderate):* Jet extends two-thirds way back into left atrium
    - *4+ (severe):* Jet extends to the back wall of left atrium.

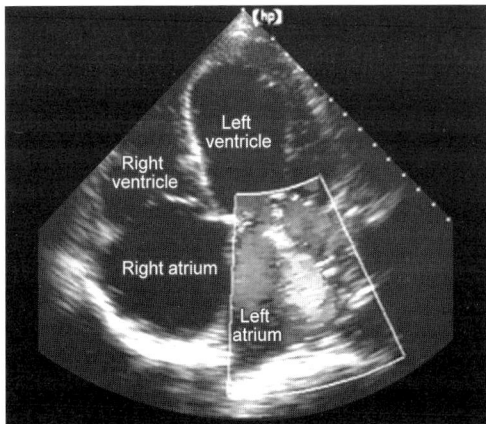

Fig. 6.5: Severe mitral regurgitation (MR) on color-flow imaging.

- *Cause of MR:* A central jet implies noncoaptation, as in functional MR. A central jet moves freely within left atrium and recruits more surrounding red blood cells (RBCs), thus MR grade may be overestimated (the "bowling ball effect"). Rheumatic MR jet is directed posteriorly (when AML is more affected) or anteriorly (when PML is more affected). Eccentric jets are obstructed by LA wall and its size is underestimated (the "Coanda effect"). In this case the regurgitation should be calculated to one grade higher than the observed grade.
- *Continuous wave Doppler:* Spectral display is holosystolic with peak flow velocity at mid. Early or late systolic peaks suggest contamination from AS flow. The greater the intensity of regurgitant jet and the more denser the continuous wave (CW) envelop, the more severe the MR **(Figs. 6.6A and B)**.

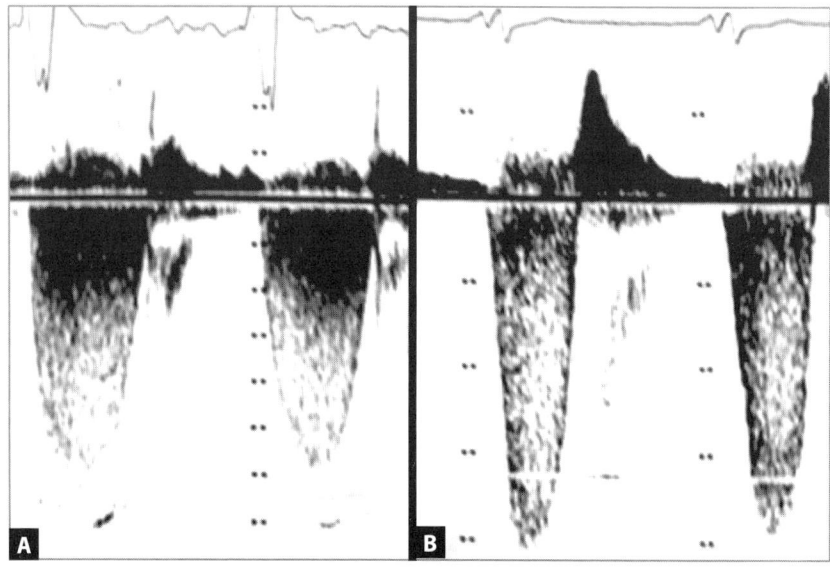

Figs. 6.6A and B: Moderate MR (A); severe MR (B) on CWD.
(MR: mitral regurgitation; CWD: continuous wave Doppler)

- *Pulsed-wave Doppler:* Study done in apical 4-chamber with sample volume within left atrium near coaptation point of mitral leaflets. It allows detection, quantification of MR. A large region of abnormal signal within left atrium suggests severe MR. Severity of MR can also be quantitated by calculating regurgitant volume and regurgitant fraction. Difference between mitral flow and aortic flow is the regurgitant volume. It is also helpful in determining the timing of regurgitation—holosystolic (classical) or late systolic, e.g., in MVP. PWD can be useful in estimation of regurgitant volume, and assessing pulmonary venous flow and severity of MR.

Q13. How does cardiac catheterization help patients having MR?
Ans.
- *Confirmation of diagnosis:* A tall 'V' wave in left atrium, or pulmonary capillary wedge pressure (PCWP) tracing is characteristic.
- *Exclusion of other valvular lesions.*
- *Assessment of LV function:* E-F slope can be assessed from LV graphy. The presence of LV dysfunction may be confirmed by finding a high left ventricular end-diastolic pressure (LVEDP).
- *Assessment of severity of MR:* The grading system from LV graphy is as follows **(Fig. 6.7)**:
    - *1+ (mild):* Contrast from left atrium clears with each beat; the entire left ventricle is never opacified
    - *2+ (moderate):* Contrast does not clear with one beat; may faintly opacify left atrium
    - *3+ (moderately severe):* Complete opacification of left atrium, equal in intensity to left ventricle.
    - *4+ (severe):* Complete opacification of left atrium in one beat; contrast material refluxes into the pulmonary veins.

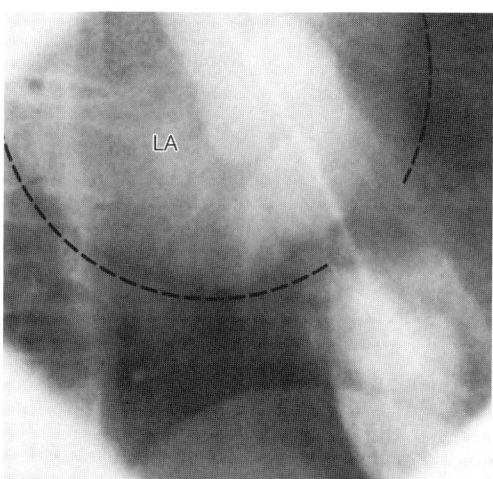

Fig. 6.7: LV graphy showing severe MR (hugely dilated left atrium outlined). (LA: left atrium; LV: left ventricle; MR: mitral regurgitation)

- *Coronary angiography:* It helps to ascertain the presence of concomitant CAD. Men older than 40 years and women older than 50 years, even in the absence of symptoms or risk factors for CAD, should undergo CAG before surgery.

Q14. When is MV repair (MVRe) indicated?
Ans. Mitral valve repair is strongly recommended whenever possible. It is most successful in the following:

- Children and adolescents with pliable valves
- Adults with MR secondary to MVP
- Cases with annular dilatation
- Cases with chordal rupture
- Cases with perforation of leaflet caused by IE.

It is less successful in older patients with rigid, calcified, deformed valves, and RHD. However, younger patients with severe rheumatic MR in the absence of active carditis may undergo MVRe.

Q15. What are the transcatheter therapies for MR?
Ans.
- *Transcatheter mitral valve repair (TMVr) with MitraClip system:* Here, mitral edge-to-edge repair is done for symptomatic patients with primary MR, who are at a high risk for surgery and have suitable anatomy. Percutaneous MVRe provides relief from severe MR in patients who would otherwise not be candidates for surgical correction, or in those who prefer a less invasive approach without the need for cardiopulmonary bypass. It provides significant and durable reduction of MR and improves outcome. MitraClip system **(Fig. 6.8)** is the best studied percutaneous MVRe providing edge-to-edge leaflet repair. Recently, transcatheter mitral valve replacement (TMVR) has shown interesting results.

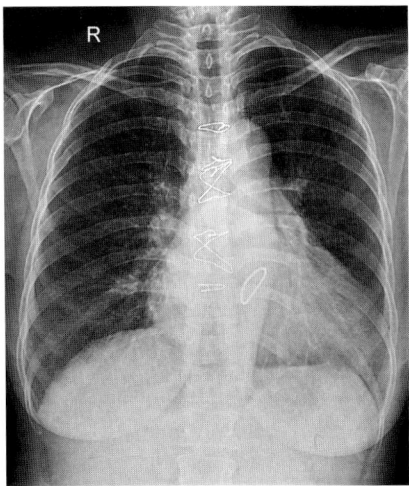

Fig. 6.8: MitraClip in situ.

- *Transcatheter mitral valve replacement:* It is rapidly evolving as a treatment option for symptomatic MR patients who present with high surgical risk and are not suitable for surgery. It is a viable alternative to traditional surgical treatment. The TMVR devices have expanded treatment options for complex MV diseases. Thus, MR, MS, and mixed MVD—all could potentially be candidates for TMVR.

Q16. Surgical repair or replacement—which one is preferred for MR?

Ans. Surgical repair is preferred over replacement in primary MR. It is the gold-standard care providing superior outcomes. It involves leaflet resection, chordal transposition, annuloplasty repair, and implantation of artificial chordae.

In secondary MR, the optimal approach is less defined. Either surgical or valve replacement may be undertaken.

Q17. When is surgery undertaken in MR?

Ans. The goal of surgery is prevention of development of irreversible changes in myocardial structure and function. Hence, MVR should be performed before LV dysfunction is severe and irreversible (E-F <30% and/or end-systolic dimension >55 mm).

It is indicated in the following:

- Patients having disabling symptoms with hemodynamically significant MR.
- Patients with progressive LV dilatation or dysfunction on echocardiographic and hemodynamic studies, even if symptom is not disabling [i.e., left ventricular internal diameter at end systole (LVIDs) >50 mm and EF <50%].
- Patients having PH (PASP >50 mm Hg) or AF with preserved LV function, even though asymptomatic.
- Acute symptomatic MR in which repair is likely to be beneficial.
- Post infarction MR—papillary muscle infarction or rupture usually require urgent MVR.

Q18. When to consider MVR and MVRe?

Ans. Without surgical treatment, the prognosis for patients with MR and HF is poor. Hence, MVRe or MVR is indicated in symptomatic patients. MVRe is strongly recommended whenever possible (e.g., annular dilatation, MVP, papillary muscle dysfunction, chordal rupture, perforation of leaflet in IE). MVRe with chordal preservation may be undertaken in severe LV dysfunction [EF <30% and/or left ventricular internal diameter at end diastole (LVIDd) >55 mm]. Young patients with severe MR may undergo repair.

■ AORTIC STENOSIS

Q1. Classify aortic valve (AV) disease.

Ans.

- *On the basis of valvular dysfunction:* AS and AR
- *On the basis of underlying pathology:* Age-related calcific AS (formerly called senile or degenerative), rheumatic, congenital, i.e., BAV.

Q2. What is calcific aortic valve diseases (CAVDs)?

Ans. It is age-related aortic valvular change with stenosis and calcification on morphologically normal **(Figs. 6.9A and B)** or congenitally BAV. It shares many pathophysiological features in common with atherosclerosis, and represents a proliferative and inflammatory change with accumulation of lipids. It may lead to bone formation analogous to vascular calcification.

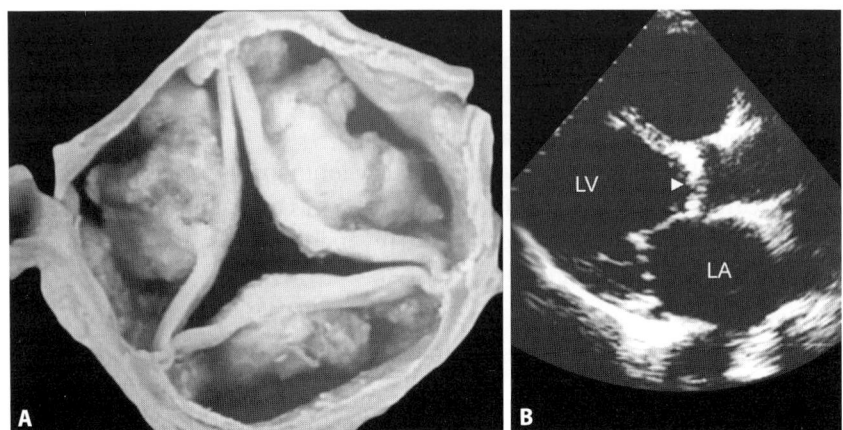

Figs. 6.9A and B: Calcific aortic valve (A); 2-D (two- dimensional) echocardiography (B). (LA: left atrium; LV: left ventricle)

CAVD has the following features:
- Involves base of leaflets, spares edges, and there is no commissural fusion (in contrast to rheumatic AS).
- Risk factors are similar to those for vascular atherosclerosis—hypertension, smoking, diabetes mellitus (DM), increased low-density lipoprotein (LDL), lipoprotein(a) [LP(a)].
- It is also linked to metabolic syndrome.
- Increases risk of cardiovascular death by 50%.

Q3. What is aortic sclerosis?
Ans. In aortic sclerosis, there is mild focal area of valve thickening without impairment of leaflet motion. It is found in 25% adults over 65 years, and in 50% over 85 years. In contrast to AS, there is no significant obstruction to outflow. Aortic sclerosis may progress over time to AS. The prevalence of aortic sclerosis increases with age. Progression from sclerosis to stenosis is 1.8–1.9% per year. With the population aging, prevalence of AS is expected to increase in the community.

Q4. What is the difference between AS and aortic sclerosis?
Ans. Aortic stenosis is an obstruction to the outflow of blood from the left ventricle to aorta. The obstruction may be at the valve (valvular), above the valve (supravalvular), or below the valve (subvalvular).

In aortic sclerosis, valve leaflets are thickened and sclerosed, but their motion is not restricted. Hence, there is no obstruction to LV outflow.

Q5. Classify AS.
Ans.
- *Etiologically:*
  - Congenital—degeneration and calcification of BAV.
  - Acquired—senile and rheumatic.
- *According to the site of stenosis:* Valvular, supravalvular, and subvalvular
- *Depending on severity (by hemodynamic study; in presence of normal COP):*
  - *Mild AS:* Valve area >1.5 cm^2, peak systolic pressure gradient across AV: <50 mm Hg
  - *Moderate AS:* Valve area >1.0 to 1.5 cm^2, gradient: 50–75 mm Hg
  - *Severe AS:* Valve area ≤1.0 cm^2, gradient: >75 mm Hg

Q6. What are the stages of valvular AS?
Ans. The 2014 AHA/ACCF guidelines are as follows:
- *Stage A (at risk of AS):* Asymptomatic BAV
- *Stage B (progressive AS):* Asymptomatic; mild (gradient: <20 mm Hg) to moderate (gradient: 20–39 mm Hg)
- *Stage C (asymptomatic severe AS):*
  - *Stage C1:* With normal LVEF
  - *Stage C2:* With LV dysfunction
- *Stage D (symptomatic severe AS):*
  - *Stage D1:* High gradient; normal LVEF
  - *Stage D2:* Low gradient with reduced LVEF
  - *Stage D3:* Low gradient with normal LVEF.

Q7. What is severe AS? What are its types?
Ans. Aortic stenosis is leveled as severe when the aortic valve area (AVA) is ≤1.0 cm^2, mean AV gradient is ≥40 mm Hg, or peak jet velocity is ≥4 m/s. Severe AS may be of the following categories:
- *Depending on symptoms:* Symptomatic (Stage D1 of AHA) or asymptomatic (Stage C of AHA)
- *Depending on gradient:* High flow, high gradient: MPG ≥40 mm Hg, and low flow and low gradient: MPG ≤40 mm Hg

Again, low gradient AS may be of two types:
1. *With reduced LVEF (EF <50%):* Stage gradient decreases with development of LV dysfunction.
2. *With preserved LVEF (EF >50%):* A paradoxical low gradient occurring in elderly patients with small, hypertrophied left ventricle, or those with concurrent hypertension (with reduced transaortic flow).

Q8. What is silent AS?
Ans. When aortic murmur is absent in severe AS with congestive HF, it is called silent AS. When failure improves, the murmur reappears. In the

meantime, characteristic carotid pulse and radiologic evidence of valvular calcification reveal the diagnosis.

Q9. How does concomitant MS affect AS?
Ans.
- *Symptom:* Patients with concomitant MS and AS are symptomatic from early on.
- *Sign:* MS decreases loudness of AS murmurs (as flow through AV is less), but unless MS is very severe, AS murmur dominates and can even cause MS murmurs to be absent. This is because of loss of compliance caused by left ventricular hypertrophy (LVH), induced by AS. It results in slow diastolic expansion of LV, and attenuates murmur of MS. When AF is found in AS, the possibility of associated MV disease should be considered. Loss of atrial contribution of ventricular filling may cause serious hypotension.

  In such conditions, mitral valvotomy is performed first as the procedure is less hazardous.

  Degree of AS may be grossly underestimated if MS is severe. Signs of AS are considerably diminished and gradient across the valve may read only 25 mm Hg in spite of severe AS.

Q10. What are the signs of severe AS?
Ans.
- *Pulsus parvus et tardus:* In carotid; thrill along carotid artery. An apparently normal carotid pulse does not exclude severe AS; coexisting hypertension or AR may alter the finding.
- *Ejection systolic murmur of grade 3 or greater:* Although with LV failure SV falls, AS murmur becomes softer; rarely disappears altogether.
- *Single S_2:* Indicating calcification and immobility, buried P_2 within prolonged aortic ejection murmur, and prolongation of LV systole making A_2 coincide with P_2.

Q11. What is pulsus parvus et tardus?
Ans. *Parvus* means "low amplitude", and *tardus* means "slow-rising", "late-peaking". In severe AS a slow-rising, late-peaking (tardus), low-amplitude (parvus) carotid pulse is a characteristic feature.

Q12. What is Gallavardin phenomenon?
Ans. It is the high frequency systolic murmur radiating to apex in AS that may be mistaken for murmur of MR. Dynamic auscultation differentiates—murmur of valvular AS is augmented by squatting [increased stroke volume (SV)] and reduced by Valsalva maneuver and standing (reduced transvalvular flow).

Q13. How does MR coexist with AS?
Ans. Aortic valve disease is present in nearly one third of patients with rheumatic MS.

Aortic stenosis often accompanies MR (organic or functional). It may be difficult to recognize two distinct systolic murmurs. The increased LV pressure secondary to left ventricular outflow tract (LVOT) obstruction may augment MR flow, whereas the presence of MR may diminish LV preload and SV. The cause and severity of AS and MR can be accurately diagnosed with echo.

Q14. How does dobutamine echo help in the assessment of AS severity?
Ans. Dobutamine echo is used to augment flow to differentiate severe AS from pseudo-severe AS, such as moderate AS with primary LV dysfunction. In severe AS, aortic velocity increases to at least 4 m/s. It can also provide evidence of myocardial contractile reserve (increase in SV >20% of baseline), which is an important predictor of operative risk and survival after AVR in these patients. Among symptomatic patients with severe AS, prognosis is worst when left ventricle fails, and COP and transvalvular gradient are low.

Q15. How is follow-up of asymptomatic AS done?
Ans. Patients are followed up clinically and with echo based on AS severity.
- *Severe AS:* Repeat imaging is performed every 6–12 months.
- *Moderate AS:* Repeat imaging is performed every 1–2 years.
- *Mild AS:* Repeat imaging performed is every 3–5 years.
  A change in signs and symptoms prompts repeat imaging sooner.

Q16. When is AVR indicated in AS?
Ans. Aortic valve replacement is recommended for the following:
- Adults with symptomatic, severe AS (even if symptoms are mild).
- Severe AS with a LVEF <50%.
- Severe asymptomatic AS undergoing coronary artery bypass grafting (CABG) or other heart surgery.
- Apparently asymptomatic severe AS, when exercise testing provokes symptoms or a fall in blood pressure (BP).
- Also considered in asymptomatic cases with very severe calcific AS.

Q17. Surgical aortic valve replacement (SAVR) or TAVR—what is the current choice of therapy in AS?
Ans. Transcatheter aortic valve replacement has become the treatment of choice for patients with degenerative AS. Previously, TAVR was indicated for cases where SAVR could not be undertaken for prohibitive risk. There has been a paradigm shift in this area. Now, SAVR is reserved for patients in whom TAVR is unsuitable. Since 2019, the number of TAVR has exceeded the number of SAVR in many countries. TAVR has also paved the way for percutaneous transcatheter treatment of mitral and TVs. Self-expandable and balloon-expandable transcatheter heart valves (THV) are now available. With aging of the population, increasing number of competent operators and centers, advancing technologies, newer indications, and affordability of the procedure, TAVR technology will expand in the near future.

Q18. When is TAVR a treatment option for AS?
Ans. Transcatheter aortic valve replacement is currently done routinely for symptomatic severe AS patients with high surgical risk, and who are ≥75 years of age. In future, it may be undertaken in patients with moderate AS and HF, moderate but symptomatic AS, asymptomatic severe AS, low flow/low gradient AS, AR, etc.

Q19. What is the prognosis of patients with AS?
Ans.
- Survival is poor once even if mild symptoms develop unless outflow obstruction is relieved. Average survival without AVR is only 1–3 years after symptom onset.
- Sudden cardiac death (SCD) risk is high with symptomatic severe AS. AVR is undertaken promptly. The risk of SCD increases dramatically once symptoms develop. Patients are advised to report promptly of any symptoms possibly related to AS.
- Among symptomatic patients with severe AS, prognosis is worst when left ventricle fails and COP and transvalvular gradient are low.

Q20. How to differentiate different grades of AS?
Ans. Although AS becomes symptomatic when severe, various grades of AS may be differentiated on the following points listed in **Table 6.8**:

TABLE 6.8: Various grades of aortic stenosis (AS)—differentiation.

		Mild	Moderate	Severe
AV area		>1.5 cm^2	>1.0–1.5 cm^2	≤1.0 cm^2
AV gradient		<50 mm Hg	50–75 mm Hg	>75 mm Hg
Symptoms		Rare	May be with unusual stress	Occur with ordinary activities—angina, syncope, heart failure
Signs		Pulse normal	Usually normal	Slow rising
		Apex beat normal	Usually normal; may be heaving	Always heaving and sustained, may be shifted
		A$_2$ present	May be present	A$_2$ absent
		Systolic thrill absent	Absent	Present
		Systolic murmur soft	Peak in early systole	Loud, harsh, with peak in late systole
		S$_4$—absent	Absent	May be present
Investigation		ECG—normal	Usually normal	LVH e-strain
		CXR—normal	Usually normal	Heart may be enlarged, valvular calcification; poststenotic dilatation
		Aortic cusp separation (on M-mode echo) >12 mm	8–12 mm	<8 mm

Contd...

Contd...

Treatment	Not needed	Avoidance of exertion and competitive sports	Aortic valve replacement
Prognosis	Excellent	Good; may progress to severe AS	Lethal, if patient is symptomatic *Mean survival:* 3–4 years in angina, 2–3 years in syncope, 1–2 years in heart failure (if AVR refused)

Q21. How does echo help in patients with AS?
Ans. Echocardiography aids in diagnosis of AS and assessment of its severity.

It may show the following:

- *M-mode echo:* Eccentric closure line in BAV, reduced aortic cusp seperation
- *2DE:* Thickening and calcification of cusps; supra- and subvalvular locations of stenosis may be apparent. LVH and assessment of LV function.
- *Doppler:* Assessment of AV gradient and determining the severity. It may obviate the need for cardiac catheterization, especially in younger patients.

Q22. How is grading of AS done on echo?
Ans.

- *Continuous wave Doppler:* High aortic jet velocity needs CWD. Severity of AS is graded by: Maximum aortic flow velocity, pressure gradient (peak and mean) across AV, and AVA measurement. Various grades of aortic stenosis are shown in **Table 6.9**.

TABLE 6.9: Grading severity of aortic stenosis (AS).

Severity	Maximum flow velocity (m/s)	MPG (mm Hg)	Aortic valve area (cm^2)
Mild	2.5	<15	1.0–1.5
Moderate	2.6–3.9	15–50	0.5–1.0
Severe	4	>50	<0.5

(MPG: mean pressure gradient)

Mean pressure gradient is more accurate than peak gradient for assessment of severity. In severe AS, there is midsystolic peaking of jet velocity, while in less severe cases peaking occurs in early systole. A correct and maximum jet has a distinctive high velocity; audible sound and spectral display show a fine feathery appearance **(Fig. 6.10)**.

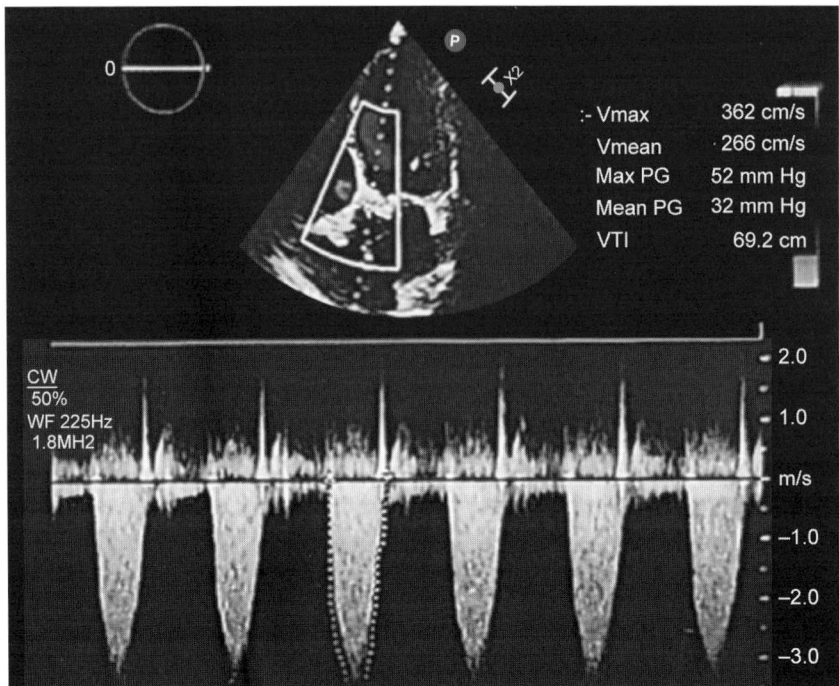

Fig. 6.10: Moderate AS (PPG: 52 mm Hg; MPG: 25 mm Hg).

- *Pulsed-wave Doppler:* LV diastolic compliance can be assessed.
- *Color-flow imaging:* It shows systolic mosaic across stenotic valve with flow acceleration in LVOT. It is a useful adjunct to Doppler. It helps in detecting direction of stenotic jet and allows accurate alignment of CWD cursor.

Q23. What is the role of cardiac catheterization in AS?
Ans. It is done to:
- *Define the degree of stenosis accurately:* Systolic pressure gradient across the stenosis is measured and AVA is calculated.
- Assess the LV function on LV graphy.
- Perform coronary angiography to document possible CAD in patients over the age of 40 years. Significant CAD should be bypassed at the time of AVR.
- Check the aortic root on aortography.

Q24. When is AVR recommended in AS?
Ans.
- Symptomatic patients with severe AS
- Asymptomatic patients with severe AS—who are undergoing CABG, surgery on aortic or other valves, and have LV systolic dysfunction.

Q25. What is the role of aortic valvotomy or balloon valvuloplasty?
Ans. These procedures may be undertaken in the following circumstances:
- In children who are symptomatic or asymptomatic with severe AS with pliable mobile cusps; it is done to allow growth, so that AVR may be done later in life.
- In patients with severe symptoms, in whom surgery may be unduly risky, such as the very elderly or those suffering from other disabling illness, e.g., malignancy.
- To buy time in patients with severe HF, in order to improve surgical risk.
- In subvalvular stenosis, corrective valvotomy to widen the orifice may be helpful.

These procedures have not replaced AVR because of the high rate of restenosis and complications.

Q26. What is transaortic valve implantation (TAVI)?
Ans. This is a new device for percutaneous replacement of stenotic AV, and is an alternative to surgical replacement. Here, the diseased aortic leaflets remain in place. A preliminary balloon aortic valvuloplasty is performed, then a prosthesis consisting of a balloon or self-expanding stent, into which a functional pericardial valve is sewn, is advanced into the aortic orifice over a special guidewire. Deployment of the stent within the diseased valve allows the new pericardial leaflets to begin functioning.

AORTIC REGURGITATION

Q1. Classify AR.
Ans.
- *Etiologically:*
  - Congenital—bicuspid valve, supracristal VSD with prolapse of right coronary cusp ruptured sinus of Valsalva aneurysm.
  - Acquired—rheumatic fever, IE, aortic dissection (Type A), cystic medial necrosis, e.g., Marfan syndrome, ankylosing spondylitis, hypertension, syphilitic aortitis.
- *Clinically:*
  - Acute, e.g., acute rheumatic fever, IE, aortic dissection, surgery, trauma, and prosthetic valve dysfunction.
  - Chronic, e.g., chronic RHD.

Q2. What are the stages of chronic AR?
Ans. The 2014 AHA/ACCF guidelines are as follows:
- *Stage A:* Asymptomatic; at risk of AR, such as BAV, RHD, IE, disease of the aorta, etc., no or trace of AR
- *Stage B:* Asymptomatic; mild (jet <25% of LVOT) to moderate (jet 25-64% of LVOT)

- *Stage C:* Asymptomatic; severe AR (jet >65% of LVOT)
  - *Stage C1:* Mild to moderate LV dilatation; LVESD ≤50%; normal LVEF (>50%)
  - *Stage C2:* Severe LV dilatation; LVESD >50 mm; depressed LVEF (<50%)
- *Stage D:* Symptomatic severe AR; jet >65%; LVESD >50 mm; mild to moderate LV dysfunction (EF <40%); exertional dyspnea, angina, or more severe HF symptoms.

Q3. What are the hemodynamic consequences of acute AR?

Ans. In acute AR, a large volume of regurgitant blood enters LV, which does not get sufficient time to dilate. There is a marked increase in LVEDP, which may approach or exceed LA pressure. As a result, mean LA pressure and pulmonary venous pressure increase and produce varying degrees of pulmonary edema. Acute AR is poorly tolerated and generally requires early surgical treatment.

In contrast to chronic AR, in acute AR the dominant pulsation in neck is venous, not arterial. Also, S_1 is soft (premature closure of MV) with no rocking motion of precordium, and short, soft early diastolic murmur. Tachycardia and low BP are characteristic features.

Q4. How can angina occur in chronic AR?

Ans. With rapid decline in diastolic pressure in the ascending aorta that occurs with severe AR, the driving force for coronary flow, which mainly occurs in diastole, is reduced. Again, late in the course of AR, LVEDP elevates because of a large regurgitant fraction. This combined with low diastolic pressure at coronary ostia, lowers pressure gradient in coronary bed. Patients with coexistent CAD may have a dramatic reduction of coronary flow, resulting in typical angina.

Q5. What are the signs of severe AR, clinically?

Ans.
- Symptoms (may have long asymptomatic period)
- *Peripheral signs:* Hill's sign—disproportionate elevation in femoral arterial systolic pressure compared to brachial: >40 mm Hg; diastolic BP: 30–50 mm Hg; pulse pressure >50% of systolic BP.
- Apex beat shifted downwards and laterally.
- Austin Flint murmur at the apex; systolic murmur in aortic area, and longer duration of early diastolic murmur.

Q6. How to differentiate murmur of AR from Graham Steell murmur?

Ans. Both AR and PR produce EDM. They are differentiated on the following clinical grounds **(Table 6.10)**:

TABLE 6.10: Murmur of aortic regurgitation (AR) and Graham Steell murmur—differences.

AR murmur	Graham Steell murmur
Evidence of rheumatic heart diseases	Evidence of pulmonary hypertension
Systolic flow murmur in aortic area	Nil
EDM in wider area	EDM localized below pulmonary area
Murmur louder in expiration	Louder in inspiration
P_2 not loud	P_2 loud
Systolic thrill in neck (due to high flow)	Nil
Feature of RVH not marked	RVH features marked
Peripheral signs of AR	Nil

Q7. What are the peripheral signs in AR?

Ans. The wide pulse pressure can produce the peripheral findings listed in **Table 6.11**, each named after the person who described it except de Musset's sign, who was the patient himself in whom it was noticed first by his attending physician who was his brother.

TABLE 6.11: Peripheral signs of aortic regurgitation (AR).

Sign	Physical findings
Water-hammer pulse (collapsing pulse)	Rapid appearance of high-volume pulse, which suddenly disappears
Corrigan's pulse	Visible carotid pulsation
Quincke's pulse	Capillary pulsation visible in the fingernail bed or lip
de Musset's sign	Head bobbing with each heartbeat
Müller's sign	Systolic pulsation of the uvula
Hill's sign	Popliteal cuff pressure more than brachial cuff pressure
Traube's sign	Pistol shot (systolic) sound over the femoral artery
Duroziez's sign	To-and-fro murmur over the femoral artery induced by light pressure over it

Q8. What are the differences in symptomatology between AS and AR?

Ans. Aortic stenosis and AR demonstrate differing symptomatology as listed in **Table 6.12**:

TABLE 6.12: Symptomatology in aortic stenosis and (AS) and aortic regurgitation (AR).

Points	AS	AR
Asymptomatic period	Shorter	Longer (in mild to moderate AR)
Chest pain	More frequent, on exertion; dev. early	Lately; prominent; nocturnal
Palpitation	Not a feature	Characteristic
Syncope	Prominent feature	Unusual
LV syst. function	Deteriorates earlier	Maintained long through dilatation and hypertrophy
SCD risk	High with severe cases	Low
AVR	Always indicated even in mild symptomatic	Not indicated in asymptomatic; severe
Prognosis	Poor (once symptomatic)	Excellent in symptomatic if normal LV function

(AS: aortic stenosis; AR: aortic regurgitation; LV: left ventricular; syst.: systolic; SCD: sudden cardiac death; AVR: aortic valve replacement)

Q9. What are the differences in semiology between AS and AR?

Ans. Physical signs in AS and AR are contrasting. Although some similarities exist as listed in **Table 6.13**:

TABLE 6.13: Semiology in aortic stenosis (AS) and aortic regurgitation (AR).

Points	AS	AR
Pulse	Low-peak, slow-rising, low volume	Rapid rise and fall (collapsing), high volume
	Anacrotic pulse	Water-hammer pulse
BP	Low-systolic, narrow-pulse pressure	High-systolic, low-diastolic, wide-pulse pressure
Apical impulse	Localized, heaving	Shifted, hyperdynamic
Thrill	Systolic in aortic area (in severe AS)	Along carotid artery (due to high flow)
Heart sounds	A_2 soft, S_4 ±, ejection click (if no calcification)	S_3 ±, no ejection clicks
Murmur	ESM harsh, no EDM, Gallavardin phenomenon ±	ESM soft (flow murmur), EDM
	Carotid shudder present	Carotid shudder—nil

(ESM: early systolic murmur; EDM: early diastolic murmur)

Q10. What are the other valvular diseases that may coexist with AR?
Ans.
- *Aortic regurgitation and mitral stenosis:* Usually, a proximal lesion-mask sign of a distal lesion on physical examination. Thus, significant AR may be missed in patients with severe MS. Wide-pulse pressure may be absent. An accentuated S_1 and an OS in a patient with AR should suggest MV disease.
- *Aortic regurgitation and mitral regurgitation:* Relatively infrequent; clinical features of AR usually dominate, and it is sometimes difficult to determine whether MR is organic or functional. With severe combined regurgitant lesions, blood may reflux into pulmonary veins. The relative severity of each lesion can be assessed by Doppler echo, especially proximal isovelocity surface area (PISA) or vena contracta methods. If severe, the MR may be corrected by annuloplasty at AVR. Functional MR often regresses after AVR alone.

Q11. What is a cor bovinum?
Ans. Patients with severe chronic AR have the largest LV end-diastolic volumes of any form of heart diseases, resulting in so-called cor bovinum (bovine heart). The adaptive response to gradually increasing chronic AR permits the ventricle to function as an effective high-compliance pump, handling a large SV often with little increase in filling pressure for a long time.
Figure 6.11 Cor bobinum in chronic AR on chest X-ray P/A view.

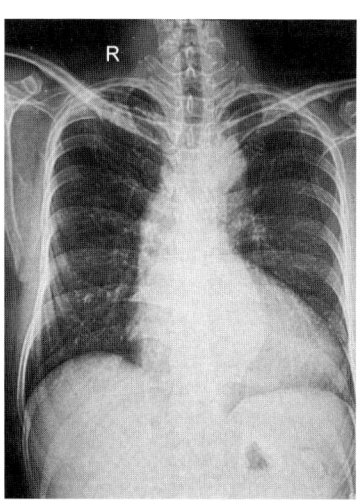

Fig. 6.11: X-ray chest showing cor bobinum in severe chronic AR.

Q12. How does echo help in AR?
Ans. Echocardiography can provide information about the etiology of AR, its severity and LV size and function. It can also exclude other valvular involvement.

- *Effect of regurgitation:*
  - Diastolic fluttering of AML—often present on M-mode and 2DE, decreased MV opening with increased E point septal seperation
  - Dilated ascending aorta, left atrium and left ventricle.

Assessment of LV systolic function—2DE is much superior to M-mode
- *Determination cause of AR:*
  - AV vegetations suggest IE
  - Premature closure of MV—acute AR
  - Prolapse of flail aortic leaflet into LVOT in congenital AR
  - Dilated aortic root with double wall in aortic dissection
- *Exclusion of other valvular lesion:* Associated mitral stenosis in patients with Austin Flint murmur.
- *Confirming the diagnosis and assessing the severity of AR:* Color Doppler imaging may confirm the presence of AR. The severity is assessed by calculating the percentage of LVOT diameter occupied by the regurgitant jet.

Q13. How can Doppler study help in the diagnosis of severity of AR?
Ans.
- *Color Doppler:* Measuring the size of regurgitant jet with CFI that involves measuring the width of regurgitant jet at the orifice of the valve and comparing that diameter with the diameter of subaortic outflow tract (measured about 0.5 cm below the valve) and expressed as a percentage. Severe AR >60%, moderate AR 30–60%, and mild AR <30% **(Figs. 6.12A and B)**.

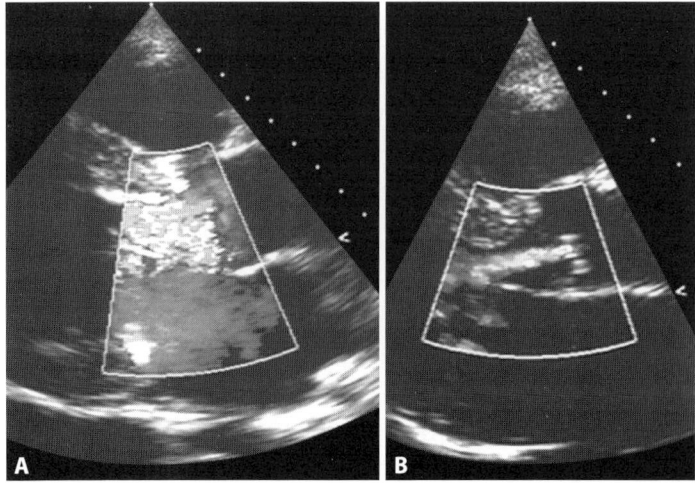

Figs. 6.12A and B: CFI showing severe AR (A) and mild AR (B).
(CFI: color flow imaging; AR: aortic regurgitation)

- *Continuous-wave Doppler:* The rate of decline of regurgitant velocity is an indicator of severity of AR. With severe AR, the gradient from aorta to left ventricle decreases rapidly, and produces a rapid deceleration in diastolic flow velocity **(Fig. 6.13)**.

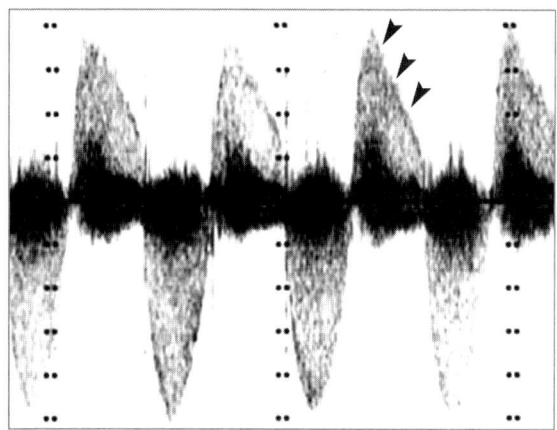

Fig. 6.13: CWD showing moderate AR (left) and severe AR with steep deceleration slope (arrowed). (CWD: Continuous-wave Doppler; AR: aortic regurgitation)

- *Pulsed-wave Doppler:* Tracing in the descending aorta can show holodiastolic flow resulting from the regurgitant, reversed flow.

Q14. What is the role of cardiac catheterization in AR?

Ans. Cardiac catheterization is done to document the following:
- *Severity of AR; done by aortography* **(Fig. 6.14)**:
  - *Grade I:* Faint and incomplete opacification of LV
  - *Grade II:* Faint and complete opacification
  - *Grade III:* LV opacification equal to that of aortic
  - *Grade IV:* Opacification greater than aortic opacity which clears slowly.

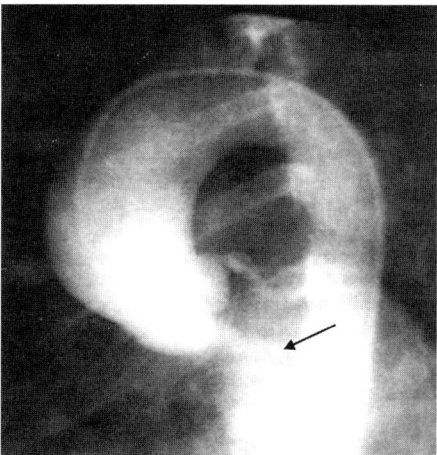

Fig. 6.14: Aortography showing moderate aortic regurgitation (AR) (arrowed).

- Dilatation of aortic root and to exclude rupture sinus of Valsalva, dissection or other rare congenital defects mimicking AR.
- LV function—calculation of LV volume and EF from LV graphy.
- To exclude additional valve lesions—MS, AS, MR, etc.
- Coronary lesions by CAG in patients older than 40 years.

Q15. What are the indications of AVR in patients with AR?
Ans. Asymptomatic patients with severe AR and normal LV function do not require prophylactic operation. They have an excellent prognosis.

In the absence of obvious contraindication or serious comorbidity, AVR is advisable for the following:
- Symptomatic patients (NYHA class III or IV) with preserved LV systolic function
- Patients with progressive LV dilatation or dysfunction on serial studies (even though mildly symptomatic—NYHA class II)
- Patients with mild to moderate LV dysfunction (EF: 25–49%) whether symptomatic or asymptomatic.
- Acute AR—urgent AVR may be needed.
- Rupture sinus of Valsalva aneurysm with AR.
- Sometimes considered when severe LV dilatation (LVIDs >55 mm) occurs in asymptomatic patients with normal LV systolic function.

Surgery should be carried out before severe LV dysfunction has developed as NYHA class III or IV symptoms and LVEF <50% are independent risk factors for poor postoperative survival.

Even after a successful AVR, persistent cardiomegaly and LV dysfunction may persist. Therefore, surgical intervention is highly desirable before irreversible LV changes have occurred.

Aortic valve replacement in severe AR needs a larger prosthetic valve as the aortic annulus is larger; mild postoperative LVOT obstruction is less than that in AS.

Q16. How to follow up a patients with severe AR done?
Ans. Patients with severe AR are known to have a long asymptomatic period. Predictors of development of symptoms are: LV systolic dysfunction and/or an increased LV size (LVIDd ≥70 mm and LVIDs ≥50 mm). Irreversible LV dysfunction may occur when patients are symptomatic, which may preclude valve replacement. Hence, patients with severe AR must be followed carefully with the following:
- Chest X-ray—done every year to see any increase in cardiothoracic ratio.
- Electrocardiogram—done in every 6 months interval to see LVH with or without ST-T changes (strain pattern). This strain pattern indicates deterioration in LV function.
- Echocardiography—done to see progressive LV dilatation and any LV dysfunction (i.e., LVEF). If LVIDs is <50 mm, echo is done yearly, and if LVIDs is 50–54 mm, echo is done every 6 months. AVR is recommended if LVIDs is >55 mm.

TRICUSPID VALVE DISEASE

Q1. What are the causes of TR? Give its treatment.
Ans.
- *Secondary or functional:* Most frequent; due to RV dilatation resulting from PH due to left heart diseases, cor pulmonale, RV infarction, etc.
- *Primary:* RHD, endocarditis in IV drug abusers, Ebstein anomaly.

Treatment includes:
- Treatment of the failure state; often TR improves
- TV repair with an annuloplasty ring to bring the leaflets closer together in patients undergoing MVR.
- TV replacement in those with rheumatic damage.

Q2. When is a TV replacement needed?
Ans.
- In organic diseases of TV with severe TR—Ebstein anomaly, carcinoid, IE, etc.
- Patients with severe functional TR; satisfactory result not achieved by ring annuloplasty at operation table [as assessed by transesophageal echo (TEE)].

The risk of thrombosis of mechanical prosthesis is greater in the tricuspid than in the mitral or aortic position because of low pressure and flow in the right side of the heart. For this reason, a bioprosthesis is the valve of choice for the tricuspid position in adults. Postoperative vitamin-K antagonist is recommended in patients with carcinoid heart disease.

Mild TR without annular dilation does not require surgical treatment. PH reduces after successful MV surgery. However, even mild TR should be repaired if there is a dilation of tricuspid annulus, because it progresses if left untreated.

PROSTHETIC VALVE DISEASES

Q1. What are the types of prosthetic valves?
Ans. There are two types—bioprosthetic and mechanical prosthetic.
1. *Bioprosthetic:* Carpentier-Edwards porcine valve (only the three cloth-covered wire stents are radio-opaque) and valves manufactured from pericardium mounted on a frame. Homograft (cadaveric aortic or pulmonary valves) can be used in a young patient requiring an AVR. In young women who want to have children, a homograft is the valve of choice in the aortic position, accepting the need for a valve replacement in 10 years. In mitral position, however, mechanical valve is better, as a redo MVR carries twice the risk of an AVR redo, and a mitral xenograft deteriorates faster in younger patients, particularly during pregnancy.
2. *Mechanical prosthetic:* Major groups are: Bileaflet (St. Jude's medical)—low bulk, flat profile, low transvalvular gradient, and less thrombogenic (in mitral position). CarboMedics valve is similar and avoids interference

of disc excursion by subvalvular structures. Tilting-disc valve (Bjork—Shiley disc valve), pyrolite carbon discs (not radio-opaque) swing to an angle of 80°, providing a large central orifice. Starr–Edwards ball valve—high profile valve, which has four struts in case of mitral and three in aortic prosthesis. The silastic ball is not seen radiologically.

Q2. What are the normal and abnormal auscultatory findings in prosthetic valves?
Ans.
- *Normal findings:*
  - In Starr–Edwards, tilting disc, and bileaflet-opening click and closing click heard in all three
  - Systolic ejection murmur in aortic position and diastolic murmur in mitral. Diastolic murmur also in aortic position with Bjork–Shiley or Medtronic Hall
  - Starr–Edwards cause mild obstruction; systolic murmur in both aortic and mitral position
- *Abnormal auscultatory findings:*
  - In both bileaflet and tilting disc—decreased intensity of closing clicks in both aortic and mitral position
  - Aortic diastolic murmur in St. Jude's in aortic position and high frequency holosystolic murmur in mitral position for both St. Jude's and bileaflet
  - Starr–Edwards—decreased intensity of opening or closing click in aortic position
  - Aortic diastolic murmur in aortic position
  - High frequency holosystolic murmur in mitral position.

Q3. Compare and contrast between bioprosthetic and mechanical valves.
Ans. Both bioprosthetic and metallic prosthetic valves are indicated in different situations. Also, they differ in durability and complications **(Table 6.14)**:

TABLE 6.14: Bioprosthetic and mechanical prosthesis—comparison.

Bioprosthetic	*Mechanical*
Material—biological (porcine)	Metallic
No need for endothelialization	Needed
Degenerates; need replacement after 8–12 years	No
Long-term anticoagulation not needed	Needed
Risk of infective endocarditis—less	More; prophylaxis needed
Indication—very old, before pregnancy	Widespread

Q4. What are the indications of bioprosthetic valves?
Ans.
- Patients in whom anticoagulation carries risk, e.g., young women who wish to have future pregnancies.

- In older patients whose lifespan is otherwise limited, and in whom risk of anticoagulation is high.

Q5. What are the things to consider during double valve replacement (DVR) in patients with multivalvular disease?
Ans.
- Double valve replacement is associated with increased short- and long-term risks; BMV can be the first procedure if MS is the predominant lesion, with subsequent AVR when needed. Surgical valvotomy undertaken if BMV is not an option, or if concurrent AVR is needed.
- Preoperative identification of significant AV disease in patients who have to undergo BMV is vital. The procedure may prove hazardous as it can impose a sudden load on left ventricle that was previously protected by MS and may lead to acute pulmonary edema.
- Patients are advised not to undergo multivalvular surgery until they reach late NYHA class II or III, unless they exhibit evidence of declining LV function. The decision to treat more than one valve finally depends on findings of direct inspection or palpation, or the findings of intraoperative TEE.

Q6. What are the strategies for anticoagulant therapy in artificial valves?
Ans.
- In case of MVR—long-term anticoagulation with warfarin with target INR: 3.0–3.5.
- In AVR—warfarin dose adjusted with target INR: 2.0–2.5.
- In bioprosthetic valve—short-term anticoagulation suffices.

Q7. How to investigate artificial valve function?
Ans.
- *Chest X-ray:* It shows types of valves and their location **(Fig. 6.15)**.

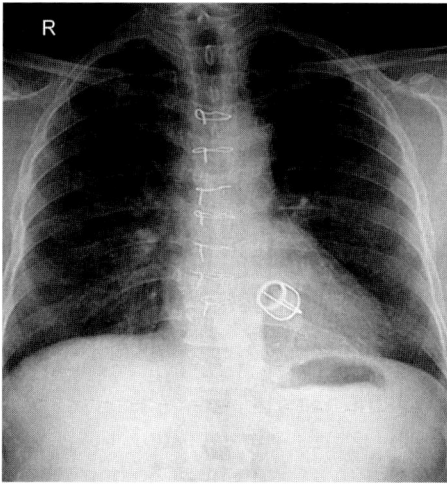

Fig. 6.15: Starr-Edwards metallic prosthesis in mitral position.

- *Echocardiography:* Obstruction or stenosis created by pannus (fibrous tissue between prosthetic material and native tissue) and thrombus (less echogenic, more mobile; may protrude outside sewing ring). Pannus is more common in aortic prosthesis, and thrombus is more common in mitral. Vegetation may also produce stenosis (clinical findings differentiate). In prosthetic obstruction, leaflets show restricted mobility.
- *Doppler study:* This study shows high mean and peak gradients (in comparison with baseline gradients) in prosthetic obstruction. CWD recording of normally functioning mechanical AV is V-shaped (in place of U-shaped in stenotic valve). In stenosis of prosthetic valve, it becomes rounded. In prosthetic-patient mismatch, effective orifice area of prosthesis is too small in relation to patient's body surface area, resulting in abnormally high postoperative transprosthetic gradient.
- *Color flow imaging:* Normally, mild regurgitation prevents thrombus formation ("the washing jet"). Pathological valvular regurgitation jet is wider and demonstrates more turbulence. Paravalvular regurgitation in mechanical prosthesis results, owing to suture not holding onto a degenerated and calcified annulus. IE destroying portions of annulus may also produce regurgitation. It is less common with bioprosthetic valves, which thicken and degenerate over time to produce severe regurgitation. When several sutures are dehisced, severe paravalvular leaks develop with rocking movement of prosthesis. Severe regurgitation also leads to LV dilatation, increase in PASP, and increased gradient across prosthetic valve with preserved motion (compared to baseline).

Q8. What precautions are to be taken in pregnancy with an artificial valve?
Ans. During pregnancy, warfarin can cause fetal hemorrhage, teratogenicity, and spontaneous abortion, because warfarin crosses placenta, but vitamin K-dependent clotting factors do not, and fetal liver cannot manufacture them.
- After an effective warfarin control, pregnant patients must be switched from warfarin to heparin at about 36 weeks. Dose: 1000 units/h IV, initially after being admitted to hospital, then 10,000–12,500 units subcutaneous (SC) 12 hourly.
- Second stage of labor should be shortened; the cesarean section is undertaken, and heparin is stopped about 6 hours prior to delivery. It is restarted as soon as possible after delivery, with warfarin being restarted at 2 days postpartum.
- In pregnancy, heparin has to be started very early to avoid the teratogenic effect of warfarin in the first trimester and continued up to delivery. The typical embryopathy occurs with exposure at 6–12 weeks' gestation. The switch from warfarin to heparin must be immediately on obtaining a positive pregnancy test.

- Heparin does not cross the placenta and hence does not cause fetal malformation or fetal hemorrhage. Retroplacental bleeding and spontaneous abortion can still occur.

SUGGESTED READING

1. Bonow RO, Carabello BA, Kanu C, de Leon AC Jr, Faxon DP, Freed MD, et al. ACC/AHA Guidelines for management of patients with valvular heart disease. Circulation. 2006;114:e84-231.
2. Grubb NR, Newby DE. In: Grubb NR (Ed). Churchill's Pocketbook of Cardiology, 2nd edition. Edinburg: Churchill Livingstone; 2006.
3. Julian DG, Campbell-Cowan C, McLenachan JM. Disorders of the cardiac valves. In: Julian DG (Ed). Cardiology, 8th edition. Philadelphia: Saunders; 2005.
4. Manchanda O. Valvular heart disease. In: Manchanda SC (Ed). Oram's Clinical Heart Disease, 3rd edition. New Delhi: CBS Publishers and Distributor; 1999.

7 Congenital Heart Diseases

"The credit for the first accurate description of any congenital heart disease goes to Leonardo da Vinci, who described a case of atrial septal defect with sets of brilliant drawing in 1513 AD."

—History of Cardiology

INTRODUCTION

Congenital heart diseases (CHDs) are abnormalities in cardiovascular structure or function that are present at birth, even if it is discovered much later. The heart is the first organ to develop in utero. The entire development of the heart and great vessels occurs between the third and eighth week. Because of the complex embryonic development of the heart CHD is common and is either due to altered development or failed progression to the adult normal form. The incidence is about 0.8% of live births excluding bicuspid aortic valves and mitral valve prolapse (excluding bicuspid aortic valve and mitral valve prolapse). Of the CHD cases, small ventricular septal defect (VSD), atrial septal defect (ASD), mild pulmonary stenosis (PS), bicuspid AV, and MVP are incidentally diagnosed. More than 85% of CHD patients survive to adulthood and live a productive life—the entity called adult CHD. Interventional treatment has largely replaced surgery as the treatment of choice in secundum ASD, coarctation of the aorta, persistent ductus arteriosus (PDA), and PS.

Q1. Define congenital heart disease.
Ans. Congenital heart diseases are abnormalities in cardiocirculatory structure or function that are present at birth, even if they are discovered much later. It results from the altered embryonic development of a normal structure. Incidence is about 1% of live birth (not included are bicuspid AV and MVP).

Q2. What are the causes of CHD?
Ans.
- Genetic (by chromosomal aberration or single gene mutation or transmission)—familial ASD, congenital heart block, situs inversus, long QT, Holt-Oram syndrome, and hypertrophic cardiomyopathy (HCM). At present, <15% of all cardiac malformations can be accounted for genetic cause. Most are not inherited in a simple manner.
- Environmental—maternal rubella causing PDA, PS, and ASD; fetal alcohol syndrome causing VSD; and lithium causing tricuspid regurgitation (TR).

- Multifactorial—combination of a hereditary predisposition (abnormality in genetic code) and an environmental trigger. Most CHDs were thought to be multifactorial.
  More recent advances in molecular biology suggest that a much higher percentage are caused by point mutations.

Q3. How to classify CHD?
Ans.
- *On cyanosis (as presentation):*
  - *Acyanotic:*
    - L-R shunt—ASD, VSD, PDA, partial anomalous pulmonary venous connection (PAPVC), aortopulmonary (AP) window, and rupture sinus of Valsalva aneurysm
    - Obstructive—aortic stenosis (AS), PS, and coarctation of the aorta
    - Valvular regurgitation—Ebstein's anomaly and corrected transposition of great artery (TGA)
    - Miscellaneous—HCM, prolonged QT, congenital complete heart block (CHB), coronary artery abnormalities, and right ventricular (RV) dysplasia
  - *Cyanotic:*
    - Increased pulmonary flow—total anomalous pulmonary venous connection (TAPVC), TGA, double outlet right ventricle (DORV), persistent truncus, AV septal defect, and single ventricle
    - Decreases pulmonary flow—tetralogy of Fallot (TOF), pulmonary atresia, severe PS with ASD, and Ebstein's anomaly
    - Miscellaneous—pulmonary arteriovenous fistula

Congenital heart disease is also classified as follows: CHD may manifest clinically in pediatric age or in adult life (i.e., adult CHD).
- *According to severity, adult CHD may be:*
  - Simple (can be cared in the general medical community), e.g., small ASD, isolated patent foramen ovale (PFO), VSD (isolated, small), isolated valvular AS, mild PS, ligated PDA, repaired ASD, and VSD
  - Moderately severe (should be seen periodically at a special center), e.g., aneurysm of sinus of Valsalva or rupture, primum ASD, PDA, moderate to severe PS, sinus venosus ASD, VSD with aortic regurgitation (AR), coarctation of aorta, right ventricular outflow tract (RVOT) obstruction, subaortic AS, and sub- or supravalvular AS
  - Complex (should be seen regularly at a special center), e.g., all cyanotic CHD, DORV, Eisenmenger's syndrome, single ventricle (double inlet, outlet, and common or primitive), pulmonary atresia, pulmonary vascular obstructive disease (PVOD), TGA, tricuspid atresia, trances arteriosus, etc.

Q4. What is complex CHD?
Ans. These are critical congenital malformations that are severe enough to result in cardiac catheterization, cardiac surgery, or death within the first year

of life. Complex CHD should be seen regularly at CHD centers and monitored throughout life.

Q5. How does time influence the clinical manifestations of CHD?
Ans. Anatomical and physiological changes in the cardiovascular system can continue indefinitely from prenatal to adulthood. Thus, time influences markedly the manifestations of CHD.
- Many CHDs are not symptomatic till adulthood—hence, called adult CHD, e.g., ASD.
- Some are manifested in pediatric age, e.g., moderate to large VSD and complex CHD.
- Some CHD may improve with time during postnatal life, e.g., Ebstein's anomaly of the tricuspid valve (TV) may improve after birth due to the fall of pulmonary vascular resistance (PVR) and a decrease in TR.
- Tetralogy of Fallot, severe PS, and pulmonary atresia may not become cyanotic until normal closure of the ductus arteriosus.
- Ventricular septal defect, if small, may close spontaneously or may lead to the development of RVOT obstruction and/or AR or PVOD.
- Ductal constriction many days after birth, in some infants, may lead to the development of coarctation of the aorta.
- The pattern of many lesions' changes in adult life due to the development of chamber enlargement, ventricular dysfunction, arrhythmia, pulmonary hypertension, and comorbidities.

Q6. Who are the caregivers for adult CHD?
Ans. The pattern of many lesions changes in adult life due to anatomical and physiological changes and the development of comorbidities. Hence, adult CHD is treated by a physician or a team familiar with both pediatric and adult cardiology issues—including personnel with congenital heart surgery and interventional catheterization procedures.

Q7. What are the transcatheter therapies available for patients with CHD?
Ans. Percutaneous catheter-based therapies are applied in the following conditions **(Box 7.1)**:

> **BOX 7.1:** Percutaneous interventions in congenital heart disease.
> - Balloon atrial septostomy-life saving for neonates with TGA; an atrial communication is created by tearing a hole in the atrial septum using a balloon catheter
> - Pulmonary valvuloplasty—done for pulmonary valvular stenosis by balloon inflation with a diameter of 100–120% of the pulmonary valve annulus
> - Aortic valvuloplasty—may be undertaken in adult AS with pliable, noncalcified valves
> - Atrial septal defect—done by Amplatzer septal occluding device; secundum ASD, up to 40 mm in size with sufficient rims (>5 mm) to pulmonary veins and mitral valve (MV) attachments and a pulmonary artery pressure (PAP) <70 mm Hg. Antiplatelets are given for 3–6 months until the device is completely endothelialized

Contd...

Contd...

- Persistent ductus arteriosus—small- or medium-sized patent ductus with no pulmonary hypertension (PH) can be occluded with a variety of transcatheter occluding devices or coils
- VSD—only undertaken in acquired VSD due to acute myocardial infarction (AMI)
- Coarctation of the aorta—transcatheter balloon dilatation and stenting

(AS: aortic stenosis; ASD: atrial septal defect; TGA: transposition of the great arteries; VSD: ventricular septal defect)

Q8. What is dextrocardia? What are the types?
Ans. It is the congenitally right-sided heart (regardless of the position of abdominal viscera).

Two types:
1. Dextrocardia with situs inversus—mirror image of normal. The incidence of CHD is only 5%.
2. *Dextrocardia with situs solitus (formerly termed dextroversion):* The ventricles fail to swing from the primitive right-sided position to the normal left-sided position, resulting in an abnormal relationship between the ventricles and the rest of the cardiovascular structures. Both the abdominal viscera and atria are in normal position. The incidence of CHD is 98%.

Q9. What is levocardia? What are the types?
Ans. It is the congenitally left-sided heart.

Two types:
1. Levocardia with situs solitus—entirely normal
2. *Levocardia with situs inversus:* This is a mirror image of dextroversion (hence, formerly termed levoversion). The incidence of CHD is nearly 100%.

Q10. How does adult CHD differ from that in infants and children?
Ans. Ventricular septal defect is the most common congenital defect in infants and children, but most children who survive to adulthood without surgical correction will have spontaneous closure of the defect. Hence, bicuspid AV and ASD are the most common adult CHDs. Again, adults are much less likely than infants and children to have complex congenital lesions; the lesions are either corrected in childhood or cause death before childhood. Adults with corrected CHD are increasingly more common.

Q11. How to prevent CHD?
Ans.
- Avoid the use of teratogenic agents and drugs during pregnancy
- Avoid radiation
- Prenatal detection of genetic abnormalities—amniocentesis, chorionic villous biopsy to obtain fetal cells, and detection of genetic abnormalities

- Fetal echocardiography—when chromosomal abnormalities are diagnosed
- Immunization for rubella.

ATRIAL SEPTAL DEFECT

Q1. What is ASD? How does ASD differ from PFO?
Ans. An ASD is a through-and-through communication between two atria resulting from a deficiency of tissue in the septum.

Patent foramen ovale is due to the failure of the septum primum and secundum to fuse completely. There is a probe patency of the septum, and communication is not through and through. Here, the septum primum is not adherent to the superior limbic band of the septum secundum.

Q2. What are the types of ASD?
Ans.
Anatomical types of ASD are:
- *Ostium secundum defect:* At the region of the fossa ovalis; most common (70%); septal tissue separates the defect from AV valves. PAPVC is present in a few cases.
- Ostium primum defect—also called partial atrioventricular defect; defect of the AV septum lying inferior to the fossa ovalis. It is part of the common atrioventricular canal defects.
- Sinus venosus defect—represents a biatrial connection of the superior vena cava (SVC), which straddles the otherwise normal intact atrial septum. PAPVC more common; one or more of right-sided pulmonary veins drain into the vena cava or directly to the right atrium near its junction with vena cava (**Fig. 7.1**).
- Coronary sinus defect—rare; it is part of a complex defect consisting of the absence of the coronary sinus and entry of the left SVC directly into the right atrium.

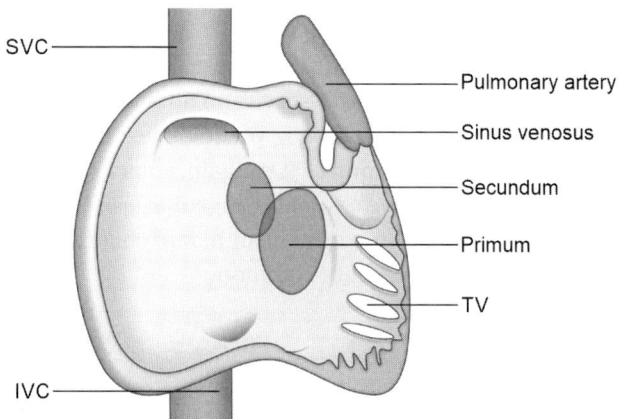

Fig. 7.1: Locations of defects in ASD seen from the RA side.
(IVC: inferior vena cava; RA: right atrium; SVC: superior vena cava; TV: tricuspid valve)

Q3. How does ASD differ from PFO?
Ans. In 15–20% of cases, septum primum and septum secundum do not fuse, resulting in PFO and occasionally permitting R-L shunting, depending on transseptal pressure gradients. In secundum ASD, underdevelopment of the septum secundum results in a true opening in the interatrial septum (IAS).

Q4. How does ostium secundum defect differ from other varieties of ASD?
Ans. Ostium secundum defects are the only true ASDs; all others are L-R shunts at the atrial level, not being surrounded by true atrial septal tissue. Thus, device closure is feasible and is the preferred strategy in secundum ASD. Patients with sinus venosus defects are at risk of developing caval and/or pulmonary vein stenosis even after surgical correction and should be kept under intermittent review. Ostium primum defect is an atrioventricular septal defect (endocardial cushion defect) rather than an ASD. Coronary sinus septal defects occur when there is a partial or complete deficiency of the roof of the coronary sinus; atrial level shunting at the mouth of the coronary sinus occurs, but the true IAS is intact.

Q5. What is a sinus venosus type defect?
Ans. Sinus venosus defect of SVC type is due to deficiency between the SVC and, usually right upper and middle pulmonary veins, but the true IAS is intact. They have an SVC-pulmonary vein-left atrial connection.

Inferior sinus venosus defects result from a breakdown between the right atrial wall and the inferior right-sided pulmonary veins.

Q6. What are the causes of cyanosis in ASD?
Ans. Causes are shunt reversal and Eisenmenger syndrome, a prominent Eustachian valve directing the inferior vena cava (IVC) flow to left atrium (LA) via a secundum ASD, and sinus venosus ASD of IVC type.

Q7. Why is splitting of S_2 in ASD wide and fixed?
Ans.
- Wide—pulmonary valve has to remain open for a longer time because of increased RV stroke volume and right bundle branch block (RBBB)
- Fixed—the septal defect equalizes the left and right atrial pressure throughout the respiratory cycle.

Physiological splitting narrows during expiration and widens during inspiration as more blood goes to the right-side during inspiration. Due to high pressure aortic component normally precedes the pulmonary.

Q8. Does the defect in ASD produce any murmur?
Ans. There is no murmur through the defect, as there is almost no gradient across it. The ejection systolic murmur heard at the second or third left intercostal space is secondary to increased flow to the pulmonary arteries. Rarely, a continuous murmur may be produced across ASD in the presence of a small defect plus mitral stenosis (MS) (Lutembacher's syndrome) or mitral

regurgitation (MR), which raises the pressure in the LA considerably higher than RA.

Q9. How may ASD mimic mitral stenosis on clinical examination?
Ans.
- S_1 is loud in MS—tricuspid component of S_1 may be loud in ASD.
- A split S_2 of ASD may be confused with an opening snap in MS.
- Mid-diastolic murmur (MDM) in MS may be confused with a similar murmur resulting from high flow through the TV in ASD.
- Palpable P_2 due to PH in MS may be confused with a palpable pulmonary artery in ASD due to high flow.

Also, a left parasternal lift due to right ventricular hypertrophy (RVH) in MS may be confused with a hyperdynamic RV in ASD.

Q10. When is PAPVC suspected?
Ans. If the size of ASD is out of keeping with the size of RV, an associated abnormality of pulmonary venous drainage is suspected. Clinical findings in PAPVC are similar to those of ASD. The primary diagnosis is ASD, with subsequent investigations identifying the diagnosis. Pulmonary angiography is the most helpful procedure to identify anomalous venous drainage in the catheterization laboratory.

Surgery is not needed when a single anomalous vein does not produce RV volume overload.

Q11. What are the associations of ASD?
Ans.
- *Mitral valve disease:* MVP in secundum type, cleft posterior leaflet in primum type that may produce MR, which exaggerates L-R shunt. A thrill in the pulmonary area is common; MDM at the tricuspid area is predominant. Acquired rheumatic MS with ASD is called Lutembacher's syndrome. L-R shunt increases due to MS. MDM is masked as flow across the MV is reduced. Systolic murmur is heard at the septal defect.
- Partial anomalous pulmonary venous drainage (PAPVD) into right atrium—it is present in 15% of all ASD (65% of sinus venosus ASD) and increases the amount of L-R shunt. In TAPVD (total anomalous pulmonary venous drainage), ASD with R-L shunt is essential for survival.
- Skeletal deformity—Holt–Oram syndrome, a familial disorder consisting of ASD and deformity of the upper limb (polydactyly, triphalangeal or fingerized thumb, radial deformity, etc.), kyphoscoliosis, and pigeon chest.
- Pulmonary stenosis—thrill present in the pulmonary area.
- Tetralogy of Fallot—a combination of TOF with ASD is called pentalogy of Fallot.
- Pulmonary hypertension—results from a high PVR. Eisenmenger's syndrome may supervene.

- Infective endocarditis—rare with secundum type and suggests ostium primum defect or concomitant PS.

Q12. What is the importance of the presence of PFO?
Ans. Patent foramen ovale has been implicated in cryptogenic stroke by paradoxical embolism or in-situ thrombus formation. The presence of an IAS aneurysm in combination with a PFO increases the adverse events. Device closure is warranted in patients with PFO and atrial septal aneurysm who have had a stroke.

Q13. When is closure indicated in ASD?
Ans.
- Closure is done for hemodynamically significant ASD (Qp/Qs >1.5, ASD associated with RV volume overload), especially if device closure is available and appropriate.
- In patients with PH and hemodynamically significant ASD (PA pressure more than two-thirds of systemic arterial pressure, or PVR more than two-thirds of SVR) with evidence of pulmonary artery reactivity when challenged with a pulmonary vasodilator [e.g., 100% O_2 or nitric oxide (NO)].
- Device closure is the therapy of choice for secundum ASDs when there are adequate rims (0.5 mm and the stressed diameter is <36–40 mm). Presence of an anomalous pulmonary venous connection or proximity of the defect to the AV valve, or coronary sinus or systemic venous drainage usually precludes the use of the device. After device closure, patients require 6 months of anticoagulation and endocarditis prophylaxis until the device is endothelialized. It improves functional status in symptomatic patients no matter what their age; it has proven to be safe and effective with better preservation of RV function and lower complications than surgery.
- Surgery is the option for those with sinus venosus or ostium primum defects or with secundum defects with unsuitable anatomy.

Q14. How radiologic findings of MS differ from those of ASD?
Ans. Clinical signs of both the conditions may overlap. Radiological findings differentiate **(Table 7.1)**.

TABLE 7.1: Radiological findings in mitral stenosis and atrial septal defect.

Points	Mitral stenosis	ASD
Cardiomegaly	Not present	Usually present
LA enlargement	Double contour right border and straightening of left border	Nil
RA, RV enlargement	Occurred lately (after development of PH)	Early

Contd...

Contd...

Rightward shift of cardiac silhouette	Nil	Yes
Pulmonary conus	Full (in PH)	Bulged
Pulmonary plethora	Nil	Present
Pulmonary congestion	Present	Nil
Pulmonary vasculature	Upper lobe prominent (i.e., cephalization)	Lower lobe dilated (i.e., caudalization)
Dilated right PA (inverted comma sign)	Present	Absent
Pulmonary edema	May develop	Never develop

(ASD: atrial septal defect; LA: left atrium; PA: pulmonary artery; PH: pulmonary hypertension; RA: right atrium; RV: right ventricular)

Q15. How is echocardiographic assessment done in ASD?
Ans.
Things to look for are:
- Location of the defect (superior, inferior, anterior, and posterior)
- Size of the defect
- Identification of multiple defects
- Adequacy of rims (superior, inferior, anterior, and posterior).

Q16. How to differentiate the three types of ASD on echocardiography?
Ans.
- Parasternal long-axis view—RV volume overload—with dilatation of RV and abnormal motion of IVS (brisk anterior movement in early systole or flattening in diastole, i.e., paradoxic septal motion) in otherwise healthy young patient is an indirect finding on M-mode echocardiography [other causes are pulmonary regurgitation (PR), TR, and anomalous pulmonary venous return].
- Parasternal short-axis view—abnormal ventricular septal geometry (in parasternal short-axis view)—leftward displacement or flattening of interventricular septum (IVS) in diastole (in systole, it becomes more rounded).
- Apical four-chamber view—visualization of ostium primum ASD may be done. Secundum defect may be diagnosed if "T-sign"—a bright horizontal echo produced by the edge of the true defect giving an inverted T appearance is present.
- Subcostal four-chamber view—presence and approximate size of secundum defect assessed **(Figs. 7.2A and B)**. Ostium primum, and sinus venosus type ASD may be assessed in apical four-chamber view **(Fig. 7.3)**. Most superior and posterior portion of atrium needs to be visualized to detect smaller sinus venosus defect. Also entrance of SVC and pulmonary veins can be done to detect anomalous pulmonary venous drainage.

Ostium primum defect may occur alone (partial atrioventricular canal) or in association with defect in inlet ventricular septum (complete atrioventricular canal or endocardial cushion). Absence of most inferior portion of atrial septum, at level of insertion of septal leaflets of AV valve is diagnostic (in apical four-chamber view). Both AV valves are at the same plane in AV canal defect.

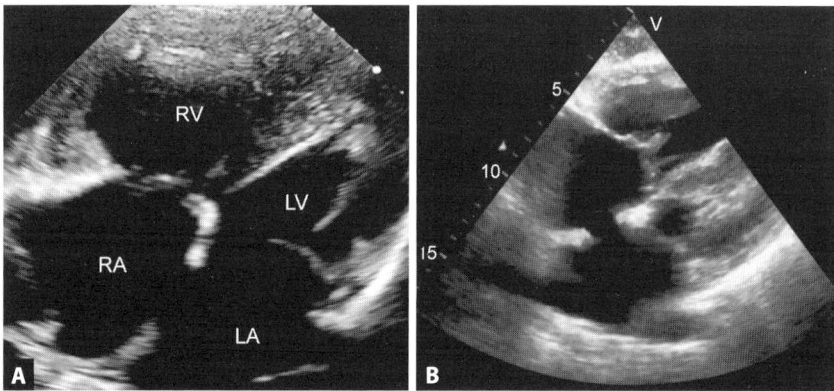

Figs. 7.2A and B: Secundum ASD seen in apical four-chamber (A) and subcostal four-chamber (B) view. (ASD: atrial septal defect; LA: left atrium; LV: left ventricular; RA: right atrium; RV: right ventricular)

- Transesophageal echo—most accurate technique due to proximity and orientation of septum relative to esophagus.
- Contrast echo and/or Doppler—when diagnosis is in doubt. Pulsed Doppler shows low-velocity left-to-right flow extending from mid systole to mid-diastole. Color flow imaging can confirm presence of trans-septal flow, can differentiate echo dropout from a true anatomic defect. Quantification of shunt size can be done with the Doppler technique.

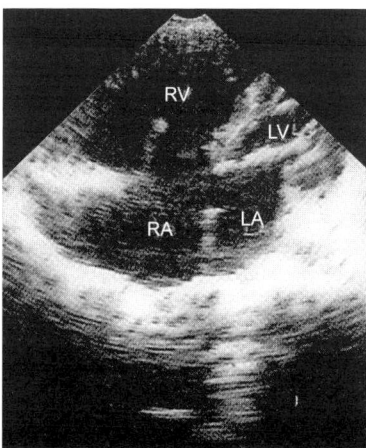

Fig. 7.3: Ostium primum defect in apical four-chamber view. (LA: left atrium; LV: left ventricular; RA: right atrium; RV: right ventricular)

Q17. Does spontaneous closure occur in ASD?
Ans. Spontaneous closure of secundum ASD beyond the first 2 years of life is rare.

Q18. What are the factors that contribute to high mortality and morbidity in ASD if closure is not done?
Ans. Congestive heart failure (CHF) due to irreversible PH and shunt reversal (Eisenmenger's syndrome) is the most common cause. Also, pulmonary embolism or paradoxical embolism with brain abscess in patients with atrial fibrillation (AF) and infective endocarditis (virtually only in ostium primum type) may be responsible.

Q19. When should atrial septal defect be surgically repaired?
Ans. Surgical closure is recommended even in asymptomatic patients to avoid the development of pulmonary hypertension, AF. The ideal age for closure is preschool age (5–10 years). Mortality in adults and low risk of surgical closure in young children mandates surgery in preschool age, but excellent results have been obtained even over the age of 60 years, although mortality increases. If the pulmonary to systemic flow ratio exceeds 1.5:1 it may be assumed that the defect is sufficiently large to cause symptoms in later life, hence to be repaired (small ASD can be left alone). PVR should preferably be <10 units (a high PVR increase operative mortality).

Q20. Is cardiac catheterization needed for ASD patients?
Ans. Cardiac catheterization is typically not required for diagnostic purposes, except to assess PVR, to assess for coronary artery disease prior to planned surgical closure in adult patients, or as part of transcatheter device closure. Most young patients with a secundum ASD now undergo repair without cardiac catheterization. It may also be avoided in selected patients with a primum ASD if PAP, papillary muscle architecture, and atrioventricular valve morphology can be adequately assessed with ultrasound.

Q21. Differentiate between secundum and primum ASD.
Ans. Secundum type defects are true ASD bounded by atrial septal tissue on both margins. Primum defects are atrioventricular defects. The differences between the two are mentioned in **Table 7.2**.

TABLE 7.2: Difference between secundum and primum defect.

Points	Secundum ASD	Primum ASD
Prevalence	About 90%	About 8%
Sex	Female > Male	Female = Male
Age of presentation	Usually adult	Usually childhood
MV	Usually normal, occasionally prolapsing	AML may be cleft, varying degree of MR

Contd...

Contd...

Pansystolic murmur	Nil	Due to MR
Apex beat	Normal	Forceful, shifted (if MR)
Infective endocarditis	Rare	Not uncommon
CXR	LA, LV not enlarged	Enlarged
ECG	RBBB + RAD	RBBB + LAD
Echocardiography	Echo dropout at fossa ovalis or at midseptum (needs subcostal view for confirmation)	Echo dropout at the lower portion of IAS (apical four-chamber view is enough)
Intervention	Device closure may be done in some	Cannot be done; the MV may need repair or replacement

(AML: anterior mitral leaflet; ASD: atrial septal defect; CXR: chest x-ray; ECG: electrocardiogram; IAS: interatrial septum; LA: left atrium; LAD: left anterior descending artery; LV: left ventricular; MR: mitral regurgitation; MV: mitral valve; RAD: right axis deviation; RBBB: right bundle branch block)

Q22. What are PAPVC and TAPVC?

Ans. Here, one or more pulmonary veins drain into the right atrium either directly or via the SVC. The condition is physiologically similar to that of an ASD with an L-R shunt. Sinus venosus ASD commonly coexists, but is not invariably present, as in TAPVC.

In TAPVC, all the blood from the lungs enters the right atrium by one route or another. To enable oxygenated blood to reach the systemic side, an ASD or patent foramen ovale is essential. O_2 saturation in all four chambers of the heart, and also the pulmonary artery and aorta, may be identical.

Q23. What are the factors favoring device closure of ASD?
Ans.

- Device closure is possible only in secundum ASD. There should be adequate tissue margins at the superior and inferior rims of the defect for secure snapping of the closure device to the tissue. However, despite persistent shunting in ASDs with insufficient rims, late closure may produce a satisfactory outcome.
- Avoids potential surgical complications, reduces length of hospital stay, and eliminates the midline sternotomy scar.

  Criteria for closure are: Pulmonary-to-systemic shunt with flow ratios >1.5:1. Also, patients with smaller ASDs (flow ratios <1.5:1) in the settings of paradoxical embolism (morbidity associated with closure is low). It is contraindicated in those patients with a pulmonary-to-systemic shunt ratio as low as 0.7:1, which signifies severe pulmonary vascular disease.

VENTRICULAR SEPTAL DEFECT

Q1. What are the components of the IVS?
Ans. Seen from the RV aspect, IVS has a membranous and a muscular part, which again has an inlet (or posterior), trabecular, and an outlet (or infundibular) part **(Fig. 7.4)**.

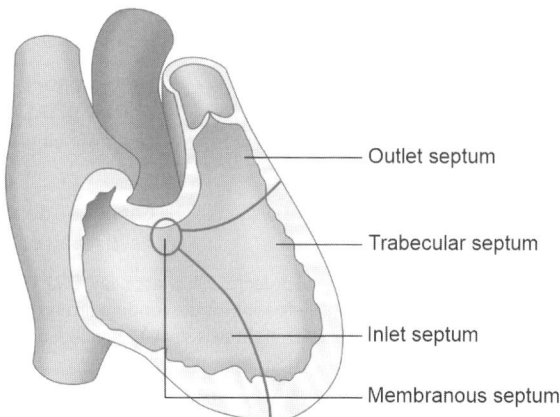

Fig. 7.4: Components of IVS (viewed from RV).

The membranous septum is contiguous with portions of inlet, trabecular, and outlet septum, i.e., all these three converge on membranous septum. Also, perimembranous defects encroach upon inlet, trabecular, or outlet septum. Exact boundaries are determined by extension into one or all three components of muscular septum. It is located directly beneath AV (subaortic). Membranous IVS has a right atrial-left ventricular component that contains AV-conducting tissue and remains intact in perimembranous VSD. A defect in such a location is called Gerbode defect. His bundle and bundle branch remain beneath deficient septum and close to free edge of perimembranous defect. Inlet septum occupies inlet portion of RV and has chordae tendineae attached to septal leaflet of TV. Outlet septum is beneath aortic and pulmonary valves. Trabecular part occupies the major part of muscular septum and is in between the two.

Q2. Classify ventricular septal defects.
Ans.
- *Etiologically:*
  - Congenital
  - Acquired—as a complication of AMI, usually muscular
- *According to the anatomical location of the defect:*
  - Membranous (infracristal); most common: 80%
  - Inlet (posterior): 5%
  - Trabecular: 10%
  - Outlet (supracristal) or infundibula: 5%

Trabecular VSD may be single or multiple, small or large. Outlet defect is located in cephaloid portion of infundibular septum. Roof of the defect is either a remnant of infundibular septum or the contiguous aortic and pulmonary valve (doubly committed and subarterial). Left and right coronary cusp of AV sometimes prolapse into outflow tract of RV. Uncommonly, a pulmonary cusp may prolapse through the defect. Outlet defect may also be due to developmental malalignment of infundibular septum relative to trabecular septum as in TOF.

- *According to the size of the defect:* Small (<0.5 cm^2/m^2), moderate (0.5–1.0 cm^2/m^2), and large (>1.0 cm^2/m^2)
- *Pathophysiologically it may be:*
  - Restrictive—when resistance to L-R shunt is at the level of the defect; RV systolic pressure is normal or less than LV systolic pressure
  - Nonrestrictive—when resistance to L-R shunt is at the pulmonary vascular bed and not at the VSD; right ventricular systolic pressure (RVSP) = left ventricular systolic pressure (LVSP).

Q3. How does congenital VSD exist?
Ans. Ventricular septal defect may occur in the following forms:
- Isolated VSD
- As an integral part of a syndrome—e.g., Fallot's tetralogy, DORV, and truncus arteriosus
- As an association—pulmonary atresia, TGA, coarctation, etc.

Q4. How heart failure (HF) develops in infancy in large VSD? What are the manifestations?
Ans. In the first few days after birth, pulmonary venous pressure (PVR) falls, and RV pressure falls below LV pressure. This allows gradually increasing L-R shunt of blood through the defect, the lung, and back to LA and LV. But with a large VSD, PVR cannot fall because of the large shunt. The LV volume overload eventually leads to LV failure and pulmonary edema.

Typical features of HF in infancy:
- Tachypnea with intercostal recession (↑work of respiration with stiff lung)
- Failure to thrive
- Feeding problems—sweating on feeding, failure to suck adequately
- Hepatomegaly
- Frequent chest infection and chronic ill health—due to persistent high pulmonary blood flow. Irreversible pulmonary veno-occlusive disease (PVOD) starts from the age of 1 year, if not closed.

Q5. What are the findings in different degrees of VSD?
Ans. Size of the defect in VSD determines the clinical findings, management, and outcomes **(Table 7.3)**.

TABLE 7.3: Various degrees of VSD—findings.

Points	Small	Moderate	Large
Definition:			
Defect size	<0.5 cm^2/m^2	0.5–1.0 cm^2/m^2	>1.0 cm^2/m^2
L-R shunt	Insignificant (<2:1)	>2:1	>2:1
PAH	Nil	Nil or mild	Moderate to severe
Symptoms:			
Growth retardation	–	±	+
CHF	–	–	+
IE	+	+	±
Sign:			
Precordium	Normal	Increased activity (LV, slight RV)	Increased activity (LV and RV)
S$_2$	Normal	Wide and variably split, P$_2$ normal or loud	Splitting close, P$_2$ load
Murmur	Loud pansystolic harsh (ejection type in muscular), no MDM	Harsh pansystolic MDM in the apex	Ejection systolic or decrescendo MDM; disappears with development of PVOD
Investigation:			
ECG	Normal	LV+LA+LAD	LV+LA+RV+
CXR	Normal	Pulmonary plethora, LV enlargement ± LAE ±	Cardiomegaly (biventricular, pulmonary plethora, large PA c̄ peripheral pruning when PVOD develops
Echocardiography	LV, LA—normal; no RVH RV systolic pressure—N	LV volume overload, LA—mildly enlarged, no RVH, estimated RV systolic pressure <50% LV systolic pressure	LV volume overload, LA enlarged, RVH. Estimated RV systolic pressure >50% LV systolic pressure
Treatment	Observe for spontaneous closure; prophylaxis for IE	Surgery	Surgery
Prognosis	Excellent, life span normal	PVOD occurs if not closed	Heart failure may develop in infancy, with high mortality. PVOD develops in survivors after infancy

(CHF: congestive heart failure; CXR: chest X-ray; ECG: electrocardiogram; IE: infective endocarditis; LA: left atrium; LAD: left axis deviation; LAE: left atrial enlargement; LV: left ventricle; MDM: mid-diastolic murmur; PAH: pulmonary arterial hypertension; PVOD: pulmonary veno-occlusive disease; RV: right ventricle; RVH: right ventricular hypertrophy; VSD: ventricular septal defect)

Q6. What factors influence the spontaneous closure of VSD?
Ans.
- Size of VSD—80% of small VSDs close spontaneously by late childhood. For those that persist, their restrictive nature protects the patient from pulmonary vascular injury. 10% of large VSDs close spontaneously, and another 50% show a decrease in size.
- Type of VSD—closure common in trabecular-type muscular and perimembranous variety (its location behind the medial papillary muscle of the TV opposes it and helps to close spontaneously). Closure occurs by ingrowth of fibrous tissue, endocardial proliferation. Prolapse of an aortic cusp through the defect may contribute closure. On closure, an aneurysm of the membranous septum may occur. It does not occur in defects adjacent to valves—in infundibular (supracristal), inlet (posterior), or malalignment defect., i.e., TOF, DORV, etc.
- Age of patients—the likelihood of spontaneous closure diminishes with age while progression of PVOD in large VSD increases.

Q7. How does the size of the defect determine prognosis in VSD?
Ans. The single most important variable influencing the natural history of VSD is its size. Small perimembranous VSD closes spontaneously. Thus, a disturbing loud and harsh precordial holosystolic murmur is not alarming but rather is a reassuring thing. Again, a small VSD after 20 years of age is unlikely to close.

Spontaneous closure is less likely in large defects. Large nonrestrictive VSD, if not corrected within 2 years, PVOD develops. Increased mortality due to HF and pulmonary infection is usually encountered.

Q8. What is the clinical differential diagnosis of VSD?
Ans.
- An innocent systolic murmur—in infants and children in the left parasternal region, ejection in type, not accompanied by a thrill
- Pulmonary stenosis—left parasternal heave, occasional ejection click, and wide, variable splitting of S_2; P_2 soft
- Mitral regurgitation—pansystolic murmur best heard at the apex, radiates to the axilla
- Aortic stenosis—ejection systolic murmur best heard along the left sternal border or at apex and may be accompanied by thrill and soft S_2.

Q9. What are the complications of VSD?
Ans.
- Congestive heart failure in infancy, with large defect, and death may occur.
- Aortic regurgitation—occurs in about 5% with membranous or infundibular defects.

- Infective endocarditis—may occur with any VSD. Antibiotic prophylaxis is needed for dental procedures, etc., and antibiotic coverage for 3 months after patch closure is needed (until the patch is endothelialized).
- Right ventricular outflow tract obstruction—subvalvular obstruction owing to progressive hypertrophy of crista supraventricularis, occurs in moderate to large L-R shunt. It is common in those who had PA banding. It decreases pulmonary flow and flooding of the lung but may ultimately cause shunt reversal and cyanosis.
- Eisenmenger's syndrome—shunt reversal owing to irreversible PH from longstanding exposure to pulmonary vasculature to L-R shunting across VSD. The term Eisenmenger's complex is used when VSD is associated with shunt reversal.

It produces cyanosis and its associated complications.

Q10. How to detect various types of VSD on echocardiography?
Ans.
- Perimembranous and outlet VSD—perimembranous defects are visible in the parasternal long-axis view (with slight medial angulation) but not from four-chamber views). The defect is located superior to and just below the AV **(Fig. 7.5)**.

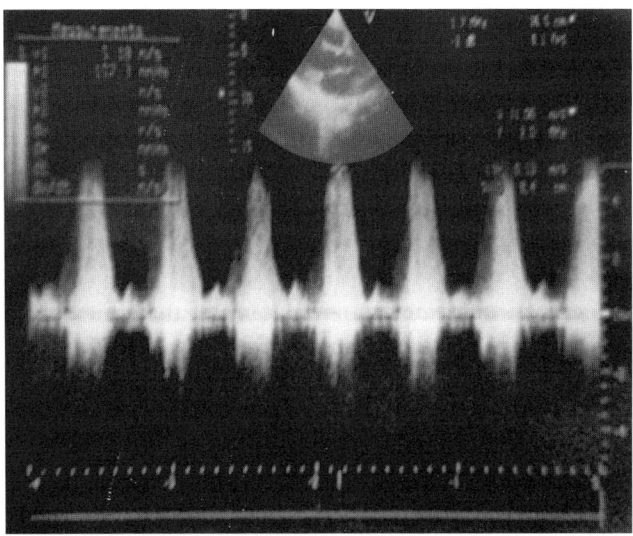

Fig. 7.5: CWD showing restrictive perimembranous VSD (gradient 107 mm Hg).

- Outlet VSD—outlet defect may be above and below crista supraventricularis in location. Supracristal (defect often small and may be missed, particularly if color flow imaging is not used) is detectable from a high parasternal long-axis view or parasternal short-axis view. Slight lateral angulation and rotation visualize both the aortic and pulmonic valve, with a defect adjacent to both. This should be differentiated from perimembranous by a short-axis view at great vessel level. Perimembranous defects are located more medially, usually near the septal leaflet of the TV (at the 11 o'clock position of aortic annulus). Outlet defects are more anterior and leftward (at the 2 o'clock position of aortic annulus). Outlet defects are differentiated as supra- or infracristal in location. Infracristal defects are to the right of the midline, whereas supracristal defects are far leftward and adjacent to the pulmonic valve.

- Inlet VSD—visualized by apical four-chamber view by inferior tilting of the scanner plane, inlet defect being imaged in the area between atrioventricular valves. If both AV valves are seen at the same plane, an atrioventricular canal defect is said to be present.
- Trabecular defect—apical four-chamber view may permit visualization but is difficult to detect with two-dimensional echocardiography (2DE). Trabecular defects may appear as multiple narrow, irregular channels through the muscular septum. Detection is facilitated by the simultaneous use of color Doppler imaging.

Q11. How is screening for the presence of VSD done on echocardiography?

Ans. If VSD is suspected but cannot be visualized directly with 2DE, the defects are either small or located in a part of the septum that is difficult to assess. In this situation Doppler study may detect a high velocity systolic jet crossing the septum from left to right in a small restrictive VSD. CFI is preferred, although continuous-wave Doppler (CWD) or pulsed wave Doppler (PWD) can also be utilized. Larger defects produce wider jets when imaged with color Doppler. The RV septal surface is systematically interrogated using multiple views—left parasternal, apical, and subcostal windows.

In addition to detecting VSD, Doppler can assess the magnitude and direction of the shunt.

Q12. What is the treatment for VSD?
Ans.
- *Treatment of HF:*
  - Digoxin
  - Diuretics
  - Correction of anemia—if any
  - Treatment of infection—if any
- Surgery—when the defect is large and medical therapy is unsuccessful; surgery is done at 3 months (some wait up to 1 year).

Q13. What are the indications of closure in VSD?

Ans.

- *Large, hemodynamically significant defect:* L-R shunt ($Q_p:Q_s$) >2:1, and RVSP >65% of LVSP, if the PVR is <8 Woods units. Closure is done very early in life, when pulmonary vascular resistance (PVR) is still reversible or has not developed. Elective closure of a large shunt should be done during preschool age (to minimize any subsequent distinction of the patient from their normal classmates).
- *Increasing AR:* AR is repaired along with closure of VSD only if moderate AR exists.
- Failure to thrive in infancy, despite medical treatment.
- Previous endocarditis complicating VSD. Such patients or those with residual lesions following repair warrant continuous antibiotic prophylaxis postoperatively.
- The presence of a perimembranous or outlet VSD with more than mild AR or a history of infective endocarditis is also a relative indication **(Figs. 7.6A and B)**.

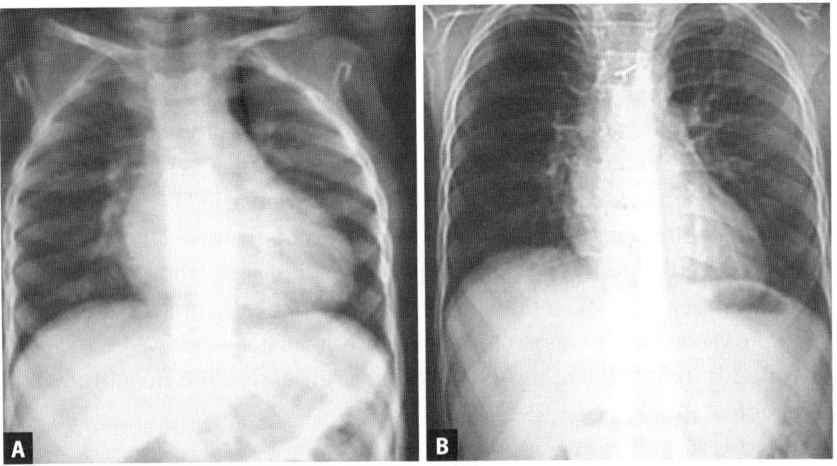

Figs. 7.6A and B: Chest radiograph of a child with nonrestrictive VSD and AR—before (A) and after (B) surgical closure.

Q14. Is transcatheter device closure possible in VSD?

Ans. Small muscular defects located apically either congenital or postinfarction, may be closed by a double clamshell device that have not closed spontaneously, and where surgical risk is exceedingly high. Unfortunately, the device is not suitable for the commoner perimembranous type as the device may interfere with aortic or TV or cause left ventricular outflow tract (LVOT) obstruction. The long-term outcome of this approach is yet to be determined.

■ PERSISTENT DUCTUS ARTERIOSUS

Q1. How does physiologic closure of the ductus arteriosus occur? How does the ductus remain patent?
Ans. Several changes occurring at birth initiate normal functional closure of the ductus within the first 15–18 hours of life. With the onset of spontaneous respiration, blood O_2 tension increases. This is coupled with a decrease in circulating prostaglandins (removal of the placenta, the primary source, along with increased metabolism by pulmonary circulation). The functional closure is followed by eventual fibrosis and anatomic closure by the second or third week of life. The fibrotic remnant of the ductus persists in the adult as ligamentum arteriosum. Failure of this process by 3 months of age results in PDA.

Q2. What are the types of PDA?
Ans. Persistent ductus arteriosus may be short or long, narrow or wide (width varying from a few mm to 2 cm). Pathophysiologically, it may be restrictive or nonrestrictive. In restrictive variety, a narrow ductus is the site of resistance to L-R shunt. In nonrestrictive type, a wide ductus allows large flow into the pulmonary vasculature with consequent early development of PH and shunt reversal.

Q3. Describe the hemodynamic alterations in PDA.
Ans. In PDA, the blood, which has just been oxygenated, passes from the aorta to the pulmonary artery and goes through the lung once again. From the lungs, blood flows into the LA, left ventricle, aorta, and ductus again. The left ventricle has to cope with this augmented flow and left ventricular overload results if the shunt is large. The large flow may produce a mid-diastolic murmur near the mitral area. Also, an aortic ejection systolic murmur is not uncommon (often hidden by the Gibson murmur).

Q4. How PDA can be handled pharmacologically?
Ans.
- *Helping closure of PDA:* By using prostaglandin inhibitor (aspirin and indomethacin). This can be undertaken in premature infants with PDA and neonates with PDA and left ventricular failure.
- Helping to keep the ductus patent—prostaglandin (PGE_1) infused via an umbilical artery catheter in neonates may keep the ductus patent. It may be undertaken in neonates with pulmonary atresia.

Q5. What is Gibson's murmur?

Ans. Continuous murmur (described by G.A. Gibson in 1900), loudest toward the end of systole and early part of diastole—the time when the pressure difference between the aorta and pulmonary artery is maximal, is the cardinal sign of PDA. It is uncommon to be found below 3 years of age. It is also called machinery murmur (also sometimes called train in tunnel) murmur. It is best heard near the pulmonary area, but sometimes heard rather lower, and occasionally under the left clavicle.

Persistent ductus arteriosus is commonly detected in infancy because of the presence of this characteristic murmur.

Q6. What is the differential diagnosis of PDA?
Ans.
- Clinically—other conditions associated with continuous murmur, e.g., ruptured sinus of Valsalva aneurysm, coronary arteriovenous fistula. VSD with AR produces a to and fro murmur (not continuous); diastolic component is high-pitched and the murmur is not a machinery one.
- On catheterization—other causes of increased O_2 saturation in pulmonary artery compared with right ventricle: AP septal defect*, sinus of Valsalva rupturing into pulmonary artery, ALCAPA (aberrant left coronary artery arising from pulmonary artery).

Q7. What is silent PDA and differential cyanosis?
Ans. Both are features of a large PDA, with raised PVR may lead to a silent PDA. With a progressive increase in pulmonary vascular resistance, first the diastolic component of continuous murmur disappears, followed by the systolic component, leaving a silent ductus. When PVR increases further, shunt reversal occurs. The patient develops differential cyanosis, i.e., cyanosis (and clubbing) of toes but no cyanosis in fingers. This is due to deoxygenated blood from lungs going to the arteries of the lower limb via PDA (ductus is connected to the aorta just beyond the left subclavian artery).

Q8. What are the echocardiographic findings of PDA? What are the differential diagnoses?
Ans.
- Direct visualization of the ductus in high left parasternal short-axis view at the level of the pulmonary artery bifurcation.
- Doppler study—Turbulent flow within the main pulmonary artery throughout the cardiac cycle on CWD **(Fig. 7.7)**.

Similar findings may also be found in aortopulmonary window, PR, and ALCAPA.

---

*It more commonly simulates a large VSD with PH than a PDA; unlike VSD murmur is ejection type, and pulse is bounding.

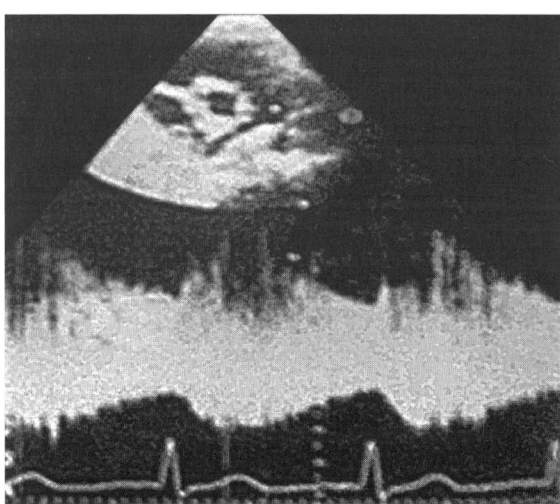

Fig. 7.7: CWD recording in left parasternal short axis at great vessel level showing PDA flow (continuous flow above baseline with late systolic peaking).

- CFI—a narrow jet of mosaic flow entering the distal pulmonary artery near the origin of the left pulmonary artery along its posterolateral border with flow acceleration in the descending thoracic aorta. With a large defect, continuous mosaic may occupy the whole of the distal main pulmonary artery.

Q9. What are the complications of PDA?
Ans.
- Infective endarteritis
- Heart failure—large ductus with high pulmonary blood flow loads the left heart, and HF may develop. It is most likely to develop in infancy. If it does not appear during this period, it is unlikely to occur before the third decade.
- Pulmonary hypertension—in a few cases, causing Eisenmenger's syndrome.

Q10. What is the medical management of PDA?
Ans.
- Treatment of HF—adequate oxygenation (particularly to premature infants), diuretics, digoxin, etc.
- Patients not responding to the above treatment, or for high-risk patients: Transfemoral catheter closure of the ductus may be undertaken.
- Pharmacologic closure—by using prostaglandin inhibitors (aspirin or indomethacin) in premature infants.
- Prevention of infective endarteritis.

- Primary prevention of PDA—obstetric measures to decrease the incidence of prematurity, widespread immunization to reduce the number of those born with rubella syndrome.

Q11. When is closure of PDA is indicated?
Ans.
Current recommendations are:
- Uncontrollable HF in infants
- Failure to grow properly in association with a large shunt with a pulmonary-to-systemic flow ratio exceeding 2:1
- Previous history of infection of the ductus
- Continued patency with any size of shunt beyond the first 6 months of life. The recommended age for elective surgical ligation is 1–2 years of age (at least in the preschool period).
- In adults, surgical ligation undertaken when pulmonary vascular resistance (PVR) is acceptable, i.e., PVR <8 Woods units.
  Patients with device occlusion or after surgical closure should be followed up periodically for possible recanalization.

Q12. What are sinus of Valsalva aneurysm and fistula?
Ans. This is a congenital failure of the aortic media to fuse with the annulus fibrosus of the AV, resulting in aortocardiac fistula. Commonly right aortic sinus communicates with the right ventricle; occasionally noncoronary sinus drains into the right atrium. Rupture occurs in the third or fourth decade. Progressive dilatation has continued since then. The patient may present with chest pain of sudden onset, dyspnea, bounding pulse, and a loud superficial continuous murmur accentuated in diastole (when opens into RV), as well as a thrill, along the right or left lower sternal border.

Q13. Compare and contrast between PDA and rupture sinus of Valsalva aneurysm.
Ans. Persistent ductus arteriosus is extracardiac, and a sinus of Valsalva fistula is an intracardiac communication. Differences between the two are shown in **Table 7.4**.

TABLE 7.4: Persistent ductus and rupture sinus—comparison.

Point	PDA	Rupture sinus of Valsalva
Age of presentation	Early	Later
Location of shunt	Extracardiac	Intracardiac
Machinery murmur	High up; left 2nd intercostal space	Lower in location
Operation	Closed surgery	Open; under cardiopulmonary bypass

(PDA: persistent ductus arteriosus)

Q14. Compare and contrast different shunt anomalies.

Ans. Atrial septal defect, VSD, and PDA are three common shunt anomalies with left-to-right shunt. Their comparative features are mentioned in **Table 7.5**.

TABLE 7.5: Shunt anomalies—comparison.

Points	ASD	VSD	PDA
Definition	Through and through communication between atria at the septal level	Opening in that part of the ventricular septum that separates the two ventricles	Persistent patency of the ductus arteriosus connecting the aorta to PA
Shunt present	Not from birth, cannot occur until normal RV resistance to filling goes below LV	From birth	From birth
Volume load falls on chamber dilatation	RV RA and RV	LV LA and LV (RA, RV late)	LV LA and LV
Symptoms: Dyspnea	Uncommon	Common	Uncommon
Heart failure in infancy	Does not occur	May occur	May occur
RV failure	May occur early	Late	Late
Infective endocarditis	Rare	Common	Common
Eisenmenger's syndrome	Rare	Common	Common
Signs: Differential cyanosis S_2	Nil Wide and fixed splitting	Nil Single (in large VSD)	Pathognomonic (if shunt reversed) closely split, and moves normally with respiration
RV lift	Always present	If present—lately (after PH develops)	May be present lately (after PH develops)
Investigations: ECG	LVH absent; RVH common; partial RBBB and P-pulmonale very common	LVH may be present; P-pulmonale, RVH common	LVH may be present; RVH may occur; P-pulmonale is rare
CXR	RAE considerable, PA enlargement extreme, aorta small	PA enlargement moderate, aorta normal, RAE absent	PA enlargement moderate, aorta enlarged, RAE absent

Contd...

Contd...

Echo	RV volume overload, echo dropout in IAS	LV volume overload echo dropout seen in a large defect	LV volume overload; the duct may be seen
O_2 step up on catheter	RA	RV	Pulmonary artery
Device closure	Yes	Muscular	Possible
Surgical closure	Always needed	Needed in moderate to large defects	Always needed

(ASD: atrial septal defect; CXR: chest X-ray; ECG: electrocardiogram; IAS: interatrial septum; LA: left atrium; LV: left ventricle; LVH: left ventricular hypertrophy; PA: pulmonary artery; PDA: patent ductus arteriosus; PH: pulmonary hypertension; RA: right atrium; RAE: right atrial enlargement; RBBB: right bundle branch block; RV: right ventricle; RVH: right ventricular hypertrophy; VSD: ventricular septal defect)

PULMONARY STENOSIS

Q1. When are pulmonary stenosis patients symptomatic?
Ans.
- Patients with mild PS at age exceeding 2 years are rarely symptomatic and rarely develop progressive obstruction (in contrast to those with AS).
- Moderate PS is also well tolerated, provided there is no other disorder.
- Patients with severe PS develop symptoms of right HF and dyspnea on exertion in their fourth or fifth decade of life. Cyanosis may occur due to an R-L shunt through the foramen ovale. Symptoms such as angina, exertional syncope, and symptoms from infective endocarditis are uncommon (unlike AS).

Q2. What are the signs of severe PS?
Ans.
- General signs—cyanosis may be present, pulse—small and blood pressure may be low, jugular venous pressure (JVP)—raised (in RV failure), and edema (RV failure)
  - Characteristic facies may be seen in Noonan's syndrome (male Turner), William's syndrome (elf-like facies), or round, plump face with isolated PS
- *Precordial signs:*
  - RV heave
  - Systolic thrill—in the pulmonary area
  - Ejection click (disappears if calcified), S_2 widely split, P_2 becomes inaudible with increasing severity, ejection systolic murmur, best heard in the third or fourth space and radiates to the left shoulder. The

murmur does not increase with inspiration (too much lung placed between the heart and the stethoscope).
- Sign of right HF—hepatomegaly and ascites may be present.

Q3. How to assess pulmonary stenosis on echocardiography?
Ans. Assessment done in parasternal short-axis view through the base of the heart.
- M-mode—depth of "a" wave is proportionate to peak pressure gradient (PPG), as measured with CWD
- 2DE—presence of RVH, increased trabeculation of RV, and subvalvular narrowing—in severe stenosis. Thickening of cusps, systolic doming, decreased excursion, and calcification (in adults) are not indicators of severity.
- Continuous-wave Doppler—peak flow velocity and maximum systolic pressure gradient show severity.

Q4. How is pulmonary stenosis classified?
Ans. Doppler study aids in grading the severity of PS. It correlates well with the catheterization data. The peak pressure gradient is measured by using continuous wave Doppler and PS is classified as:
- *Mild:* Gradient <40 mm Hg
- *Moderate:* Gradient 40–80 mm Hg
- *Several:* Gradient >80 mm Hg

Q5. What is the treatment of PS?
Ans.
- Mild to moderate PS—intervention is rarely needed.
- Severe PS—with suprasystemic RV pressure and in failing RV—the treatment of choice is balloon valvuloplasty, usually with a 75% decrement of transvalvular gradient (**Fig. 7.8**).

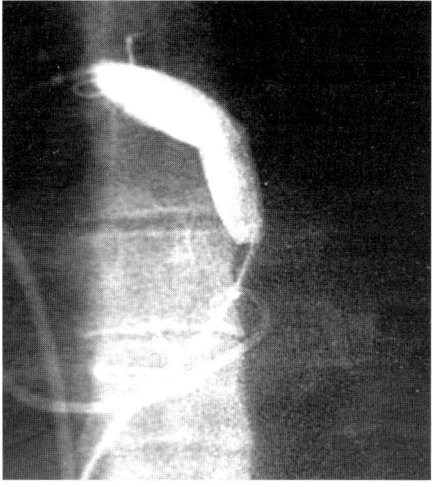

Fig. 7.8: Pulmonary balloon valvuloplasty.

Surgery: Pulmonary valvotomy—done, if balloon dilatation fails. In isolated infundibular stenosis, resection of the hypertrophic area may be required through open heart surgery.
- Pulmonary stenosis secondary to carcinoid syndrome has a poor prognosis. Balloon valvuloplasty is often unsuccessful, and valve replacement is needed.

TETRALOGY OF FALLOT

Q1. How does Fallot's tetralogy develop? What are its components?
Ans. Developmentally, there is anterior and upward displacement of the bulbus septum. Bulbus cordis fails to rotate properly, so that the aorta is more anterior and to the right than normal. Anterior displacement produces a malalignment VSD beneath the AV, as well as infundibular obstruction, which in turn leads to RV hypertrophy.

Thus, four components of TOF are:
1. Ventricular septal defect—large, usually infracristal, extending from crista to TV ring
2. Overriding of the aorta
3. Right ventricular outflow obstruction—usually infundibular
4. Right ventricular hypertrophy

Q2. What is Fallot's triad and pentad? What is a pink Fallot (or acyanotic TOF)?
Ans.
- Fallot's triad—PS with reversed interatrial shunt; RV hypertrophy occurs due to PS
- Fallot's pentad—when ASD is present along with Fallot's tetrad
- Acyanotic TOF or pink Fallot—in TOF, cyanosis may be absent if RV outflow obstruction is slight. There may be a bidirectional shunt or L-R shunt with pulmonary flow twice the systemic flow, and arterial O_2 saturation is normal.

Q3. How does squatting help patients with TOF?
Ans. The history of squatting for relief of dyspnea is the hallmark of TOF and appears at about the age the child begins to walk.

Mechanism:
- It increases peripheral resistance by compression and kinking of the femoral arteries and the aorta, which reduces the L-R shunt. RV blood is diverted into the pulmonary circulation, thus increasing more oxygenated blood going to the left side.
- It decreases venous return from the leg and reduces the volume of highly unsaturated venous blood reaching the right heart; O_2 saturation increases.
- It may also prevent dynamic infundibular obstruction by counteracting the effect of orthostatic hypotension.

Q4. How do cyanotic spells occur? Give their management.
Ans.
- Increased RV outflow obstruction due to systolic contraction of hypertrophied infundibulum. It may occur with increased exertion, activity, and drugs with inotropic action.
- Decrease in peripheral resistance increases R-L shunt; pulmonary blood flow decreases, and cyanosis increases.

In cyanotic spells, increasing cyanosis and tachypnea may progress to convulsion, unconsciousness, and death. They may last for a few minutes to several hours.

Treatment:
- O_2 inhalation
- Knee chest position—to ↓ R-L shunt
- Morphin 0.1 mg/kg—to decrease infundibular tone
- Propranolol—to relieve RVOT obstruction; a daily dose of 1-3 mg/kg may prevent or reduce cyanotic spells
- Adequate hydration with intravenous (IV) fluid
- $NaHCO_3$ in 5% dextrose—if acidosis present

Q5. Why RV failure is uncommon in TOF?
Ans. Right ventricular failure is uncommon in TOF, even in adult survivors. RV is protected from excessive pressure load because of the presence of a large nonrestrictive VSD, which permits direct decompression into the aorta. RV is well-equipped to eject at systemic vascular resistance.

Q6. What are the associations and complications of TOF?
Ans.
- Associations—right-sided aortic arch (30%), ASD, PDA, PLSVC (persistent left superior vena cava), anomalous origin of left anterior descending artery (LAD) from right coronary artery (RCA), or a prominent conal branch from RCA. These vessels cross the RV outflow tract.
- Complications—cyanotic spells, cerebral abscess (possibly by paradoxical embolism), cerebrovascular accident (due to increased blood viscosity and hypoxia), infective endocarditis, and AR—may occur naturally from dilated aortic root or after endocarditis. Following total correction, new complication may arise—RV failure, RVOT aneurysm, PR, reopened VSD, tachyarrhythmia, heart block (as His bundle is just beneath VSD), etc.

Q7. What are the physical signs of TOF?
Ans.
- Patients who have not undergone surgical repair: Developing cyanosis, clubbing, and polycythemia, quiet apex, RV heave uncommon (in spite of hypertrophy as it can freely empty into aorta), A_2 palpable (large, anterior aorta), S_2 single (A_2 only), may be loud, and ejection systolic murmurs

in pulmonary area (due to RVOT obstruction, not VSD). The intensity and duration of the systolic ejection murmur vary inversely with the severity of subvalvular obstruction—the opposite of the relationship that exists in patients with pulmonary valve stenosis. With extreme outflow tract stenosis or pulmonary atresia and during an attack of paroxysmal hypoxemia, no murmur or only a short, faint murmur may be present. With cyanotic spell, the murmur is quieter and may disappear, a diastolic murmur may appear due to AR. Sometimes a continuous murmur due to large aortopulmonary collaterals may be heard in the back.

- Patients with palliative treatment—characteristic continuous murmur of shunt may be heard.
- Patients who have undergone surgical repair—some degree of turbulence remains across RVOT, producing a variable systolic murmur at the left upper sternal border, murmur of PR may be audible in this area. Chronic volume loading of the RV may produce dysrhythmia and right HF. A residual VSD or leak in the patch may produce a systolic murmur at the left lower sternal border; a diastolic murmur of AR may also be found.

Q8. What are the aortic changes in TOF?
Ans.
- Overriding of the aorta-aorta is biventricular; aortic root diameter is the same as the ventricular defect. Aorta receives the full output of the LV and part of the RV (the remainder reaches the lung through the obstructed outflow tract).
- Aorta and AVs are bigger than normal, lie forward, and its root is uncovered. A_2 is slightly accentuated.
- Aortic arch is right sided in 25%.

Q9. How does TOF differ from DORV on echocardiography?
Ans. Clinical scenario and management of DORV are similar to those of TOF. In TOF, overriding ranges from minimal to extreme. "50% rule": On echocardiography, is that: if >50% aorta overrides LV, it is TOF; if >50% of the aorta overrides RV, it is DORV.

Q10. How does TOF differ from isolated PS?
Ans. Both are RV outflow obstructions, although, in TOF, there is an infundibular in most of the cases. The two conditions are differentiated by the following features **(Table 7.6)**.

TABLE 7.6: Differences between tetralogy of Fallot and isolated pulmonary stenosis.

Isolated PS	TOF
No cyanosis, clubbing	Cyanosis, clubbing—present
RV heave—present	Nil
Systolic thrill—present	Nil

Contd...

Contd...

S₂-soft (pulmonary component)	S₂-not soft, may be loud (aortic component)
Ejection click—may be found	Nil
Murmur—midsystolic	Ejection systolic
No change in amyl nitrate inhalation	Murmur may change

(PS: pulmonary stenosis; RV: right ventricle; TOF: tetralogy of Fallot)

Q11. How does TOF differ from Eisenmenger's syndrome?
Ans. Both are cyanotic states with the following differences **(Table 7.7)**.

TABLE 7.7: Tetralogy of Fallot and Eisenmenger's syndrome—differences.

TOF	Eisenmenger's syndrome
Cyanosis—after birth	After shunt reverses
RV heave—nil	Present
Loud P₂—nil	Present
Systolic murmur—present	Nil
Diastolic murmur—nil	EDM of pulmonary regurgitation±

(EDM: early diastolic murmur; RV: right ventricle; TOF: tetralogy of Fallot)

Q12. What are the radiologic features of TOF? How to differentiate it from isolated pulmonary stenosis?
Ans. The following characteristic radiological features differentiate TOF from PS **(Figs. 7.9A and B)**.
- Boot-shaped heart (Cœur en sabot)—cardiomegaly with apex elevated from the diaphragm (due to RV hypertrophy)
- Concave pulmonary conus—as PS is infundibular, not valvular
- Oligemic lung fields—due to infundibular PS
- Right-sided aortic arch—in 29%.

In isolated PS, there is poststenotic dilatation (pulmonary bay is convex rather than concave), and the heart is not boot shaped.

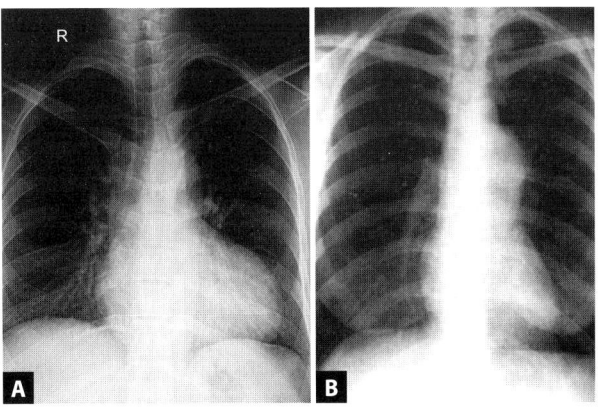

Figs. 7.9A and B: TOF (A) and pulmonary stenosis (B).

Q13. What are the echocardiographic findings of TOF? How to differentiate it from DORV?

Ans.

- M-mode—septal echo dropout, which is overridden by the anterior and posterior aortic root.
- Two-dimensional echocardiography—large malalignment VSD and aortic overriding seen in left parasternal long-axis view. VSD is nonrestrictive; discontinuity between infundibular septum and anterior aortic root apparent **(Fig. 7.10)**.

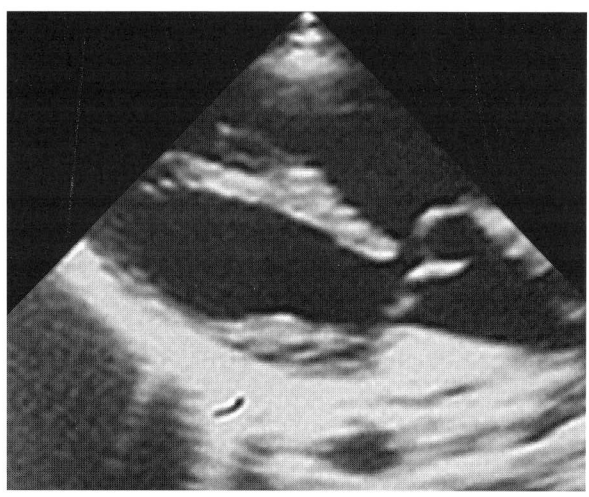

Fig. 7.10: 2DE showing malaligned VSD and aortic overriding.

Morphology of RVOT, pulmonary valve, pulmonary artery, as well as the size and extent of VSD can also be evaluated in the left parasternal short-axis view. Anomalous origin and course of LAD can also be evaluated in this view. In infants and children, a combination of subcostal coronal (long-axis) and subcostal sagittal (short-axis) views is needed.

After corrective surgery, the position and integrity of the VSD patch passing obliquely from the septum to the anterior aortic root can be assessed from the left parasternal long- and short-axis views.

- Doppler echo—PWD interrogation shows bidirectional shunt across VSD. CWD can show the site and extent of PS. It can also determine RV systolic pressure from the TR jet velocity.
- CFI—shows bidirectional shunt across the VSD; localize site of PS by observing turbulent flow across the site and flow acceleration proximal to it.

Differentiating TOF from DORV: "50 percent rule" for differentiation—in case of TOF, >50% of the aorta arises from the LV, while in DORV, >50% of the aorta arises from the RV.

Q14. When is intervention indicated in TOF?
Ans.
- Symptomatic infants are repaired at any age. Marked hypoplasia of the pulmonary arteries, small body size, and prematurity are relative contraindications for early corrective operation.
- Asymptomatic infants are advocated elective repair during the first 6 months.
- Palliation is done by balloon dilation of RVOT (with or without stenting) and pulmonary arteries or by shunt procedures.
- Surgical repair is also recommended for unoperated adults (result gratifying and operative risk is comparable to that of pediatric series).
- Palliated patients should undergo surgical repair, particularly those with increasing cyanosis and erythrocytosis (from gradual shunt stenosis or PH), LV dilatation, or aneurysm formation in the shunt. Intracardiac repair with takedown of the shunt is undertaken.
- Intervention after repair is needed if there is a residual VSD with shunt >1.5:1; residual PS with RVSP—two-thirds of systemic pressure; or severe PR associated with substantial RV dilatation or dysfunction [right ventricular ejection fraction (RVEF) ≤45%], exercise intolerance, or substantial arrhythmias. Surgery is occasionally needed for significant AR and RVOT aneurysm.

Q15. What are the interventions for TOF?
Ans.
- Surgery—closing the VSD with a dacron patch and relieving the RVOT obstruction by resection of the infundibular muscle and insertion of an RVOT or transannular patch. An extracardiac conduit is placed if an anomalous coronary artery crosses the RVOT. Patients with repaired TOF can go through pregnancy relatively safely.
- Transcatheter valve placement—percutaneous pulmonary valve (PV) replacement in selected situations. Significant branch pulmonary artery stenosis can be managed by balloon dilatation and stent placement.
- Implantable cardioverter defibrillator (ICD)—in patients presenting with aborted sudden cardiac death or substantial ventricular tachycardia (VT) (may arise at the site of right ventriculotomy, from VSD patch sutures, or from RVOT); done as a secondary preventive measure.

Q16. What is a Blalock-Taussig (BT) shunt and a modified BT shunt?
Ans. These are palliative surgical procedures undertaken for patients with TOF.

Indications: Very small infant of weight <5 kg with recurrent cyanotic spells and a size of pulmonary artery unsuitable for corrective surgery, i.e., if one of the pulmonary artery is small. Such a shunt to the smaller pulmonary artery may allow for the growth of this vessel.

In classical BT shunt, anastomosis of the subclavian artery with a homolateral branch of the PA is done. In a modified BT shunt, a tubular gore-tex graft is placed between the subclavian artery and the pulmonary artery. This preserves the patently of the subclavian artery. This is most commonly used, and it serves as a bridge to complete repair in the first year of life.

OTHER COMPLEX CONGENITAL HEART DISEASE

Q1. What is Eisenmenger's syndrome?
Ans. It is defined as PVOD that develops as a consequence of a large pre-existing left-to-right shunt such that PAP approaches the systemic level and the flow becomes bidirectional or predominantly right-to-left. The high PVR is usually established in early childhood (except in ASD) and is sometimes present from birth. Chest radiograph shows dilated central pulmonary arteries with rapid tapering of the peripheral pulmonary vasculature. Eisenmenger's syndrome due to VSD or PDA usually has a normal or only slightly increased cardiothoracic ratio. In ASD cardiomegaly, full pulmonary conus, dilated hilar pulmonary arteries with peripheral prunning are prominant features **(Fig. 7.11)**.

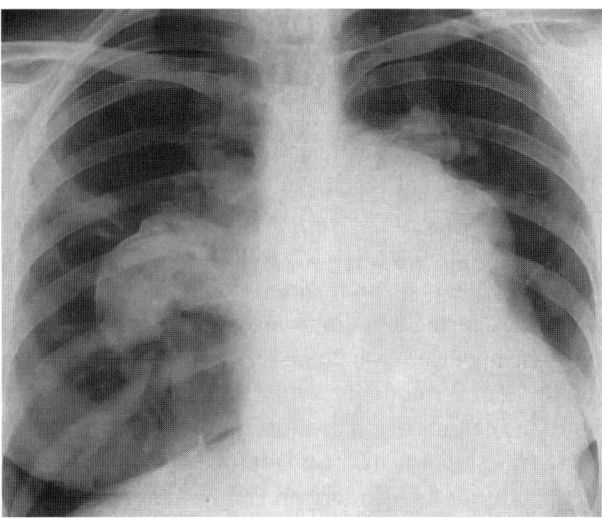

Fig. 7.11: Eisenmenger's syndrome in ASD.

Eisenmenger's syndrome due to an ASD typically has a large cardiothoracic ratio because of right atrial and ventricular dilatation, along with an inconspicuous aorta, reflecting lifelong low cardiac output. All three different pulmonary vasodilators (endothelin receptor antagonist, phosphodiesterase five inhibitors, and prostacyclins) have been shown to improve outcome.

Q2. What are the characteristic features of Ebstein anomaly?
Ans.
- Apical displacement of the septal leaflet of TV in conjunction with leaflet dysplasia. It leads to "atrialization" of the inflow tract of the RV. The anterior tricuspid leaflet may be adherent to the free wall of the RV, causing RVOT obstruction.
- Cyanosis may occur due to L-R shunting through PFO or ASD; occurs when RA pressure exceeds LA pressure and severe TR is present.
- Right-sided CHF in severe cases, with typically normal JVP because of large and compliant RA and atrialized RV.
- Widely split S_1 with loud tricuspid component (the "sail sound"); a widely split S_2 from RBBB; and a right-sided S_3. Pansystolic murmur of TR is frequently seen.
- Apical displacement of septal leaflet of TV by 8 mm/m^2 or more, combined with an elongated sail-like appearance of the anterior leaflet, confirms the diagnosis.
- Cyanosis, right-sided HF, poor functional capacity, and occurrence of paradoxical embolism are indications for intervention.

Q3. What are the chest radiographic features of Ebstein anomaly?
Ans. Cardiomegaly—highly variable in degree. A rightward convexity from an enlarged RA and atrialized RV, coupled with a leftward convexity from a dilated infundibulum. Aortic knuckle and pulmonary conus are inconspicuous; pulmonary vasculature is normal or reduced. All these give a "water bottle" appearance. This appearance is very close to that of massive pericardial effusion (here, left and right borders are not convex and the maximum diameter of the cardiac shadow is near the diaphragm).

Q4. What are TGAs and corrected TGA?
Ans. In TGA, the aorta arises from the right ventricle and is located anteriorly and to the right of the pulmonary artery, which arises from the left ventricle. The coronary arteries usually arise from the posterior aortic sinuses that face the pulmonary artery. Thus, the circulation here consists of two parallel systems. Most blood returning from systemic and pulmonary circuits returns to the same respective circuits. A variable volume mixing at various sites (ASD and PFO, VSD, and PDA) permits survival.

In corrected TGA, the TGAs (ventriculoarterial discordance) is "corrected" by arterioventricular discordance. Thus, RA is connected to morphological LV, which in turn is connected to PA. The LA communicates with the morphological RV, and this communicates with the aorta, which is anterior and to the left (L-position). An isolated corrected TGA does not usually produce symptoms unless complete heart block is present.

Q5. Name the surgical operations in complex CHD with their indications.
Ans. Most complex CHD needs corrective surgery. Some need palliative surgery before a definitive procedure **(Box 7.2).**

> **BOX 7.2:** Surgical operations in complex congenital heart disease.
> - Rastelli operation—undertaken in complex CHD, e.g., TGA with large VSD. VSD is closed by a large patch in such a way as to connect the LV to the aorta, and a conduit or homograft connects the RV to the PA
> - Arterial switch—done for TGA; aorta and pulmonary artery are relocated to their original positions, with reanastomosis of the coronary arteries to the neoaorta
> - Mustard/Senning operations (atrial switch)—involves intra-atrial redirection of oxygenated and deoxygenated blood to the systemic and pulmonary system, respectively. RV serves as a systemic subaortic ventricle. It is life-saving procedure in TGA and carries the risk of future arrhythmias, pathway obstruction, and ventricular failure
> - Fontan operation—palliative procedure for patients with effectively univentricular circulations, such as mitral or tricuspid atresia. Blood from the superior and IVC is directed to the pulmonary arteries without the benefit of a subpulmonary ventricle. Oxygenated blood returns to the systemic ventricle and is then pumped to the aorta
> - *Corrective operation in TOF:* Total correction with patch closure of nonrestrictive VSD. It is done as early as possible, but if the pulmonary artery is very small, a palliative shunt operation is done before it to allow the growth of the pulmonary artery
>
> (CHD: congenital heart disease; IVC: inferior vena cava; LV: left ventricle; PA: pulmonary artery; RV: right ventricle; TGA: transposition of the great arteries; TOF: tetralogy of Fallot; VSD: ventricular septal defect)

SUGGESTED READING

1. Canadian Adult Congenital Heart (CACH) Network. [online] Available from http://www.cachnet.org. [Last accessed May, 2025].
2. Perloff JK, Child JS. Congenital heart disease in adults. Philadelphia: WB Saunders; 1991.
3. Warner CA, Williams RG, Bashore TM, Child JS, Connolly HM, Dearani JA, et al. ACC/AHA guidelines for the management of adults with congenital heart disease: a report of the American College of Cardiology/American Heart Association Task Force on Practice Guidelines (writing committee to develop guidelines on the management of adults with congenital heart disease). Circulation. 2008;118(23):e714-e833.

8. Infective Endocarditis

*"Infective endocarditis is a primary mycotic process having two clinical variants;
an acute, fulminant and a chronic incidious form."*
—Willium Osler (Gulstonian Lecture 1885)

INTRODUCTION

A healthy heart is usually unaffected by infectious agents. When the valve is diseased or a prosthetic valve is in situ, it becomes susceptible to infection. However, a healthy right-sided valve may be affected by infective agents in intravenous (IV) drug addicts. Infective endocarditis (IE) is predominantly a complication of rheumatic heart disease in Bangladesh. Various issues involving pathogenesis, diagnosis, and treatment are discussed.

Q1. What is endocarditis?
Ans. Endocarditis is the inflammation of the endocardium, the inner lining of the heart. It may be infective or noninfective. IE is due to invading microorganisms such as bacteria, fungi, chlamydia, or Coxiella. Noninfective causes are rheumatic fever, systemic lupus erythematosus, etc.

Infective endocarditis is the infection of the heart valve (native or prosthetic), the lining of a cardiac chamber, blood vessel, or a congenital anomaly.

Q2. How to classify IE?
Ans. Infective endocarditis is classified on the basis of its clinical course, type of involved valve, and result of blood culture **(Box 8.1)**.

BOX 8.1: Classification of infective endocarditis.
- *According to the natural course of the disease (when untreated):*
  - *Acute:* Duration <6 weeks
  - *Subacute:* Duration >6 weeks
- *According to valvular involvement:*
  - Native valve endocarditis—involving diseased or healthy native valves
  - Prosthetic valve endocarditis:
    - *Early:* Within 2 months of valve implantation (i.e., perioperative infection)
    - *Late:* After 2 months (i.e., after the valve is endothelialized) of implantation
- *Depending on blood culture results:*
  - *Culture positive:* Organism identified on culture
  - *Culture negative:* No organism isolated on culture

Q3. What is the difference between acute and subacute IE?
Ans. Besides the clinical course, the two conditions differ in the following aspects **(Table 8.1)**.

TABLE 8.1: Difference between acute and subacute infective endocarditis.

	Acute	Subacute
Duration	<6 weeks	>6 weeks
Valves involved	Healthy valves; right-sided valves are more involved in intravenous drug abusers	Commonly involves left side; regurgitant lesions are more involved, mitral valve is more frequent
Organisms	Caused by virulent organisms, particularly *Staphylococcus*, that can involve healthy valves	Caused by relatively avirulent organisms (i.e., indigenous streptococci), lacking invasiveness to initiate infection in the normal heart
Symptoms and signs	Embolic features are more common; features of overwhelming sepsis are present	Immunologic phenomena such as arthritis, glomerulonephritis, Osler's node, and Janeway lesion are more common
	Changing murmur may be found	Rarely found
Complication	Heart failure and neurologic complications such as convulsion and hemiplegia are more common	Less common
Treatment	Promptly needed before C/S result available	Less urgency
	Nafcillin plus gentamicin	Penicillin plus gentamicin
	Surgery may be required	Seldom required

Q4. What is the clinical hallmark of IE?
Ans. All patients with a heart murmur and a fever of unknown origin should be considered as having IE until proved otherwise. The change in character of an existing murmur or the appearance of a new murmur is particularly suggestive of endocarditis.

The appearance of a new murmur is highly suggestive of further valvular involvement and sometimes perforation of the valve cusp. A soft apical systolic murmur is of little diagnostic value if tachycardia, pyrexia, and anemia are already present. However, fever may be absent in the elderly and patients previously treated with antibiotics or in uremic patients. Murmur may be absent with mural infections or right-sided infections.

Q5. What is a vegetation?

Ans. Vegetation composed of platelets, fibrins, and infective microbial agents is the morphologic feature of IE **(Flowchart 8.1)**.

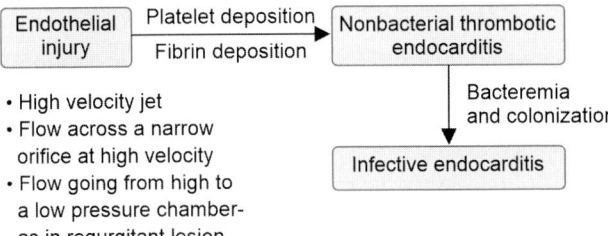

Flowchart 8.1: Infective endocarditis: Pathogenesis.

Just as the endothelial damage occurs most commonly in the high-pressure system, left-sided valves are more commonly affected than right-sided one, and regurgitant lesions are more prone to infection than stenotic lesions. A vegetation of significant size can easily be demonstrated on echocardiography **(Fig. 8.1)**.

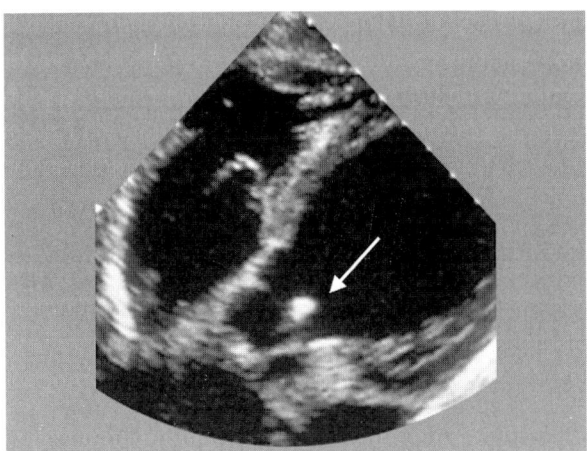

Fig. 8.1: Large vegetation on aortic valve (arrowed).

Q6. What is culture-negative endocarditis? Give its causes.

Ans. Repeatedly, negative blood culture in a patient of IE is called culture-negative IE. The causes are as follows:
- Previous antibiotic therapy
- Fastidious organisms (requiring special culture media) with peculiar growth requirements, e.g., anaerobes (require anaerobic culture), HACEK *(Haemophilus, Actinobacillus, Cardiobacterium hominis, Eikenella,* and *Kingella)* organisms (CO_2 incubation), and *Candida* (need special media)
- Cell-dependent organisms, e.g., *Coxiella burnetii* and Chlamydia that cannot be cultured from blood

- *Incorrect diagnosis:* There may be noncardiac infection in a patient who has a heart murmur, or conditions mimicking IE, e.g., rheumatic fever, atrial myxoma, nonbacterial thrombotic endocarditis, sarcoid, drug reaction, etc.
- Bacteria-free phases due to excess circulating antibody, producing resting forms
- Culture-negative endocarditis occurs in about 10% of patients with IE.

Q7. What are the characteristic features of endocarditis in intravenous drug abusers?
Ans.
- Patients are usually younger, male.
- Endocarditis in the absence of an underlying cardiac lesion is common. Tricuspid valve involvement is most common (50%), mitral and aortic valve involvement are uncommon, and involvement of the pulmonary valve is rare.
- The patient may present with pneumonia or multiple septic pulmonary emboli.
- Skin is the most frequent source of infection; *Staphylococcus* is the most common organism. Some may have more than a single microorganism isolated from blood.
- May be recurrent in some cases.

Q8. What are the predisposing risk factors for IE?
Ans.
- *Cardiac conditions:* Rheumatic and other acquired valve disease, congenital heart disease [except secundum atrial septal defect (ASD), pulmonary stenosis (PS), divided patent ductus arteriosus (PDA), prosthetic valves, hypertrophic cardiomyopathy (HCM), mitral valve prolapse (MVP) with regurgitation, and tricuspid valve in drug addicts].
- Dental and surgical interventional procedures that may produce bacteremia:
  - Dental procedures, including gingival or mucosal bleeding
  - Tonsillectomy or adenoidectomy
  - Surgical operations involving intestinal or respiratory mucosa, gallbladder operation, urinary tract surgery [if urinary tract infection (UTI) is present], prostatic surgery, incision and drainage of infected tissue, vaginal hysterectomy, and delivery (in the presence of infection)

  Bronchoscopy (with rigid bronchoscope), cystoscopy and urethral dilatation, esophageal dilatation, and sclerotherapy for esophageal varices

  Prophylactic antibiotics are recommended for persons at risk during these procedures.
- *General risk factors:* Advanced age, male gender, diabetes mellitus, and IV drug abuse

Q9. What are the cardiac conditions associated with the highest risk for IE?
Ans.
- These are prosthetic valve, history of previous IE, cyanotic congenital heart disease (including those with palliative shunt and conduit), those repaired with prosthetic material or device (during first 6 months), residual defect adjacent to patch or device (inhibiting endothelialization), and cardiac transplant recipient developing valvopathy).

Q10. What are the peripheral manifestations of IE?
Ans.
- *Petechiae:* Most common in palpebral conjunctiva, buccal and palatal mucosa, and extremities
- *Splinter hemorrhage:* Linear streaks in the proximal nail bed
- *Osler nodes:* Small tender subcutaneous nodes in the pulp of the digit
- *Janeway lesions:* Small erythematous or hemorrhagic macular nontender lesions on the palm or soles; consequence of septic embolic events
- *Roth spot:* Oval retinal hemorrhage with pale center
- *Digital infarct:* Embolic; in *Staphylococcus aureus* IE

Q11. What are the general principles of the treatment of IE?
Ans. The aim of treatment is to eradicate the infecting agent as soon as possible.
- *Isolation of the causative organism from the blood:* Bacteremia in IE is usually continuous; isolation of the organism from culture is an important prerequisite to drug therapy. In acute cases, because of its fulminant nature, treatment is needed prior to isolation of the agents. A delay until culture results are available can have deleterious consequences.
- *Selection of antibiotics:* The antibiotics must eradicate the organism completely without the help of phagocytes; hence, bacteriostatic antibiotics should be avoided. Synergistic combinations are favored for certain pathogens.
- *Adequate doses of antibiotics:* The individual dosage of antibiotics chosen should exceed the minimum bactericidal concentration (MBC) for that organism.
- *Route:* Intravenous therapy is essential. Peripheral lines should be changed every 72 hours if possible. Dilute antibiotic solution is used and a heparin flush (500 U in 5 c.c. 5% dextrose), given after each infusion, helps preserve the vein. The giving set should be changed daily.
- *Long duration of treatment:* Cure requires complete sterilization of vegetations. Bacteria are found in very high concentrations inside it and are eliminated very slowly in response to antibiotics. Therefore, treatment should be continued long enough to ensure that relapses do not occur. Most cases of endocarditis require 6 weeks of parental antibiotics.

However, certain cases of endocarditis due to penicillin-sensitive *Streptococcus viridans* and right-sided IE by *S. aureus* can be cured in 2–4 weeks.

Q12. When is empiric therapy given in IE?
Ans.
- It is often started and continued until the etiologic agent is identified and antibiotic sensitivity is known.
- Occasionally started as a therapeutic trial to help confirm a diagnosis
- Culture-negative IE, unless clinical and epidemiologic clues suggest an etiology
- In acute IE, broad-spectrum therapy that covers *S. aureus* as well as many species of streptococci and Gram-negative bacilli: Nafcillin 2 g IV 4 hourly plus ampicillin 2 g IV 4 hourly plus gentamicin 1.5 mg/kg IV every 12 hourly
- In subacute IE, ampicillin 2 g IV every 4 hourly plus gentamicin 1.5 mg/kg IV every 8 hourly (or 12 hourly)

or

Penicillin 4 million units IV 4 hourly plus gentamicin 1.5 mg/kg every 8 hourly
- For early prosthetic valve endocarditis, vancomycin 1.0 g IV 12 hourly plus gentamicin 1 mg/kg IV 8 hourly

Q13. How is blood culture done in a suspected case of IE?
Ans.
- Blood culture can be obtained in the absence of fever spikes as IE being an intravascular infection leads to continuous bacteremia.
- After antiseptic skin cleaning, blood is drawn from the vein by entering with a single movement (blood obtained with difficulty is more likely to be contaminated). 10 mL of blood is withdrawn and 5 mL of this is injected into two flasks: One containing an aerobic medium and the other an anaerobic medium.
- Three sets of the paired culture should be drawn over a period of 24 hours at three venipuncture sites. Because contamination of skin bacteria may ruin a single sample.
- The laboratory should be alerted if any fastidious infecting agent is suspected or if the patient is receiving or has received any antibiotic. For example, if a fungus is suspected, 6% sucrose should be added to the media to accelerate the growth, and prolonged incubation of up to 21 days may be needed for the HACEK group of organisms.
- The most common pathogens grow within 48 hours and incubated bottles are inspected and subcultured after 24 and 48 hours, then usually at further intervals of a week or more.

- In cases of culture-negative IE, serology for Brucella, Coxiella, and Chlamydia may be useful.

  Arterial blood offers no advantage over antecubital vein blood.

Q14. How to monitor response to antibiotic therapy in IE?

Ans.

- Temperature usually falls after 3–7 days of successful antimicrobial therapy. Persistent or recurrent fever may be a manifestation of therapeutic failure (due to the emergence of the resistant organism, superinfection with another organism, or development of an abscess) or development of a reaction to the antibiotic.
- A rising hemoglobin and falling erythrocyte sedimentation rate (ESR) are a useful sign of therapeutic success. A falling CRP (C-reactive protein), an acute phase protein released by the bacterial infection, is a good sign of infection coming under control.
- *Electrocardiogram (ECG) and chest X-ray weekly:* Enlarging heart on X-ray indicates complications, like congestive heart failure (CHF). Prolonged PR interval on ECG may suggest an aortic root abscess.
- *Echocardiography:* Vegetations are not visualized until the size is >2 mm. Weekly echocardiography showing a shrinking vegetation during antimicrobial therapy suggests therapeutic success. Significant enlargement of a vegetation indicates possible treatment failure. Vegetations of 10 mm or more in size are associated with a greater risk of emboli. The degree of valvular destruction, its hemodynamic consequences, and complications like aortic root abscess, aneurysm, and myocardial abscess can be detected by echocardiography and Doppler study. Transesophageal echocardiography (TEE) is more sensitive than transthoracic echocardiography (TTE).
- Blood culture should be obtained during therapy to ensure the eradication of the organism.

Q15. How do you suggest prophylaxis for IE?

Ans. In deciding the need for antibiotic prophylaxis, two factors are considered: Underlying cardiac lesions and the procedures to be performed. Prophylaxis is advised when the combination of cardiac lesion and the procedure seems to pose a substantial risk of IE.

- *Cardiac lesions:* High-risk conditions are prosthetic heart valve, previous IE, cyanotic congenital heart disease [tetralogy of Fallot (TOF), transposition of the great arteries (TGA), single ventricle], and surgically constructed systemic-pulmonary shunt [e.g., Blalock-Taussig (BT) shunt]. Intermediate risk conditions are acquired rheumatic valvular disease, most congenital heart disease (noncyanotic) except secundum ASD, HCM, and MVP with regurgitation.

- *Procedures likely to induce bacteremia:* Oropharyngeal procedures, dental procedures known to induce gingival or mucosal bleeding, tonsillectomy and/or adenoidectomy, bronchoscopy with a rigid bronchoscope, gastrointestinal procedures, surgical operations involving intestinal mucosa, sclerotherapy for esophageal varices, dilatation of esophageal stricture, biliary surgery and endoscopic retrograde cholangiopancreatography (ERCP) with biliary cannulation, genitourinary procedures, cystoscopy, urethral dilatation, and prostatic surgery. Others include incision and drainage of the infected tissue.

Bacteremia is highest for events that traumatize the oral mucosa, followed by those that traumatize the genitourinary tract.

It is relatively low for gastrointestinal diagnostic procedure. In orodental procedures, prophylaxis is primarily directed against viridans streptococci, and in the latter situations, it is directed against enterococci.

Therapy may need to be individualized in a given clinical setting.

High-risk cardiac patients may need prophylaxis prior to low-risk procedures such as endoscopy (with or without biopsy), TEE, vaginal hysterectomy and delivery, and bronchoscopy with flexible bronchoscope (with or without biopsy).

Prophylaxis in gastrointestinal procedures is recommended for high-risk cardiac lesions but optional for intermediate-risk cases.

Q16. What regimens are used for prophylaxis of IE?
Ans. Depending on the procedures to be undertaken, antibiotic prophylaxis is mentioned in **Box 8.2**.

BOX 8.2: Regimens for prophylaxis of infective endocarditis.
- For dental, oral, respiratory tract, or esophageal procedures: Oral amoxicillin 2 g 1 hour before the procedure (also given for minor GI or GU procedure)

    Ampicillin 2 g IV/IM within ½ hours before the procedure (for those unable to take oral agent)
    - Clindamycin 600 mg 1 hour before the procedure or cephalexin 2 g 1 hour before the procedure or azithromycin 500 mg 1 hour before the procedure (oral), or vancomycin 1.0 g IV slowly plus gentamicin 1.5 mg/kg IV/IM (for patients who are allergic to penicillin)
- For genitourinary/gastrointestinal (excluding esophageal) procedures:
    - Ampicillin 2 g IV/IM plus gentamicin 1.5 mg/kg IV/IM ½ hour before procedure; after 6 hours, ampicillin 1 g IV/IM or amoxicillin 1 g orally (for high-risk patients), or vancomycin 1 g IV over 1–2 hours plus gentamicin 1.5 mg/kg IV/IM within ½ hour of starting the procedure (for high-risk patients with penicillin allergy)
    - Ampicillin 2 g orally 1 hour before the procedure or ampicillin 2 g IV/IM within 1½ hours of starting the procedure (for moderate-risk patients)

    Vancomycin 1 g IV over 1–2 hours (for moderate-risk patients with penicillin allergy)
- After incision and drainage of soft tissue infection: Antistaphylococcal penicillin or first-generation cephalosporin is an appropriate choice of prophylaxis

(GI: gastrointestinal; GU: genitourinary; IM: intramuscular; IV: intravenous)

Q17. How is the selection of an antimicrobial agent done in the treatment of IE?

Ans. Infective endocarditis needs antibiotic treatment with a combination of drugs for long duration **(Box 8.3)**.

BOX 8.3: Selection of antibiotics for infective endocarditis.
- Penicillin-sensitive streptococci (*Streptococcus viridans*): Penicillin G 4 million units IV every 6 hours for 4 weeks or penicillin G 4 million units every 6 hours plus gentamicin 1.0 mg/kg IV/IM every 12 hours for 2 weeks or ceftriaxone 2 g IV/IM daily for 4 weeks or vancomycin (if penicillin allergy): 30 mg/kg IV daily in two divided doses for 4 weeks
- Penicillin-resistant streptococci (*Enterococcus faecalis*, etc.): Penicillin G 18–30 million units/day IV (continuous or divided) plus gentamicin 1 mg/kg IV/IM every 8 hours or ampicillin 2 g/d IV (continuous or divided) plus gentamicin 1.0 mg/ kg IV every 8 hours or if penicillin allergy-vancomycin 15 mg/kg IV 12 hours plus gentamicin 1.0 mg/kg IV every 8 hours. Duration of therapy: 4–6 weeks (4 weeks for patients with symptoms <3 months)
- *Staphylococcus* (in the absence of PVE): Nafcillin 2 g IV every 4 hours for 4–6 weeks, or nafcillin plus optional gentamicin 1 mg/kg IV 8 hours for the initial 3–5 days, or in penicillin-allergic patients, vancomycin 15 mg/kg IV every 12 hours for 4–6 weeks
- *Staphylococcus* (in PVE): Nafcillin 2 g IV every 4 hours plus gentamicin 1 mg/kg IV every 8 hours, plus rifampicin 600 mg orally four times a day

In methicillin-resistant cases, vancomycin 15 mg/kg IV every 12 hours plus gentamicin 1.0 mg/kg IV/IM every 8 hours plus rifampicin 300 mg orally every 8 hours. Duration: ≥6 weeks

- Right-sided endocarditis (involving tricuspid valve): Nafcillin 2 g IV every 4 hours and gentamicin 1 mg/kg twice a day for 2 weeks. For methicillin-resistant cases, vancomycin 15 mg/kg IV every 12 hours for 4–6 weeks
- HACEK group organisms: Ceftriaxone 2 g IV/IM daily for 4 weeks or ampicillin 12 g/day IV (continuous or divided) plus gentamicin 1 mg/kg IV/IM every 12 hours. Duration: 4 weeks
- *Pseudomonas aeruginosa* and other Enterobacteriaceae-extended spectrum penicillin (ticarcillin or piperacillin) or third-generation cephalosporin or imipenem plus aminoglycoside for 4–6 weeks
- *Neisseria species:* Penicillin G 2 million units IV every 6 hours for 3–4 weeks or ceftriaxone 1 g IV/IM daily for 3–4 weeks

SUGGESTED READING

1. Habib G, Hoen B, Tornos P, Thuny F, Prendergast B, Vilacosta I. Guidelines on the prevention, diagnosis, and treatment of infective endocarditis (new version 2009): the Task Force on the Prevention, diagnosis, and Treatment of Infective endocarditis of the European Society of Cardiology (ESC). Endorsed by the European Society of Clinical Microbiology and Infectious Diseases (ESCMID) and the International Society of Chemotherapy (ISC) for Infection and Cancer. Eur Heart J. 2009;30(19):2369-413.

2. Halder SM, O'Gara PT. Infective endocarditis. In: Hurst's The Heart, 13th edition. McGraw Hill; 2011.
3. Wilson W, Taubert KA, Gewitz m, Lockhart PB, Baddour LM, Levison M, et al. Prevention of infective endocarditis: guidelines from from the American Heart Association: a guideline from the American Heart Association Rheumatic Fever, Endocarditis, and Kawasaki Disease Committee, Council on Cardiovascular Disease in the Young, and the Council on Clinical Cardiology, Council on Cardiovascular Surgery and Anesthesia, and the Quality of Care and Outcomes Research Interdisciplinary Working Group. Circulation. 2007;116(15):1736-54.

9. Diseases of Myocardium

"It is a reality that no past, present, or future classification of cardiomyopathy is likely to satisfy the purpose of all interested patients."
—BJ Mason and G Thiene

■ INTRODUCTION

Inflammation of the heart muscle, i.e., myocarditis, is due to infection or by an immune process. In myocarditis, if the host response is overwhelming or inappropriate, it may lead to cardiac remodeling and dilated cardiomyopathy (DCM) with ventricular dilatation as a consequence of inflammation-induced myocyte loss and interstitial fibrosis. About one third of DCMs are attributed to a single gene mutation. Hypertrophic cardiomyopathy (HCM) is the most common genetic cardiovascular disorder caused by a mutation of genetic mesenchyme characterized by thickening of the left ventricle.

Q1. What are the diseases that primarily involve the myocardium?
Ans. These include:
- *Myocarditis:* Inflammatory disorder of the myocardium due to infections or toxins
- *Cardiomyopathies:* Heart muscle diseases of unknown cause

These are:
- DCM
- HCM
- Restrictive cardiomyopathy (RCM)

Q2. What are the causes of myocarditis?
Ans. Myocarditis results from a number of agents, including infection, toxin, chemical agents, and radiation **(Box 9.1)**.

> **BOX 9.1:** Etiology of myocarditis.
>
> - *Infective:*
>   - *Viruses:* Coxsackie B, cytomegalovirus, and infectious mononucleosis
>   - *Bacteria:* Diphtheria, *Streptococcus* (in rheumatic fever), meningococcus, Whipple's disease, Weil's disease, and psittacosis
>   - *Parasites:* Chagas disease (*Trypanosoma cruzi*)
>   - *Others:* Fungus, rickettsiae, and mycoplasma
> - *Toxic agents:* Alcohol and heavy metals
> - *Pharmacologic agents:* Doxorubicin, cyclophosphamide, sulfonamides, lithium, and emetine
> - Radiation
> - *Allergic reaction:* Hypersensitivity state and insect stings

Q3. How do myocarditis and myocardial damage occur by infective agents?

Ans. There are three basic mechanisms:
1. *Immunologically mediated:* Most important way of myocardial damage, e.g., in viral myocarditis. Postulated mechanisms include the creation of a new cell surface antigen by the virus or antigen–antibody complex formation. DCM develops as a result of immunologic damage. In rheumatic fever, myocarditis occurs by an autoimmune mechanism induced by a streptococcal antigen.
2. Toxin production, e.g., diphtheria
3. Direct invasion of the myocardium, e.g., Chagas disease

Q4. What is the presentation, treatment, and outcome of viral myocarditis?

Ans.
- May be asymptomatic
- Antecedent flu-like symptoms
- Chest pain, sometimes palpitation, arrhythmias, and heart block, occasionally sudden cardiac death (SCD)
- Sometimes features of congestive heart failure (CHF)

Treatment: No specific treatment; bed rest, treatment of complications, such as arrhythmias and heart failure (HF). Corticosteroids for progressive symptoms

Outcome: Self-limiting in most cases, with complete recovery. Minority progress to DCM by immunologic damage

Q5. Define cardiomyopathy. Classify it.

Ans. Cardiomyopathies are a heterogeneous group of diseases of the myocardium associated with mechanical and/or electrical dysfunction, usually (but not invariably) accompanied by inappropriate ventricular dilatation or hypertrophy, and are due to a variety of etiologies that are frequently genetic in origin.

Cardiomyopathies are classified as primary (i.e., primary myocardial involvement) and secondary (as part of the generalized disease). Cardiomyopathies often lead to progressive disability and death.

The World Health Organization (WHO)/International Society and Federation of Cardiology (ISFC) classification of primary cardiomyopathy (1995): It is based on systolic and diastolic chamber dimensions and the genetic determinants [as stated by the American Heart Association (AHA)], i.e., mutation of contractile proteins **(Box 9.2)**.

Secondary cardiomyopathies are entities developing as part of generalized diseases, e.g., toxins (drugs, chemicals, and heavy metals), endocrine diseases [hypothyroidism and diabetes mellitus (DM)], nutritional (beriberi, carnitine deficiency), sarcoidosis, amyloidosis, storage diseases (e.g., hemochromatosis), and muscular dystrophy (e.g., Duchenne type).

BOX 9.2: Classification of cardiomyopathies.

- *Genetic:* HCM (autosomal dominant), arrhythmogenic right ventricular (RV) dysplasia, left ventricular (LV) noncompaction, ion channelopathies [long QT syndrome (LQTS), Brugada syndrome (BrS), and short QT syndrome (SQTS)], and glycogen storage disease
- *Mixed (genetic and acquired):* DCM and RCM
- *Acquired:* Peripartum cardiomyopathy, following myocarditis, tachycardia induced [after prolonged supraventricular tachycardia (SVT) or ventricular tachycardia (VT)], and Takotsubo cardiomyopathy (stress induced)

(DCM: dilated cardiomyopathy; HCM: hypertrophic cardiomyopathy; RCM: restrictive cardiomyopathy)

The term *specific cardiomyopathy* has been abandoned, and valvular, hypertensive, and ischemic cardiomyopathy are excluded from the current classification.

Q6. What are the various limitations in the terminology of cardiomyopathies?
Ans.
- The original WHO classification defining cardiomyopathies as "heart muscle disease of unknown cause" is obsolete with an advancement of cardiovascular knowledge and diagnosis (i.e., molecular genetics).
- Popular hypertrophic, dilated, RCM classification has major limitations, as mixed anatomic varieties exist.
- The end-stage phase of HCM may incorporate hypertrophic and dilated, as well as restrictive components.
- Etiologic classification has limitations as the same cardiomyopathy may be due to different etiologies.

Q7. What is DCM? What are the types?
Ans. These are cardiomyopathies exhibiting increased systolic and diastolic volumes and a low ejection fraction (EF: <45%). DCM may result from unknown cause (idiopathic), or known causes **(Box 9.3)**.

BOX 9.3: Dilated cardiomyopathy—types.

- Idiopathic DCM
- Ischemic cardiomyopathy
- Valvular cardiomyopathy (MR and AS)
- Hypertensive cardiomyopathy in chronic hypertension
- Peripartum cardiomyopathy
- Toxin induced—ethanol, drugs, heavy metals, cocaine, and cobalt
- Metabolic—thiamine deficiency, protein energy malnutrition, and carnitine deficiency
- Infective—postmyocarditis
- Infiltrative—hemochromatosis, sarcoidosis, and amyloidosis
- Autoimmune—SLE and RA

(AS: aortic stenosis; DCM: dilated cardiomyopathy; MR: mitral regurgitation; RA: rheumatoid arthritis; SLE: systemic lupus erythematosus)

Q8. What are specific cardiomyopathies?
Ans. These are cardiac muscle diseases associated with known cardiac or systemic processes. Known cardiac diseases such as ischemia and hypertension produce ischemic and hypertensive cardiomyopathy. Ischemic cardiomyopathy is related to previous myocardial infarction (MI) with subsequent remodeling and dilatation producing a DCM. A hypertensive cardiomyopathy may be either dilated or restrictive, depending on the chamber dimensions. Systemic disorders producing cardiomyopathy are metabolic diseases (e.g., DM and uremia), nutritional disorders (e.g., thiamine deficiency), infiltrative diseases (e.g., sarcoidosis and amyloidosis), and connective tissue diseases.

Q9. What is peripartum cardiomyopathy and its sequelae?
Ans. It is a form of DCM that occurs during the last 3 months of pregnancy and up to 6 months of delivery in the absence of a previous history of myocardial disorder. The cause is not clearly known. Some factors contributing are hemodynamic load of pregnancy, hypertension of pregnancy, myocarditis, and familial factors. Approximately half of the patients completely recover, and most others improve. The risk of recurrence is about 25% and increases with succeeding pregnancies. The mortality is high on the second recurrence. Hence, subjects who have developed peripartum cardiomyopathy should never become pregnant, even if myocardial function has fully recovered.

Q10. How does alcoholic cardiomyopathy develop? How to treat it?
Ans. Excessive alcohol consumption may produce DCM. This is by the following:
- Direct myocardial damage by the toxic effect of alcohol or its metabolites
- The toxic effect of additives, e.g., cobalt sulfate being added to stabilize froth, may produce severe cardiac failure of sudden onset (if a very large quantity of beer is ingested)
- *Nutritional deficiency:* Particularly thiamine deficiency; HF is of the beriberi type.
- Atrial fibrillation (AF) developing in alcoholics aggravates the failure.

Treatment:
- Cessation of alcohol consumption halts the progression and improves ventricular function.
- Thiamine administration in patients with thiamine deficiency.

Q11. Why is the left ventricular outflow tract (LVOT) obstruction in HCM called dynamic?
Ans. Dynamic LVOT obstruction is one of the hallmarks of HCM. Obstruction may not be present at rest:
- Outflow gradient is increased by increased myocardial contractility by exercise or inotropic agents like digitalis and isoproterenol, and decreased by agents decreasing contractility, e.g., beta-blockers.

- Decreased preload by hypovolemia, diuretics, Valsalva and standing (by decreasing venous return), and hand grip (by decreasing venous return) increases the obstruction. Increased preload or ventricular volume by squatting decreases the obstruction.
- Decreased afterload or arterial pressure by vasodilator agents, e.g., nitrates and Valsalva, increases the obstruction and increased afterload and arterial pressure by vasoconstrictor agents, e.g., phenylephrine and squatting, decreases or abolishes the obstruction.

Q12. How does mitral regurgitation (MR) occur in HCM?
Ans. Mitral regurgitation is frequent in HCM.
- Systolic anterior motion (SAM) interferes with normal valve closure—the degree of MR is directly related to the severity of obstruction and lack of leaflet cooptation.
- Primary abnormalities of mitral valve (MV): About 60% of patients with HCM have structural abnormalities of MV, including increased leaflet area, elongation of leaflets, and anomalous insertion of papillary muscles directly into the anterior mitral leaflet (AML). This may also contribute to MR.

Q13. What are the common symptoms in HCM? How do they occur?
Ans. Patients with HCM may be asymptomatic and are identified during family screening of patients with known diseases.

Common symptoms are as follows:
- *Dyspnea:* Due to LV diastolic dysfunction, impaired ventricular filling, and elevation of left atrial and pulmonary venous pressure
- *Angina pectoris:* Imbalance between O_2 supply and demand with greatly increased myocardial mass, compromised coronary flow due to abnormal intramural coronary arteries, and prolonged diastolic relaxation resulting in increased wall tension
- *Syncope or presyncope:* Due to LVOT obstruction and inadequate cardiac output with exertion or cardiac arrhythmias
- *Sudden cardiac death:* HCM appears to be the leading cause of SCD in young competitive athletes. SCD occurs due to arrhythmias.

Q14. What are the pharmacologic therapies for HCM and their purpose?
Ans. The drug therapy is aimed at the following endpoints:
- To relieve outflow obstruction and improve LV relaxation.
  - Beta-blockers are first-line therapy for HCM regardless of the presence of LV outflow obstruction. These are effective in relieving angina, dyspnea, and syncope.
  - Calcium channel blockers such as verapamil and diltiazem are effective in reducing the symptoms among patients who are intolerant to beta-blockers.

- Disopyramide, a class IA antiarrhythmic agent, may be an effective alternative or adjunct to beta-blockers and/or calcium channel blockers.
- *To control dysrhythmias:* Beta-blocker and/or verapamil are used to control the ventricular rate. Amiodarone may induce reversion to sinus rhythm in AF. Patients with nonsustained VT are treated with amiodarone; sometimes flecainide, mexiletine, or disopyramide.
- *Others:* Anticoagulants for AF, prophylaxis for infective endocarditis (in patients with outflow obstruction), and digoxin should only be prescribed when AF is irreversible or LVOT obstruction is not present, or considerable cardiac enlargement occurs in the late stage. Diuretics should be used judiciously in patients with progressive CHF secondary to impaired systolic function (i.e., end-stage HF).

Q15. How does HCM differ from aortic valve (AV) stenosis?
Ans. Both conditions produce left ventricular outflow tract obstruction. The differentiating features are mentioned in **Table 9.1**.

TABLE 9.1: Difference between hypertrophic cardiomyopathy and aortic stenosis.

Points	HCM	Aortic valve stenosis
Site of obstruction	Subvalvular; muscular IVS	Aortic valves
Factor producing obstruction	Hypertrophy of anterobasal septum, increased size and length of MV, anterior displacement of MV and papillary muscle, and Venturi effect (pulling of mitral leaflets toward septum by the high-velocity jet)	Aortic valvular stenosis ± calcification
Nature of LVOT obstruction	Dynamic; systolic anterior motion of MV with ventricular septal contact is responsible (increased by LV contraction, tachycardia, etc.)	Static
Symptoms	• SCD common • Heart failure is rare	• Less common • More common
• Signs—carotid pulse • Apex beat • Thrill	• Jerky • Tripple beat may be found • Lower left sternal area	• Anacrotic • Heaving character • Aortic area
Ejection click	Absent	May be present (if no calcification)
• Systolic ejection • Murmur	At left, sternal border; radiates to lower sternal border, but not to the neck or axilla	At right, sternal edge may radiate to the neck and apex

Contd...

Contd...

Points	HCM	Aortic valve stenosis
Effect of Valsalva, amyl nitrate inhalation, and standing on murmur	↑	↓
Effect of squatting and hand grip	↓	↑
Murmur of MR	Usually present	Absent
Early diastolic murmur	Rare	Often present (if coexistent AR)
Investigation:		
C_xR	May show LVH, no poststenotic dilatation ↓	Poststenotic dilatation is often seen
ECG	3T sign (widespread T, upright T in aVR T in II, avF) in apical variety	LVH with strain
Echocardiography	Asymmetric septal hypertrophy IVS >15 mm. septal to posterior wall ratio >1.3–1.5, systolic anterior motion of MV, midsystolic closure of AV	Concentric LV hypertrophy, ACS, AV orifice, and calcification of AV ±

(ACS: acute coronary syndrome; AR: aortic regurgitation; AV: aortic valve; CxR: chest X-ray; ECG: electrocardiogram; HCM: hypertrophic cardiomyopathy; IVS: interventricular septum; LV: left ventricle; LVH: left ventricular hypertrophy; LVOT: left ventricular outflow tract; MR: mitral regurgitation; MV: mitral valve; SCD: sudden cardiac death)

Q16. What are the predictors of sudden death in patients with HCM?
Ans. Sudden death in patients with HCM is presumed to be due to a ventricular arrhythmia. Both patients with and without outflow obstruction may die suddenly **(Box 9.4)**.

BOX 9.4: Markers of increased risk of sudden death.
- Age ≤30 years at diagnosis
- Previous cardiac arrest
- Family history of HCM and sudden death
- Recurrent syncope
- Nonsustained VT on Holter monitoring, particularly when multiple and repetitive
- Marked LV wall thickness (>35 mm)
- Abnormal decrease in exercise blood pressure

(HCM: hypertrophic cardiomyopathy; LV: left ventricular; VT: ventricular tachycardia)

Q17. How does sudden death occur in HCM?
Ans. It is most common in children and young adults (≤30 years). Most patients are asymptomatic prior to sudden death. Some patients die while

sedentary or performing mild exertion. A substantial number die during or just after vigorous physical activity. During sudden death, VT usually occurs which is precipitated by LVOT obstruction, LV diastolic dysfunction, and ischemia. Exercise-induced hypotension and activation of ventricular baroreceptors produce bradyarrhythmia and asystole.

Q18. What are the echocardiographic findings of hypertrophic obstructive cardiomyopathy (HOCM)?
Ans.

- M-mode echo asymmetrical septal hypertrophy; interventricular septum (IVS) is thicker than posterior LV free wall (≥1.5:1), feature of LVOT obstruction, e.g., SAM of MV, midsystolic closure of AV, and narrowing of LVOT. SAM is the dragging of AML by the Venturi effect of robust septum. LVOT obstruction is classically dynamic.
- Two-dimensional echocardiography (2DE)—asymmetric septal hypertrophy (ASH) leading to outflow obstruction; sometimes concentric or apical hypertrophy. The LV cavity may be obliterated (banana shape in apical four-chamber view), LA enlargement due to decreased LV compliance **(Fig. 9.1)**.

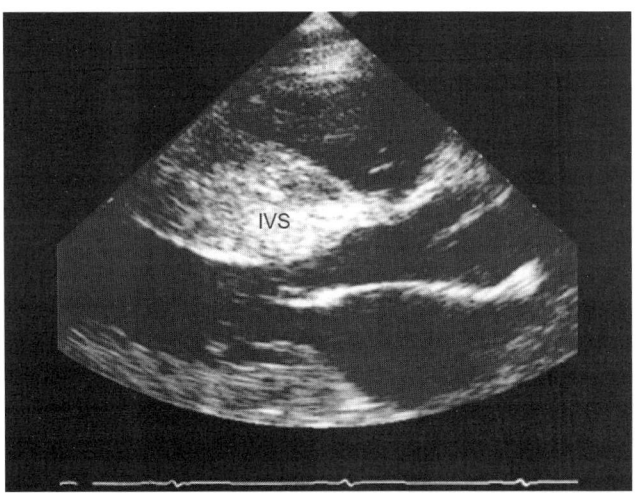

Fig. 9.1: Severely hypertrophied IVS in HOCM (2DE parasternal long axis view).

- Doppler echo-pulsed-wave Doppler (PWD) shows diastolic dysfunction of LV: reversed E/A ratio and prolonged deceleration time. It is helpful in determining flow velocity at different levels of the LV cavity. An outflow obstruction is likely if there is a significant acceleration of flow between the midcavity and LVOT. Continuous-wave Doppler (CWD) detects LVOT obstruction and its severity. It records pressure gradient at LVOT obstruction and shows spectral display with a relatively slow increase in velocity in the early systole, followed by a more gradual increase in the outflow tract velocity and a late peaking giving rise to dragger-shaped configuration. In severe cases of LVOT obstruction, the velocity curve becomes holosystolic.

Color flow imaging (CFI) helps to identify the location of obstruction-LVOT or midventricle. A turbulent or mosaic flow is seen distal to the obstruction. It can document the presence of MR, which is predominantly mid- or late-systolic. Regurgitant jet is directed posteriorly in HOCM.

Q19. What is SAM? How does it occur?
Ans. SAM is systolic anterior motion of the AML during midsystole. The most accepted explanation of SAM is that high flow velocity caused by the narrowed outflow tract draws the MV anteriorly toward the septum, resulting in subaortic obstruction and flow gradient. This suctioning effect on the mitral leaflet has been called the Venturi effect.

Other factors contributing are as follows:
- Pulling of MV against the septum by the contraction of the anomalous papillary muscle, which is located and oriented abnormally
- Pushing of the anomalous MV against the septum by the posterior wall because of its abnormal size, area, and position.

Systolic anterior motion is the echocardiographic hallmark of LVOT obstruction in HCM. The closer the leaflet comes to the septum and the longer it remains in apposition to the septum, the more severe the obstruction.

It is best identified with M-mode echocardiography **(Fig. 9.2)**.

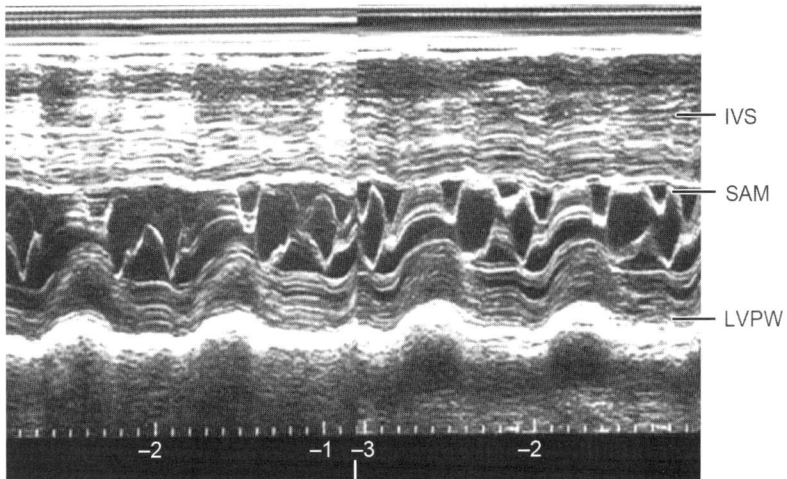

Fig. 9.2: M-mode echo in parasternal long-axis view showing ASH and SAM in HCM.

As the outflow obstruction in HCM is dynamic and may not always be present at rest, SAM may also be absent at rest and may appear with Valsalva maneuver or use of amyl nitrate.

Q20. What are the interventional treatments available for HCM patients?

Ans.

- *Surgical (septal myotomy-myomectomy, "Marrow procedure"):* Muscular resection from the basal ventricular septum is the gold standard, reserved for severely symptomatic patients who become refractory to drug treatment, with a basal peak systolic LVOT gradient of at least 50 mm Hg.
- *Dual chamber pacing:* Alternative to surgery; depolarization from the RV apex alters septal motion (i.e., IVS moves away from outflow tract) and reduces the SAM and subaortic gradient. The pacemaker should be programmed with a short AV delay to ensure that every ventricular complex is paced. Dual chamber pacing is safer and cheaper than surgery and may be considered as the initial procedure in patients with symptoms resistant to drug therapy, particularly in older and frail persons and those with MR.
- *PTSMA (percutaneous transseptal myectomy):* Alcoholic septal ablation by injecting absolute alcohol down the first septal perforator of LAD at catheterization has been shown to reduce the outflow gradient in a few cases.

Q21. When is ICD indicated in HCM?

Ans. The American College of Cardiology (ACC)/AHA guidelines recommend implantable cardioverter defibrillator (ICD) for patients with prior documented cardiac arrest, ventricular fibrillation (VF), or hemodynamically significant VT (class I). In addition, it may be reasonable to consider an ICD under the following circumstances (class IIa recommendation):

- Sudden death presumably caused by HCM in one or more first-degree relatives
- Maximal LV wall thickness 30 mm or greater
- One or more recent, unexplained syncopal episodes
- Nonsustained VT (particularly before 30 years of age), in the presence of other SCD risk factors
- Abnormal blood pressure (BP) response to exercise, in the presence of other SCD risk factors.

Q22. What is athlete's heart?

Ans. Normal physiological changes in cardiac size, structure, and autonomic tone that occur after years of intense exercise training are known as athlete's heart. Long-term athletic training can produce a physiological increase in LV cavity dimensions, wall thickness, and LV mass. Cardiac myocytes are enlarged in length and width. Thus, it is a balanced enlargement of the heart with both LV hypertrophy and an increase in end-diastolic volume. In endurance training, the repetitive and intermittent increase in the stroke volume and BP stimulates volume and pressure signals, resulting in an eccentrically enlarged heart that is both hypertrophied and dilated. In athletes who are involved in a predominantly pressure-inducing exercise, such as weight lifting or rowing, concentric hypertrophy dominates. Increased cardiac mass, chamber dimensions, and wall thickness are responsible for changes in electrocardiogram (ECG). When exercise training stops (4-6 weeks), hypertrophy regresses whereas some dilatation persists.

Q23. What are the differences between physiological and pathological hypertrophy?

Ans. Left ventricular hypertrophy occurs in pathological conditions producing LV outflow obstruction. Physiological conditions such as exercise training may also lead to LV hypertrophy. They have difference on pathogenesis **(Table 9.2)**.

TABLE 9.2: Difference between physiological and pathological hypertrophy.

Points	Physiological	Pathological
Signaling pattern	Prosurvival	Proapoptotic or profibrotic
Interstitial fibrosis	Nil	Yes
Myocyte apoptosis	No	+
Systolic contraction	N or increased	Decreased
Diastolic relaxation	N or increased	Decreased

Q24. How to differentiate athlete's heart from HCM?

Ans. Physiological hypertrophy takes place in the athlete's heart. In HCM, there is pathological hypertrophy of LV. They differ from each other in pathogenetic background and prognosis **(Table 9.3)**.

TABLE 9.3: Difference between athlete's heart and hypertrophic cardiomyopathy.

Points	Athlete's heart	HCM
Genetics	No protein mutation	Sarcomeric protein mutation
Family history	–ve	+ve
Hypertrophy pattern	Symmetric	Asymmetric
LV cavity diameter	Decreased	Increased
Diastolic function	Decreased	Normal
Doppler velocity	Normal	Abnormal
Deconditioning	Regress hypertrophy	No effect

(–ve: negative; +ve: positive; HCM: hypertrophic cardiomyopathy; LV: left ventricular)

- Most common DCM in Bangladesh—ischemic DCM (occurring after MI), valvular DCM, hypertensive DCM, idiopathic DCM, and peripartum DCM.

Q25. What is RCM?

Ans. Restrictive cardiomyopathies are diseases of myocardium characterized by abnormal diastolic function with normal or near normal systolic function associated with decreased ventricular compliance, impaired ventricular filling, and reduced diastolic volume of either or both ventricles.

Severe hypertensive heart disease, aortic stenosis, and some cases of HCM exhibit restrictive pathophysiology but are not classified as RCMs.

Q26. Classify RCM.

Ans. Pathologically, RCMs may be myocardial and endomyocardial.
- *Myocardial: Infiltrative and noninfiltrative:*
  - *Infiltrative:* Amyloidosis, sarcoidosis, hemochromatosis, glycogen storage disease, Gaucher's disease, Hurler–Scheie disease, Fabry disease, and fatty infiltration
  - *Noninfiltrative:* Idiopathic RCM, familial, scleroderma, and diabetic cardiomyopathy
- *Endomyocardial:* Endomyocardial fibrosis, hypereosinophilic syndrome, radiation, and drug toxicity.

Q27. How do you differentiate constrictive pericarditis from RCM?

Ans. Both lead to restriction in cardiac function, but they can be differentiated on the points shown in **Table 9.4**.

TABLE 9.4: Difference between constrictive pericarditis and restrictive cardiomyopathy.

Points	Constrictive pericarditis	Restrictive cardiomyopathy
Kussmaul's sign	+ve	–ve
Pericardial knock	+ve	–ve
Regurgitant murmur	–ve	±
Biatrial enlargement (ECG)	Rare	Typical
Atrial dilatation (echo)	–ve	Typical
Pericardial thickening	Present	Absent
Pressure on left and right side	Not equal	Equal (RA = PCWP; RVEDP = LVEDP)
Dip and plateau sign	Maybe present	Absent
Myocardial biopsy	Normal	Abnormal

(–ve: negative; +ve: positive; ECG: electrocardiogram; LVEDP: left ventricular end-diastolic pressure; PCWP: pulmonary capillary wedge pressure; RA: right atrium; RVEDP: right ventricular end-diastolic pressure)

Constrictive pericarditis is an important differential diagnosis of RCMs; thickened pericardium on echocardiography, computed tomography (CT), or cardiac magnetic resonance (CMR) in a patient with HF and preserved left ventricular ejection fraction (LVEF) without LV wall thickening suggest constrictive pericarditis.

Q28. When to suspect RCM?
Ans. Echocardiographic findings of biatrial enlargement, nondilated ventricles **(Fig. 9.3)** with a normal LVEF and LV wall thickness, and evidence of severe diastolic dysfunction suggest the diagnosis of RCM. The patient presents with symptoms and signs of biventricular failure, palpitation, and fatigue. AF and S_3 are common.

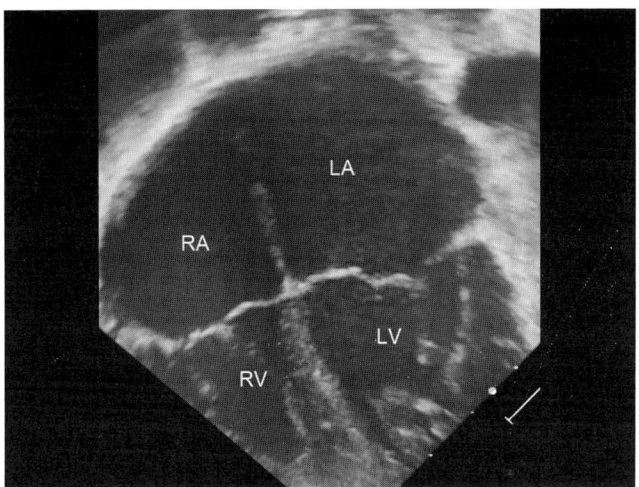

Fig. 9.3: 2DE showing dilated LA and RA.

Q29. What are the infiltrative cardiomyopathies?
Ans. Infiltrative cardiomyopathy due to infiltration of myocardium occurs in amyloidosis, sarcoidosis, hemochromatosis, and glycogen storage disease. Amyloidosis produces RCM, and sarcoidosis manifests as DCM. Amyloidosis, unlike idiopathic RCMs, shows increased LV wall thickness and subtle abnormality of LV systolic function.

Q30. What is Takotsubo syndrome (TTS)? How does it mimic acute coronary syndrome (ACS)?
Ans. Takotsubo syndrome presents with acute HF mimicking ACS with transient wall motion abnormality of LV, usually following an emotional or physically stressful event. The wall motion abnormalities extend beyond the territory of one coronary artery, and coronary angiography (CAG) reveals normal epicardial coronaries. There is acute ballooning of apical LV assuming the shape of Japanese octopus trap-pot called takotsubo with narrow apex and round dilated bottom **(Fig. 9.4)**. Troponin is mildly elevated with marked

elevation of N-terminal pro b-type natriuretic peptide (NT-proBNP). There is myocardial stunning with regional wall motion abnormality (RWMA) and reduced EF. The prognosis is generally good. Treatment includes beta-blocker and low-molecular-weight heparin (LMWH), sometimes levosimendan and mechanical circulatory support.

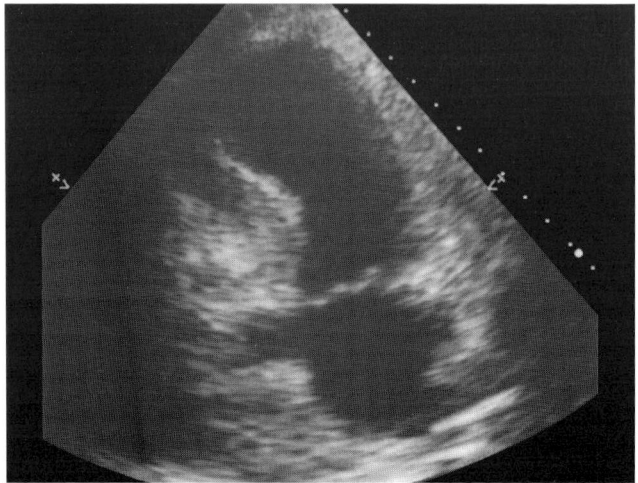

Fig. 9.4: 2DE showing apical ballooning in Takotsubo syndrome.

Q31. What is commotio cordis?
Ans. It is the SCD by blunt, nonpenetrating chest blows during athletic or recreational activities in the absence of underlying cardiovascular disease. It is now recognized as the second leading cause of death in youth sports. Most common sports are those in which projectiles are integral to the game, e.g., baseball, ice hockey, football and softball, cricket, etc. Sudden cardiac death is due to VF induced by chest wall blow resulting from ion channel activated by increased LV pressure.

■ SUGGESTED READING

1. Maron BJ, Towbin JA, Thiene G, Antzelevitch C, Corrado D, Arnett D, et al. Contemporary definitions and classification of the cardiomyopathies: an American Heart Association Scientific Statement from the Council of Clinical Cardiology, Heart Failure and Transplantation Committee; Quality of Care and Outcome Research and Functional Genomics and Translational Biology Interdisciplinary Working Groups; and Council on Epidemiology and Prevention. Circulation. 2006;113(14):1807-16.
2. Richardson P, McKenna W, Bristow M, Maisch B, Mautner B, O'Connell J, et al. Report of the 1995 World Health Organization/International Society and Federation of Cardiology Task Force on the Definition and Classification of Cardiomyopathies. Circulation. 1996;93:841-2.

3. Hara JM. The dilated, restrictive, and infiltrative cardiomyopathies. In: Libby P, Bonow RO, Mann DL, Zipes DP (Eds). Braunwald's Heart Disease. A Textbook of Cardiovascular Medicine, 8th edition. Philadelphia, PA: Saunders; 2008.
4. Gersh BJ, Maron BJ, Bonow RO, Dearani JA, Fifer MA, Link MS, et al. 2011 ACCF/AHA Guideline for the Diagnosis and Treatment of Hypertrophic Cardiomyopathy: a report of the American College of Cardiology Foundation/American Heart Association Task Force on Practice Guidelines. Circulation. 2011;124:e783-831.
5. Maron BJ. Hypertrophic cardiomyopathy. In: Libby P, Bonow RO, Mann DL, Zipes DP (Eds). Braunwald's Heart Disease. A Textbook of Cardiovascular Medicine, 8th edition. Philadelphia, PA: Saunders; 2008.

CHAPTER 10

Pericardial Diseases

"Tuberculosis should be considered in patients with fever and pericardial effusion in communities where tuberculosis is still prevalent."

—Author of the book

■ INTRODUCTION

The pericardium may be affected by infectious, neoplastic, immunologic, metabolic, and iatrogenic causes. Pericardial heart disease includes pericarditis, i.e., acute pericarditis and its sequelae, pericardial effusion (PE), cardiac tamponade, and constrictive pericarditis.

Q1. What is pericarditis? Classify it.

Ans. It is a clinical syndrome resulting from inflammation of the pericardium and is associated with chest pain, a friction rub, and characteristic electrocardiogram (ECG) changes. Classification is done on the basis of its etiology, pathological manifestation, and duration **(Box 10.1)**.

> **BOX 10.1:** Classification of pericarditis.
> - *Clinically:* Acute: <6 weeks, and chronic, i.e., chronic constrictive pericarditis
> - *Etiologically:* Primary (viral, rheumatic fever, and tubercular) and secondary (MI, pyogenic, uremic, cancer, surgery, and connective tissue diseases)
> - *Pathologically:* Serous, fibrinous, purulent, hemorrhagic, constrictive, etc.
>
> (MI: myocardial infarction)

Q2. What are the causes of pericarditis?

Ans. Causes of pericarditis include:
- Primary (as a primary manifestation)
  - *Viral infection:* Coxsackie B virus, influenza, mumps, measles, chicken pox, and human immunodeficiency virus (HIV)
  - Rheumatic fever
  - Tuberculosis (TB)
- Secondary (involvement secondary to other diseases)
  - Myocardial infarction (MI) and post-MI syndrome
  - Pyogenic and fungal infections
  - Uremia
  - *Connective tissue diseases:* Rheumatoid arthritis and systemic lupus erythematosus (SLE)
  - Trauma
  - Cardiac surgery
  - Neoplastic invasion

Q3. Classify PE.
Ans.
- *Transudative:* Congestive heart failure (CHF), nephrotic syndrome, and beriberi (wet)
- *Exudative:* Viral, tubercular, pyogenic, and uremic
- *Hemorrhagic:* Acute myocardial infarction (AMI), neoplastic invasion, dialysis, and trauma
- *Fibrinous:* Pericardium covered with adherent fibrins
- *Purulent:* Polymorphs, sometimes along with fibrin, cover pericardium.

Q4. How to quantify PE?
Ans. Quantification of PE is done according to the amount of fluid accumulated. Normally, there is usually a small amount of pericardial fluid. In mild effusion, 50–100 mL; moderate, 100–500 mL; and large, >500 mL.

The quantitative assessment of the amount of pericardial fluid is done by echocardiography, i.e., size of the echo-free space surrounding the heart:
- *Small (mild) PE:* Echo-free space posteriorly (usually 1 cm or less in width); no space anteriorly
- *Moderate PE:* Echo-free space posteriorly (>1 cm in width) with an anterior space, especially during systole
- *Large PE:* Large echo-free space around the heart throughout the cardiac cycle (at least 1 cm in width).

Q5. What is pulsus paradoxus? How is it produced?
Ans. It is an exaggeration of the normal inspiratory fall in systolic blood pressure (BP) that exceeds 10 mm Hg. Cardiac tamponade may produce pulsus paradoxus. An increased venous return on inspiration limits ventricular filling and causes the interventricular septum to bulge into the left ventricle (LV). The least ventricular filling is possible with increasing right ventricle (RV) volume, occupying more space in the rigid box. As a result, the stroke volume drops and BP decreases as a consequence.

Measurement:
- Determine the systolic BP by palpation and then inflate the BP cuff 30 mm Hg above it.
- Deflate the cuff slowly until Korotkoff sounds are heard intermittently (only on expiration).
- Then, the cuff is further slowly deflated until all beats and sounds appear to be heard (representing sound during inspiration). Now, sounds are heard during inspiration as well as expiration. The difference in systolic BP recorded at the start of Korotkoff sounds in inspiration and expiration is the estimation of pulsus paradoxus. If it is >10 mm Hg, it is taken as significant. For example, if Korotkoff sounds are heard initially at 140 mm Hg during expiration only and the sound appears to double at 120 mm Hg during inspiration, the pulsus paradoxus is 20 mm Hg.

Q6. How to differentiate acute MI from pericarditis?

Ans. The two conditions may share some features. The following points differentiate the two conditions **(Table 10.1)**:

TABLE 10.1: Differentiating acute MI from pericarditis.

Points		AMI	Pericarditis
Symptom	Chest pain (onset and duration)	Sudden onset, constant for 30–60 minutes (may last intermittently for days)	Gradual onset, hours or days
	Quality	Heavy pressure and squeezing	Sharp and pleuritic
	Radiation	Left arm	Ears, shoulder
	Aggravating factors	↑O_2 demand (i.e., exertion)	Supine, twisting the thorax or lying on the left side, deep inspiration, coughing, and swallowing
	Relieving factor	Morphine, beta-blockers, and compilation of MI	Sitting up and leaning forward, shallow respiration, and anti-inflammatory drug
	Associated symptom	Nausea, vomiting, diaphoresis, and symptoms of complications of MI	Fever and dyspnea
	Pyrexia	Often precedes the pain	Takes at least 12 hours to develop
Sign	Pericardial rub	Takes at least 20 hours to appear; transient; also may appear after 1 week in post-MI syndrome	Friction rub is diagnostic; appears early, persistent
Investigation	CxR	Normal (unless complicated by LVF and CHF)	Cardiomegaly is usual (due to effusion)
	ECG	ST elevation with convexity upward (in involved leads) followed by T inversion, dev. of Q (occurs when ST has returned to normal)	Diffuse ST elevation 8–12 leads with concavity upward (not >5 mm) and often with reciprocal depression (except aVR), no Q dev. (after normalization of ST segment)

Contd...

Pericardial Diseases

Contd...

Points		AMI	Pericarditis
	Echocardiography	Decreased myocardial contractility (in the involved area)	Pericardial effusion
	Cardiac enzymes	Increased	Normal (may increase mildly in extensive epicarditis)

(AMI: acute myocardial infarction; aVR: augmented vector right; CHF: congestive heart failure; CxR: chest X-ray; ECG: electrocardiogram; LVF: left ventricular failure; MI: myocardial infarction)

Q7. What is cardiac tamponade? What are the causes?

Ans. It is cardiac compression by rapidly accumulating PE interfering with diastolic filling, leading to a reduction in the stroke volume.

Cardiac tamponade is related to the rapidity of fluid accumulation. Sudden accumulation of <200 mL fluid can cause tamponade as in trauma; whereas, a large quantity of fluid may accumulate slowly in tuberculous or carcinomatous pericarditis without producing tamponade.

Causes: Trauma to chest, cardiac surgery, dissecting aortic aneurysm, neoplasm, acute MI with rupture of free wall, complication of percutaneous transvenous mitral commissurotomy (PTMC), etc.

Q8. What are the causes of pulsus paradoxus other than tamponade?

Ans. Pulsus paradoxus may occur in patients without cardiac tamponade:
- Status asthmaticus (abnormal pressure swings within the thorax transmitted to the aorta)
- Right ventricular infarction
- Pulmonary embolism.

Q9. When may pulsus paradoxus be absent in cardiac tamponade?

Ans.
- When left ventricular end-diastolic pressure (LVEDP) is elevated by the coexisting LV disease
- Atrial septal defect (ASD) coexists—reciprocal inspiratory change equalizes on two sides of the heart
- Coexistent aortic regurgitation.

Q10. How is cardiac tamponade diagnosed clinically? What is Beck's triad?

Ans. Sign of falling arterial pressure and cardiac output and a rising venous pressure and heart rate raises the possibility of tamponade and pulsus paradoxus strongly.

Beck's triad includes:
- Decline in systemic arterial pressure
- Elevation in systemic venous pressure
- A small, quiet heart.

These three features are typical of acute cardiac tamponade developing from trauma or invasive cardiac procedures. When the pericardium is suddenly filled with blood from trauma or therapeutic procedures, there is no time for pericardial stretching, and <200 mL of fluid can produce cardiac tamponade.

In contrast, slowly developing effusions become very large before signs of tamponade develop and do not fill the criteria of Beck's triad.

Q11. What are the characteristic radiologic features of pericardial effusion?

Ans. Pericardial effusion produces an enlarged cardiac silhouette on the chest X-ray with the following characteristic features **(Fig. 10.1)**.
- Pear- or pitcher-shaped cardiac silhouette—mirror image heart borders (right and left border look almost similar).
- Hilar overlay—hilar vascular markings are not visible, as these are covered by pericardial fluid.
- Enlarged cardiac silhouette—moderate to massive.

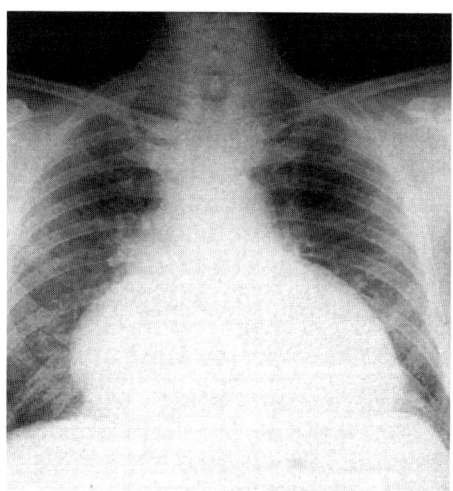

Fig. 10.1: Large pericardial effusion on chest X-ray.

Q12. What is the role of echocardiography in the diagnosis of PE?

Ans. It is the most sensitive test for the detection of pericardial effusion and is the procedure of choice. As little as 15 mL of fluid can be detected by two-dimensional echocardiography (2DE). It is seen as an echo-free space between the walls of the heart and the pericardium. Fluid collects initially within the oblique sinus. Hence, echo-free space is found behind the LV posterior wall in small effusion. With continued accumulation, fluid spreads circumferentially around the heart. For circumferential PE, the echo-free space measuring <5 mm is termed as minimal, 5–10 mm as small, 10–20 mm as moderate, and >20 mm as large effusion **(Fig. 10.2)**.

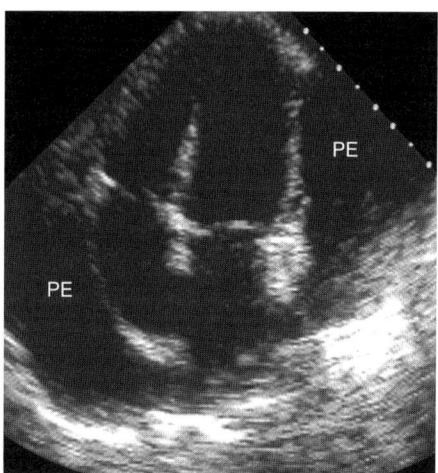

Fig. 10.2: 2DE (apical four-chamber view) showing large pericardial effusion.

Q13. What are the conditions that may be confused with PE on echocardiography?
Ans.
- *Left-sided pleural effusion:* It tracks behind the left atrium (LA) and separates the descending thoracic aorta from it, while PE in the left parasternal long axis view tapers as it approaches the LA and does not extend behind it.
- *Epicardial fat:* In obese elderly females, it may be confused as PE anterior to RV. Unless loculated, the anterior PE is always accompanied by effusion in the posterior pericardial space.

Q14. What are the echocardiographic findings of cardiac tamponade?
Ans.
- *Collapse of the RV during diastole:* Right ventricular outflow tract (RVOT) collapse is the earliest sign, seen more easily on the M-mode [timing of collapse made with the mitral valve (MV) closure and aortic valve (AV) opening]. It is more easily detected on 2DE in the left parasternal long-axis view. Right atrial diastolic collapse is also a sensitive sign but less specific. An abrupt increase in the RV size may occur during inspiration. In cardiac tamponade, diastolic collapse of the right atrium (RA) and RV is virtually diagnostic **(Fig. 10.3)**. The most common and early finding is a diastolic invagination of the RV and/or RA wall during diastole. A swinging heart on echocardiography is a more specific but late feature.

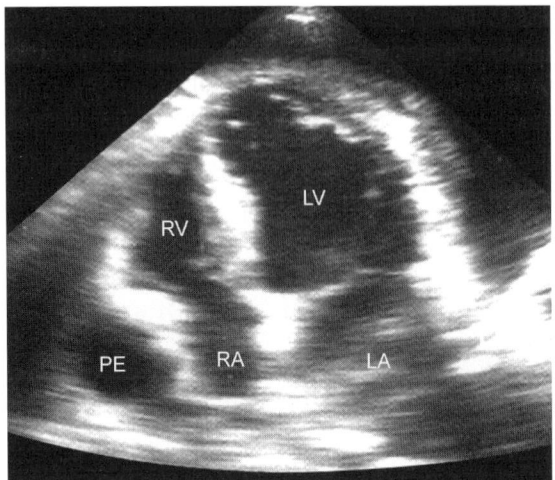

Fig. 10.3: Diastolic collapse of RV and RA in the apical four-chamber view.

- Dilated inferior vena cava, which fails to collapse during inspiration, seen on 2DE. There is an exaggerated increase in right-sided filling and decrease in left-sided filling that may be detected on pulsed wave Doppler (PWD) recording of mitral, tricuspid, and systemic venous flows. A pronounced inspiratory increase in the tricuspid flow and a concomitant decrease in the mitral flow can be demonstrated on color flow imaging (CFI).

Points to ponder: After cardiac surgery, RA and RV may adhere to the pericardium. Large PE may be loculated behind the LV wall, compressing it. Typical RA and RV collapse may be absent.

Q15. What are the indications and complications of pericardiocentesis?
Ans. *Indications*:
- *Diagnostic:* When there is doubt as to the cause of an effusion and it is large enough to be safely approached by a person doing it and also when a purulent PE is suspected.
- *Therapeutic:* Cardiac tamponade in which systolic BP has fallen to <30 mm Hg from the baseline level, or when it is immediately life-threatening and when it is producing progressive hemodynamic deterioration.

Complications: It varies according to the location and size of the pericardial fluid. The risk decreases and the chance of success increases with the increasing size of the effusion.

The risk and possible complications are as follows:
- Cardiac laceration leading to massive PE and death. This is much less likely with the apical approach as puncture of the thick-walled LV is better tolerated than puncture of the RV by the subxiphoid approach.

- *Syncope:* Due to a vasovagal reaction, it may occur at the time of pericardial puncture. Atrial and ventricular arrhythmias can occur with the puncture of cardiac chambers.
- *Acute pulmonary edema:* Sudden ventricular dilatation can occur if the tamponade is decompressed too quickly. Pulmonary edema may occur, especially if more fluid infusion is also done. Instead, drainage should be done over about 20 minutes.
- *Laceration:* Internal mammary, coronary, and pericardial artery may be involved.

Q16. What is constrictive pericarditis? What are the causes?

Ans. It is a chronic inflammation of the pericardium with fibrous thickening and calcification producing constriction of the heart leading to features of chronic heart failure **(Fig. 10.4)**.

Causes of constrictive pericarditis are:
- Tuberculosis (most common)
- Pyogenic infection of pericardium
- Following hemopericardium
- Radiotherapy of the mediastinum and/or malignancy
- Collagen disease
- *Miscellaneous:* Late complication of coronary artery bypass grafting (CABG), drug (methysergide, etc.).
  In many patients, no definite cause is found.

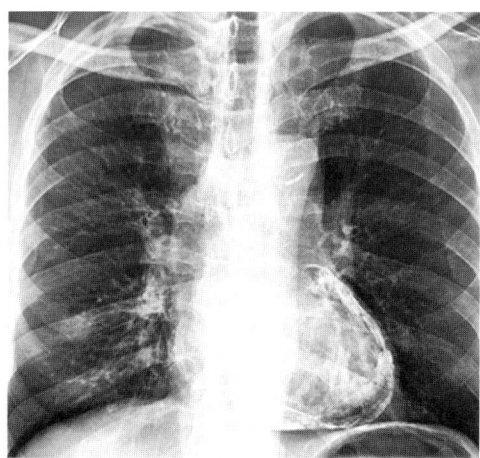

Fig. 10.4: Chest X-ray showing pericardial constriction following tubercular pericarditis.

Q17. How does constrictive pericarditis differ from cardiac tamponade hemodynamically?

Ans. In both tamponade and constrictive pericarditis, diastolic pressure in all four cardiac chambers is in equilibrium. However, they differ in the following respects **(Table 10.2)**:

TABLE 10.2: Difference between cardiac tamponade and constrictive pericarditis.

Points	Cardiac tamponade	Constrictive pericarditis
JVP/RA pressure	Prominent X descent	Prominent X and Y descent present
Kussmaul's sign (JVP increases on inspiration)	Usually absent	Present
Friedreich's sign (rapid Y descent followed by ascent)	Absent	Present
Pulsus paradoxus	Invariable	Uncommon
Square root sign (diastolic "dip and plateau" on catheterization)	Absent	Present

(JVP: jugular venous pressure; RA: right atrium)

Q18. What is cardiac cirrhosis?

Ans. The presence of ascites and splenomegaly in patients of chronic constrictive pericarditis resembles that of cirrhosis. Fibrotic obliteration of the pericardial space and a small heart due to extension of the fibrotic process resembles hepatic cirrhosis. Hence, constrictive pericarditis is also called cardiac cirrhosis.

Q19. How does constrictive pericarditis differ from CHF?

Ans. Chronic constrictive pericarditis produces some features similar to those of CHF. The differences are shown in **Table 10.3**.

TABLE 10.3: Difference between chronic constrictive pericarditis and CHF.

Chronic constrictive pericarditis	CHF
Dyspnea-nil	Prominent, orthopnea±
Ascites-gross	Edema more
JVP-higher; Kussmaul's sign +ve	JVP-prominent V; no Kussmaul's sign
Apex-impalpable	Always palpable
Murmur-nil	May be present
PH-not a feature	Usual
Splenomegaly-usual	Unusual
CxR-clear lung, calcification±	Cardiomegaly; lung-congested
Echo-EF normal, IVC-dilated	EF-reduced
Cath-diastolic pressure is identical in the four chambers	Not
Treatment-pericardiectomy	Antifailure therapy

(+ve: positive; Cath: catheterization; CHF: congestive heart failure; EF: ejection fraction; IVC: inferior vena cava; JVP: jugular venous pressure)

Q20. How TB is related to pericardial effusion?

Ans. In areas with a high prevalence of TB, a PE is often considered to be tubercular in origin, unless an alternative diagnosis is obvious. Here, empirical anti-TB chemotherapy is recommended for exudative PE before a bacteriological diagnosis is established, provided other causes such as malignancy, uremia, and trauma have been excluded. In two third cases of PE, diagnosis is based on bacteriological, histology, or analysis of pericardial fluid. In the rest, an adequate response to anti-TB serves as support for diagnosis.

Also, TB is the most frequent cause of constrictive pericarditis in Asia. It occurs in 30–60% of patients suffering from tubercular pericarditis despite prompt anti-TB and the use of corticosteroid.

Q21. How do you diagnose a case of tubercular pericardial effusion?

Ans. Diagnostic clues are as follows:
- Onset is insidious and may be huge at the time of diagnosis.
- Constitutional symptoms—fever, weight loss, anorexia, anemia, night sweat, and pressure symptoms—constriction and dyspnea.
- There is often no other evidence of TB, and the lung is rarely affected.
- *Investigation:* Aspiration of pericardial fluid: Exudative; often blood-stained, the presence of AFB (acid-fast bacilli) on staining or culture is confirmatory, occasionally, pericardial biopsy using a Vim-Silverman needle or open biopsy may be needed for diagnosis.

Treatment:
- Aspiration
- Anti-TB chemotherapy
- Surgery-early pericardiectomy, if doubt exists concerning constriction. Pericardiectomy is easier in the early stage with excellent results.

Q22. What is percutaneous balloon pericardiotomy?

Ans. Percutaneous balloon pericardiotomy (PBP) consists of creating a parietal pericardial window with a balloon-dilating catheter under fluoroscopic guidance in the catheterization laboratory. It is an effective therapy for recurrent, free-flowing, and hemodynamically significant PE, especially if associated with neoplastic disease. PBP consists of creating a parietal pericardial window with a balloon-dilating catheter under fluoroscopic guidance. It is a less invasive alternative to the surgical pericardial window. Diagnostic techniques in the pericardial space include epicardial mapping and ablation, intrapericardial echocardiography, etc. Intrapericardial delivery of drugs is also done by this technique.

SUGGESTED READING

1. Cheitlin MD, Alpert JS, Armstrong WF, Aurigemma GP, Beller GA, Bierman FZ, et al. ACC/AHA Guidelines for the Clinical Application of Echocardiography. A report of the American College of Cardiology/American Heart Association Task Force on Practice Guidelines (Committee on Clinical Application of Echocardiography). Developed in collaboration with the American Society of Echocardiography. Circulation. 1997;95(6):1686-744.
2. Maisch B, Seferovic PM, Ristic AD, Erbel R, Rienmüller R, Adler Y, et al. Guidelines on the diagnosis and management of pericardial diseases executive summary: the task force on the diagnosis and management of pericardial diseases of the European Society of Cardiology. Eur Heart J. 2004;25:587-610.

CHAPTER 11

Hypertension

"Hypertension is a condition that can claim a number of 'firsts': it is the most common chronic condition in the United States, no. 1 reason for a visit to physician, condition accounting for most drug prescription, major risk factor for CAD and stroke, and no. 1 attributable risk for death worldwide."
—JNC 7 report on Hypertension (JAMA 2003)

■ INTRODUCTION

Hypertension (HTN) is the most common, readily identifiable, and reversible risk factor for myocardial infarction (MI), stroke, heart failure (HF), atrial fibrillation, aortic dissection, and peripheral arterial disease. It is both preventable and treatable in majority of patients, and it accounts for the most drug prescriptions worldwide. Queries relating to detection and treatment are discussed here. Various issues on target organ damage (TOD), particularly hypertensive heart disease (HHD), are highlighted.

Q1. Define HTN. Classify it.
Ans. Hypertension is defined as a usual blood pressure (BP) of 140/90 mm Hg, the level of BP at which the benefit of pharmacologic treatment has been definitely established.

The risk of MI and stroke is continuous and graded down to levels as low as 115/75 mm Hg.

Classification:
- *Etiologically:* Primary (essential) and secondary
- *Type of BP rise:* Diastolic (classical essential HTN), systolic [isolated systolic HTN (ISH)], and combined (systolic and diastolic)

Other specific types:
- *Pre-HTN:* Normal or high normal BP [a systolic blood pressure (SBP) of 120-139 mm Hg and a diastolic blood pressure (DBP) of 80-89 mm Hg] which may progress to HTN if lifestyle modification is not adopted
- *Transient HTN:* Rise of BP for short periods in acute physiological stress (e.g., anxiety and tension)
- *Episodic HTN:* Sudden very high BP with restlessness, palpitation, sweating as in pheochromocytoma
- *White coat HTN:* Persistently elevated BP in physician's office with normal recording at home
- *Masked HTN:* Office readings less than home readings

- *Nocturnal HTN:* Paradoxical rise in BP at night instead of falling, occurs in renal failure
- *Malignant HTN:* Severely elevated BP (≥220/130 mm Hg) along with evidence of TOD. 5-year survival is 1% (if untreated), like malignant disease.
- *Resistant HTN:* Failure to reach goal BP in patients adhering to the full dose of an appropriately three-drug regimen that included a diuretic
- *Refractory HTN:* Failure to reach goal BP due to confounding factors involved, such as excess salt, inadequate drug, or inappropriate combination of drugs, excess alcohol intake, concomitant use of nonsteroidal anti-inflammatory drug (NSAID), steroids, amphetamine, oral pill, nasal decongestant, cyclosporine, tacrolimus, cocaine abuse, and volume overload for kidney disease
- *Borderline HTN:* BP sometimes but not always in the hypertensive range

Q2. What are the categories of HTN?
Ans. The International Society of Hypertension (ISH) and World Health Organization (WHO) categorized HTN as shown in **Table 11.1**.

TABLE 11.1: Categories of hypertension (by ISH–WHO).

Category	SBP (mm Hg)		DBP (mm Hg)
Blood pressure:			
Optimal	<120	and/or	<80
Normal	<130	and/or	80–84
High normal	130–139	and/or	85–89
Hypertension:			
Grade 1 (mild)	140–159	and/or	90–99
Grade 2 (moderate)	160–179	and/or	100–109
Grade 3 (severe)	≥180	and/or	≥110
Isolated systolic hypertension:			
Grade 1	140–159	and	<90
Grade 2	160–179	and	<90
Grade 2	≥180	and	<90

(DBP: diastolic blood pressure; ISH: International Society of Hypertension; SBP: systolic blood pressure; WHO: World Health Organization)

Q3. What is new in the 2024 European Society of Cardiology (ESC) guidelines on the management of elevated BP and HTN?
Ans. The European Society of Cardiology in their guidelines for the management of elevated BP recommended the following:
- It is recommended that BP be categorized into nonelevated BP, elevated BP, and HTN to aid treatment decisions. Elevated BP is an office SBP of 120–129 mm Hg or DBP of 70–89 mm Hg.

- Target SBP is 120–129 mm Hg among adults receiving BP-lowering drugs, provided that drugs are well tolerated. A more lenient BP target is recommended for symptomatic orthostatic hypotension, those aged ≥85 years, moderate to severe frailty, and low life expectancy. Here, BP is as low as reasonably achievable targeted.
- For a Class I recommendation for antihypertensive drugs benefit on cardiovascular disease (CVD) outcome (not only BP lowering) is needed.
- Risk-based approach in the treatment of elevated BP. In case of moderate-to-severe chronic kidney disease (CKD), established CVD, hypertension mediated organ damage (HMOD) diabetes mellitus (DM), or familial hypercholesterolemia. BP-lowering treatment is warranted.
- Systemic coronary risk evaluation 2 (SCORE2) is recommended for assessing the 10-year risk of fatal and nonfatal CVD among individuals aged 40–69 years with elevated BP who are not already considered at increased risk due to moderate-to-severe CKD, established CVD, HMOD, DM, or familial hypercholesterolemia.
- Systemetic Coronary Risk Evaluation 2 Older Persons (SCORE2-OP) is recommended for assessing the 10-year risk of fatal and nonfatal CVD among individuals aged ≥70 years with elevated BP who are not already considered at increased risk.
- Individuals with elevated BP and a SCORE2 or SCORE2-OP CVD 10-year predicted risk of ≥10% are considered at increased risk.
- Systematic coronary risk evaluation 2 diabetes should be considered to estimate CVD risk among type 2 diabetes mellitus (T2DM) (particularly in age <60 years).
- History of HTN complications, e.g., gestational diabetes and HTN, are risk modifiers considered for up classification in borderline increased 10-year CVD risk (5–10%).
- High-risk ethnicity, e.g., south Asians, family history of increased CVD, socioeconomic deprivation, autoimmune inflammatory disease, human immunodeficiency virus (HIV), and mental illness are risk modifiers for up classification in borderline increased 10-year risk (5% to <10% risk).
- If risk-based BP lowering treatment decision remains uncertain, increasing coronary artery calcium (CAC) score, carotid-femoral plaque by ultrasonography (USG), troponin or B-type natriuretic peptide (BNP) or arterial stiffness by pulse wave velocity may be considered to improve risk stratification (in borderline cases of 5% to <10% risk).
- In adults with elevated BP and low/medium CVD risk (<10% over 10 years), BP lowering with lifestyle measures is recommended and can reduce the risk of CVD.
- In adults with elevated BP and sufficiently high CVD risk after 3 months of lifestyle intervention, BP lowering with pharmacologic treatment is recommended for those with confirmed BP ≥130/80 mm Hg to reduce CVD risk.

- It is recommended that in hypertensive patients with confirmed BP ≥140/90 mm Hg, irrespective of CVD risk, lifestyle measures and pharmacological BP-lowering treatment are initiated promptly to reduce CVD risk. It is recommended to maintain BP-lowering drug treatment life-long, even beyond the age of 85 years, if well tolerated.
- In cases where BP-lowering treatment is poorly tolerated (and achieving an SBP of 120–129 mm Hg is not possible), it is recommended to target an SBP "as low as reasonably achievable". Such situations include: Pretreatment symptomatic orthostatic hypotension, age >85 years, clinically significant moderate-to-severe frailty, and limited predicted lifespan (<3 years).
- Once BP is controlled and stable under BP-lowering therapy, at least a yearly follow-up for BP and other CVD risk factors should be considered.

Q4. How BP is classified in the ESC 2024 guidelines?
Ans. In ESC 2024 guidelines, BP is categorized as given in **Table 11.2**.

TABLE 11.2: Categories of blood pressure.

Nonelevated BP	Elevated BP	Hypertension
Office BP SBP <120 mm Hg And DBP <70 mm Hg	Office BP SBP 120–139 mm Hg Or DBP 70–89 mm Hg	Office BP SBP ≥85–140 mm Hg Or DBP ≥85–90 mm Hg
HBPM SBP <120 mm Hg And DBP <70 mm Hg	HBPM Daytime SBP 120–134 mm Hg Or DBP 70–84 mm Hg	HBPM Daytime SBP ≥135 mm Hg Or DBP ≥85 mm Hg
ABPM Daytime SBP <120 mm Hg And Daytime DBP <70 mm Hg	ABPM Daytime SBP 120–134 mm Hg Or Daytime DBP 70–64 mm Hg	ABPM Daytime SBP ≥135 mm Hg Or Daytime DBP ≥85 mm Hg

Diagnosis of HTN and elevated BP requires confirmation using out-of-office measurements [home blood pressure monitoring (HBPM) or ambulatory blood pressure monitoring (ABPM)] or at least one additional subsequent office measurement.
(BP: blood pressure; DBP: diastolic blood pressure; SBP: systolic blood pressure)

Points to ponder:
- Among hypertensives, cardiovascular risk is sufficiently high to merit antihypertensive drugs.
- In elevated BP cases, risk stratification is done to identify individuals with high cardiovascular (CV) risk for antihypertensive drug use.

Q5. Why HTN is called a silent killer?

Ans. Hypertension is an asymptomatic chronic disorder that, if undetected and untreated, damages the blood vessels, heart, brain, and kidneys. Hence, it is called a silent killer.

Q6. What is white coat and masked HTN?

Ans.
- White coat HTN—consistently elevated BP reading in physician's office despite normal home or ambulatory BP measurements. There is no TOD. It is due to a transient adrenergic response to the measurements of BP only in the physician's office. Up to 30% of elevated BP at the office may have white coat HTN.
- *Masked HTN:* It is the mirror image of white coat HTN. Here, office readings underestimate out-of-office BP, presumably because of sympathetic overactivity in daily life caused by job or home stress, tobacco and alcohol consumption, or other adrenergic responses.

Q7. What is the diurnal variation of BP?

Ans. Blood pressure level is highest in the early morning ("morning surge" of BP), decreases somewhat during daytime, and lowest during sleeping hours. This is in accordance with the level of stress hormones in blood. A paradoxical rise of BP at night instead of falling is called nocturnal HTN.

Q8. What is malignant HTN? Which HTN is benign?

Ans. Severely elevated BP (≥220/130 mm Hg) along with evidence of TOD, i.e., retinal hemorrhage and papilledema, is designated as malignant HTN. If untreated the patient has a 5-year survival rate of 1%, that is equivalent to that of other malignant diseases. Hence, it is called malignant. Treatment has a dramatic effect on survival.

No HTN is benign. If untreated, all may lead to TOD. There is a graded and positive relationship between the level of BP and the risk of CVDs down to BP levels as low as 115/75 mm Hg. From the age of 40–70 years, each 20 mm Hg increase in systolic, and 10 mm Hg increase in diastolic pressure is associated with a doubling of the risk of stroke.

Q9. What is pre-HTN? What is its significance?

Ans. Pre-HTN is a high normal BP, which may progress to HTN if lifestyle modification measures are not adopted. An SBP of 120–139 mm Hg and a DBP of 80–89 mm Hg is said to be pre-HTN. After the age of 60 years, the prehypertensives are more likely to develop ISH. There is an increased likelihood of the development of vascular complications among prehypertensives. Lifestyle modification (e.g., low salt and weight reduction) is strongly recommended.

Q10. What is ISH? What is the importance?
Ans. Isolated systolic HTN is defined as an elevated SBP in conjunction with a normal DBP (<90 mm Hg). An SBP >140 mm Hg is leveled as ISH. Three grades of ISH are in **Table 11.3**.

TABLE 11.3: Isolated systolic hypertension classification.

Systolic blood pressure (SBP)	Grade
Grade 1	140–159 mm Hg
Grade 2	160–179 mm Hg
Grade 3	>180 mm Hg

(SBP: systolic blood pressure)

The presence of ISH indicates not only the presence of HTN but also the presence of diseased blood vessels. Hence, the prognosis is worse here. Elevated SBP has consistently been shown to be a better predictor of cardiovascular events including stroke and MI.

Q11. What is the target BP for antihypertensive drug therapy?
Ans. With antihypertensive drug therapy target BP to be achieved in different clinical situations as shown in **Table 11.4**.

TABLE 11.4: Target BP for drug therapy.

Patient status	Goal BP
Prevention of HHD and other TOD	<140/90 mm Hg
CAD with stable angina and ACS (UA and MI)	<130/80 mm Hg
Heart failure	<130/80 mm Hg (consider 120/70 mm Hg)
Diabetes mellitus	<130/80 mm Hg
Chronic kidney disease (CKD)	<115/75 mm Hg
Cerebrovascular disease	Controlled reduction done
Blacks	DBP <85 mm Hg
Elderly >80 years	<150/80 (DBP not <65 mm Hg)

(ACS: acute coronary syndrome; BP: blood pressure; CAD: coronary artery disease; DBP: diastolic blood pressure; HHD: hypertensive heart disease; MI: myocardial infarction; TOD: target organ damage; UA: unstable angina)

Q12. What is the relationship between the kidney and HTN?
- Kidneys are the target organs of HTN—uncontrolled HTN causes CKD. In 90% of cases of CKD, an elevated BP is found.
- Chronic kidney disease may also be a cause of HTN. Long-standing uncontrolled BP produces vascular changes and renal ischemia, releasing renin, and increasing BP in turn. A vicious cycle may thus be established— i.e., a raised BP leads to a still more raised BP. This condition is called

accelerated HTN. When papilledema develops, the condition is called malignant HTN.
- Kidney may be the cause of secondary HTN (e.g., renal artery stenosis and polycystic kidney diseases).

Q13. Hypertension begets HTN. Explain.
Ans. An elevated BP, if not controlled, produces more increase in BP by:
- A raised level of angiotensin-II, acting on the AT-1 receptor, produces vascular remodeling and release of aldosterone and noradrenaline.
- Renal ischemia in uncontrolled HTN releases renin that increases angiotensin-II in turn. Angiotensin-II raises BP in turn.

Thus, a vicious cycle is established and HTN produces more HTN. If BP is kept controlled within desirable limits with multiple drugs, the cycle can be broken and it may be possible to control BP and decrease the number and dose of antihypertensive drugs afterward.

Q14. What is HHD?
Ans. The term HHD is generally applied to heart diseases that are caused by the direct or indirect effect of chronically elevated BP.

HHD: HTN + Evidence of heart diseases

Hypertensive heart disease are:
- Left ventricular hypertrophy (LVH)
- Heart failure [diastolic, systolic, and chronic heart failure (CHF)]
- Coronary artery diseases (CADs)
- Arrhythmias—atrial fibrillation, ventricular ectopics, ventricular tachycardias, and sudden cardiac death
- Miscellaneous—aortic regurgitation (AR), mitral regurgitation (MR), etc.

Q15. What is essential HTN? Is it really essential?
Ans. Patients with primary or idiopathic HTN were previously leveled as having essential HTN. It was thought that with increasing age and stiffness of the arterial wall, a raised pressure is essential to maintain cerebral blood flow. So, the condition was designated as essential HTN. But, now it is clear that increased BP is not an essential consequence of aging and a raised BP is not essential to maintain cerebral flow. Hence, essential HTN is not essential in that sense. Any BP >140/90 mm Hg at any age is HTN requiring pharmacologic therapy.

Q16. What is drug-induced HTN?
Ans. Several drugs may cause de novo HTN, worsening of preexisting HTN, and even hypertensive crisis. Besides prescribed drugs, over-the-counter medications and herbal preparations may cause it. These are systemic steroids, analgesics, sex hormones, some chemotherapeutics, and immunosuppressants, like cyclosporine, recombinant human erythropoietin,

amphitamine, and other sympathomimetics, tricyclic antidepressants, illicit drugs like cocaine, nasal decongestants (pseudoephedrine), appetite suppressants, e.g., sibutramine, caffeine, and alcohol. Abrupt withdrawal of antihypertensive drugs like α-methyl dopa, clonidine, guanethidine, nifedipine, minoxidil, etc., may induce rebound HTN.

Q17. How is BP lowering done in ACS and acute LVF?
Ans. In hypertensive patients with ACS, BP should be lowered with intravenous (IV) nitroglycerine after administration of a β-blocker such as IV metaprolol to prevent reflex tachycardia. IV esmolol lowers BP more rapidly whose action also reveres rapidly and predictively. IV nitroglycerine alleviates angina more reliably than lowering BP. Nitroprusside can cause coronary steal and should be avoided, and hypotension must be avoided in ACS patients to avoid infarct extension.

Acute HF—nitroprusside is the drug of choice to treat hypertensive crises and acute HF. Concomitant loop diuretics both decrease acute pulmonary edema and further lower BP.

Q18. How is BP lowering done in acute stroke?
Ans. In acute ischemic stroke, BP should be lowered cautiously to avoid ischemic insult to potentially salvageable tissue (termed the ischemic penumbra), which would extend the infarct. American Heart Association (AHA)/American Stroke Association 2013 guidelines recommend the following: (1) If the stroke cannot be treated with thrombolytic therapy, BP should be treated if it remains higher than 220/120 mm Hg and initially lowered by no more than 15%, and (2) if the stroke can be treated with thrombolytic therapy, BP needs to be lowered to <185/110 mm Hg. In acute hemorrhagic stroke intensive treatment to lower SBP to <140 mm Hg showed improved functional outcome INTERACT2 (intensive BP reduction in acute hemorrhage trial 2). For either ischemic or hemorrhagic stroke, agents of choice to lower BP include nicardipine, labetalol, or urapidil. Nitroprusside and hydralazine are avoided, because they may increase intracranial pressure.

Q19. What is the usefulness of diuretics as an antihypertensive agent?
Ans. Low-dose diuretics should be the initial choice for most, if not first, it should certainly be the second drug. In more severe HTN or HTN with renal damage, a larger dose of thiazide or a loop diuretic is needed. Diuretics are indicated in elderly, ISH, and HF, in combination with other agents.

Q20. What is the position of β-blockers as antihypertensives?
Ans. Beta-blockers lower BP by decreasing cardiac output (COP); decrease brachial BP but aortic BP less well. These are less protective for primary prevention but important for secondary protection (CAD and HF). They should not remain as the first choice for primary HTN. Specific recommendations are HTN with CAD (particularly post-MI, angina), CHF, and tachyarrhythmias.

Side effects are fatigue, impotence, increased incidence of DM, masking hypoglycemia in DM, and increase in stroke incidence.

Q21. What are the factors that determine the benefits of lowering BP?
Ans. Benefit of reducing BP correlates with the extent of BP rather than from how it is reduced (with few exceptions). Benefit of treatment is more in age >65 years than those for younger, as they are at much greater risk. Benefit more from treatment of moderate-to-severe HTN than from mild HTN. All those younger than 80 are benefited with antihypertensives.

Q22. What are the things to consider in the selection of antihypertensive drugs?
Ans. Efficacy, tolerability, presence of concomitant diseases, like DM, presence of TOD, and cost-effectiveness are to be considered.
- Caution during vigorous BP reduction—patient with acute stroke susceptible to BP <160/100 mm Hg and patient with CAD to DBP <80 mm Hg.
- α-blockers do not decrease COP; patient remains physically active, no change in lipid and sugar; may improve prostatism in benign prostatic enlargement. Combined α- and β-blockers (labetalol and carvedilol) are used in hypertensive crisis and pregnancy.
- Centrally acting drugs, like methyldopa, decrease peripheral resistance with little effect on COP. Renal flow remains normal. It is safe in pregnancy.
- Calcium channel blockers are preferred in the elderly, ISH, and angina [rate-limiting calcium channel blocker (CCB)].
- Angiotensin-converting enzyme inhibitors (ACEIs) are preferred drugs in HF, CAD, post-MI, and DM; angiotensin receptor blockers (ARBs) are the same as ACEI and used for those intolerant to ACEI.
- Direct vasodilators are used as an adjunct to the above and in resistant HTN.

Recent randomized controlled trial (RCT) and expert opinion show (1) ACEI are more potent antihypertensives, (2) dual renin-angiotensin system (RAS) blockers (ACEI plus ARB) are dangerous, (3) ACEI/ARB, CCBs, and thiazide diuretics are the three first-line drugs, (4) most effective two-drug combinations are ACEIs/ARBs with diuretics or ACEI/ARB and CCB. They have additional effect when used in combination, (5) β-blockers are the first-line drug for angina and HF, experts disagree to use it as a first-line drug for uncontrolled HTN of their inferior stroke prevention and increased risk for incident DM, and (6) in order of potency, CCBs are dihydropyridines > diltiazem > verapamil.

Q23. What are the major TOD caused by hypertension?
Ans. These are:
- Hypertensive heart disease
- Hypertensive CVD

- Hypertensive kidney disease
- Hypertensive vascular diseases and retinopathy

Q24. A hypertensive developed acute myocardial infarction (AMI)—what are the special features?
Ans. A very high BP in the case of AMI is a hypertensive emergency. BP should be controlled rapidly, otherwise, there is a risk of further increase in infarct and development of acute LVF. Caution is needed not to lower DBP <80 mm Hg to decrease coronary flow, which occurs mainly in diastole.

Q25. A hypertensive developed stroke—what are the special attributes?
Ans. A controlled reduction of BP is needed here. Caution is needed not to lower BP below 160/100 mm Hg to avoid the risk of cerebral ischemia by lowering BP. Cerebral flow is maintained at a higher pressure in hypertensives, and a quick reduction may precipitate cerebral ischemic damage.

Q26. What are the mechanisms of HF in HHD?
Ans. Risk of HF increases two- to threefold in HTN. Long-standing uncontrolled HTN produces pressure overload, LVH, and diastolic dysfunction. Also, by producing coronary atherosclerosis and rupturing the plaque, it leads to MI, decreased myocardial contractility, and systolic dysfunction. CHF results as a consequence as shown in **Flowchart 11.1**.

Flowchart 11.1: Mechanism of heart failure in HHD.

(CHF: chronic heart failure; HHD: hypertensive heart disease; HTN: hypertension; LVH: left ventricular hypertrophy; MI: myocardial infarction)

Q27. Left ventricular hypertrophy in HTN—what is its importance and prognosis?
Ans. Left ventricular hypertrophy develops in long-standing uncontrolled HTN. LVH, if it continues leads to the development of diastolic HF and subsequently to systolic HF. Chest pain may manifest due to relative ischemia of hypertrophied myocardium. If BP is controlled adequately, LVH is still reversible.

Q28. What is myocardial remodeling in HTN?
Ans. Long-standing and uncontrolled HTN produces myocardial remodeling. It involves loss of myocytes and fibrosis with consequent change in cardiac

morphology. Myocardial remodeling results in loss of normal conical form with impairment of pumping capacity. HF develops as a result. Myocardial remodeling is the consequence of loss of regulation between proremodeling and antiremodeling factors.

Increased proremodeling factors: Noradrenaline, aldosterone, reactive O_2 species, troponin-I, and transforming growth factor-beta (TGF-β).

Decreased antiremodeling factors: Nitric oxide (NO), prostacyclin (PGI_2), insulin-like growth factor 1 (IGF_1), and tumor necrosis factor-alpha (TNF-α)

Q29. What is an HTN continuum?
Ans. Hypertension, if not controlled, leads to LVH, diastolic, followed by systolic HF. HTN is a risk factor for CAD and MI. Through insulin resistance, HTN increases the risk of development of noninsulin-dependent diabetes mellitus (NIDDM). Thus, uncontrolled HTN leads to death called an HTN continuum.

Q30. What is "rule of halves" in HTN?
Ans.
- Only about half of the hypertensive subjects in the general population are aware of the condition.
- Only half of those aware of the problem are being treated.
  and
- Only half of those treated are considered adequately treated.

This was evident in the 1970s among the general populations of most developed countries. Thus, HTN is an "iceburg" disease.

Q31. Which HTN is more important to treat systolic or diastolic?
Ans. The Framingham Heart Study showed that in subjects younger than the age of 50 years, the best predictor of cardiovascular risk is a high diastolic pressure, but in older subjects aged more than 60 years, systolic pressure is the best predictor.

Q32. What are the advantages of diuretics as an antihypertensive agent?
Ans. Diuretics, especially thiazides, are the first-line antihypertensive drugs. It is equally effective in systolic as well as diastolic HTN. It is:
- Low cost
- Efficacious and effective with a wide range of renal function
- Can be combined with other classes. It potentiates the action of β-blockers, ACEI, and ARB and is available in combination.
- Antihypertensive effect persists indefinitely. Lower pressure may lead to Na^+ retention with the use of others, which does not occur with diuretic use.
- It is the drug of choice in HTN with heart and renal failures.

Q33. What is the current status of β-blockers as an antihypertensive agent?

Ans. They lower BP by decreasing COP. β-blockers lower brachial BP but aortic BP less well. They are less protective for primary prevention but important for secondary prevention (CAD and HF). They are not the first choice for primary HTN, and may increase stroke and the incidence of diabetes. They are specifically indicated in post-MI, CHF, and tachyarrhythmias.

Q34. Which antihypertensive drugs should not be stopped suddenly? What is rebound HTN?

Ans. These are β-blockers, α-methyldopa, reserpine, clonidine, and prozosin. A rise in BP with the sudden stopping of antihypertensive drugs is rebound HTN.

Q35. What are the drugs that can be used in HTN with pregnancy?

Ans. These are the following drugs used in HTN with pregnancy: α-methyl dopa, CCBs, α–β blockers (labetalol), and sometimes diuretics.

Q36. What are the causes of elevated BP in a renal transplant patient?

Ans. Successful renal transplantation may cure primary HTN but 50% of recipients become hypertensive within 1 year.

Causes are renal artery stenosis (at the site of anastomosis), rejection reaction, high-dose steroids and cyclosporins or tacrolimus, and excess renin release from the retained diseased kidney.

Hypertension is more common with donors having a family history of HTN.

Q37. What is the importance of ambulatory BP monitoring? When is it done?

Ans.
- Average level of ambulatory BP records predicts the risk of morbid events better than clinic BP.
- It is the only way of recording BP during sleep. Normal ambulatory BP values for adults are <135/85 mm Hg while awake and <120/75 mm Hg during the night.

Ambulatory recordings of BP are done in the following situations: White coat HTN, masked HTN, refractory HTN, episodic HTN, and nocturnal HTN. Nighttime BP is usually lower than daytime BP. Individuals with <10% reduction from night to day appear to be at increased risk of TOD.

Q38. What is resistant HTN?

Ans. It is the failure to reach goal BP in patients who are adhering to full doses of an appropriate three-drug regimen that includes a diuretic. It is usually found in patients when a secondary cause is not explored. Refractory HTN is an almost similar condition with some confounding factors involved. These are excess sodium intake, inadequate dose or inappropriate combinations of antihypertensives, excessive alcohol intake, concomitant use of NSAIDs, steroids, amphetamines, antidepressants, cocaine abuse, oral contraceptives, nasal decongestants, cyclosporine, tacrolimus, volume overload from kidney disease, etc.

Q39. What are the interventional treatments available for HTN?
Ans.
- Medical
  - Renal denervation therapy (RDN)—transcatheter denervation of afferent renal artery by lesser in cases of resistant HTN
  - Balloon dilatation and bare metal stent placement in renal artery stenosis
  - Stenting in coarctation of the aorta, etc.
- Surgery: In coarctation of the aorta and renal artery stenosis (some cases)

Q40. Antihypertensive drugs need to be continued lifelong—Justify.
Ans. Hypertension is a disease that needs to be controlled lifelong. Hence, antihypertensive drugs need to be continued lifelong on most occasions. However, after a period of well-controlled numbers and dose of antihypertensives may be reduced and BP controlled with the minimal amount of antihypertensive drugs. In some situations, BP decreases, such as after AMI, and HF. This is due to loss of myocardial contractility. In such situations, antihypertensives need to be reduced or even discontinued temporarily or permanently.

SUGGESTED READING

1. Chobanian AV, Bakris GL, Black HR, Cushman WC, Green LA, Izzo JL Jr., et al. The seventh report of the Joint National Committee on Prevention, Detection, Evaluation, and Treatment of High Blood Pressure: the JNC 7 report. JAMA. 2003;289:2560.
2. Chowdhury MA, Uddin MJ, Haque MR, Ibrahimou B. Hypertension among adults in Bangladesh: evidence from a national cross-sectional survey. BMC Cardiovasc Disord. 2016;16:22.
3. Mancia G, De Backer G, Dominiczak A, Cifkova R, Fagard R, Germano G, et al.; Management of Arterial Hypertension of the European Society of Hypertension; European Society of Cardiology. 2007 guidelines for the management of arterial hypertension: the Task Force for the Management of Arterial Hypertension of the European Society of Hypertension (ESH) and of the European Society of Cardiology (ESC). Eur Heart J. 2007;28(12):1462-536.
4. McEvoy JW, McCarthy CP, Bruno RM, Brouwers S, Canavan MD, Ceconi C, et al.; ESC Scientific Document Group. 2024 ESC guidelines for the management of elevated blood pressure and hypertension. Eur Heart J. 2024;45(38):3912-4018.
5. Park K (Ed). Epidemiology of chronic noncommunicable diseases and conditions. In: Parks's Textbook of Preventive and Social Medicine, 19th edition. 2007. p. 311.
6. Whitworth JA. 2003 World Health Organization (WHO)/International Society of Hypertension (ISH) statement on management of hypertension. J Hypertens. 2003;21(11):1983-92.

CHAPTER 12

Heart Failure and Cardiogenic Shock

"There is but one meaning for the term cardiac failure-it signifies inability of the heart to discharge its contents adequately."
—Sir Thomas Lewis (1933)

▪ INTRODUCTION

Heart failure (HF) is more common as coronary artery disease (CAD) prevalence increases and patients survive longer with modern treatment of myocardial infarction (MI). Also, increases in life expectancy and population aging add to the total burden of HF cases. The HF syndrome initially starts with impaired ability of the pumping function of the heart, ultimately involving almost all organs of the body by neurohormonal and circulatory changes. HF, when severe enough, leads to organ hypoperfusion and features of shock, the entity called cardiogenic shock.

Q1. How HF is defined? What is circulatory failure?
Ans. Heart failure may be defined as a pathophysiologic state in which the heart is unable to pump adequate blood to meet the metabolic needs of the body at normal filling pressure or can do so at raised filling pressure.

Circulatory failure is a general term that refers to an inadequacy of the cardiovascular (CV) system in performing its basic functions of providing nutrition to the cells of the body and removing metabolic products from cells. It may be due to cardiac (i.e., HF) or noncardiac (peripheral) conditions, e.g., inadequate blood volume, peripheral vascular abnormalities, etc.

Q2. Is HF and myocardial failure synonymous?
Ans. Heart failure is frequently but not always caused by a defect in myocardial contraction. The term myocardial failure is appropriate here. Occasionally, HF may occur in the presence of normal myocardial function, e.g., impaired left ventricular (LV) filling in mitral stenosis (MS) or sudden LV overload in acute aortic regurgitation (AR) can produce HF in the presence of normal myocardial function.

Q3. Define congestion. What is congestive HF?
Ans. Congestion or circulatory overload is a general term referring to excess blood volume from either cardiac (i.e., congestive HF) or noncardiac causes. Noncardiac causes of congestion include excess parenteral fluid administration. Congestive HF is a clinical syndrome in which systemic and pulmonary congestion occurs due to systolic and/or diastolic HF.

- Pulmonary venous congestion results from disordered function of the left ventricle or left atrium. It results in dyspnea, paroxysmal nocturnal dyspnea, and orthopnea.
- Systemic venous congestion is due to the disorder of the right ventricle (RV) and atrium but is often the end result of left-sided HF. It produces raised jugular venous pressure (JVP), enlarged tender liver, and peripheral edema.

Q4. What are the forms of HF?
Ans.
- *Right-sided versus left-sided HF:*
  - In right HF, there is a reduction in RV output for any right atrial pressure. There are features of systemic venous congestion (i.e., raised JVP, enlarged liver, and dependent edema)
  - In left HF, there is a reduction of LV output and/or an increase in the left atrial (LA) or pulmonary venous pressure (manifested as dyspnea and basal pulmonary crepitations).
  - In biventricular HF, both right- and left-sided HF coexists because the disease, e.g., dilated cardiomyopathy (DCM) and ischemic heart disease (IHD), affects both ventricular or because the left-sided failure leads to chronic elevation of LA pressure, pulmonary hypertension, and subsequent right HF.
- *Forward versus backward HF:*
  - Forward failure implies an inadequate cardiac output (COP) by the failing ventricle, while backward failure implies that it is due primarily to venous congestion with fluid retention behind the failing ventricle, causing pulmonary and systemic congestions.
- *Diastolic versus systolic HF:*
  - In systolic HF, there is an impaired myocardial contractility, i.e., systolic dysfunction **(Figs. 12.1A and B)**. In diastolic HF, ventricular dysfunction results from excessive stiffness of the myocardium. The noncompliant LV develops a high-pressure during diastole, causing an elevation in pulmonary capillary wedge pressure (PCWP). Also, preload decreases as less blood fills the ventricle, which in turn reduces COP.
  - Patients with systolic LV dysfunction invariably have diastolic dysfunction, although isolated diastolic dysfunction may remain in the absence of systolic dysfunction.
- *High output versus low output HF:* The COP is often depressed in patients with HF due to IHD, hypertension, valvular heart disease, and cardiomyopathies but tends to be elevated in patients with HF and hyperthyroidism, anemia, pregnancy, and beriberi.

- *Acute versus chronic HF:* In acute heart failure (AHF), symptoms of severe congestive HF develop over a period of minutes to hours. Here, myocardial dysfunction develops suddenly, e.g., in acute MI, acute myocarditis, acute AR, or mitral regurgitation (MR) (due to infective endocarditis, etc.). Chronic HF develops gradually, and a variety of compensatory changes take place with progressive impairment of cardiac function.

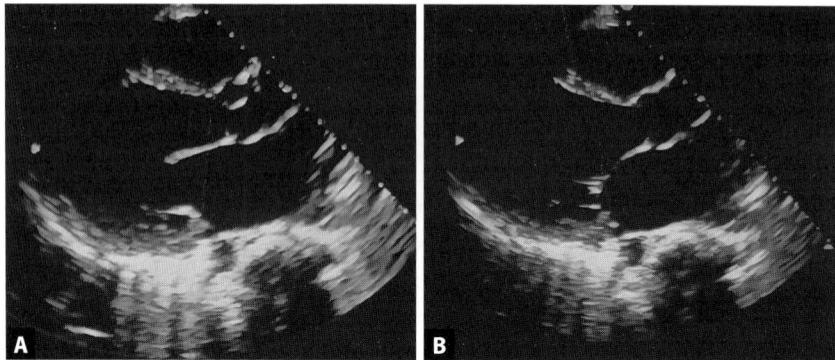

Figs. 12.1A and B: 2DE showing poor LV function in diastole (A) and systole (B).

- Acute on chronic HF—sudden deterioration of cardiac function in patients having chronically depressed cardiac function. Intercurrent illness (infection, etc.), increased metabolic demand (anemia, pregnancy, and thyrotoxicosis), arrhythmia [e.g., atrial fibrillation (AF)], development of myocardial ischemia, and noncompliance with antifailure therapy may produce acute on chronic HF.
- Heart failure with reduced ejection fraction (HFrEF) and HF with preserved EF (HFpEF): Clinical HF with a left ventricular ejection fraction (LVEF) of <40% is HFrEF, and that with an LVEF of >50% is HFpEF. Nearly half of patients with HF have HFpEF. With increasing comorbidities such as obesity, hypertension, metabolic syndrome, and aging of the population, the incidence of HFpEF is increasing.

Patients with LVEF 40–50% are leveled as HF with midrange EF. In the revised HF definition, an LVEF of 41–49% is leveled as HF with mildly reduced EF (HFmrEF).

Q5. What are the common causes of left HF and right HF?
Ans. Causes of left HF include:
- Ischemic heart disease—MI and chronic IHD (producing ischemic cardiomyopathy)
- Hypertensive heart disease—systemic hypertension
- Valvular diseases—MS (produces LA failure), MR, and aortic valvular disease [aortic stenosis (AS) and AR]
- Congenital heart disease—ventricular septal defect (VSD) and patent ductus arteriosus (PDA)
- Cardiomyopathy

Causes of right HF include:
- Secondary to left HF (most common)
- Chronic obstructive pulmonary diseases (COPDs)
- Right ventricular infarction
- Congenital heart disease—pulmonary stenosis, atrial septal defect (ASD), etc.
- Cardiomyopathy

Q6. What are the stages of HF?

Ans. American College of Cardiology and American Heart Association (ACC/AHA) guidelines have classified HF in stages that emphasize the evolution and progression of HF across a continuum **(Table 12.1)**.

TABLE 12.1: Stages of heart failure.

Stage A	Patients are at high risk of developing heart failure, as patients with hypertension, diabetes, and dyslipidemia
Stage B	Patients have structural heart diseases but without symptoms of heart failure, e.g., patients with previous MI and asymptomatic LV dysfunction
Stage C	Patients with structural heart disease who have developed symptoms of heart failure, e.g., patients with previous MI with shortness of breath and fatigue
Stage D	Patients with refractory heart failure requiring special intervention, e.g., patients waiting for cardiac transplantation

(LV: left ventricular; MI: myocardial infarction)

Q7. What is the functional classification for HF?

Ans. The New York Heart Association (NYHA) functional classification is widely applied in HF classification **(Table 12.2)**.

TABLE 12.2: NYHA functional classification.

Class I	Patients have heart disease but without any limitation of ordinary physical activity
Class II	Patients have a slight limitation of physical activity. Ordinary physical activity causes symptoms (fatigue, palpitation, dyspnea, and anginal pain)
Class III	Patients have marked limitations of physical activity. Less than ordinary activity causes symptoms
Class IV	Patients are unable to carry on any physical activity without discomfort. Symptoms are present even at rest

(NYHA: New York Heart Association)

Q8. What is the hemodynamic (Forrester) classification of HF in MI?

Ans. Forrester's hemodynamic subsets are based on data obtained from invasive monitoring of patients with acute myocardial infarction (AMI), i.e., cardiac index (CI) and PCWP **(Table 12.3)**.

TABLE 12.3: Forrester hemodynamic classification (of myocardial infarction).

Class I	Normal PCWP (<18 mm Hg) and normal CI (>2.2 L/min/m²)
Class II	PCWP >18 mm Hg and normal CI >2.2 L/min/m². Clinically, there is a backward failure with pulmonary congestion. Mortality: 10.2%. Treatment includes the use of vasodilators (e.g., nitrates) ± diuretics
Class III	PCWP <18 mm Hg and low CI (<2.2 L/m/m²). Clinically, the patient has forward failure with peripheral hypoperfusion. Mortality: 22.4%. Patients usually respond to the administration of plasma expanders
Class IV	PCWP >18 mm Hg and CI low (<2.2 b/m/m²). Clinically, patients have both pulmonary congestion and hypoperfusion. Mortality: 55.5%. Drugs to increase contractility (inotropes) and reduce LV afterload (dilators) are useful

(CI: cardiac index; LV: left ventricular; PCWP: pulmonary capillary wedge pressure)

Q9. What is the Killip classification of HF?

Ans. The Killip classification is based on clinical signs that correlate the degree of HF with mortality in patients with acute coronary syndrome **(Table 12.4)**.

TABLE 12.4: Killip classification of heart failure.

Class I	No evidence of left ventricular failure; mortality is 5%
Class II	Bibasilar rales, S_3 gallop; mortality is 20%
Class III	Patients are in pulmonary edema; mortality is 40%
Class IV	Patients are in cardiogenic shock defined by: Systolic BP < 80–90 mm Hg with evidence of hypoperfusion; mortality is 80% (improved to 50% with current therapy)

(BP: blood pressure)

Q10. What are the features of diastolic LV dysfunction?

Ans. It refers to impairment of diastolic filling resulting from excessive stiffness and diminished compliance of the myocardium.
- Mechanism of HF in diastolic dysfunction:
  - Left ventricular diastolic pressure, causing an elevation of LA pressure and pulmonary capillary pressure (PCP).
  - Preload, due to diminished filling of noncompliant LV, which in turn reduces COP.

Common causes are:
- Severe LV hypertrophy—hypertensive heart disease and AS
- Hypertrophic cardiomyopathy (HCM)
- Restrictive cardiomyopathy

Investigation findings are:
- Chest X-ray—heart is usually normal in transverse diameter, and features of pulmonary venous hypertension are usual.

- Electrocardiogram (ECG)—left ventricular hypertrophy (LVH) is the most common finding.
- Echocardiographic findings—LVH with normal ejection fraction (EF decreased in systolic failure). On the Doppler study, a low E/A ratio (i.e., ratio of early transmitral flow to atrial contraction): <1.0 (normal 2:1), a long deceleration time (i.e., time from peak filling velocity of the E-wave to baseline), and long isovolumetric relaxation time (IVRT) [i.e., interval between aortic valve (AV) closure and mitral valve (MV) opening] are consistent with impaired relaxation of the ventricle.
- Endomyocardial biopsy—occasionally, if there is suspicion of infiltrative myocardial disease, e.g., sarcoidosis and amyloidosis.

Q11. What is the difference between acute left ventricular failure (LVF) and pulmonary edema?

Ans. Pulmonary edema may occur in patients with acute LVF, but both conditions are not synonymous. Besides LVF, pulmonary edema may result from noncardiac causes **(Figs. 12.2A and B)**.

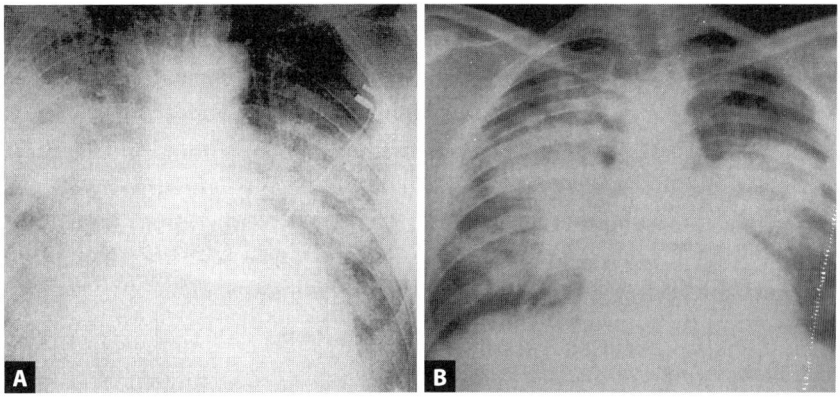

Figs. 12.2A and B: Pulmonary edema in AMI (A) and acute renal failure (B).

Afterloading conditions, e.g., acute renal failure (ARF) may produce it. Noncardiogenic pulmonary edema can occur with surgery, trauma, and sepsis, which is probably inflammatory in origin and known as adult respiratory distress syndrome (ARDS).

Q12. How does acute pulmonary edema develop HF?

Ans. Conditions that raise LV end-diastolic pressure or LA pressure may result in elevated pulmonary venous pressure. Such processes include diseases that reduce LV contractility, e.g., IHD or cardiomyopathy, as well as processes that decrease LV compliance, such as IHD, AS, and hypertension. MS results in elevated LA pressure. An elevated pulmonary venous pressure leads to an elevated PCP. Pulmonary lymphatics become engorged in an attempt to drain fluid from the pulmonary interstitium, thus preventing the formation of edema. When PCP is more than that, the lymphatics reach their limit, and interstitial edema develops. Subsequently, alveolar flooding or pulmonary edema develops when pressure is >25 mm Hg.

Q13. What is the universal definition of HF?
Ans. Heart failure is a clinical syndrome with symptoms and/or signs caused by a structural and/or functional cardiac abnormality and corroborated by elevated natriuretic peptide levels and/or objective evidence of pulmonary or systemic congestion.

Q14. What are revised staging for HF?
Ans. The 2021 European Society of Cardiology (ESC) guidelines revised stages of HF as follows:
- At-risk for HF (Stage A)—patients at risk for HF but without current or prior symptoms or signs of HF and without structural or biomarker's evidence of heart disease
- PreHF (Stage B)—patients without current or prior symptoms or signs of HF, but evidence of structural heart disease or abnormal cardiac function, or elevated natriuretic peptide levels
- HF (Stage C)—patients with current or prior symptoms and/or signs of HF caused by a structural and/or functional cardiac abnormality
- Advanced HF (Stage D)—patients with severe symptoms and/or signs of HF at rest, recurrent hospitalization despite guideline-directed management and therapy (GMDT), refractory or intolerance to GDMT, requiring advanced therapies such as consideration for transplantation, mechanical circulatory support (MCS), or palliative care

Q15. What is the revised classification of HF?
Ans. New ESC 2021 recommended revised classification of HF done according to LVEF:
- Heart failure with reduced EF (HFrEF)—HF with an LVEF of ≤40%
- Heart failure with mildly reduced EF (HFmrEF)—HF with an LVEF of 41–49%
- Heart failure with preserved EF (HFpEF)—HF with an LVEF of ≥50%
- Heart failure with improved EF (HFimpEF)—HF with a baseline LVEF of ≤40%, a ≥10-point increase from baseline LVEF, and a second measurement of LVEF of >40%

Q16. What is the difference between HFrEF and HFpEF?
Ans. Elevated filling pressure, pulmonary hypertension, and impaired COP reserve are common in both conditions. Also, reduced exercise tolerance and poor quality of life are common to both.

Differentiating points are given in **Table 12.5**.

TABLE 12.5: HFrEF and HFpEF—differences.

Points	HFrEF	HFpEF
Demographic	Any age, male > female	Older, female > male
LV size	Dilated	Normal
LV systolic dysfunction	Decreased severely	Mildly
LV diastolic dysfunction	+	+++
Pulmonary hypertension	++	+
BNP level	Increased	Normal or decreased
Response to therapy	Effective	Less effective
Benefit of treatment	Proved	Not well proved

(BNP: B-type natriuretic peptide; HFpEF: heart failure with preserved ejection fraction; HFrEF: heart failure with reduced ejection fraction; LV: left ventricular)

Q17. What are the common causes of HF in South Asian people?
Ans.
- Ischemic heart disease
- Hypertensive heart disease
- Dilated cardiomyopathy
- Rheumatic heart disease (RHD)
- Cor pulmonale
- Nonrheumatic valvular diseases
- Congenital heart disease
- Peripartum cardiomyopathy
- Endocrine and metabolic
- Hypertrophic cardiomyopathy

Q18. What are the nutritional causes of HF?
Ans. Deficiency of micronutrients may contribute to HF in developing countries, including Bangladesh. These are deficiencies of thiamine, iron, L-carnitine, selenium, coenzyme Q10, phosphate, and calcium.

Q19. What are the special attributes of HF in South Asian people?
Ans.
- Patients are younger and sicker and get less medication compared to what is recommended by guidelines.
- Ischemic heart disease, RHD, hypertension, DCM, and coronary heart disease (CHD) are the main causes.
- Heart failure patients comprise 20–30% of patients attending the cardiac OPD
- Mortality is high; one third die within 1 year of follow-up
- More hospital readmission; <30% receive angiotensin-converting enzyme inhibitor/angiotensin receptor blocker (ACEI/ARB) and β-blocker.

Q20. What is acute HF? What are the clinical presentations?

Ans. Acute HF refers to the rapid or gradual onset of symptoms and/or signs of HF, severe enough for the patient to seek urgent medical attention, leading to an unplanned hospitalization or an emergency department visit. AHF may be the first manifestation of HF, or more frequent be due to an acute decompensation of chronic HF. Clinical presentations are mainly based on the presence of signs of congestion and/or peripheral hypotension.

Four clinical presentations are:
1. Acute decompensated HF
2. Acute pulmonary edema
3. Isolated RV failure
4. Cardiogenic shock

Q21. What is advanced HF?

Ans. Advanced HF is characterized by persistent symptoms despite maximal therapy. It has the following features: Severe, persistent symptoms (NYHA class III or IV), severe cardiac dysfunction (LVEF ≤30%), isolated RV failure, nonoperable severe valve abnormalities, nonoperable severe congenital abnormalities, persistently high b-type natriuretic peptide (BNP) or N-terminal pro-b-type natriuretic peptide (NT-proBNP) with severe LV diastolic dysfunction, episodes of pulmonary or systemic congestion or episodes of low output or malignant arrhythmia, and severe impairment of exercise capacity.

Q22. What are the ESC recommendations in HF management?

Ans.
- Sodium-glucose cotransporter-2 (SGLT2) inhibitors (dapagliflozin, empagliflozin, and sotagliflozin) are recommended for patients with HFrEF to reduce the risk of HF hospitalization and death.
- Sodium-glucose cotransporter-2 inhibitors (canagliflozin, dapagliflozin, empagliflozin, ertugliflozin, and sotagliflozin) are recommended in patients with type 2 diabetes mellitus (T2DM) at risk of CV events, end-stage renal dysfunction, and CV death.
- Patients with HF and chronic coronary syndrome-coronary artery bypass grafting (CCS-CABG) should be considered as the first choice revascularization strategy, in patients suitable for surgery, especially if they have diabetes mellitus (DM) and for those with multivessel disease, percutaneous coronary intervention (PCI) may be considered as an alternative, considering coronary anatomy, comorbidities, and surgical risk.
- In patients with HF and valvular heart disease–aortic valve intervention [transcatheter aortic valve replacement (TAVR) or surgical aortic valve replacement (SAVR)] is recommended in HF with severe high-gradient

AS to reduce mortality and improve symptoms. Percutaneous edge-to-edge MV repair should be considered in selected patients with secondary MR not eligible for surgery and not needing CABG, who are symptomatic despite optimal medical therapy (OMT) in order to improve symptoms and reduce morbidity and mortality.
- Vericiguat may be considered in patients in NYHA class II–IV who have had worsening HF despite treatment with an ACEI [or angiotensin receptor-neprilysin inhibitor (ARNI)], a β-blocker, and a mineralocorticoid receptor antagonist (MRA) to reduce the risk of CV mortality or HF hospitalization.
- For HFmrEF, an ACEI or ARB, a β-blocker, an MRA, and sacubitril/valsartan may be considered to reduce the risk of HF hospitalization and death.
- For HFpEF, screening and treatment of etiologies and comorbidities are recommended.
- Influenza and pneumococcal vaccination should be considered in order to prevent HF hospitalization.
- Home-based and/or clinic-based programs and self-management strategies are recommended to reduce the risk of HF hospitalization and mortality.
- Supervised, exercise-based, cardiac rehabilitation program should be considered in patients with more severe disease, frailty, or with comorbidities.
- Noninvasive home telemonitoring (HTM) can be considered in order to reduce the risk of recurrent CV and HF hospitalization and CV death.
- Patients with advanced HF—continuous inotropes and/or vasopressors may be considered in patients with low COP and evidence of organ hypoperfusion as bridge to MCS or heart transplantation. Heart transplantation is recommended for patients with advanced HF, refractory to medical/device therapy, and who do not have absolute contraindications.
- Intravenous (IV) iron supplementation with ferric carboxymaltose should be considered in symptomatic HF patients with LVEF ≤50% and iron deficiency (serum ferritin <100 ng/mL, or serum ferritin 100–299 ng/dL with transferring saturation <20%, to reduce the risk of HF hospitalization).
- Heart failure with AF—long-term treatment with an oral coagulant should be considered for stroke prevention in patients with a CHA_2DS_2-VASc score of 1 in men or 1 in women.
- Acute pulmonary edema is characterized by dyspnea with orthopnea, respiratory failure (hypoxemia-hypercapnia), tachypnea (>25 breaths/min), and increased work of breathing. Routine use of opiates is not recommended; it may be considered to relieve dyspnea and anxiety or intractable pain.

- Intravenous vasodilators may be considered to relieve AHF symptoms when systolic blood pressure (SBP) is >110 mm Hg in acute HF to improve symptoms and reduce congestion.
- Among the vasopressors, norepinephrine, a prominent arterial vasoconstrictor, is preferred in patients with severe hypotension. It increases perfusion to the vital organs at the expense of an increased LV afterload. A combination of norepinephrine and inotropic agents may be considered, especially in patients with advanced HF and cardiogenic shock.
- Computed tomography (CT) coronary angiography (CAG) should be considered in patients with a low to intermediate pretest probability of CAD or those with equivocal noninvasive stress tests in order to rule out coronary artery stenosis. Invasive CAG may be considered in patients with HFrEF with an intermediate to high pretest probability of CAD and the presence of ischemia in the noninvasive stress test.
- An implantable cardioverter-defibrillator (ICD) should be considered to reduce the risk of sudden cardiac death (SCD) and all-cause mortality in patients with symptomatic HF (NYHA class II–III) of a nonischemic etiology, and an LVEF ≤35% despite OMT, provided they are expected to survive substantially longer than 1 year with good functional status.
- Cardiac resynchronization therapy (CRT) should be considered for symptomatic patients with HF in sinus rhythm and a QRS duration of 130–149 ms and left bundle branch block (LBBB) and with LVEF ≤35%. Patients with an LVEF ≤35% who have received a conventional pacemaker or an ICD and subsequently develop worsening HF despite OMT and who have a significant proportion of RV pacing should be considered for "upgrade" to CRT.

Q23. How do cardiologic findings correlate with raised pulmonary venous pressure in PCWP recording in HF?
Ans. Pulmonary venous pressure leads to elevation of pulmonary capillary pressure. Long-standing raised PCP produces changes in pulmonary vasculature and raises pulmonary arterial pressure (i.e., pulmonary hypertension).

Left HF ›–› raised LA pressure or LVEDP ›–› pulmonary venous pressure ›–› PCP ›–›pulmonary artery pressure (PH)
When PCP is 18–20 mm Hg, pulmonary venous congestion with redistribution of fluid to the upper zone occurs (i.e., upper lobe diversion). The lower zone vessels undergo active vasoconstriction to prevent accumulation in the interstitium. Hence, fluid is diverted to the upper zone.

As PCP >20 mm Hg, interstitial edema occurs with peribronchial cuffing and Kerley's B lines.

Pulmonary capillary pressure: 25–30 mm Hg frank pulmonary edema occurs, with flooding of the alveolar space, most prominent in perihilar areas (bat wing distribution)

When pulmonary arterial hypertension supervenes pulmonary artery in dilated, pulmonary conus is full, and peripheral attenuation of pulmonary vasculature occurs (due to sclerotic changes). The tendency to develop pulmonary edema decreases.

Q24. What are the compensatory changes in HF?
Ans. These are some cardiac and circulatory changes that take place which for a time may maintain an adequate circulation in HF.

- Cardiac—dilation of the heart in response to volume load; hypertrophy of the heart in response to pressure load and increased heart rate.
- *Circulatory:* These are the neuroendocrine responses in HF. Sympathetic activation increases heart rate and augments cardiac contractility, vasoconstriction of arteries and veins. Activation of renin-angiotensin-aldosterone system:
    - Leads to vasoconstriction, sodium retention, and expansion of blood volume
    - Release of antidiuretic hormone leads to urinary retention

Although these are compensatory to start with, they eventually prove counterproductive and embarrass the circulation. The clinical manifestation are largely the effects of these mechanisms.

Q25. How does pleural effusion develop in HF?
Ans. The parietal pleura is supplied by the systemic circulation, and the visceral pleura is supplied by the pulmonary circulation. Normally, net filtration from the parietal pleura into the pleural space is absorbed by the visceral pleura and true accumulation does not occur. An increase is systemic venous pressure as occur in right HF increase fluid formation. An increase in pulmonary pressure as in left HF impedes fluid resorption. When pleural effusion develops effusion in HF are usually bilateral but when unilateral, they accumulate frequently on the right side.

Q26. What is cardiac asthma? How does it differ from bronchial asthma?
Ans. It is the dyspnea and wheezing due to elevated pulmonary venous pressure developing in patients with acute LVF or raised LA pressure as in MS. Here, increased airway resistance is due to engorged venules, edema, and increased responsiveness of the bronchial tree. It is important to distinguish the two conditions as management is significantly different **(Table 12.6)**.

TABLE 12.6: Cardiac and bronchial asthma—differentiating points.

Points	Cardiac asthma	Bronchial asthma
History	Angina, MI, hypertension, valvular disease	Paroxysmal attack of dyspnea, allergic disease
Symptoms	Cough with frothy, pinkish sputum	Usually a dry cough or with mucoid expectoration
	Features of sympathetic activation (sweating, pallor, and cold extremities)	Features of RTI present
Signs	Cyanosis—peripheral; pulsus alternans (in severe LVF)	Cyanosis—central; pulsus paradoxus (in severe cases)
Heart	Signs of underlying heart diseases—MI and hypertension are present	Absent
Lung	Inspiratory crepitation bilateral, initially basal—typical	Coarse crepitations (both inspiratory and expiratory) may be present; rhonchi are typical
	No feature of hyperinflation	A feature of hyperinflation usually
Investigations: ECG	Features of underlying heart disease—MVD, IHD, etc.	P-pulmonale (RAE) may be seen in chronic cases
X-ray chest	Cardiomegaly, bilateral hilar haze, sometimes, Kerley's B-line, pleural effusion	No cardiomegaly, features of hyperinflation and RTI
Echocardiography	Diagnostic feature of the underlying cardiac disease	Normal
Respiratory function test	Normal	Abnormal
Treatment	Morphine, furosemide IV, nitrate S/L	Nebulized salbutamol and steroid

(ECG: electrocardiogram; IHD: ischemic heart disease; IV: intravenous; LVF: left ventricular failure; MI: myocardial infarction; MVD: microvascular dysfunction; RTI: respiratory tract infection)

Q27. Outline the treatment of HF.

Ans. Principles of treatment of HF are:
- Removal of the precipitating causes—anemia, infection, and pregnancy
- Correction of underlying causes by medical or surgical means, e.g., hypertension, valvular disease, congenital heart disease, and infective endocarditis.
- Control of congestive failure state:
  - Reduction of cardiac workload, including both preload and afterload—bed rest, control excess salt and water intake, and use of diuretics

- Vasodilators—to decrease preload and afterload
- Enhancement of myocardial contractility–by inotropic drugs such as digitalis.

Q28. What is the use of digoxin in congestive HF?
Ans. In congestive HF by stimulating myocardial contractility, digitals improves pulmonary and systemic congestion. Indications in congestive HF are:
- Congestive HF with AF—its effect on AV node slows the ventricular response to fast AF; it is the classic indication
- Heart failure in children—it is the mainstay of therapy
- Congestive HF with sinus rhythm when bed rest, diuretics and vasodilators do not produce satisfactory result, when a large heart with S_3 gallop present, one where there is no valvular stenotic lesion, digoxin is likely to be beneficial. Once failure is controlled and heart is smaller, digoxin can be withdrawn.

Q29. What is the role of vasodilators in the treatment of HF?
Ans.
- *Improvement of failure:* In HF neurohumoral activation increases preload and afterload by contraction of arteries and veins. Vasodilators, by decreasing the preload and the afterload, improve the failure state. Vasodilators are useful in both acute and chronic HF. In acute failure, sodium nitroprusside with a rapid and brief duration of action, is the ideal agent.
- Improvement of survival: Controlled trials show that vasodilators, e.g., angiotensin-converting enzyme (ACE) inhibitors, improve survival. This is probably by reducing plasma norepinephrine levels, correcting hypokalemia and hyponatremia, thus preventing life-threatening arrhythmias.

Q30. How do β-blockers help in HF? How is it given?
Ans.
- Used carefully in patient with stable HF with NYHA functional class II–III, β-blockers can improve symptoms and improve survival. Symptomatic improvement by β-blockers are due to improvement in diastolic compliance of LV. Also, it counters the excessive peripheral vasoconstriction and afterload induced by sympathetic activation in chronic HF. Vasodilatory β-blockers such as carvedilol are preferable here. It causes upregulation of cardiac β-receptors (which are downregulated by sympathetic activation of HF). Survival benefits of β-blockers in HF is by reducing SCD by its antiarrhythmic action.

Beta blockers are started in low dose and increased gradually, because tolerability is highly dependent on the level of cardiac reserve and severity of baseline symptoms. LV EF reduces during first few weeks of initiation of therapy, even when started at a low dose. It should not be attempted in unstable ambulatory patients with CHF or in patients hospitalized for decompensated HF. Carvedilol 3.125 mg b.d. started, increasing gradually to 25 mg b.d., if tolerated or the drug is withdrawn. The drug may need to be reduced or stopped if the patient decompensates.

Q31. What is the difference between acute and chronic HF?
Ans. Besides, the duration of the two conditions differs in pathogenesis, clinical features, and management strategies **(Table 12.7)**.

TABLE 12.7: Acute and chronic heart failure—differentiating points.

Points	Acute	Chronic
Duration of the symptom	Minutes to hours	Long standing
Sympathetic overactivity	More	Less
Neurohumoral activation	Less	More
Pulmonary congestion	More	Less
Edema	Nil or less	More
Sign	BP normal or high	Usually low
S3 gallop	More	Less
CxR	Heart not enlarged	Enlarged
Rx	Morphin useful	Not usually

(BP: blood pressure; CxR: chest X-ray)

Q32. What are the mainstay of treatment of acute LVF?
Ans.
- Oxygen—high flow (60–100%), using nasal prong
- Morphine IV: Dose 10–15 mg (in aliquot doses)—it reduces sympathetic drive, produces venodilation, and reduces preload. It also reduces anxiety and distress.
- Diuretics—furosemide 40–80 mg IV, the acute effect is venodilation, thus reducing LA pressure, and intravascular volume reduction occurs later.
- Nitrates—produce venodilation; fluid is redistributed into capacitance vessels and LA pressure acutely reduces. Upward titration done every 10–20 minutes until SBP <110 mm Hg or limited improvement is observed. Dose: sublingual glyceryl trinitrate (GTN) 2–5 mg or IV GTN 0.6–12 mg/min.

Other measures:
Sodium nitroprusside (IV) in hypertensive crisis; dose: 10–200 µg/kg/min
  Digoxin—in atrial fibrillation; dose: 0.5 mg (oral) repeated after 6 hours.
  Treatment of triggering factors.

Q33. How does morphine help in acute LVF?
Ans. Morphine decreases ventricular afterload—by decreasing arterial resistance and pressure secondary to a reduction of centrally mediated sympathetic tone. It decreases preload by increasing the capacity of the peripheral vascular bed and venous pooling—sometimes called pharmacologic phlebotomy perhaps aided by a decrease in respiratory pump or depression of respiratory center activity. It also decreases anxiety and distress, thus decreasing work to breathe.

Q34. What is BNP? Give its importance.
Ans. B-type natriuretic peptide is a biomarker secreted in response to increased cardiac wall tension and/or circulating neurohormone. It is an useful adjunctive tool in diagnosis of patients with HF. In systolic HF, BNP levels are directly related to wall stress, EF and functional class of patients. A raised BNP distinguishes cardiac from noncardiac cause in a patient with dyspnea [e.g., HF from pulmonary embolism (PE)]. In general, a BNP of <100 pg/mL is considered to have a high negative predictive value, whereas concentration >400 pg/mL is considered to have a high positive predictive value for HF as the etiology of dyspnea. Nesiritide, a recombinant human BNP is used therapeutically and indicated for acutely decompensated CHF patients who has dyspnea at rest or with minimal activity. It also provides prognostic information. Level of NT-BNP (large, biologically inactive N-terminal fragment of BNP) predict response to treatment in HF. A normal serum BNP level has a high negative predictive value of 95% to exclude the diagnosis of HF.

In a patient at risk for HF, serum BNP level may facilitate earlier identification of those who would benefit from initiation of therapy to prevent or delay progression to over HF.

Q35. What drugs increase survival in patients with HF?
Ans. These are angiotensin-converting enzyme inhibitors/angiotensin receptor blockers (ACEIs/ARBs), and β-blockers.

Q36. How is renin–angiotensin system (RAS) inhibition achieved in HF with reduced EF?
Ans. Renin–angiotensin system inhibition can be done by:
- Angiotensin-converting enzyme inhibitors—RCT clearly established the benefits of ACEI in patients with mild, moderate, or severe symptoms of HF and in patients with or without CAD
- Angiotensinogen receptor blockers were developed with the rationale that angiotensin-II production continues in the presence of ACE inhibition, driven through alternative enzyme pathways. ARBs do not inhibit kinase and are associated with much lower incidence of cough angioedema than ACEIs. ARB use reduces morbidity and mortality, especially in ACEI-intolerant patients.

- Angiotensin receptor-neprilysin inhibitor—an ARB combined with an inhibitor of neprilysin (enzyme that degrades natriuretic peptides, bradykinin, adrenomedullin, and other vasoactive peptides) reduced CV death or HF hospitalization significantly. The first approved ARNI is valsartan/sacubitril. ARNI has been found to be superior to ACEI. For those in whom ARNI is not appropriate, continued use of an ACEI for all classes of HFrEF remains strongly advised. Again, for those in whom an ACEI or ARNI is inappropriate, use of an ARB remains advisable.

Q37. What is new in the management of HF? What was the updated strategy for the management of HF?

Ans. In 2016, ACC/AHA/HFSA (Heart Failure Society of America) updated the management of HF as shown in **Box 12.1**.

BOX 12.1: ACC/AHA/HFSA update for HF management.

- RCTs have shown the benefit of angiotensin receptor neprilysin inhibitor (ARNI) and ivabradine in treating HFrEF
- Inhibition of RAS with ACEI, ARB and ARNI-all reduce morbidity and mortality in HF patients-all class I recommendation
- β-blockers continue to be a mainstay of pharmacological agents in the management of HFrEF
- ARNI has been approved for patients with symptomatic HFrEF and is intended to be substituted for ACEI or ARBs and should replace ACEI or ARBs when stable patients with mild to moderate HF on these agents have an adequate BP and are otherwise tolerating standard therapies
- Ivabradine, a sinoatrial node inhibitor (selective for if receptors), can be beneficial in reducing HF hospitalization for patients with NYHA class II–III HF or stable chronic HF (LVEF <35%) receiving evidence-based heart rate reducing medications(with class IIa recommendation)

(ACC/AHA/HFSA: American College of Cardiology/American Heart Association/Heart Failure Society of America; ACEI: angiotensin-converting enzyme inhibitor; ARB: angiotensin receptor blocker; BP: blood pressure; HFrEF: heart failure with reduced ejection fraction; HF: heart failure; LVEF: left ventricular ejection fraction; NYHA: New York Heart Association; RAS: renin–angiotensin system; RCTs: randomized controlled trials)

A full update is in process, including more options for pharmacological treatment of HF that will provide more hope for better outcomes for morbidity and mortality related to HF.

Q38. What are the interventional HF therapies?

Ans. These are device-based therapies directed to HF patients who remain highly symptomatic despite current guideline-directed drug and electrophysiologic device therapies. These targets the primary and secondary valve diseases, LV dilation or remodeling, elevated LA and PAP, and reduced COP. These include:

- Transcatheter aortic valve replacement
- Percutaneous MV repair (e.g., MitraClip system)

- Pulmonary artery (PA) pressure monitoring
- Interatrial shunt device, etc.

Q39. What are the device therapies for HF?
Ans. These are devices implanted to improve LV EF:
- Cardiac resynchronization therapy
- Left ventricular assist device (LVAD)

Q40. What are the surgical treatments available for patients with HF?
Ans.
- As treatment of underlying cause of heart failure with mitral valve regurgitation (HF-MVR) for mitral regurgitation, CABG for CAD, LV aneurysmectomy in LV aneurysm following MI, correction of congenital lesions, etc.
- Dynamic cardiomyoplasty (latissimus dorsi) is wrapped around the heart to augment its function. This may be employed in the end stage if cardiac transplantation is not available.
- *Left ventricular volume reduction (Batista operation):* A segment of the free wall of the dilated. LV is resected; LV volume and wall stress are reduced.
- Cardiac transplantation is the therapy of choice in patients with end-stage heart disease who are unlikely to survive the next 6–12 months.

Q41. When is heart transplantation indicated?
Ans. Heart transplantation remains the gold standard for the treatment of advanced HF in the absence of contraindications and comorbidities. It significantly improves the quality of life and functional status. Indications are advanced HF, and no other therapeutic option, except for LVAD as a bridge to transplantation.

Q42. How can HF care be improved?
Ans. The following strategies may be beneficial:
- Use guideline recommendation—all should receive vasodilator, ACEI preferred, and ARB as alternative. If neither can be given, a combination of hydralazine-nitrate should be used. If the patient is still symptomatic on ACEI/ARB, then the patient should be started on ARNI. These are started after stopping ACEI/ARB and at low dose.
- Diuretics are used in an adequate dose to reduce shortness of breath and eliminate pedal edema. Torsemide and metolazone are sometimes more useful. Torsemide is better absorbed and can be used in high doses. Spironolactone or eplerenone is added to all.
- β-blockers are given to all and up-titrated. Ivabradine is used if an adequate heart rate could not be achieved.
- Diet-restricted salt and water
- Weight monitoring by increasing diuretics and restricting water

- Influenza and pneumococcal vaccination
- Setting up HF clinic to improve patient follow-up and reduce hospitalization
- Beyond drugs patients assessed for device therapy (ICD and CRT) for those with LBBB, and an EF <35%.
- Patients with multiple, frequent hospitalizations, those who are in end-stage HF, LVAD or heart transplantation are a practical option and should be offered.

Q43. What is cardiogenic shock? What are the causes?
Ans. It is the syndrome resulting from systemic hypoperfusion with widespread cellular and organ dysfunction caused by severe acute or chronic LV dysfunction.

Causes:
- Acute MI—massive MI with >40% of myocardium involved, complicated MI—VSD, MR, RV infarction, and ventricular rupture. Cardiogenic shock complicates 5–15% of acute MI.
- Inadequate ventricular function—DCM and severe myocardial dysfunction in end-stage valvular heart disease
- Cardiac obstruction or compression—cardiac tamponade, PE, tension pneumothorax, severe HCM, and LA myxoma
- Hypovolemia—rupture of aortic aneurysm and dissecting aneurysm

Q44. What are the features of cardiogenic shock? How do they differ?
Ans. These are:
- Evidence of hypoperfusion altered mental status—restlessness, agitation, obtundation, cold, clamy skin, and approximately urine output <20 mL/h.
- Hypotension—systolic BP <80–90 mm Hg, may be associated with sinus tachycardia with weak, thready pulse. Raised LV end-diastolic pressure or PCWP >18 mm Hg. Low cardiac output: CI <1.8 L/min/m^2.
- Evidence of primary cardiac disease, e.g., acute MI.

The hemodynamic abnormalities in cardiogenic shock are similar to those in LVF without cardiogenic shock, except that arterial pressure is low and cardiac index is reduced. For example, in acute MI, when 30% of the myocardium is destroyed, LV dysfunction and pulmonary congestion develop, i.e., acute LVF (EF 30–40%); when >30% myocardium is destroyed, decompensation occurs with resultant cardiogenic shock (EF <20–30%).

Q45. What is the mechanism of cardiogenic shock in acute MI?
Ans.
- In acute MI, it is the result of pump failure due to massive myocardial damage.
- Old infarction—manifestation of extensive earlier myocardial damage
- Infarct extension or infarct expansion with associated ischemic dysfunction

- Underlying metabolic derangement or dysrhythmias
- Mechanical defects—ventricular septal rupture (VSR), papillary muscle rupture with MR, and free wall rupture
- Extensive RV infarction

Pump failure initiates a positive feedback loop as follows, which accounts for the high mortality (80%) in cardiogenic shock **(Flowchart 12.1)**.

Flowchart 12.1: Mechanism of cardiogenic shock

```
         ┌──────────── Pump failure ◄────┐
         ▼                                │
  ↓ Myocardial perfusion                  │
         │                                │
         ▼                                │
  • ↓ Coronary perfusion    ↓ Tissue hypoperfusion
    pressure
  • ↓ Arterial pressure
  • Metabolic acidosis,
    arrhythmia
         │                                │
         └──────► ↑ Infarct size ─────────┘
```

Q46. How does hypotension and shock develop in patients with RV infarction?

Ans. Right ventricular infarction is a variant of acute MI in which there is an extensive RV involvement. It usually accompanies inferior or inferoposterior MI, presumably when right coronary artery (RCA) is occluded. Usually, there is also a localized area of LV involvement along with RV. In RV infarction, lung perfusion decreases; hence, less blood comes to left side of the heart in turn. There is a net reduction in the left heart filling with hypotension and shock. This condition can be managed by IV volume expansion with normal saline-aliquots of 100–200 cc of saline and the patient examined frequently for signs of pulmonary congestion. Several liters of fluid may be required to increase output by increasing LV filling and to reverse shock. Risk of developing pulmonary edema is minimal as LV involvement is localized and global LV function is reasonably maintained. Inotropic support with dobutamine undertaken if COP fails is increased after volume expansion.

Q47. What are the indications of invasive monitoring in AMI?

Ans. Invasive monitoring is indicated in the management of complicated AMI

- *Cardiogenic shock:* To distinguish inadequate ventricular filling pressure from inadequate systolic function. The former is treated with volume expansion and the latter with inodilators. Also, to differentiate VSR from acute MR.
- Cardiac failure not responding to therapy, to monitor response to vasodilator and β-blocker, or to differentiate severe lung disease from LVF

- Miscellaneous—refractory ventricular tachycardia, assessment of cardiac tamponade, temporary pacing, intra-aortic balloon pump (IABP), etc.

Q48. What are the components of invasive monitoring?
Ans. Invasive monitoring consists of:
- Insertion of balloon flotation (Swan-Ganz) catheter for the measurement of pulmonary arterial, PA occlusive pressure (equivalent to pulmonary wedge pressure), RA pressure (or central venous pressure), and COP by the thermodilution method
- Arterial monitoring through the radial artery; it is done for patients in shock and for those receiving vasopressor agents
- Folley's catheter for measurement of urine output

The goal of hemodynamic monitoring in AMI is to maintain ventricular performance, support BP, and protect jeopardized myocardium.

Q49. Outline the treatment of cardiogenic shock.
Ans.
- Establishment of effective ventilation and oxygenation. O_2 via face mask or ventilator. Arterial PaO_2 should be above 70 mm Hg.
- Restoration of adequate COP; arterial pressure should be above 70 mm Hg.

Dopamine: 5–10 µg/min
- Treatment of associated conditions: Hypotension—IV infusion of volume expander; pain (in AMI)—morphine.
- Antiarrhythmic agents, direct current (DC) shock, and correction of acid-base abnormality.
- Intra-aortic balloon counter pulsation—if drug treatment is ineffectual, especially in AMI with cardiogenic shock. IABP provides temporary circulatory support before doing percutaneous transluminal coronary angioplasty (PTCA) or CABG.
- PTCA to salvage myocardium with assistance of IABP
- Surgical—CABG for patients with suitable anatomical and mechanical complications, e.g., acute MR VSD in AMI

Q50. How does cardiogenic shock occur in PE and tension pneumothorax?
Ans. Massive PE reduces the cross-sectional area of the pulmonary outflow when the cross-sectional area is reduced by 50% or more, shock occurs. The RV cannot increase its systolic pressure to overcome the increased resistance. Blood flow is reduced, and shock results

In tension pneumothorax, the heart is compressed from outside. It cannot produce effective stroke output; hence, shock results.

Q51. What are the key therapeutic options for patients with cardiogenic shock?

Ans. Five therapies are frequently used to treat patients with cardiogenic shock:
1. Inotropes/vasopressors
2. Fibrinolytics
3. PCI
4. CABG
5. Mechanical circulatory support

Revascularization appears to improve survival. Patients who are potential candidates for revascularization of the culprit artery should be revascularized. Routine revascularization of the nonculprit may be associated with worsened outcome. In patients with STEMI and shock in whom PCI or CABG is not suitable, fibrinolytics can be given unless they have a contraindication.

Q52. Give the use of sympathomimetic amines in various circulatory failure states.

Ans. These provide short-term hemodynamic support in various circulatory failure states.

- Dobutamine—useful in HF without hypotension. It decreases blood pressure (vasodilatation via β_2-receptor), and does not cause excessive tachycardia. It can be used in conjunction with IV dopamine in acute circulatory failure.
- Dopamine—produces renal vasodilatation directly in low dose (2.5–5 μg/kg/min) and has a beneficial effect in circulatory shock. Higher doses (5–10 μg/kg/min) have more inotropic effect but tend to cause tachycardia and vasoconstriction.
- Adrenaline—its vasoconstrictor effect (via α-receptor) makes it more suitable for patients with low systemic vascular resistance. It is more arrhythmogenic than dopamine. Dose: 1–10 mg/min.
- Noradrenaline—predominantly an α-agonist and is mainly used in septic shock to increase systemic vascular resistance.

Q53. What are the MCS devices used in cardiogenic shock?

Ans. These are circulatory support devices undertaken in cardiogenic shock when rapid augmentation of COP and reduction of ventricular filling pressure are required to sustain life. Two categories are:
1. *Temporary:* (1) IABP—most commonly used; increases diastolic blood flow, decreases afterload, decreases myocardial O_2 consumption, increases coronary perfusion, and modestly enhances COP. (2) Extracorporeal membrane oxygenation (ECMO)—provides cardiopulmonary support for patients whose heart and/or lungs can no longer provide adequate physiologic support. It is similar to a cardiopulmonary bypass (CPB) circuit used in cardiac surgery. It is either venovenous (for oxygenation

only) or venoarterial (for oxygenation and circulatory support as in biventricular failure). Cannulation of the femoral artery and vein is done here. Concomitant IABP may be needed to unload LV. (3) Impella—continuous, microaxial pump that sends blood from LV with a flexible pigtail loop into the ascending aorta. The proximal end of the catheter is connected to the external pump.
2. *Long term:* LV assisted devices (LVAD). Here, devices are placed under operation, and they use continuous flow technology instead of pulsatile one as in temporary MCS.

■ SUGGESTED READING

1. Griffin BP, Topol EJ. Heart failure and transplantation. In: Griffin BP, Topol EJ (Eds). Manual of Cardiovascular Medicine, 3rd edition. Philadelphia: Lippincott Williams & Wilkins; 2009.
2. Hunt SA, Abraham WT, Chin MH, Feldman AM, Francis GS, Ganiats TG, et al.; American Heart Association Task Force on Practice Guidelines; American College of Chest Physicians; International Society for Heart and Lung Transplantation; Heart Rhythm Society. ACC/AHA 2005 guideline update for the diagnosis and management of chronic heart failure in the adult: a report of the American College of Cardiology/American Heart Association Task Force on Practice Guidelines (Writing Committee to Update the 2001 Guidelines for the Evaluation and Management of Heart Failure): developed in collaboration with the American College of Chest Physicians and the International Society for Heart and Lung Transplantation: endorsed by the Heart Rhythm Society. Circulation. 2005;112(12):e154-235. [online] Available from https://pubmed.ncbi.nlm.nih.gov/16160202/ [Last accessed May, 2025].
3. Otto MH, John DC. Clinical assessment of heart failure. In: Libby P, Bonow RO, Mann DL, Zipes DP (Eds). Brunwald's Heart Disease: A Textbook of Cardiovascular Medicine, 8th edition. Philadelphia: Saunders; 2008.
4. Yancy CW, Jessup M, Bozhurt B, Butler J, Casey Jr. DE, Colvin MM, et al. 2016 ACC/AHA/HFSA focused update on new pharmacological therapy for heart failure: an update of the 2013 ACCF/AHA guideline for the management of heart failure. J Am Coll Cardiol. 2016;68(13):1476-88.

13 Cardiac Arrhythmias

"Devices and radiofrequency ablation have revolutionized the therapy of life-threatening and symptomatic arrhythmias."

—Lionel H Opie

■ INTRODUCTION

Cardiac arrhythmias may result from a disturbance in the formation of the cardiac impulse or its conduction. A disturbance of the formation of impulse may lead to an abnormality in its rate or rhythm. A disturbance in the conduction of cardiac impulse may be sinoatrial (SA), atrioventricular (AV), and those involving the right and left bundle.

Q1. What are cardiac arrhythmias? Classify it.

Ans. Cardiac arrhythmia is defined as a disturbance of rhythm resulting from abnormalities in impulse formation or its conduction.

Classification:
- According to the heart rate (HR), arrhythmias may be bradyarrhythmia (rate <60 beats/min) and tachyarrhythmia (rate >100 beats/min).
- According to the site of origin, arrhythmias may be supraventricular (arising in the atrium and AV junctional area, i.e., AV node and adjacent specialized tissues) and ventricular.
    - Supraventricular arrhythmias: Sinus arrhythmia, sinus bradycardia and tachycardia, atrial ectopics, supraventricular tachycardias (SVTs), atrial tachycardia, atrial flutter, atrial fibrillation (AF), junctional ectopics, accelerated junctional rhythms, and junctional tachycardia
    - Ventricular arrhythmias: Ventricular ectopics, ventricular tachycardias (VTs), and ventricular fibrillation (VF)
- Etiologically, it may be primary, which is independent of a significant change in hemodynamic function, and secondary, where hemodynamic deterioration or a metabolic abnormality initiates the electrical disturbance.
- Based on the duration, arrhythmias (tachyarrhythmias) are of three types: Paroxysmal, persistent, and chronic. In paroxysmal tachyarrhythmia, the duration is short (seconds to hours) and it tends to be recurrent. Persistent ones last for days or weeks, and chronic ones last for months to years.

Q2. What is the mechanism of tachyarrhythmias?

Ans.
- Disturbance of impulse formation: Deranged automaticity and triggered activity. Deranged automaticity may result from inappropriately rapid

firing from the normal pacemaker due to ischemia, metabolic disturbance, or drugs (e.g., inappropriate sinus tachycardia). It may also result from abnormal automaticity of a later or ectopic focus under conditions of ischemia or pharmacologic manipulation (e.g., ventricular extrasystoles and idioventricular rhythm). A triggered activity refers to the pacemaker activity that is dependent on afterdepolarization from a prior impulse or series of impulse. It may occur by (1) early afterdepolarizations (EAD): Occurring before repolarizations of cardiac tissue, e.g., arrhythmias of long QT syndrome and torsades de pointes produced by class I and class III antiarrhythmics and (2) delayed afterdepolarizations (DAD): Occurring after the repolarization of the surrounding tissue is complete, e.g., arrhythmias of digitalis toxicity; an increase in intracellular calcium is associated. Afterdepolarizations are oscillations in the membrane potential. If these reach the threshold level for the surrounding cardiac tissue, they may trigger an action potential, thus precipitating further afterdepolarizations, perpetuating the pacemaker activity.
- Disorders of impulse conduction, i.e., re-entry. In order for re-entry to occur, three conditions must be met: Two functionally distinct conduction pathways, unidirectional conduction block in one of the pathways, and a difference in the conduction rates in the pathways (i.e., slow conduction via one and return of conduction via the other), e.g., SVTs and VT. SVT occurs due to the presence of two distinct pathways, e.g., AV nodal re-entrant tachycardia (AVNRT) or accessory pathway in AV re-entrant tachycardia (AVRT). VT occurs due to myocardial ischemia or scar that conducts imputes inhomogeneously. Thus, the impulse can spread into an area that has already repolarized after being previously depolarized. This sets up a circular movement of the impulse, resulting in sustained arrhythmias such as VT.

Both mechanisms may be involved in some tachycardias.

Q3. What is the mechanism of bradyarrhythmias?
Ans. Bradyarrhythmias are either due to abnormalities of cardiac impulse formation or AV conduction. The abnormality of impulse formation occurs in sick sinus syndrome, most commonly due to idiopathic degeneration. Abnormalities of conduction [first-, second-, and third-degree or complete heart block (CHB)] are most commonly due to idiopathic fibrosis, ischemic heart disease (IHD), and drugs.

Q4. What are the causes of an irregular pulse?
Ans.
- *Regularly irregular:* Sinus arrhythmia and second-degree heart block (Wenckebach's phenomenon)
- *Irregularly irregular:* AF, multifocal atrial tachycardia (MAT), second-degree heart block with irregular dropped beat, SA block with irregular

dropped beat, paroxysmal atrial tachycardia (PAT) with variable AV block, and atrial flutter with variable AV conduction
- Occasionally irregular: Ectopic beats (atrial and ventricular)

Q5. What do you mean by SVT?

Ans. The term "SVT" is used when the tachycardia focus is above the bifurcation of the bundle of His and thus may be atrial or junctional (as opposed to ventricular).

Based on the duration of tachycardia, SVTs are of three groups: Paroxysmal, persistent, and chronic. In paroxysmal SVT, the duration is short (seconds to hours) and it tends to be recurrent. Persistent SVT lasts for days or weeks and may be associated with specific contributing factors, e.g., chronic obstructive pulmonary disease (COPD), electrolyte disturbance, drug toxicity, etc. Chronic SVT lasts for months to years.

Q6. What are the common types of paroxysmal supraventricular tachycardia (PSVT)?

Ans.
- *Atrioventricular nodal re-entrant tachycardia (AVNRT):* It is the most common form of SVT.

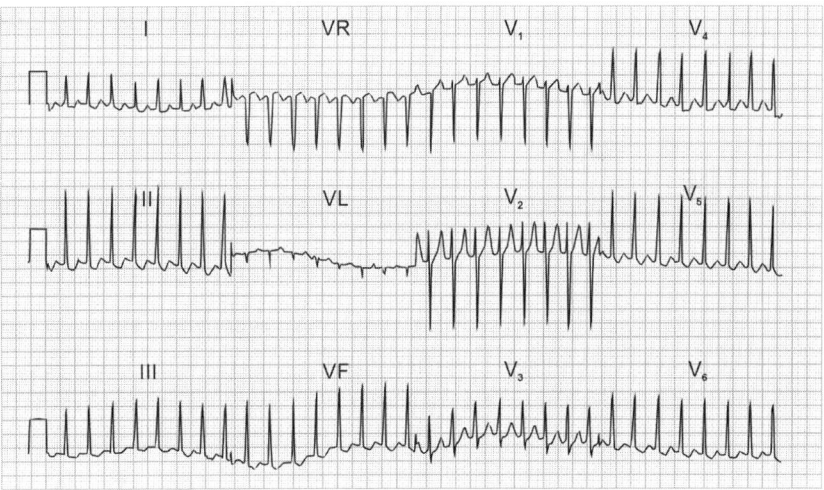

Fig. 13.1: SVT-AVNRT (P wave not identifiable).

Features:
- It is generally seen with subjects without underlying heart disease.
- Ventricular rate (VR) typically 150–250 beats/min
- The P wave cannot be identified on a standard electrocardiogram (ECG) **(Fig. 13.1)**—the atrial activity begins soon after ventricular activation (P wave is hidden within QRS).
- The resting ECG is normal.

- Atrioventricular re-entrant tachycardia (AVRT)—due to the accessory pathway [Wolff-Parkinson-White (WPW) syndrome]

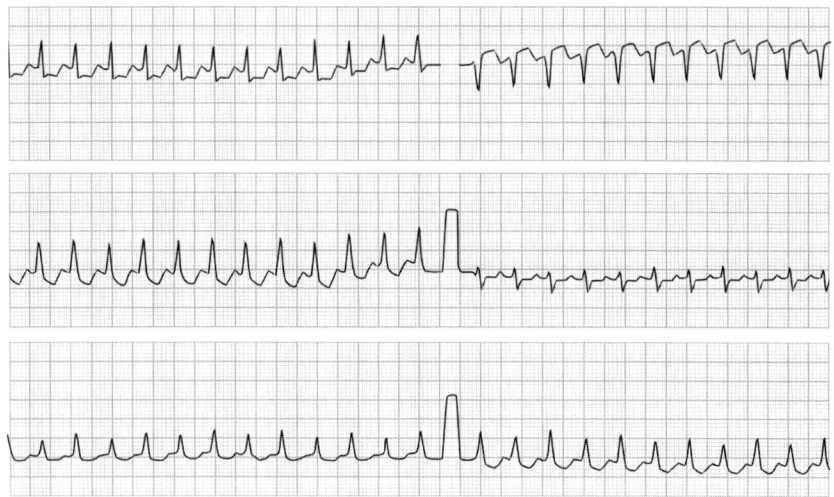

Fig. 13.2: SVT-AVRT with retrograde P after QRS.

Features:
- Seen with patients having accessory pathway bypassing the AV node with orthodromic conduction
- The VR may be faster >200 beats/min.
- The retrograde P wave may be present after the QRS—since atrial activation must follow ventricular activation **(Fig. 13.2)**.
- Resting ECG shows pre-excitation cause: Short PR interval (<0.12 seconds) and broad QRS (>0.12 seconds) with delta wave in some leads.

Besides the AV node and the extra AV node, bypass tract re-entry may be localized to the SA node and atrium.

Q7. What are narrow complex tachycardias?
Ans. Narrow complex tachycardias are cardiac rhythms >100 beats/min, with a QRS duration of <0.12 seconds. These may be regular or irregular.
- Irregular narrow complex tachycardias include:
  - AF
  - Atrial flutter with variable AV block
  - MAT
- Regular narrow complex tachycardias include:
  - Sinus tachycardia (physiologic or pathological)
  - Atrial flutter with regular AV block
  - PAT
  - AVNRT
  - Accessory pathway (AV) reentry tachycardia

Q8. What is the difference between paroxysmal atrial tachycardia (PAT) and multifocal atrial tachycardia (MAT)?

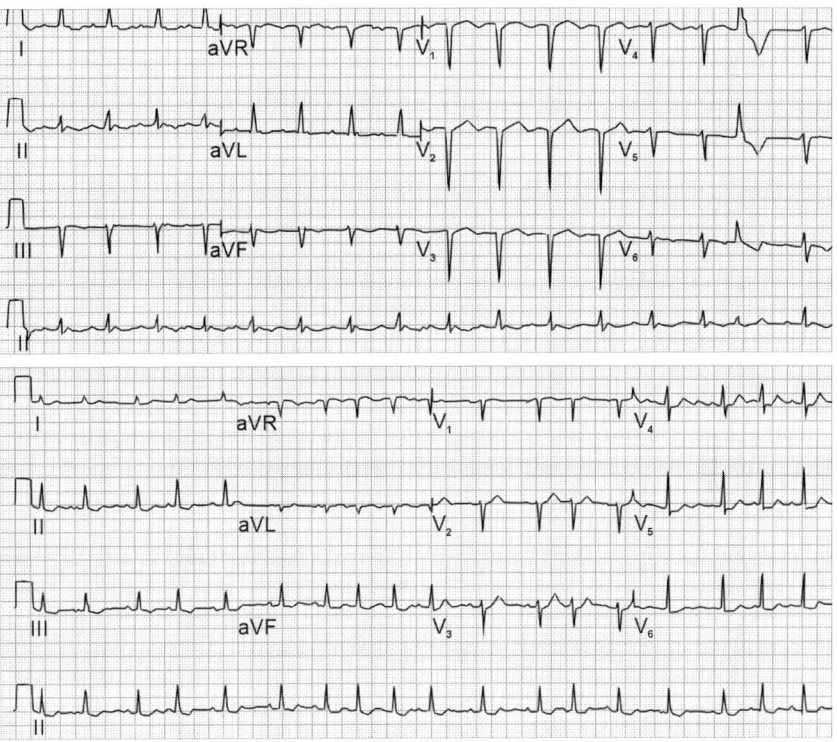

Fig. 13.3: PAT (upper) and MAT (lower).

Ans.

- *Paroxysmal atrial tachycardia:* It is a run of atrial ectopic beats due to rapid discharge of an ectopic focus. A series of three or more rapidly occurring regular and consecutive atrial extrasystoles occurs. The rate is usually 150–200 beats/min. The PR interval is often prolonged.
- Causes include thyrotoxicosis **(Fig. 13.3)**.
- *Multifocal atrial tachycardia:* It is also called chaotic atrial tachycardia, and it is due to ectopics arising from multiple different atrial foci. It is characterized by marked variation in P wave morphology (at least three P wave contours should be present to make the diagnosis), variable PR intervals, and totally irregular PP and RR intervals. The atrial rate is generally 100–130 beats/min. Loss of AV conduction of each P wave is infrequent, making it possible to distinguish MAT from AF. It is commonly seen in COPD and severe congestive heart failure (CHF) and may precede the onset of AF. It is important to recognize MAT, as it is easily confused with AF, yet does not respond to digitalis, which may mistakenly be given in toxic doses in an attempt to slow the VR **(Fig. 13.3)**.

Q9. Outline the treatment of cardiac arrhythmias.
Ans.
- *Pharmacologic:* Antiarrhythmic drugs
- *Electronic:* Cardioversion and defibrillation in acute cases; implantable cardioverter-defibrillator (ICD) and permanent pacemaker (PPM) in chronic cases
- *Catheter ablation:* Radiofrequency (RF) ablation of specific foci involved, e.g., in PSVT and VT
- *Surgical:* Aneurysmectomy and coronary artery bypass grafting (CABG)

The availability of catheter ablation and implantation devices (pacemaker and ICDs) to treat a wide variety of arrhythmias has relegated drug treatment to a secondary role.

Q10. What is AF? Classify AF.
Ans. Atrial fibrillation is atrial arrhythmia due to multiple re-entry circuits in atria that beat rapidly, ineffectively, and in an uncoordinated manner.

Atrial fibrillation is classified on the basis of its etiology, duration, morphology of its wave, and ventricular response **(Box 13.1)**:

BOX 13.1: Classification of atrial fibrillation.

- *Etiologically:*
  - Primary or lone: No structural heart diseases
  - Secondary: In the presence of structural heart disease and other diseases, e.g., mitral valvular disease, hypertension, coronary artery disease, cardiomyopathy, pericarditis, myocarditis, thyrotoxicosis, respiratory infection, etc. The most common correctable cause is thyrotoxicosis
- *Duration of AF:*
  - Paroxysmal
  - Persistent
  - Permanent
- *According to the VR in response to AF (if untreated):*
  - Fast—rate as high as 200 beats/min
  - Slow–as low as 50 beats/min
- *According to the morphology of the fibrillatory wave:*
  - Fine: Wavy baseline in ECG
  - Coarse: Large, defined, and irregular atrial waves **(Fig. 13.4)**

(AF: atrial fibrillation; ECG: electrocardiogram; VR: ventricular rate)

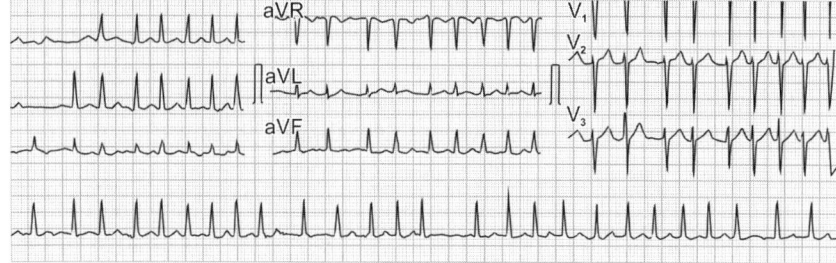

Fig. 13.4: Atrial fibrillation: ECG showing a wave replaced by fibrillatory wave, irregular R-R interval.

Q11. What are the AF types based on their duration?
Ans.
- *Paroxysmal:* AF that terminates spontaneously within 7 days
- *Persistent:* AF that persists for >7 days; those persisting for longer than 1 year is termed longstanding persistent
- *Permanent:* Longstanding AF refractory to cardioversion (although it may be successfully eliminated by surgical or catheter ablation)

Some patients with paroxysmal AF occasionally can have episodes of persistent AF, and vice versa. The predominant form of AF determines how it should be categorized. A confounding factor in AF classification is cardioversion and antiarrhythmic drug therapy. Generally, classification should not be altered on the basis of the effects of electrical cardioversion or antiarrhythmic drug.

Q12. What are the causes of AF with a regular VR?
Ans. The VR during AF can appear more regular when a junctional tachycardia independently controls the ventricles, when there is a high-degree AV block with a regular escape rhythm, or when QRS complexes are fully paced.

Q13. What are the hemodynamic consequences of AF?
Ans.
- *Loss of atrial systole:* May impair left ventricle (LV) function and decrease cardiac output
- *Rapid VR:* Decreases diastolic filling of LV and coronary flows
- *Thromboembolic phenomena:* Increase the long-term risk of stroke. Risk more with mitral valve disease (MVD), age >65 years, diabetes mellitus (DM), hypertension, heart failure, echo findings of LV dysfunction, left atrium (LA) enlargement, mitral annular calcification, and prosthetic valve.

Q14. What are the objectives of management in AF?
Ans.
- *Control of the HR (in all three types):* Digoxin, β-blocker, rate-limiting ca-channel blocker, RF ablation of the AV node followed by PPM (for drug-resistant cases with no structural heart diseases), overdrive atrial pacing in sinus node disease (bradycardia-related AF)
- *Control of rhythm (in persistent and chronic):* By chemical or electrical cardioversion
- *Prevention of recurrence:* β-blocker, class IC drugs [avoided in coronary artery disease (CAD) and LV dysfunction], amiodarone (when others fail)—in paroxysmal AF
- *Prevent thromboembolism:* Heparin, warfarin, aspirin in persistent, chronic AF, and frequent prolonged >24 hours of episodes of paroxysmal AF

Q15. How is control of the VR achieved in AF?
Ans. The ventricular response is generally controlled through drugs that slow conduction through the AV node.

- Digoxin, frequently used as a first-line drug, is much less effective in acute rate control than others. The onset of action is slow (1–4 hours). Digoxin is effective at controlling the resting HR; however, it is less effective at suppressing the ventricular response to activity and exercise (when circulating catecholamine level increases). It is the agent of choice for rate control in patients with CHF or severe impairment of LV function. It is also the preferred agent in situations that contraindicate β blockers or calcium channel blockers (e.g., asthma and hemodynamic instability).
- β-blockers have a rapid onset of action as well as short half-lives in both oral and intravenous (IV) forms. Onset of action of IV propranolol, metoprolol, and esmolol has their onset of action in approximately minutes. These are agents of choice in AF associated with elevated catecholamine levels (i.e., postoperative patients). Oral agents, e.g., propranolol, atenolol, and metoprolol, can also be used for rate control.
- Calcium channel blockers include diltiazem and verapamil. The IV forms are rapidly effective in controlling acute AF and have a short duration of action. Both drugs are also used as short-acting and sustained-release oral preparation.

A β-blocker or a calcium channel blocker may be added to digoxin if adequate rate control cannot be achieved by one drug.

Q16. How is risk stratification for thromboembolic prevention and susceptibility to hemorrhage done in AF?
Ans. Risk stratification for thromboembolic prevention is done by the $CHADS_2$ (cardiac failure, hypertension, age ≥75 years, diabetes, and prior stroke) score. Each of the first four risk factors counts as 1 point, and a prior stroke or transient ischemic attack (TIA) as 2 points. There is a direct relationship between the $CHADS_2$ score and annual risk of stroke in the absence of aspirin or warfarin therapy. The $CHADS_2$ score has been superseded by the CHA_2DS_2-VASc score, because it more accurately discriminates low-risk patients from intermediate-risk patients. Here, age (A_2) carries 2 points; VASc (vascular disease, age 65–74 years, and sex category, e.g., female) carries 1 point. The maximum score is 9.

Hemorrhagic complication following warfarin use (also other anticoagulant uses) is done by the HAS-BLED score. The components are hypertension, abnormal renal or liver function, stroke, bleeding history or predisposition, labile international normalized ratio (INR), elderly (>75 years), and concomitant drug [antiplatelet or nonsteroidal anti-inflammatory drug (NSAID)] or alcohol use. Each of these components scores 1 point. As the score increases from 0 to 9, there is a stepwise increase in bleeding risk with warfarin.

Q17. What is the position of nonvitamin K oral anticoagulants (NOACs) in thromboembolic prevention in AF?

Ans. Randomized clinical trials (RCTs) show that NOACs are noninferior or superior to warfarin in efficacy and safety in patients with nonvalvular AF who had risk factors for stroke. The risk of intracranial hemorrhage is about 50% lower with NOACs compared to warfarin.

Nonvitamin K oral anticoagulants lose most of their effect by 24 hours after discontinuation. The onset of action of dabigatran, rivaroxaban, and apixaban is approximately 1.5–2 hours after a dose. The rapid onset of action and washout eliminates the need for bridging therapy with heparin before surgical or invasive procedures.

Aspirin does not prevent thromboembolic complications as effectively as warfarin or NOACs in patients with AF.

Q18. What HR is appropriate in patients with chronic AF? When to stop the drug?

Ans. The average ventricular response over a 24-hour period (evaluated by Holter monitoring) should be similar to that in a patient of comparable age without AF. A resting HR of 70–90 beats/min is generally appropriate. The ventricular response associated with exertion should be appropriate for the level of exercise (i.e., rates of 90–100 beats/min for modest activity, 100–120 beats/min for more vigorous, and 120–170 beats/min for very vigorous activity). Elderly sedentary patients may require digoxin only for control of the ventricular response at rest and with modest activity. However, in more active patients of all ages, a combination of digoxin with a β-blocker or a long-acting calcium channel blocker will result in better 24-hour control of the HR.

Q19. What are the indications of cardioversion in AF? How is it done?

Ans. In AF, cardioversion is done to restore and maintain sinus rhythm. If AF is of <3 months' duration, in young patients, and in those with no structural heart disease.

Cardioversion is done:
- Chemically by class IC antiarrhythmic agents (flecainide and propafenone) and class III agents (amiodarone and sotalol)
- Electronically by direct current (DC) shock.

Cardioversion in AF—indications:
- Emergency DC shock—in fast AF with hemodynamic compromise. Thrombus in LA appendage is excluded by transesophageal echocardiogram (TEE), and IV heparin is given before shock.
- In AF of <48 hours duration, immediate DC shock is given (after IV heparin). Flecainide IV can be given following an attack of an identifiable cause of AF.

- In AF of >48 hours duration, shock deferred until the patient established on warfarin for 3 weeks and underlying condition dealt with warfarin continued for 1-6 months with INR 2-3.

Q20. What are the contraindications of cardioversion in AF?
Ans.
- Long-standing AF with a dilated LA
- When underlying cause of AF cannot be eliminated.
- Electrolyte imbalance
- Coronary artery disease, where the patient has lost angina
- Atrial fibrillation with low VR (without digoxin)

Q21. How is cardioversion done for AF?
Ans. For restoration and maintenance of sinus rhythm, cardioversion is done in two ways:
1. *Chemical cardioversion:* It is usually attempted first. Any patient who fails chemical cardioversion should be considered electric cardioversion by DC shock. Drugs used are class IA agents [quinidine, procainamide, and disopyramide (procainamide is the drug of choice if the conduction over an accessory pathway with WPW syndrome)], class IC agents (flecainide and propafenone), and class III agents (amiodarone and sotalol). Class IC and class III drugs have an added advantage of slowing the ventricular response when AF does occur. Amiodarone therapy probably has a higher likelihood of maintaining sinus rhythm, although even low-dose therapy (200 mg/day) increases the risk of pulmonary toxicity.
2. *Electrical cardioversion:* When it is determined that restoration of sinus rhythm should be attempted, this is most efficiently carried out with direct electrical cardioversion. The defibrillator should be synchronized on the QRS complex (so that it does not induce VF), starting at 100 joules and progressing to 300 joules.

Q22. What are the conditions that increase the risk of thromboembolism and stroke in AF?
Ans. Permanent AF presents a considerable risk for thromboembolism and stroke. Patients with AF have >5-fold increase in risk of stroke; among patients with heart disease, the risk exceeds 17 times. Conditions increasing the risk are age >65 years, DM, hypertension, CHF, history of previous stroke or TIA, prosthetic heart valve, CAD, and hyperthyroidism. In these high-risk patients, warfarin is given (target INR 2.0-3.0). The risk of embolic events tends to cluster around changes in rhythm; the highest incidence occurring within the first year after the onset of chronic AF, and on the first few days after conversion to the sinus rhythm.

Q23. What is the relationship of stroke risk with AF types?
Ans. Paroxysmal, persistent, or permanent forms of AF increase stroke risk to a similar degree. Even subclinical AF of ≥6 minutes duration has

been associated with an increased risk of ischemic stroke or systemic embolism.

Guideline recommendation for anticoagulation is the same in patients with paroxysmal and persistent AF, although the burden of AF is greater in persistent AF than in patients with paroxysmal AF.

Q24. What are the indications of anticoagulants in AF? How is it done?
Ans.
- In all cases of AF of >24 hours duration (regardless of its etiology) to decrease the risk of LA thrombus formation
- Prior to elective cardioversion of AF >48 hours duration. Warfarin given for 3 weeks (INR 2-3) and continued for 1-6 months
- Prior to emergency cardioversion—IV heparin
- Anticoagulation for an indefinite period—when the patient cannot be successfully cardioverted and the cause of AF cannot be eliminated in chronic AF and in frequent paroxysmal AF

Q25. Warfarin or aspirin—which one is more effective for thromboembolism in AF? What are the contraindications of warfarin therapy in AF?
Ans. A number of major trials have attempted to compare the benefits of aspirin and warfarin in minimizing the stroke risk in patients with AF. Overall, warfarin has shown an annual average 68% reduction in the relative risk of stroke, with aspirin showing a reduction of around 30%.

Contraindications of warfarin include: Inability to monitor prothrombin time (INR), prior major bleeding events on warfarin, history of major gastrointestinal (GI) bleeding, serious liver disease, uncontrolled hypertension in an elderly patient, history of falls, or unstable gait.

Q26. What is the treatment of a first episode of AF?
Ans. These include:
- Determination of etiology—whether due to an organic heart disease. In a patient with advanced heart disease of any etiology and dilated LA, the first episode heralds a chronic fibrillatory state. If these are absent, removal of precipitating factors (e.g., pneumonia, thyrotoxicosis) and observation for recurrence are done.
- In the presence of significant heart disease, therapy for the particular condition is done, e.g., interventions for mitral stenosis (MS) and closure of atrial septal defect (ASD).
- Control of VR is achieved with digoxin, a β blocker, and a calcium channel blocker.
- Cardioversion—done if the patient requires the benefit of slowing the VR to prolong the diastolic filling (e.g., MS) or atrial contribution to contribute to ventricular filling [e.g., aortic stenosis (AS)].

Q27. What is the risk of cardioversion in patients of AF getting digoxin?

Ans. Patients getting a toxic dose of digoxin may have an increased risk of VF following DC cardioversion. DC cardioversion may be performed safely in patients receiving a usual dose of digitalis. If there is a question of digitalis toxicity, it is generally recommended that lower energy levels be utilized. Alternatively, prophylactic lignocaine should be administered if increased ectopy is noted.

Q28. What is the importance of left atrial appendix in thrombus formation in AF?

Ans. Approximately 90% of LA thrombi form in the LA appendage and have been described as "our most lethal human attachment." Successful excision or closure of left atrial appendage (LAA) greatly reduces the risk of thromboembolic complication in patients with AF. Percutaneous LAA occlusion devices are now used as an alternative to surgical closure techniques.

Q29. What are the causes of temporary AF?

Ans. Temporary or reversible AF may occur with excessive alcohol intake ("holiday heart" syndrome), open heart or thoracic surgery, myocardial infarction (MI), pericarditis, myocarditis, and pericardial effusion.

Q30. What are SVT and PSVTs?

Ans. Supraventricular tachycardias are all tachyarrhythmias that either originate or incorporate supraventricular tissue in a re-entrant circuit. Supraventricular includes atria, AV node, and His bundle.

Paroxysmal supraventricular tachycardias are rapid, regular tachycardias with an abrupt onset and termination.

Causes of PSVT:
- Atrioventricular nodal re-entrant tachycardia—two third
- Atrioventricular re-entrant tachycardia, including WPW syndrome—one third
- Atrial tachycardia: 5% only

Q31. What is Wolff Parkinson-White (WPW) syndrome? Explain the ECG findings. What conditions may mimic it?

Ans. The term WPW syndrome is applied to conditions comprising both ventricular pre-excitation on ECG and paroxysmal tachyarrhythmia. Ventricular pre-excitation means ventricular activation occurs earlier than would be expected from activation via the AV node—His bundle system due to the presence of an accessory pathway of conduction.

Electrocardiogram findings of WPW syndrome are:
- Short PR interval, typically <0.12 seconds. The QRS complex exceeds 0.12 seconds with some leads showing the characteristic slurred upstroke and

wave (the so-called Eiffel Tower appearance and a normal terminal QRS portion **(Fig. 13.5)**.

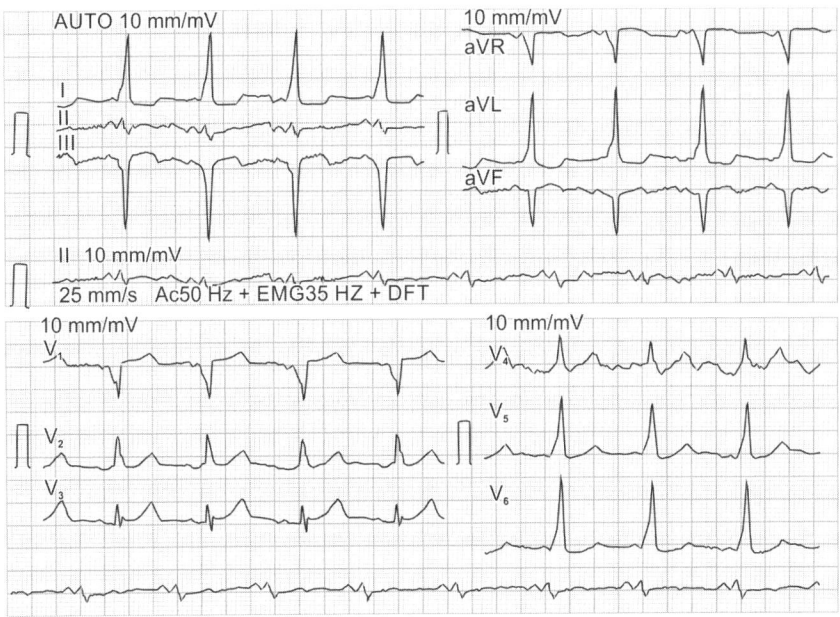

Fig. 13.5: WPW syndrome (short PR interval, delta wave, broad QRS).

The ST-T segment is directed opposite to the major δ and QRS vector. A short PR interval is due to the early activation of part of one ventricle by the rapidly conducting accessory pathway (bundle of Kent) bypassing the AV node. A wide QRS is analogous to a fusion beat—a portion of the ventricle is activated via the accessory pathway, and the remainder is activated by the normal pathway. δ wave results at the junction of two portions of the QRS complex. Here an impulse from the atrium is conducted down both the accessory pathway and AV node, arriving at the ventricle at nearly the same time.
- ST-T segment changes are secondary.

Electrocardiogram pattern in WPW conduction may mimic:
- *Myocardial infarction:* The δ wave may be oriented superiorly, producing Q in II, III, aVF, and simulating inferior infarction. Anterior orientation of δ wave produces R in V_1, simulating posterior MI, and rightwardly oriented δ wave produces Q in aVL, mimicking anterior MI. Ventricular depolarization is abnormal in WPW syndrome; hence, myocardial infarction cannot be read from the ECG. Conversely, an infarction pattern present during normal AV conduction can be masked by the development of WPW syndrome.

- *Ventricular hypertrophy:* An anteriorly oriented δ wave can produce as tall R in V_1 mimicking right ventricular hypertrophy (RVH). Similarly, a left and posteriorly oriented δ can inscribe deep QS wave in V_{1-3} and tall R in I, avL, V_{5-6} mimicking left ventricular hypertrophy (LVH).
- *Bundle branch block:* Wide QRS complex along with a tall, slurred R wave in V_1 and deep S wave in V_6 resulting from an anteriorly oriented δ wave may mimic right bundle branch block (RBBB). Again, wide QRS along with tall, slurred R in V_6 and wide S with notch in the down stroke, resulting from a posteriorly oriented δ may mimic left bundle branch block (LBBB).

Q32. What are the arrhythmias seen in patients with WPW syndrome?
Ans.
- *Atrioventricular re-entrant tachycardia:* 80–85%, usually precipitated by an atrial premature beat. In the usual form, impulse is conducted antegradely through the AV node and retrogradely through the accessory pathway (orthodromic tachycardia). In antidromic tachycardia, impulse is conducted antegradely through the accessory pathway and retrogradely through the AV node, which is uncommon.
- *Atrial fibrillation:* 15–30%, it may cause sudden cardiac death (SCD). If the accessory pathway has a short refractory period and is able to conduct rapidly, a very fast VR may cause hypoxia (as the protection by the gating effect of the AV node is lost) or VF may be precipitated by an impulse falling in the vulnerable period **(Fig. 13.6)**.

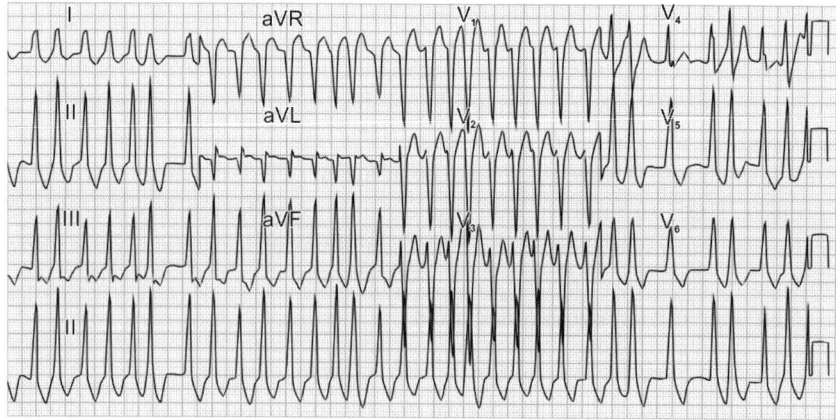

Fig. 13.6: Atrial fibrillation in WPW syndrome.

- *Other arrhythmias:* Atrial flutter 5%, VF (rarely).

Q33. What are the associations and prognosis of WPW syndrome?
Ans. Congenital lesions associated with WPW syndrome are: Ebstein's anomaly, hypertrophic cardiomyopathy, and mitral valve prolapse. Paroxysmal tachycardias are a common problem in these conditions. WPW

syndrome may be concealed and not obvious on the surface ECG. In this situation, the accessory pathway only conducts retrogradely. About three quarter of adults have no evidence of heart disease. The prognosis is excellent in patients without tachycardia or without associated cardiac anomaly. For most patients with recurrent tachycardia, the prognosis is good. Sudden death occurs rarely among those manifesting AF with very rapid VR. Some children and adults can lose their tendency to develop tachyarrhythmia as they grow older (due to fibrosis).

Q34. How to treat tachyarrhythmias due to WPW syndrome?
Ans.
- *Termination of acute episode:* Patients demonstrating hemodynamic instability should be cardioverted rapidly. Stable patients may be treated medically.
    - Supraventricular tachycardia with narrow QRS: Attempts to slow the AV nodal conduction by vagal maneuvers—carotid sinus massage, Valsalva. Drugs—IV adenosine (6-12 mg), verapamil (5-10 mg), diltiazem (20-25 mg), and esmolol (0.5 mg/kg)—are all effective.
    - Supraventricular tachycardia with wide QRS: IV, procainamide is recommended. Amiodarone IV is useful. Ca-channel blockers, β-blockers, and digoxin should be avoided as their efficacy is low and may accelerate the ventricular response rate and precipitate VF. If the tachycardia persists, synchronized DC shock is the treatment of choice.
    - Atrial fibrillation: IV procainamide, as it slows accessory pathway conduction and frequently converts AF to sinus rhythm.

    Atrioventricular node blocking drugs (verapamil, adenosine, β-blockers, and digoxin) should not be used. These drugs can slow conduction through AV node and paradoxically accelerate the ventricular response by increasing the conduction over the accessory connection. Furthermore, hypotension resulting from drug-induced vasodilatation may result in increased catecholamine release and increased accessory pathway conduction. It is in this setting that VF is likely to occur. Ablation of the accessory pathway as the definitive therapy often results in termination of AF.
- *Long-term management:*
    - Medical therapy—avoidance of drugs that shorten the refractory period of the accessory pathway, e.g., digoxin. Oral administration of class IC drugs (flecainide or propafenone) or class III drugs (amiodarone or sotalol). These drugs work to slow conduction in both the accessory pathway and the AV node. A combination of drugs that work on the AV node (calcium channel blockers and β-blockers) with drugs that work exclusively on the accessory pathway (class IA drugs) can be effective.

- Percutaneous intervention—by RF ablation is considered for: Patients at high risk—family history of sudden death, patients who are competitive athletes or are in high-risk occupations, patients with a history of AF or aborted SCD, and patients with tachycardia refractory to medical therapy or those who are intolerant to medical therapy.

Q35. What are broad complex tachycardias?
Ans. Broad complex tachycardias are any cardiac rhythm >100 beats/min, with a QRS duration of ≥0.12 seconds. Most of these arrhythmias are ventricular in origin, involving an automatic focus or re-entry circuit within the ventricles. Occasionally, SVT can have broad complexes because of a pre-existing conduction defect (e.g., LBBB or RBBB), aberrant conduction (due to rapid rate or ischemia), or antegrade conduction through an accessory pathway.

Q36. What is VT? What are the types?
Ans. Ventricular tachycardia is defined as three or more QRS complexes of ventricular origin at a rate >100 beats/min (usually 120–220 beats/min) **(Fig. 13.7)**.

There are two main types of VT:
1. Sustained—duration >30 seconds; it may be monomorphic or polymorphic
2. Nonsustained—duration up to 30 seconds

Other special types of VT:
3. Slow VT—an accelerated idioventricular rhythm at rate of 60–100 beats/min
4. Short run of VT—salvos of 3–5 consecutive ventricular impulse

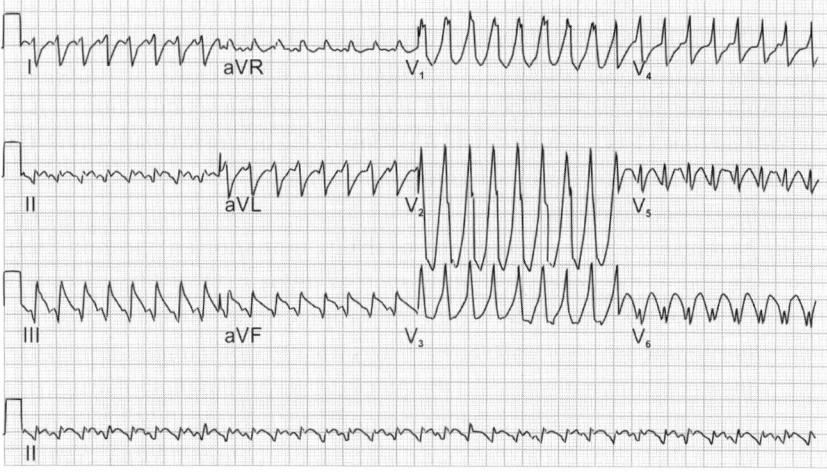

Fig. 13.7: Ventricular tachycardia (broad QRS, RSr pattern in V_1, AV dissociation).

Q37. What is the difference between SVT and VT?

Ans. Both are arrhythmias with fast VR. The following features are helpful in differentiating the two **(Table 13.1)**.

TABLE 13.1: Differences between supraventricular tachycardia and ventricular tachycardia.

SVT	VT
Age: Younger	Older
No structural disease	Yes—MI, cardiomyopathy, LVH
Ventricular rate >170 beats/min	<170 beats/min
Cardiac arrest—nil	VF, cardiac arrest—may develop
AV dissociation—nil	Yes—cannon wave
QRS <0.14 seconds; discordant, RBBB, triphasic V_1	>0.14 seconds; concordant, bizarre, monophasic
Capture* and fusion† beat—nil	May be present
Independent P wave—nil	May be present
CSM‡, IV adenosine—slow ventricular rate	No effect

(AV: atrioventricular; CSM: carotid sinus massage; LVH: left ventricular hypertrophy; MI: myocardial infarction; RBBB: right bundle branch block; SVT: supraventricular tachycardia; VF: ventricular fibrillation; VT: ventricular tachycardia)
*Capture beat—sinus impulse conducted to ventricle and captures it
†Fusion beat—ventricular depolarization results in part from sinus impulse and in part from ventricular foci
‡Carotid sinus massage

In troublesome cases, treatment should be directed toward VT; lignocaine with or without DC shock is helpful in both SVT and VT. When QRS is wide and VT is mistakenly diagnosed as SVT with aberrant conduction, IV verapamil frequently causes a clinically significant fall in BP and is a potentially lethal event.

Q38. What is VF? What are the types?

Ans. Ventricular fibrillation is defined as chaotic electrical disturbance of ventricle with uncoordinated and ineffective contraction that eventually proceeds to cardiac arrest.

Types:
- *Etiologically:* Primary [as primary cardiac manifestation, as a complication of acute myocardial infarction (AMI)] and secondary (occur preterminally in most illnesses)
- *Mode of origin:* De novo and VT degenerating to VF, e.g., VF developing from R on T **(Fig. 13.8)**
- Depending on ECG finding—fine VF (<0.2 mv) and coarse VF (responds better to defibrillation)

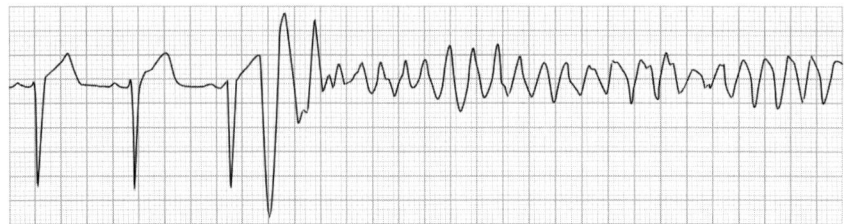

Fig. 13.8: Ventricular fibrillation (developing from R on T).

Q39. What is the clinical significance of ventricular premature complexes (VPCs)?

Ans. Ventricular premature complexes occur frequently in health, incidence increases with age. Emotional stress and consumption of tea, coffee, alcohol, and tobacco may induce them. Electrolyte disturbance, e.g., hypocalcemia, and drugs (e.g., digoxin) are common causes of VPCs. These may appear in AMI or chronic IHD and are possible markers of the extent of myocardial damage. These do not necessarily cause VF and sudden death. Suppression is considered in patients with: Multifocal VPCs, frequent VPCs, salvos of three, recurring over hours, and R on T-phenomenon. Such VPCs are best treated with a β-blocking agent. Amiodarone has been shown to be effective in reducing arrhythmic death post-MI in patients with poor LV function. In chronic IHD, the prognosis of patients depends on the severity of LV dysfunction.

Q40. What is long QT syndrome and torsades de pointes?

Ans.

In long QT syndrome, the QT interval is prolonged to 0.50–0.60 seconds (normal: 0.38–0.42 seconds).

Normal QT interval corrected for HR, i.e.,

$$QTc = \frac{QT}{\sqrt{R\text{-R interval}}} = 0.38 - 0.425$$

A long QT interval may be congenital (genetic) or acquired (drug or electrolyte effect)

Common drugs responsible are: Class IA and class III antiarrhythmics, tricyclic antidepressants, chlorpromazine, erythromycin, quinine, chloroquine, cisapride, and terfenadine. Electrolyte disturbances—hypokalemia, hypomagnesemia, and hypocalcemia. β-blockers are used in congenital QT prolongation.

Torsades de pointes (twisting of the points): Torsades de pointes is nonsustained, polymorphic VT that usually occurs in the presence of a prolonged QT interval. ECG shows irregular RR intervals and varying amplitude of QRS complexes, which appear alternatively above and below the baseline (i.e., twisting of the points). The VR varies from 200 to 300 beats/min. It is repetitive and may degenerate into VF **(Fig. 13.9)**.

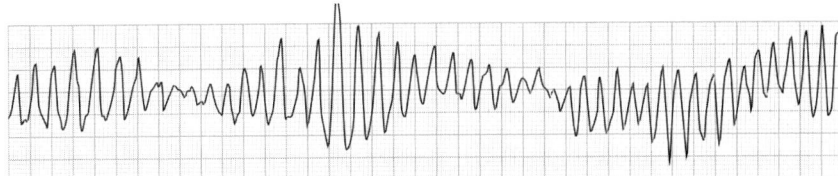

Fig. 13.9: Torsades de pointes.

It is treated by agents that shorten the QT interval, such as isoproterenol or temporary cardiac pacing.

Q41. What is channelopathy?
Ans. These are inherited arrhythmogenic disorders of the heart characterized by altered excitability, in the absence of significant structural cardiac lesions. Ion channels and other proteins involved in the control of cardiac excitability are affected here. A genetic mutation affecting the genes that control cardiac excitability is responsible for it. These are manifested with syncope, sudden death in young, otherwise healthy individuals, and peculiar ECG findings, like long QT syndrome (abnormally prolonged QT interval with abnormal T wave), Brugada syndrome (BrS), short QT syndrome, etc.

Q42. What is Brugada syndrome?
Ans. Brugada syndrome is characterized by syncope, cardiac arrest, and sudden death occurring at rest or during sleep with peculiar ECG findings of ST-segment elevation in leads V_1-V_3 and RBBB (incomplete or complete 0 in the absence of acute myocardial ischemia. Physical conditions (fever, overeating, and alcohol) and drugs (local anesthetics, cocaine, β-blockers, tricyclic antidepressants, propofol, and alfa-agonists) may trigger syncope and cardiac arrest. ICD implantation is the only effective treatment.

Q43. What is RF ablation?
Ans. Here, catheter ablation is done by delivering RF energy (400–500 Hz) over electrodes on the catheter placed next to the area of the endocardium integrally related to the arrhythmia. Thus, it permanently destroys the local tissue (atrial or ventricular) that plays a critical role in the generation and maintenance of the arrhythmia. RF energy is currently the preferred procedure as it is precise and produces minimal cardiac damage, no barotrauma, needs no general anesthesia, and allows performing electrophysiology (EP) study and ablation in one procedure.

Uses:
- Wolff–Parkinson–White tachycardias—ablation of accessory connection is curative.
- Atrioventricular nodal re-entrant tachycardia (AVNRT)—slow component of the pathway can be safely ablated.

- Chronic fast AF—direct AV node ablation; permanent pacing will be needed.
- Atrial flutter—to destroy the area of slow conduction
- Others—as treatment of ectopic atrial tachycardia, some VT [right ventricular outflow tract (RVOT) pattern], etc.

Here, the cardiac electrophysiologist first performs a diagnostic EP study to uncover the mechanism of the underlying tachyarrhythmia. Then specialized mapping catheters are used to locate precisely and destroy the area responsible.

Q44. What is proarrhythmia?
Ans. Proarrhythmia is defined as a new, higher form of arrhythmia, especially with hemodynamically important symptoms occurring early after the drug use (<30 days), and not due to other obvious causes. Two basic mechanisms of proarrhythmias are (1) prolongation of QT interval and action potential duration that occur with class I and class III agents and (2) alteration is re-entry substrates with incessant wide complex tachycardia after terminating VF, which occurs with class IC agents. Also, the patient's own tachycardia, previously paroxysmal, becomes incessant (by class I and IC agents).

The cardiac arrhythmia suppression trail (CAST) study showed that proarrhythmic sudden death can occur even when ventricular ectopics are apparently eliminated. Continuous vigilance is required throughout the therapy with antiarrhythmic agents to detect proarrhythmia. Measures that are helpful: (1) Not treating arrhythmias unless the overall effect will clearly be beneficial, (2) trying to avoid the use of class I, especially class IC agents, and (3) defining subjects at high risk for proarrhythmia and arrhythmic death.

Q45. What is a symptomatic bradycardia?
Ans. These are pathologic bradycardias that place the patient at risk of syncope or cardiac arrest or produce hemodynamic compromise in the patient.

Bradycardia (i.e., HR <60 beats/min) may be present without symptoms in many healthy individuals and patients with heart disease as a result of medications.

Symptomatic bradycardias other than CHB do not require emergency intervention.

Q46. What are the causes of symptomatic bradycardia?
Ans.
- Complete heart block
- Second-degree AV block (Mobitz type-2)
- Sick sinus syndrome
- Atrial fibrillation with slow VR
- Sinus bradycardia with rate <42 beats/min

- Junctional rhythm—HR: 40-60 beats/min, arising from the area surrounding the AV node that serves as an escape mechanism to prevent ventricular asystole in case of complete AV block. The QRS complex is narrow, and P wave is absent.

Q47. What is sick sinus syndrome? What are the types?
Ans. It is an abnormality of the sinus node associated with extensive degeneration within and around it.

Types include:
- Persistent spontaneous sinus bradycardia not caused by drugs and inappropriate for the physiological circumstance
- Sinus arrest or SA exit block
- Combination of SA or AV conduction disturbances
- Bradycardia-tachycardia syndrome (paroxysmal regular or irregular tachyarrhythmia alternating with periods of slow atrial or VRs)
   More than one can be present in the same patient on different occasions (Fig. 13.10).

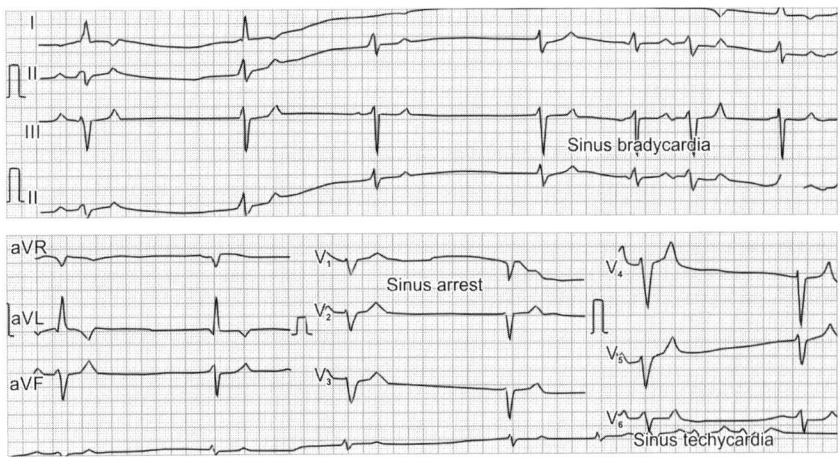

Fig. 13.10: Sick sinus syndrome.

Q48. What is heart block? What is AV block?
Ans. Heart block is the transient or permanent disturbance of impulse conduction due to functional or anatomical impairment of the AV conducting tissue. Types of heart block are—SA block, AV block, intra-atrial, and intraventricular conduction defects (LBBB and RBBB).

Atrioventricular block: Here, atrial impulses are conducted with delay or not conducted at all to the ventricle (when the AV junction is not physiologically refractory). The sites of block are nodal (AV node) and infranodal (His bundle or bundle branch).

Q49. What is CHB? Classify CHB.

Ans. It is a type of AV dissociation where no atrial activity is conducted to the ventricular and atria, and ventricles are controlled by independent pacemakers **(Fig. 13.11)**. It is classified on the basis of its etiology, site of block, and onset **(Box 13.2)**.

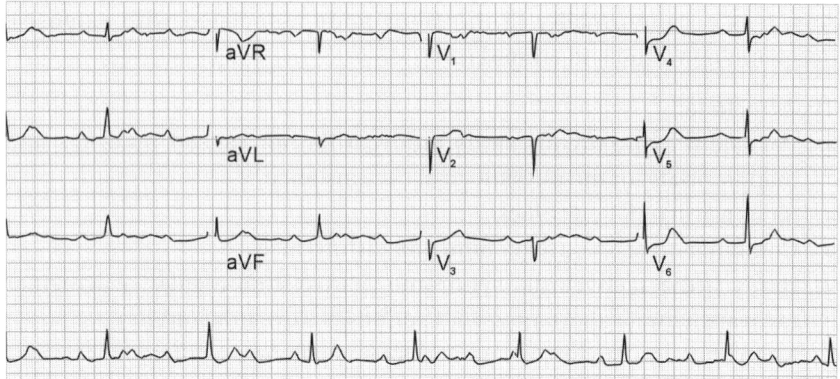

Fig. 13.11: Complete heart block (P and QRS occurring without any relation to each other; PR interval completely changing).

BOX 13.2: Complete heart block—classification.

- *Etiologically:*
  - Congenital (isolated or in combination with other lesions)
  - Acquired, e.g., AMI, idiopathic fibrosis, drug-induced, infection (infective endocarditis), and traumatic (surgery)
- *Clinically:*
  - Acute, e.g., AMI, drug induced
  - Chronic, e.g., idiopathic fibrosis
- *Site of block:*
  - Nodal (in AV node)-QRS narrow, HR: 40–60 beats/min
  - Infranodal (at His bundle or distal to it)-QRS broad, HR <40 beats/min

Q50. What is AV dissociation?

Ans. Atrioventricular dissociation means that atrial and ventricles activate independently of each other. It occurs when the intrinsic VR speeds up above the sinus rate, e.g., accelerated idioventricular rhythm or when the sinus rate slows below the intrinsic VR, e.g., extreme sinus bradycardia.

Atrioventricular dissociation is not a form of complete AV block and does not require pacing. In AV block, atrial impulse cannot be conducted to the ventricles despite the temporal opportunity for this to occur. In contrast, in AV dissociation, atrial impulse may be conducted to stimulate the ventricle if the temporal opportunity is provided. Hence, VR may not be regular in AV dissociation **(Fig. 13.12)**. In CHB, atrial rate usually exceeds the ventricular escape rate. Because of AV nodal failure, P wave and QRS complexes are dissociated.

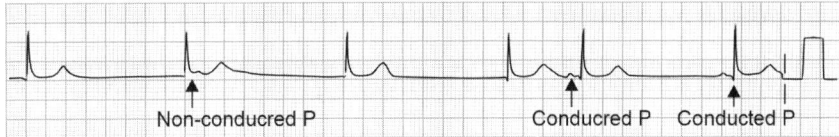

Fig. 13.12: AV dissociation (intrinsic ventricular rate exceeds atrial rate; at times P wave conducted to ventricles).

Q51. What are the differences between CHB and AV dissociation?
Ans. In CHB, there is always AV dissociation, but AV dissociation can occur without CHB. They differ from each other in the aspects mentioned in **Table 13.2**.

TABLE 13.2: Difference between CHB and AV dissociation.

CHB	AV dissociation
Often permanent	Usually transient
Syncope—common	Uncommon
Atrial rate > ventricular	Slower than ventricular
QRS—ventricular or supraventricular	Usually supraventricular
P after T—may occur	Does not occur

(AV: atrioventricular; CHB: complete heart block)

Q52. What is an accelerated junctional rhythm? How does it differ from CHB?
Ans. Junctional rhythm that is faster than the sinus rhythm is referred to as accelerated junctional rhythm (also called slow VT). Here, HR varies from 70 to 130 beats/min **(Fig. 13.13)**.

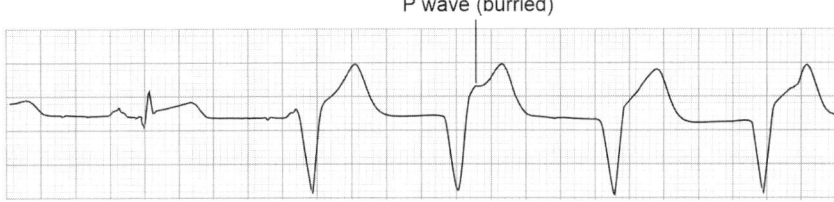

Fig. 13.13: Accelerated junctional rhythm (slow VT).

Causes are: Acute MI (inferior > anterior), digitalis toxicity, valve surgery, acute rheumatic fever, dc cardioversion, cardiac catheterization, etc.

Difference from CHB: In both conditions, there is AV dissociation with changing PR interval. VR is faster than the atrial rate in accelerated junctional rhythm and slower than the atrial rate in CHB. The QRS complex has a normal duration in accelerated junctional rhythm, whereas, in CHB, it is usually broad. P wave of normal morphology is present in both conditions.

Q52. What is high-grade AV block? How does it differ from CHB?

Ans. When two or more consecutive atrial impulses fail to be conducted to the ventricle, it is defined as high-grade AV block, i.e., AV conduction is 3:1 or greater **(Fig. 13.14)**.

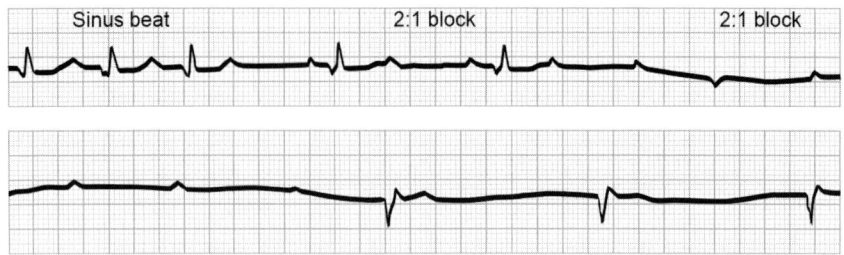

Fig. 13.14: Sinus rhythm progressing to 2:1 block and a 4:1 (high grade) AV block.

Occasionally, runs of consecutive atrial impulses may fail to conduct to the ventricles for up to 10–20 seconds with or without an escape rhythm, resulting in ventricular asystole and syncope. In CHB, all P waves fail to conduct to the ventricle, resulting in complete dissociation of P waves and QRS complexes. A PPM is indicated in both conditions.

Q53. What is an Adams-Stokes attack? How does it differ from epilepsy?

Ans. It is the episodic cardiac arrest and syncope with failure of normal and escape pacemakers, with or without VF resulting from severe heart block (CHB, or Mobitz type II second-degree block).

The attack usually lasts some 10–30 seconds. A prolonged Adams-Stokes episode may produce convulsions from cerebral hypoxia. The attacks may occur in series or may be separated from one another by months. An artificial pacemaker prevents the attack. Although convulsions may occur in both, an Adams-Stokes attack differs from epilepsy **(Table 13.3)**.

TABLE 13.3: Adams-Stokes attack and epilepsy—difference.

Adams-Stokes attack	*Epilepsy*
No aura or warning	Aura often present
Unconsciousness transient	May be prolonged
Pale or cyanosed during an attack	Tonic–clonic state during an attack
The patient is pulseless during an attack	Not pulseless
Recovery is rapid and complete	Recovery prolonged with drowsiness
Flushing (as blood courses through dilated capillaries) occurs on recovery	Absent

SUGGESTED READING

1. Blomstorm-Lundqvist C, Scheinman MM, Aliot EM, Alpert JS, Calkins H, Camm AJ, et al. ACC/AHA/ESC guidelines for the management of patients with supraventricular arrhythmias-executive summary: a report of the American College of Cardiology/American Heart Association Task Force on Practice Guidelines and the European Society of Cardiology Committee for Practice Guidelines (Writing Committee to Develop Guidelines for the Management of Patients With Supraventricular Arrhythmias). Circulation. 2003;108(15):1871-909.
2. Epstein AE, DiMarco JP, Ellenbogen KA, Estes NA 3rd, Freedman RA, Gettes LS, et al. ACC/AHA/HRS 2008 guidelines for device-based therapy of cardiac rhythm abnormalities. J Am Coll Cardiol. 2008;51:e1-62.
3. Fuster V, Ryden LE, Cannom DS, Crijns HJ, Curtis AB, Ellenbogen KA, et al. ACC/AHA? ESC 2006 guidelines for the management of patients with atrial fibrillation: a report of the American College of Cardiology/American Heart Association Task Force on Practice Guidelines and the European Society of Cardiology Committee for Practice Guidelines (Writing Committee to Revise the 2001 Guidelines for the Management of Patients with Atrial Fibrillation). Eur Heart J. 2006;27:1979-2030.
4. Goldschager N, Goldman MJ. Normal cardiac rhythm & the supraventricular arrhythmias. In: Goldschager N, Goldman MJ (Eds). Principles of Clinical Electrocardiography, 13th edition. USA: Appleton & Lange; 1989.

CHAPTER 14

Cardiac Arrest and Sudden Cardiac Death

"90% of natural sudden deaths are sudden cardiac death (SCD), and 50% of CHD deaths are SCD."
—Author of the book

■ INTRODUCTION

Abrupt cessation of cardiac function and the ensuing circulatory collapse are commonly due to ischemic heart disease (IHD). It may also occur in valvular heart disease, congenital heart disease, and cardiomyopathies. Unless promptly resuscitated by basic life support (BLS) and advanced life support (ALS) measures, death occurs. Death occurring unexpectedly within 1 hour of the onset of the event is designated as sudden cardiac death (SCD). About 90% of sudden deaths are cardiac in origin, i.e., cardiac arrest.

Q1. What is cardiac arrest? Classify it.

Ans. Cardiac arrest is defined as the sudden and complete cessation of effective cardiac function, leading to a precipitous decrease in cardiac output and the ensuing cardiac collapse. Cardiac arrest is due to ventricular fibrillation (VF), pulseless ventricular tachycardia (VT), ventricular asystole, or electromechanical dissociation (EMD). The patient loses consciousness as cerebral blood flow is lost and irreversible cerebral damage results if the circulation is not re-established within 3 minutes. Cardiac arrest is classified depending on its cause, electrical mechanism, and place of occurrence of the event **(Box 14.1)**.

> **BOX 14.1:** Classification of cardiac arrest.
>
> - *Etiologically:*
>   - Primary, i.e., due to primary cardiac involvement, e.g., in CAD
>   - Secondary, i.e., secondary to respiratory arrest as in drowning, drug overdose, suffocation, carbon monoxide poisoning, and airway obstruction. Respiratory arrest leads to arterial hypoxemia, myocardial hypoxia, and consequent secondary cardiac arrest
> - *According to electrical mechanism:*
>   - *Tachyarrhythmic:* It is due to VF or sustained VT. These are initiating events in most cardiac arrests. After a variable period, fibrillation may cease and asystole or PEA emerges. In significant minorities, asystole and PEA may be the initial recording
>   - *Bradyarrhythmic:* It is due to asystolic, i.e., inability to generate a mechanical event because of complete absence of electrical activity (asystole) or dissociation between abnormal spontaneous electrical activity and mechanical function (in PEA)

Contd...

Contd...

- *According to the place of occurrence of the event:*
  - *Out-of-hospital cardiac arrest (OHCA)*
  - *In-hospital cardiac arrest (IHCA)*

(CAD: coronary artery disease; PEA: pulseless electrical activity; VF: ventricular fibrillation; VT: ventricular tachycardia)

Q2. What are the causes of cardiac arrest?

Ans. Depending on the electrical mechanisms of arrest, the causes are:

- *Ventricular fibrillation and pulseless VT:* Extensive acute myocardial infarction (AMI), advanced chronic IHD, cardiomyopathy, atrial fibrillation (AF) with fast ventricular rate in Wolff–Parkinson–White (WPW) syndrome, and R-on-T phenomenon.
- *Ventricular asystole:* Late manifestation of VF, profound vagal stimulation (surgery, anesthesia, diagnostic procedure, Stokes–Adams attack, and metabolic disturbances) **(Fig. 14.1)**.
- *Pulseless electrical activity (PEA):* Cardiac rupture in AMI, hypovolemia in severe hemorrhage, cardiac tamponade, pneumothorax, etc.

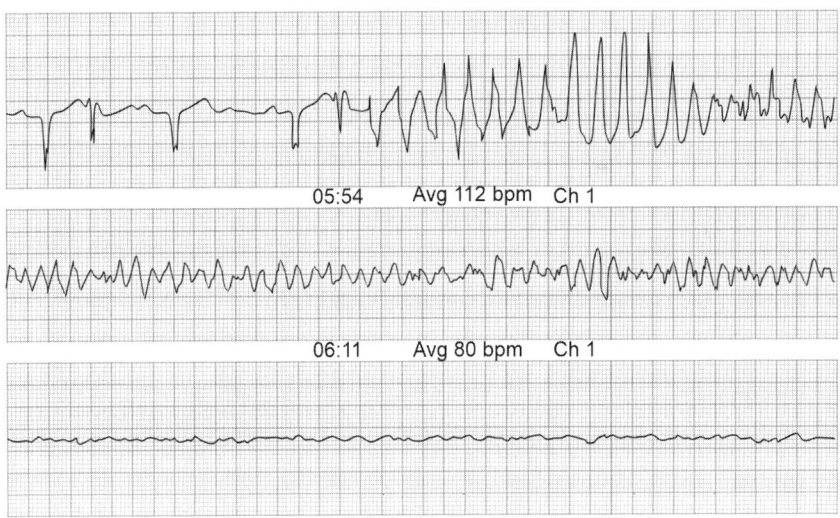

Fig. 14.1: Holter recording showing sinus rhythm proceeding to polymorphic VT, VF, and asystole.

Q3. How does cardiac arrest differ from cardiogenic shock?

Ans. Cardiac arrest is an electrical event, whereas cardiogenic shock is a mechanical state of the heart, hence the difference in clinical features and treatment **(Table 14.1)**.

TABLE 14.1: Difference between cardiac arrest and cardiogenic shock.

Points	Cardiac arrest	Cardiogenic shock
Mechanism	Electrical—ventricular fibrillation or asystole	Mechanical—loss of myocardial contractility
Onset	Sudden	Gradual
Loss of cardiac function	Complete	Not complete (complete only terminally)
Patient's level of consciousness	Unconscious	Conscious, restless, agitated, obtunded
Vital signs (pulse, BP, and respiration)	Absent	Present (pulse—rapid, BP—low)
Treatment	Immediately needed—basic and advanced life support measures	Hemodynamic support (inotropic agent and mechanical), treatment of the underlying cause
Prognosis	Survival depends on rapidly with which BLS and ALS are undertaken	Depends on the extent of myocardial dysfunction

(ALS: advanced life support; BLS: basic life support; BP: blood pressure)

Cardiac arrest is the terminal event in all cardiac diseases including conditions leading cardiogenic shock.

Q4. What is a chain of survival in cardiac arrest? What are its components?
Ans. These are sequences of events necessary to maximize the chance of cardiac arrest victims to survive **(Fig. 14.2)**.

Components of a strong chain of survival:
- *Early access:* Arrest should be witnessed and help called immediately.
- Basic life support [cardiopulmonary resuscitation (CPR)] should be started immediately.
- Defibrillation within a few minutes, aiming at restoring normal circulation
- *Early advanced cardiac care:* Venous access, intubation, ventilation, antiarrhythmic drugs, etc.

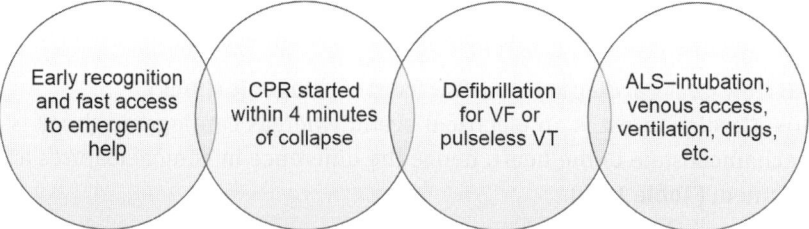

Fig. 14.2: Chain of survival. (ALS: advanced life support; CPR: cardiopulmonary resuscitation; VF: ventricular fibrillation; VT: ventricular tachycardia)

Successful resuscitation depends on a rapid sequence of steps undertaken with minimal delay.

Q5. What are BLS and ALS? What are their purposes?
Ans. Basic life support and ALS are measures undertaken to overcome cardiac arrest. The aim of BLS is to maintain an oxygenated blood supply to the vital organs, especially the brain. It is a holding measure until the definitive treatment of the patient's underlying rhythm disturbance can restore circulation, i.e., by ALS. BLS includes (*ABC* of resuscitation):
- *A*irway: To open by head-tilt/chin-lift technique
- *B*reathing: If no breathing or breathing is ineffective, mouth-to-mouth or mouth-to-airway
- Circulation: External cardiac massage by chest compression, 15:2 (15 compressions and two ventilations when two rescuers); 100 compressions/minute

As there is usually no time to call an expert, everyone should know it, and hence called BLS.

Advanced life support includes defibrillation (for VF), airway management (endotracheal intubation or artificial ventilation), administration of appropriate drugs (adrenaline and lignocaine for VF, adrenaline and atropine for ventricular asystole, etc.), and pacing (in ventricular asystole). BLS alone rarely resuscitates without immediate defibrillation and ALS. Arrest victims should have cardiac monitoring as soon as possible to allow immediate defibrillation in VF. However, CPR is essential to improve survival if there is any delay in defibrillation or arrest is not due to VF, but rather due to asystole or EMD. Thus, it may be a life-saving measure in cardiac arrest.

Q6. What are the evolutionary changes in CPR?
Ans.
- Early CPR is done more for drowning than true SCD—mouth-to-mouth resuscitation done for drowning victims. The first equivocally performed chest compression in humans was done in 1891 by Dr Friedrich Maass.
- In 1960, the American Heart Association (AHA) started a CPR program to acquaint physicians and train the general public. CPR algorithms for BLS were: A (airway), B (breathing), and C (chest compression).
- Advanced life support was developed at the third national conference on CPR held in 1979.
- In 2005, the AHA started the bystander CPR, i.e., bystanders who witness a sudden collapse should provide high-quality chest compression by pushing hard and fast on victim's midchest and call for emergency assistance.
- In 2010 (at the 50th anniversary of CPR), a change in the BLS sequence of steps from A-B-C to C-A-B (chest compression, airway, and breathing) was

recommended. Chest compression of adequate rate and depth, allowing complete recoil after each compression, minimizing interruptions in compressions, and avoiding excess ventilation, was emphasized.

Q7. What is cardiocerebral resuscitation (CCR)?

Ans. Cardiocerebral resuscitation advocates continuous chest compressions without mouth-to-mouth ventilations for witnessed cardiac arrest, developed by the University of Arizona Sarver Heart Center Resuscitation Group. It advocates prompt defibrillation and early venous access. Endotracheal intubation is delayed, excessive ventilation is avoided, and early administration of epinephrine is advocated. CCR is not recommended for individuals with respiratory arrest.

Q8. What is the thump version and cough CPR?

Ans.

- *Thump version:* A vigorous blow to the mid sternum may sometimes restart the heart in ventricular asystole of short duration or revert VT if done within a few seconds of the arrest. This is called the thump version. Rhythmic blows may maintain limited perfusion and can be continued in ventricular asystole (if it fails, CPR is started followed by other ALS measures). The efficacy of the thump version is variable in patients with VT and may rarely cause VF. It is generally ineffective in VF, and hence should not be used in a patient with VT and a pulse unless a defibrillator is immediately available.
- *Cough CPR:* Continuous and early initiation of coughing in an alert and responsive patient with VT may maintain the conscious state as a result of a rise in intrathoracic pressure. The induced increase in aortic pressure leads to flow to the carotid system and the brain. In the same way, patients with VF can maintain consciousness as long as the cough is continued. Cough CPR is practiced by the patient himself when alone. There is probably no cardiac compression on coughing.

Q9. What is the difference between defibrillation and cardioversion?

Ans.

- Defibrillation and cardioversions are electrical countershocks that depolarize a critical mass of myocardium, thereby allowing the establishment of a normal rhythm in both supraventricular tachycardia (SVT) and VT. Defibrillation is the process where asynchronized countershocks are given to depolarize a critical mass of myocardium in an effort to terminate VF. External cardiac defibrillation for VF is an emergency procedure and the only successful form of treatment.
- Cardioversion is the means by which synchronized electrical countershocks are used to terminate cardiac arrhythmias other than VF.

The principal danger of cardioversion is the production of VF by delivery of a shock during the vulnerable period. To avoid this, all defibrillators have a control mechanism that allows synchronization of the electrical shock on the R wave of the electrocardiogram (ECG). Synchronization must be used for cardioversion of supraventricular arrhythmias (e.g., AF and SVT) and ventricular arrhythmias (e.g., VT). On the contrary, defibrillators placed in a synchronized mode in VF may fail to discharge during the event because they may not detect an ECG deflection large enough to allow synchronization.

Q10. What are the indications and contraindications of cardioversion and defibrillation?

Ans. Direct current (DC) shock for cardiac arrhythmias can be emergent or elective. Defibrillation is always indicated for VF or pulseless VT.

Indications:
- *Emergency:* Any arrhythmia resulting in hemodynamic instability, myocardial ischemia, and congestive heart failure (CHF)
- *Elective:* VT, SVT, AF, or flutter, where the ventricular rate is high with hemodynamic compromise and the patient is intolerant

Contraindications:
- Atrial or atrial appendage thrombi
- The patient does not desire to be resuscitated.

Q11. What energy output and mode of countershocks are needed in different situations?

Ans. The mode and amount of countershocks vary in different cardiac conditions **(Table 14.2)**.

TABLE 14.2: Countershocks in different conditions.

Arrhythmia		Energy output	Mode (i.e., synchronization)
Ventricular fibrillation:	• Initial • Subsequent	• 100 J (biphasic) • 100 J, 150 J	No
Ventricular tachycardia:	• Initial • Subsequent	• 100 J (biphasic) • 100 J, 150 J	Yes
Supraventricular tachycardia:	• Initial • Subsequent	• 50 J • 100 J, 200 J	Yes
Atrial fibrillation:	• Initial • Subsequent	• 100 J • 200 J, 300 J, 360 J	Yes
Atrial flutter:	• Initial • Subsequent	• 30–50 J • 50 J	Yes

Q12. What are the potentially reversible causes of cardiac arrest?

Ans. These are 4*H*s: *H*ypoxia, *h*ypovolemia, *h*ypo/*h*yperkalemia and metabolic disorders, and *h*ypothermia and 4*T*s: *t*ension pneumothorax, *t*amponade, *t*oxic/therapeutic effect, and *t*hromboembolic/mechanical obstruction.

Q13. How can cardiac arrest be prevented?
Ans.
- *In surgical patients:* Careful preoperative assessment, use of atropine in premedication (block vagal reflexes), avoiding precipitating factors, e.g., hypoxia, etc.
- Adequate earthing of electronic appliances during catheterization (to avoid electrocution)
- Desensitization, inquiry to be made regarding sensitivity to drugs
- Training radiological staff, as it is common with radiologic investigations

Q14. What are the drugs used in the management of cardiac arrest?
Ans.
- *Ventricular fibrillation:* An unsynchronized DC shock is required immediately, and between shocks, external cardiac compression and mouth-to-mouth ventilation are performed. If these are unsuccessful, the following drugs may help, particularly if hypoxia and acidosis can be controlled:
  - Lignocaine
  - Adrenaline 1 mg intravenous (IV) results in more vigorous and coarse fibrillation that is more responsive to defibrillation; it is by improving coronary flow.
  - Bretylium tosylate IV if lignocaine fails
  - Amiodarone IV may be of short-term benefit in patients with recurrent VT or VF.
  - Propranolol IV for recurrent VT/VF in the setting of ischemic ventricular asystole
  - Atropine 0.5–1.0 mg IV (up to 2 mg) is effective in asystole due to vagal activation associated with anesthesia, diagnostic procedures, and surgery
  - Calcium gluconate IV 2–4 mg/kg or 0.5–1.0 g of oral dose if calcium channel blockers, hypocalcemia, or hyperkalemia is the cause.
- *Electromechanical dissociation:*
  - Epinephrine 1 mg IV in 5 minutes
  - Calcium chloride IV has been used, but with doubtful benefit.
  - *Drugs for precipitating factors:* For acidosis, $NaHCO_3$, dose 1 mEq/kg, is repeated once every 15 minutes. In asystole, DC shocks have not been demonstrated to have any benefit and may, in fact, produce a stunned myocardium, leading to a delay in the return to rhythm.

Q15. Does $NaHCO_3$ help in cardiac arrest? What is the risk in its administration?
Ans. Acidosis often complicates cardiac arrest that may be corrected by $NaHCO_3$.

Dose: Amount required = 5 × weight (in kg) × deficit of $NaHCO_3$ (in mEq/kg) 8.4% solution of $NaHCO_3$ contains 1 mEq/mL of $NaHCO_3$ 1 mg/kg given, and repeated every 15 minutes, acid–base status should be assessed before further injection. Risk: Excessive quantity of $NaHCO_3$ may overload the circulation and pulmonary edema may result.

Q16. What are the ALS measures for different electrical events causing cardiac arrest?
Ans.
- *Ventricular fibrillation:* CPR and defibrillation as early as possible; if unsuccessful after three shocks, injection adrenaline 1 mg IV followed by CPR for 1 minute, and then defibrillation is repeated (up to three cycles)
- *Sustained VT:* CPR and defibrillation
- *Asystole:* CPR, atropine, adrenaline, and pacing
- *Pulseless electrical activity:* CPR and look for reversible causes

Q17. What is SCD? How does death occur in SCD?
Ans. Sudden cardiac death refers to any natural death from a cardiac cause occurring within an hour of the onset of acute symptoms. Pre-existing heart disease may have been known to be present, but the time and mode of death are unexpected. SCD is therefore always nontraumatic and should be unexpected and instantaneous. Most episodes occur in persons with structural heart diseases, most commonly coronary artery disease (CAD). 80% of episodes of SCD are primary, i.e., without any precipitating factor. The risk of recurrence is high for these patients. A secondary episode of SCD is one in which a precipitating factor can be identified, such as acute myocardial ischemia or AMI, drug toxicity or proarrhythmia, decompensated CHF, or severe electrolyte imbalance. The risk of recurrence is less here. Controlling the precipitating factors prevents recurrence.

A quarter of SCDs may be due to noncardiac causes such as pulmonary embolism, aortic rupture, intracranial bleeding, etc.

The cause of death in SCD is cardiac arrest. Most episodes are due to malignant ventricular arrhythmia-VF and sustained VT, usually rapidly degenerating to VF. Asystole and EMD are some causes found in increasing proportion as the time since arrest increases.

Q18. What are the etiologies of SCD?
Ans. *Ischemic heart disease*: AMI and chronic IHD. 85% cause of SCD is IHD.
- Non-IHD
  - *Cardiomyopathies:* Dilated and hypertrophic
  - *Valvular heart diseases:* Aortic stenosis, mitral valve prolapse (MVP), aortic regurgitation (AR), and infective endocarditis
  - *Congenital heart diseases:* Tetralogy of Fallot (TOF) and transposition of the great arteries (TGA) (post-Mustard or Senning)

- *Primary electrical abnormalities:* Long QT syndrome (LQTS), WPW syndrome, complete heart block (CHB), and Brugada syndrome (BrS)
- *Electrolyte abnormalities:* Hypokalemia, hypomagnesemia, and hypocalcemia
- *Drugs:* Antiarrhythmic agents (Class Ia), erythromycin, terfenadine, tricyclic antidepressants, cisapride, cocaine, alcohol, and organophosphates

Q19. What is the "rule of the 50s" in SCD?
Ans.
- Sudden cardiac death accounts for 50% of all cardiovascular (CV) deaths
- Approximately, 50% of all SCDs are the unexpected first expression of a cardiac disorder
- Sudden cardiac death often strikes during the victim's productive years, accounting for up to 50% of years of potential life lost from heart diseases.

Q20. What are the causes of SCD in patients without structural heart diseases?
Ans. In 5–10% of SCD victims, no structural heart disease can be found at autopsy. Genetic ion channel disorders ("channelopathies") may be responsible. These are:
- *Long QT syndrome:* It is a heterogeneous disorder with genetic variations of different potassium and sodium channels characterized by delayed cardiac repolarization and a propensity to syncope and SCD. Torsades de pointes (TdP), a self-limiting ventricular tachyarrhythmia, sometimes degenerating into VF and SCD, is the mechanism. SCD is usually precipitated by sympathetic stimuli such as physical activity (particularly swimming and diving into cold water) or emotional stress. A number of drugs, such as erythromycin, anti-Parkinsonian, antidepressants, and cisapride (removed from the market), can induce LQTS.
- *Brugada syndrome:* It is caused by a genetically determined loss or reduction of Na+ channel. There is a coved ST-segment elevation in the right precordial leads (V1 and V2). There is a loss of action potential dome in the epicardium but not in the endocardium. It generates a transmural gradient that predisposes to re-entry, premature ventricular contractions (PVCs), polymorphic VT, and VF. It may be triggered by sodium channel blockers, fever, vagotonic agents, betablockers, antidepressants, hypokalemia, etc. SCD typically occurs during sleep or at rest.
- *Catecholaminergic polymorphic VT:* It is an inherited disorder characterized by adrenergically mediated polymorphic VT in a setting of physical or emotional stress.
- *Short QT syndrome (SQTS):* It is a rare inherited channelopathy associated with SCD and AF. A QTc interval shorter than 0.36 seconds shortens ventricular refractory periods, increases the dispersion of repolarization, and predisposes to re-entry.

Q21. What are the causes of SCD in young persons?
Ans. Sudden cardiac death is by far the first manifestation of underlying cardiac disease in the majority of young persons. The most common causes during the first and second decades of life are:
- *Coronary artery disease:* Congenital anomalies of the coronary arteries, atherosclerotic CAD, and aortic dissection involving coronary arteries
- *Myocardial disease:* Myocarditis and hypertrophic cardiomyopathies (HOCMs)
- *Congenital heart disease:* Aortic stenosis and surgically corrected TOF and TGA
- *Others:* Arrhythmias associated with MVP, congenital arrhythmogenic disorders, and conduction system abnormalities

Q22. Who are the survivors of SCD? How does it occur?
Ans. In the true sense, a victim of SCD cannot survive (as nobody returns to life after death). The survivors of SCD are actually those surviving an episode of cardiac arrest, i.e., the condition that may produce death of a person with SCD if he or she has not been resuscitated. These are cases of "aborted SCD."

The most important determinant of successful resuscitation is the time interval from cardiac arrest to initiation of intervention. Early institution of BLS and ALS measures provides survival in such situations. Since most patients are found in VF, the time to successful defibrillation is a key element to survival. Again, the earlier the CPR is performed, the greater the proportion of patients to be found in VF as opposed to asystole or EMD. Thus, successful defibrillation is likely when early CPR is performed.

Q23. What are the risk factors for SCD? How to identify them?
Ans. Factors that increase the risk for SCD are:
- Coronary artery disease: Active or provocable ischemia, more than one previous myocardial infarction (MI)
- Left ventricular (LV) dysfunction with ejection fraction (EF) <30% and CHF
- *Cardiac rhythm disturbances:* Complex ventricular ectopy, inducible VT, and autonomic dysfunction
- Survivors of SCD
- Cardiac syncope
- Left ventricular hypertrophy
- *Lifestyle factors:* Cigarette smoking (increase myocardial O_2 demand and decrease coronary flow), alcohol abuse (increase ventricular arrhythmia), emotional stress, and competitive sports in athletes with HOCM.

Survivors of SCD should have a detailed CV evaluation on reversible precipitating factors, and the underlying causes must be identified and treated.

Risks of recurrent SCD—identification:
- *Electrocardiogram:* For evidence of MI or ischemia, intraventricular conduction delay, accessory pathway (WPW syndrome), prolonged QT interval, and LV hypertrophy
- *Ambulatory ECG monitoring:* Several findings predict a higher recurrence rate of SCD—presence of atrioventricular block or intraventricular conduction defects, prolonged QT interval, increase in resting heart rate >10 beats/min, detection of nonsustained VT, and reduced heart rate variability (baroreflex sensitivity)
- *Echocardiography:* Measurement of LV function, valvular diseases, and cardiomyopathy (including HOCM)
- Stress techniques (exercise or pharmacologic) with radionuclide imaging in CAD to detect myocardial ischemia and/or viability
- *Coronary angiography:* Assessment of CAD or coronary anomalies
- *Signal-averaged ECG:* Late potentials in ECG predict the future development of sustained VT and SCD
- Electrophysiologic study in survivors of cardiac arrest may reveal the mechanism of arrest, help in the implantation of an implantable cardioverter defibrillator (ICD), and have prognostic significance

Q24. How to prevent SCD?
Ans.
- Identification of individuals at risk for SCD from history, findings of physical examination, and investigations
- *Pharmacologic agents:* As the majority of episodes of SCD occur in patients with CAD, agents that reduce myocardial ischemia, prevent or limit the extent of myocardial dysfunction or ventricular arrhythmia in patients with congenital prolonged QT syndrome, and arrhythmogenic right ventricular (RV) dysfunction are used. ICD is superior to antiarrhythmic agents in the secondary prevention of SCD. Prevention of remodeling after MI reduces the incidence of SCD. Myocardial reperfusion with a thrombolytic agent or revascularization with percutaneous intervention (PCI) decreases mortality. Drugs that help prevent SCD are:
  - Betablockers
  - Angiotensin-converting enzyme (ACE) inhibitors prevent remodeling after MI and reduce SCD in patients with CHF and LV dysfunction.
  - *Anti-arrhythmic agents:* Amiodarone has been shown to reduce SCD. In patients with CHF who are at high risk for SCD, prophylactic therapy with amiodarone has been shown to decrease mortality. Sotalol, by its beta-blocking effect, is also effective in preventing SCD.
- *Implantable cardioverter defibrillator:* It has the ability to detect lethal ventricular arrhythmias and to deliver a shock to terminate it. ICD can offer protection against both tachycardiac and bradycardiac SCD (both

primary and secondary). Pacemakers may prevent bradycardia and pauses in congenital LQTS and in patients with HOCM (dual-chamber pacing). Automatic external defibrillation (AED) is designed to be used by emergency personnel for victims of out-of-hospital SCD.
- *Surgical therapy:* Coronary artery bypass grafting (CABG) reduces SCD in patients with triple-vessel CAD and LV dysfunction (primary prevention). As secondary prevention of recurrent cardiac arrest and SCD, it is done in patients with critical CAD with significant myocardium at risk of ischemia and in patients with no inducible monomorphic ventricular arrhythmia at electrophysiology study (EPS).

SUGGESTED READING

1. 2005 American Heart Association Guidelines for Cardiopulmonary Resuscitation and Emergency Cardiovascular Care. Circulation. 2005;112:151-203.
2. American Heart Association: 2010 American Heart Association Guidelines for Cardiopulmonary Resuscitation and Emergency Cardiovascular Care. [online] Available from http://www.heart.org. [Last accessed May, 2025].
3. John J, Gordon AE. Cardiopulmonary and cardiocerebral resuscitation. In: Hurst's The Heart, 13th edition. New York City, NY, USA: McGraw-Hill; 2011.
4. Robert JM, Agustin C. Cardiac arrest and sudden cardiac death. In: Libby P, Bonow RO, Mann DL, Zipes DP (Eds). Brunwald's Heart Disease: A Textbook of Cardiovascular Medicine, 8th edition. Philadelphia, PA, USA: Saunders; 2008.

CHAPTER 15

Syncope and Hypotension

> *"Syncope was once thought to be God's curse or weird and use to be treated by people knowing witchcraft."*
> —History of Cardiology

▰ INTRODUCTION

Hypotension resulting in a reduction in blood flow to the reticular activating system of the brain stem may result in transient loss of consciousness, followed by quick recovery known as syncope. Cardiac syncope may be an early sign of sudden cardiac death.

Q1. Define hypotension. What is postural hypotension?
Ans. Hypotension in adults is defined as a blood pressure (BP) of <90/60 mm Hg. If hypotension is accompanied by features of widespread tissue hypoperfusion, such as mental obtundation, confusion, restlessness, oliguria, etc., the condition is called shock (cardiogenic shock, if the cause is cardiac). In cardiogenic shock, BP is usually <80/60 mm Hg.

A reduction of systolic BP of at least 20 mm Hg or a diastolic BP of 10 mm Hg within 3 minutes of quiet standing is defined as orthostatic hypotension.

Q2. What is syncope?
Ans. Syncope is defined as a transient loss of consciousness associated with a loss of postural tone, with spontaneous recovery due to a reduction of blood flow to the reticular activating system in the brain stem. Cessation of cerebral blood flow leads to unconsciousness within 10 seconds. Syncope may be the only warning sign before sudden cardiac death occurs.

Syncope has the following features:
- Onset is sudden.
- Loss of consciousness is complete.
- Recovery is spontaneous; there is no stupor or coma.

Q3. What are the causes of cardiac syncope?
Ans.
- *Arrhythmic:*
  - Tachyarrhythmias: Ventricular—ventricular tachycardia (VT), ventricular fibrillation (VF), long QT syndrome, and supraventricular—atrial fibrillation (AF), atrial flutter, supraventricular tachycardia (SVT), Wolff-Parkinson-White (WPW) syndrome, and pacemaker-mediated

- Bradyarrhythmias: Sinus node dysfunction (sick sinus syndrome) and atrioventricular (AV) block
- *Obstructive:*
  - Left-sided—aortic stenosis, hypertrophic cardiomyopathy (HCM), tight mitral stenosis (MS), atrial myxoma, and prosthetic valve dysfunction
  - Right-sided—pulmonary stenosis, pulmonary hypertension, tetralogy of Fallot, and pulmonary embolism
- Miscellaneous—inferior myocardial infarction (MI), mitral valve prolapse (MVP), neurocardiogenic syncope, carotid sinus syncope, etc.

Q4. What is the difference between syncope and cardiac arrest?

Ans. Both conditions lead to loss of consciousness. But cardiac arrest is a grave condition needing basic life support (BLS) and advanced life support (ALS). The differences between the two are given in **Table 15.1**.

TABLE 15.1: Differences between syncope and cardiac arrest.

Syncope	Cardiac arrest
It may be cardiac as well as noncardiac in origin, e.g., neurogenic	Cardiac cause—VT, VF, asystole
Loss of consciousness is transient and reversible	The unconscious is not reversible unless intervened with life support measures
No stupor or coma	Stupor or coma supervenes
Usually, no immediate mortality	Definite immediate mortality
Life support measures (BLS and ALS) rarely needed; spontaneous recovery occurs	BLS, ALS needed; no spontaneous recovery

(ALS: advanced life support; BLS: basic life support; VF: ventricular fibrillation; VT: ventricular tachycardia)

Q5. What are the characteristic features of arrhythmic syncope?

Ans. Arrhythmias (brady- or tachyarrhythmias) may produce a catastrophic fall in cardiac output, as a result of a very slow or very fast heart rate in a patient with limited cardiac reserve.

The features are as follows:
- Syncope occurs in patients with underlying heart disease.
- Palpitation is a frequent symptom prior to the attack of syncope.
- Syncope is not associated with postural changes.
  Some patients may develop cardiac arrest.

Q6. What is the difference between cardiac and neurogenic syncope?

Ans. In neurogenic syncope, a combination of vasodepression and vasovagal features results in fainting. There is a profound fall in BP due to vasodilatation with bradycardia due to vasovagal reaction **(Table 15.2)**.

TABLE 15.2: Differences between neurogenic and cardiac syncope.

Neurogenic	Cardiac
Structural heart disease absent	Present
Associated with postural change; usually develops when standing, rarely when sitting, and virtually never when lying or walking	Not associated with posture. Obstructive varieties may be precipitated by exertion
Precipitating circumstances—sudden severe pain, trauma, fright, emotional stress, a hot, crowded environment, usually recurrent	Nil
• Warning signs—weakness, nausea, abdominal discomfort, diaphoresis, and unsteadiness for seconds are usually present • Head up till the test is positive	Nil Not needed

Q7. How does syncope occur in ischemic heart disease?
Ans. In IHD, syncope may occur due to the following:
- *Acute MI:* Acute inferior MI may produce significant bradycardia and hypotension that predispose to presyncope or syncope [hence angiotensin-converting enzyme inhibitors (ACEIs), beta-blockers, and diuretics are to be avoided during the first few hours except if congestive heart failure (CHF) occurs]. Acute anterior MI may produce syncope due to arrhythmia—sustained rapid VT or symptomatic nonsustained VT may cause syncope.
- Reduced cardiac output (COP) by severe regional or global ischemia with pre-existing left ventricular (LV) impairment
- Drug-induced-glyceryl trinitrate (GTN) syncope due to excessive vasodilatation, beta-blockers, and calcium channel blockers producing heart block and reduced COP

Q8. How does syncope occur in obstructive cardiac lesions?
Ans. Here, syncope occurs because of restriction of COP, frequently with exertion, peripheral vascular resistance falls, but the COP is fixed, leading to hypotension. Ventricular arrhythmia frequently occurs at the time of syncope. Aortic stenosis is sometimes associated with AV block.

Q9. What are the causes of syncope in the elderly?
Ans.
- Orthostatic hypotension
- Postprandial hypotension (after 1 hour of meal)
- Medications
- Aortic stenosis
- Carotid sinus hypersensitivity
- Bradyarrhythmias—sick sinus syndrome and heart block

Q10. What is orthostatic hypotension? What drugs cause it?

Ans. A 20 mm Hg drop in systolic or a 10 mm Hg drop in diastolic BP within 3 minutes of standing, resulting in syncope, is leveled as orthostatic hypotension.

Drug causes are diuretics, alpha-adrenergic blockers (labetalol and terazosin), adrenergic neuron blockers (guanethidine), ACEI, antidepressants, alcohol, ganglion blocking agents (hexamethonium), tranquilizers (barbiturates), vasodilators (calcium blockers, hydralazine, and prazosin), and centrally acting antihypertensives (alpha-methyl dopa and clonidine).

Other causes are primary autonomic failure (Parkinsonism, Shy–Drager syndrome), aging, Guillain–Barré syndrome, etc.

Q11. How does Holter monitoring help in syncope?

Ans. It allows an arrhythmic cause of syncope to be established or excluded. Current guidelines recommend that it be used in patients who have clinical or electrocardiogram (ECG) features suggestive of an arrhythmogenic syncope or a history of recurrent syncope with injury or suggestive of an arrhythmogenic syncope to guide subsequent examination, such as an electrophysiology (EP) study. Holter monitoring is most likely to be diagnostic when used in occasional patients with frequent (e.g., daily) episodes of syncope or presyncope.

Q12. How to investigate patients with cardiac syncope?

Ans. The nature of the investigation is dictated by the history and findings of the physical examination **(Table 15.3)**.

TABLE 15.3: Investigations in syncope and their interpretation.

Investigation	Interpretation
ECG	Arrhythmias, atrioventricular block, pre-excitation, LVH, MI, or obstructive valvular lesions (AS, PS, TOF), etc.
Echocardiography	Myocardial disease and LV function (as an indicator of prognosis; before septal myomectomy or septal ablation for HOCM, repair of valve as in valvular obstruction, CABG in life-threatening arrhythmia due to ischemia
Exercise ECG	Arrhythmia and hypotension induced by exercise in arrhythmic and obstructive syncope (resuscitation equipment should be at hand). Inducible myocardial ischemia as a contributor is evaluated (HCM to be excluded prior to exercise ECG)
Ambulatory ECG	Documents arrhythmias and relates them to symptoms (by patient-activated event recorder), aids in defining therapeutic response. Sinus pause >2 seconds, Mobitz type II or complete heart block, and runs of nonsustained VT should be taken seriously

Contd...

Contd...

Investigation	Interpretation
Signal average ECG	Presence of high frequency low amplitude signals in the terminal portion of ECG (late potential) suggests a substrate for reentrant ventricular arrhythmia
Invasive electrophysiologic study	Done in patients with organic heart disease and syncope in whom noninvasive evaluation is negative. Defines conduction system disease, elicits supraventricular and ventricular tachycardias, and measures their hemodynamic effect and response to pharmacologic and pacing interventions

(AS: aortic stenosis; CABG: coronary artery bypass graft; ECG: electrocardiogram; HCM: hypertrophic cardiomyopathy; HOCM: hypertrophic obstructive cardiomyopathy; LV: left ventricular; LVH: left ventricular hypertrophy; MI: myocardial infarction; PS: pulmonary stenosis; TOF: tetralogy of Fallot; VT: ventricular tachycardia)

SUGGESTED READING

1. Gregoratos G, Abrams J, Epstein AE, Freedman RA, Hayes DL, Hlatky MA, et al. ACC/AHA task force on Practice guidelines/North American society for Pacing and electrophysiology committee to update the 1998 Pacemaker Guidelines: ACC/AHA/NASPE 2002 guideline update for implantation of cardiac pacemakers and antiarrhythmic devices: summary article: a report of the American college of Cardiology/American Heart association task force on Practice Guidelines (ACC/AHA/NASPE Committee to update the 1998 pacemaker guidelines). Circulation. 2002;106:2145.
2. Hugh C, Douglas PZ. Hypotension and syncope. In: Libby P, Bonow RO, Mann DL, Zipes DP (Eds). Brunwald's Heart disease: A Textbook of Cardiovascular Medicine, 8th edition. Saunders: Philadelphia, PA; 2008.
3. Strickberger SA, Benson DW, Biaggioni I, Callans DJ, Cohen MI, Ellenbogen KA, et al. AHA/ACCF scientific statement on the evaluation of syncope. Circulation. 2006;113:316.

CHAPTER 16

Cardiac Pacing (Including Implantable Cardioverter Defibrillator, Cardiac Resynchronization Therapy and EP Study)

"Pacemaker evolved primarily as a life saving device for patients with complete heart block, now used as an aid to alleviate symptoms in heart failure."
—History of Cardiology

■ INTRODUCTION

Pacemakers and other implantable devices for the management of cardiac arrhythmias have undergone tremendous growth and evolution since the introduction of transvenous pacing in the late 1950s. Advancement of electronics, computer technology, power source (i.e., battery), and miniaturization of pacemaker generators have contributed to the rapid development of the field of pacing. The use of implantable devices extends from bradycardia management to tachycardia (antitachycardia pacing) to management of sudden cardiac death (SCD) by implantable cardioverter defibrillator (ICD) and heart failure management by cardiac resynchronization therapy (CRT).

Q1. What is a pacemaker? What are the basic components of a pacemaker generator?

Ans. A pacemaker is a device that delivers battery-supplied electrical stimuli over leads with electrodes in contact with the heart.

Essential components of a pacemaker generator are:
- *Power source (battery):* Lithium-iodine is the chemical commonly used, having a longer end of life with more predictable behavior.
- *Circuitry:*
  - Output circuits—control programmable features of the pulse, including amplitude and pulse width
  - Sensing circuits—process the intracardiac electrocardiogram (ECG), including external electromagnetic interference (EMI)
  - Timing circuits—control the pacing intervals and sensing and refractory periods. They may be altered by input from the sensing circuits.
- *Others (present in some generators):*
  - Telemetry circuits—allow communication between an external programmer and the pulse generator for pacemaker programming and retrieval of information

- Microprocessor—computer chips with memory. These allow downloading of new features by means of telemetry and increased storage for diagnostic data.
- Sensor circuits—for rate-responsive pacing

Q2. What are the types of pacemakers?

Ans. Categories of pacemaker varies according to its duration of pacing, polarity and chamber paced **(Box 16.1)**.

BOX 16.1: Types of pacemakers.

- According to the duration of pacemaker function—temporary and permanent
- According to the polarity of the pacemaker lead:
  - *Unipolar:* Leads have one terminal (−); the device can act as the positive terminal
  - *Bipolar:* Has two terminals at the lead tip; the current path is short, and the pacing signal is small on ECG. Extracardiac potentials are less likely to interfere with function
- According to the chamber paced:
  - Single-chamber pacemakers—carry a single lead within the RA or RV. Single-chamber atrial (e.g., AAI) pacemakers are used in sick sinus syndrome. Single-chamber ventricular (e.g., VVI) pacemakers are used in atrial fibrillation with symptomatic bradycardia **(Figs. 16.1A and B)**
  - Dual-chamber pacemakers–carry two leads in the RA or RV. This allows sequential pacing of atria and ventricles (e.g., DDD) or ventricular pacing in synchrony with the patient's intrinsic atrial rhythm in CHB (VDD mode)

(CHB: complete heart block; ECG: electrocardiogram; RA: right atrium; RV: right ventricle)

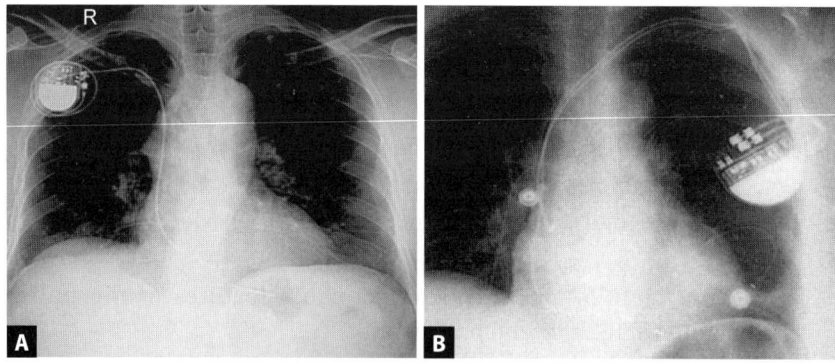

Figs. 16.1A and B: Single-chamber (VVI) pacemaker (A); dual-chamber (DDD) pacemaker (B).

Q3. How are pacemaker units coded?

Ans. Pacemaker units have been classified to enable operators to identify the capabilities of individual units. The three-letter code is now in general use:

First letter—relates to the chamber(s) paced:
    O = none
    A = atrium
    V = ventricle
    D = dual (A+V)

Second letter—relates to the chamber(s) sensed:
>O = none
>A = atrium
>V = ventricle
>D = dual (A+V)

Third letter indicates the pacemaker's response to the sensed impulse:
>O = none
>T = triggered
>I = inhibited
>D = dual (T+I)

To cope with the facilities available on new programmable units, the three-letter code has been expanded to a five-code:

Fourth letter—relates to programmability and rate modulation:
>O = none
>P = simple programmable
>in = multiprogrammable
>C = communicating
>R = rate-adaptive sensor

Fifth letter—relates to antitachyarrhythmia function:
>O = none
>P = pacing (antitachyarrhythmia)
>S = shock
>D = dual (P+S)

Q4. What are unipolar and bipolar pacemakers? Give their advantages and disadvantages?
Ans. Pacemaker may be unipolar or bipolar according to the electrode configuration of the pacing lead or the configuration of the pulse generator.

Unipolar: Cathode (negative) is on the lead tip, and the anode (positive) is the pacemaker can. It results in a large sensing antenna. A large pacemaker artifact (spikes) on the ECG is caused by the proximity of the circuit to the ECG electrodes.

Advantages: Better sensing of ventricular extrasystoles, low-amplitude signals, and shifted axis.

Disadvantages:
- Oversensing of external signals, especially myopotentials (i.e., pectoralis muscle activity)
- Skeletal muscle stimulation—twitching may occur
- Large pacemaker spikes on ECG may obscure native wave structure.

Bipolar: The electrodes are at the stimulating end of the lead—the cathode (negative) at the distal tip and the anode (positive) at the proximal ring.

It results in a smaller sensing antenna. A smaller pacemaker artifact (spikes) on the ECG results.

Advantages:
- Less myopotential oversensing
- Less skeletal muscle stimulation
- Smaller pacemaker spikes on ECG do not obscure native wave structure.

Disadvantages:
- More complex lead design is more susceptible to malfunction and failure.
- Small pacemaker spikes on ECG may be difficult to see.

Q5. Compare and contrast between temporary and permanent pacemaker.

Ans. Both are electronic devices to treat symptomatic bradycardia producing hemodynamic compromise **(Figs. 16.2A and B)**. TPMs are external devices used for short periods of time. PPMs are internally implanted devices intended for long-term control **(Table 16.1)**.

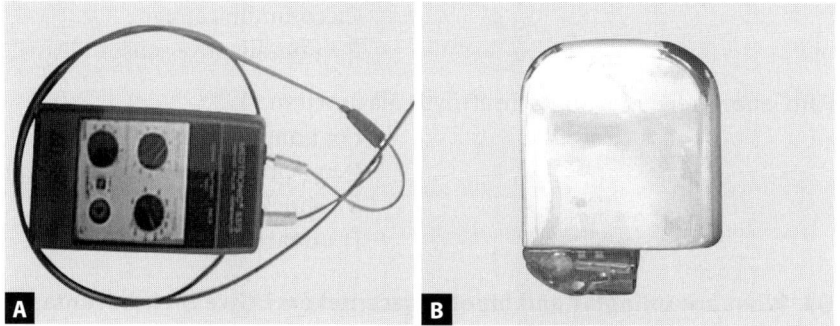

Figs. 16.2A and B: TPM generator (A) and PPM generator (B).

TABLE 16.1: Comparison between temporary and permanent pacemaker generators.

Points	TPM	PPM
Generator type	Bipolar	Unipolar or bipolar
Location of the generator	External; portable	Internal, subcutaneous pocket in subclavicular location
Route and method of insertion	Femoral vein, subclavian, internal jugular, median basilic, by Seldinger technique	Cephalic or subclavian, axillary, basilic vein (sometimes)
Chamber paced	Single chamber—RV apex	Single or dual chamber
Duration of pacing	7–14 days	>10 years (in simple demand pacemaker)- depending of battery life*

Contd...

Contd...

Points	TPM	PPM
Power source	Alkaline battery	Lithium-iodine battery
Reuse of the generator	Always done	Usually not done
Indications	As a bridge to PPM, especially for patients who are unable to undergo immediate PPM or for patients whose bradycardia is severe and hemodynamically unstable	Symptomatic bradyarrhythmias of long duration

*Depends on the current output required for capture, the requirement for incessant or intermittent pacing, and the number of chambers paced.

Q6. What are the indications for temporary pacing?
Ans.
- *In acute myocardial infarction (MI):*
  - Asystole and complete heart block (CHB)—in anterior or inferior infarction with hemodynamic instability
  - Second-degree atrioventricular (AV) block—Mobitz Type II AV block, usually in association with anterior infarction. It carries a high risk of developing complete AV block. Prophylactic pacing is done.
  - Bundle branch block—Patients with evidence of trifascicular disease* or nonadjacent bifascicular disease** complicating MI (should be prophylactically paced).
  - Others—symptomatic bradycardia (sinus pause >3.5 seconds) and transient asystole not responding to atropine
- As a bridge to permanent pacing in permanent symptomatic bradycardia, e.g., in CHB and sick sinus syndrome
- *During cardiac surgery:* Surgery adjacent to the AV node and bundle of His, e.g., aortic valve replacement (AVR) for calcific aortic stenosis (AS) (calcium extending into the site of the AV node). Tricuspid valve surgery in Ebstein's anomaly, ostium primum atrial septal defect (ASD), and AV canal defects, and corrected transposition of the great artery (TGA).
- Prophylactically—during right heart catheterization in patients with LBBB, electric cardioversion in patients with sick sinus syndrome
- Miscellaneous—drug overdose (e.g., digoxin, β-blocker, verapamil); termination of refractory tachyarrhythmias with overdrive pacing during electrophysiology (EP) study.

---

*Trifascicular disease: Right bundle branch block (RBBB) and left anterior hemiblock (LAHB) or left posterior hemiblock (LPHB) plus long PR interval, alternating RBBB and left bundle branch block (LBBB).
**Nonadjacent bifascicular disease: RBBB plus new LPHB.

Point to ponder:
Right bundle branch block in anterior myocardial infarction-left anterior descending (MI-LAD) supplies both RBBB and the anterior superior division of left bundle branch (LBB). The onset of RBBB, especially with left-axis deviation, often precedes infranodal heart block. An abrupt transition can occur from 1:1 conduction to Mobitz Type II block or complete asystole. The lack of escape rhythm makes this particularly dangerous and warrants TPM even with only the onset of RBBB in anterior MI.

Q7. What are the indications of permanent pacing?
Ans. In general, permanent pacing is instituted for persistent or intermittent symptomatic bradycardia. It is indicated in long-standing conditions resulting from the failure of impulse formation and conduction.
- Acquired chronic complete AV block—symptomatic (Stokes-Adams attack) or with ventricular rate <40 beats/min, irrespective of symptoms (asymptomatic is unusual)
- *Mobitz Type II AV block:* Progressive, predictable, and may result in Stokes-Adams attack.
- Chronic bundle branch block—symptomatic patients with bifascicular block and patients with trifascicular disease (such as RBBB with alternating LAHB/LPHB, LBBB with alternating RBBB, or LBBB plus long PR interval)
- *Post-MI:* Persistent complete AV block or Mobitz type II AV block following anterior infarction. If such a block regresses during a hospital stay, subsequent Holter monitoring may help identify subjects at risk who need permanent pacing.
- Sick sinus syndrome—when it is documented in association with symptomatic bradycardia or symptoms that arise from drug-induced bradycardia (used to control tachyarrhythmias).
- Congenital complete AV block—in the presence of rate-related symptoms, failure of the AV node to respond to exercise, or a daytime ventricular rate <50 beats/min (carries a higher long-term risk of syncope or sudden death). Asymptomatic children may survive into adult life when permanent pacing is easier to insert.
- Carotid sinus hypersensitivity with recurrent syncope

Q8. What are the indications of epicardial lead placement in PPM?
Ans. Here, a pacing wire is attached to the epicardium with a thoracotomy or by subxiphoid route. The permanent unit is usually intra-abdominal (extraperitoneal below the rectus muscle). It is less reliable in the long term; wire displacement and fracture may occur due to kinking and vigorous movement.

Epicardial lead placement is done:
- In infants weighing <7–8 kg, small children—where rapid growth makes transvenous pacing difficult
- When the chest is already open, i.e., in the course of a cardiac operation, when heart block develops during surgery
- When transvenous access cannot be obtained
- If endocardial lead placement cannot be achieved

Q9. What are the steps in PPM implantation?
Ans. The subclavian method is commonly used in PPM implantation. The subclavian vein passes over the first rib behind the medial third of the clavicle to join the internal jugular vein in forming the innominate vein. It lies just anterior to the subclavian artery and the apical pleura. The head turned to the right (for left-sided puncture). Ensure adequate hydration. The patient is not to inhale deeply with head down and do Valsalva maneuver during puncture **(Fig. 16.3)**.

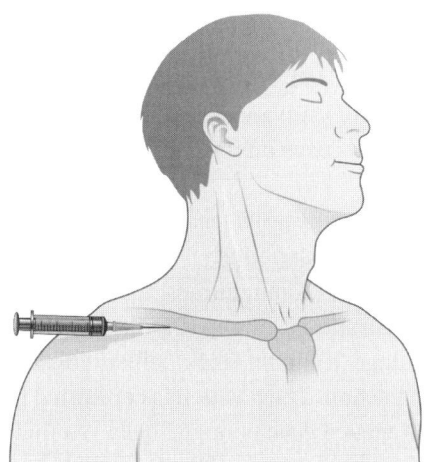

Fig. 16.3: Subclavian puncture for PPM implantation.

- Infiltrate 5–10 mL of 1% lignocaine into subcutaneous (SC) tissue 1–2 cm below the clavicle and two third distance from the sternoclavicular to the acromioclavicular joint; infiltrate toward the suprasternal notch.
- Another 5–10 mL of lignocaine 1% given SC along the line of the planned incision, the line of lead insertion, and in the area of the pacemaker pocket.
- Introduce the access needle just lateral to the midclavicular line at an angle of 15° both to the long axis of the clavicle and to the chest wall. Advance the needle slowly toward the suprasternal notch, keeping close to the underside of the clavicle (horizontally and nearly parallel to the

- clavicle) and above the first rib until the vein is entered at a depth of 4–5 cm. Vary the angle slightly if the vein is missed at the first pass.
- Flexible j-shaped guidewire is inserted (using Seldinger technique). The guidewire is left in situ and secured with the help of an artery forceps.
- Two separate punctures are done for dual-chamber pacemaker.
- Incision and pocket is made (by blunt dissection).
- Plastic sheath with a central dilator is fed over the guidewire and gently pushed to its full length into the vein to dilate it.
- Inner dilator is removed, leaving a port entry into the vein; the orifice is covered with fingertip to stop blood leakage.
- The lead is fed into the superior vena cava (SVC) immediately under fluoroscopy. The introducer sheath peeled out (after pulling it out of the vein) from the lead.
- Lead is now manipulated into the appropriate place. J-curve made at distal 3 cm of stylet (supplied with the pacemaker), fed into lead, and advanced into right atrium (RA).
- Lead advances until it passes through tricuspid and pulmonary valves.
- Stylet is taken out, and a soft, straight stylet is placed within 1–2 cm of the lead tip. Retract the lead slowly until it starts to fall toward the floor of the right ventricle (RV). Advance the lead smoothly until it reaches the RV apex. Leave enough curve on the lead that it does not straighten with deep breaths.
- In dual chamber pacing, the atrial lead (j-shaped) is positioned in the RA appendage (located anterosuperiorly)
- Lead is fed into the SVC/RA junction using a soft, straight stylet. Retract the stylet, and the lead should curl up slightly. Lead advanced until it slips into the RA appendage. It should "flick" left and right in AP view because of appendage contraction. The position is confirmed in the right anterior oblique (RAO) 45° view. Leave enough "belly" so that the lead does not straighten out or fall into the body of the RA.
- Active lead fixation is done by rotating the lead hub, braced over a stylet when passive lead fixation is unstable, the lead is displaced, or when the apical position gives inadequate electrogram or threshold values (lead thresholds are usually quite high immediately after placement owing to tissue injury, but fall over 5–10 minutes).
- Electrogram (atrial and ventricular), threshold, and lead impedance are tested to see lead stability. Pacing at 10 V ("Ten volt test") is done to exclude diaphragmatic or phrenic nerve pacing. The threshold is rechecked if lead movement is suspected during device positioning.
- Pocket is made medial to incision in plane of prepectoral fascia. The pocket should be large enough to accommodate the pacemaker and lead without allowing undue movement.

- Leads home pushed and secure appropriate screw-on device header. Coil spare leads under the pacemaker and orient the device face-up.
- Pocket is closed using a layer of dissolvable sutures between the muscle and the opposing SC layer. One or two further layers of SC suturing are used to oppose skin edges. Skin closure is ideally done using subcuticular dissolvable sutures (to give a good cosmetic result).

Q10. What is the programmability of pacemakers?
Ans. It is the noninvasive, stable, reversible change in the operating parameters of an implanted pacemaker generator. Programmability is the means by which the cardiologist chooses the particular type of pacing program that is most suitable for an individual patient. Pacemaker programming is accomplished by activation of the programming head positioned over the implanted pulse generator after making the desired changes in programmable parameters. When three or more functions are altered, the system is called multiprogrammable. A handheld programmer is necessary.

These are:
- Pacing rate
- Energy output (with an adequate safety margin, exceeding the threshold voltage)
- Sensitivity (with an adequate safety margin, exceeding the threshold voltage for detecting sensed ECGs)
- *Hysteresis:* It refers to the escape interval from the sensed beat to the next paced beat. It is longer than the pacing rate, e.g., 50–70 hysteresis indicates that pacing at a rate of 70 beats/min will occur when the sinus rate falls below 60 beats/min; the sinus rate will emerge when the rate exceeds 70/min. It is particularly useful in sick sinus syndrome with a sinus rate marginally slower than the pacing rate. It is not desirable in atrial fibrillation (AF).
- Lead polarity—unipolar may be converted to bipolar (immune to external signals)
- Others—refractory period, AV delay, etc.

Advantages of programmability: (1) Selection of the most appropriate pacing parameter or mode; (2) Noninvasive diagnosis and correction of pacing malfunctions; and (3) Extension of pulse generator longevity by reduction of energy output.

Q11. What do you mean by sensing failure and oversensing?
Ans. Sensing failure means the pacemaker fails to notice an intrinsic cardiac impulse; hence, it is not inhibited. This is because the pacing unit is too insensitive or the R wave of the intrinsic ECG is too small or the slew rate is too slow. In a programmable pacing unit, the sensitivity may be increased, e.g., R wave sensitivity increased from 2 to 10 mV. A porous tip electrode may offer better sensitivity **(Fig. 16.4)**.

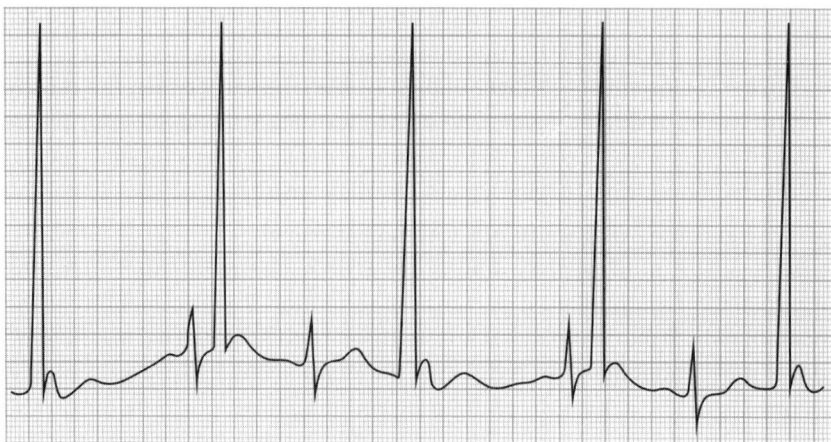

Fig. 16.4: Undersensing in VVI mode (pacemaker tries to pace because it has not sensed the intrinsic rhythm).

In oversensing, the pacemaker is inhibited by electrical signals other than the R wave, e.g., physiological myopotential signals from skeletal muscle (usually pectoral) or nonphysiological EMI, e.g., leak from microwave ovens, etc. In this setting, the pacemaker must be reprogrammed to a lower level **(Fig. 16.5)**.

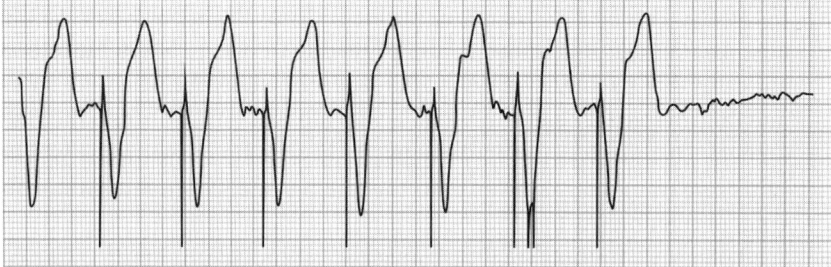

Fig. 16.5: Oversensing in VVI mode (pacemaker inhibited when it should pace).

Q12. What is pacemaker syndrome and pacemaker-mediated tachycardia (PMT)?

Ans. Pacemaker syndrome is a sign and symptom caused by inadequate timing of atrial and ventricular contractions. It is seen with VVI pacing because of an abnormal wave of depolarization. The retrograde ventriculoatrial (VA) conductions cause atrial contraction against closed mitral and tricuspid valves. The resulting low cardiac output (COP) and blood pressure (BP) produce vertigo, lightheadedness, and occasional syncope. This problem can be rectified by pacing the atrium prior to the ventricle using DVI or appropriately programmed DDD pacing. The problem can be exaggerated with VVIR pacing.

Pacemaker-mediated tachycardia—wide complex (paced) tachycardias sustained by the continued active participation of the pacemaker. PMT may appear, at first glance, to be ventricular tachycardia (VT), especially for pacemakers with bipolar leads. The pacing artifact may be difficult to discern on an ECG tracing.

PMT may be:
- When a dual chamber pacemaker attempts to track the rapid atrial rate during an atrial tachyarrhythmia, producing rapid ventricular pacing
- When oversensing occurs in the atrial channel, such as myopotential
- Endless loop tachycardia (ELT) occurs when a repetitive sequence of sensing of retrograde atrial activity triggers a ventricular pace beat.

Q13. Give the various indications of commonly used pacemaker units?
Ans.
- *VVI:* Here spontaneous QRS potentials are sensed by the pacemaker, and subsequent pacing stimulus is inhibited. A pacing stimulus then occurs at a set rate unless further spontaneous QRS potentials fall within that period **(Fig. 16.6)**. Devices are cheap. VVIR devices are suitable for those with AF (heart rate responds to activity and exercise).

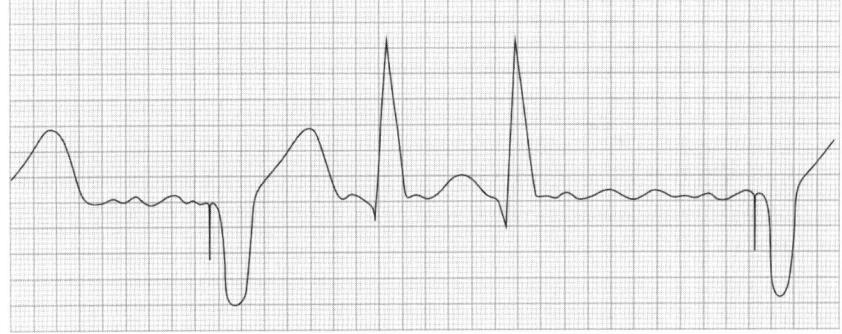

Fig. 16.6: ECG tracing in VVI mode.

It is the unit of choice in patients with AV block and AF, and sick sinus syndrome with atrial paralysis. It may be used in symptomatic bradycardia. Patients with AV block and persistent sinus node function will lose atrial contribution to ventricular filling as the atrium often contracts against closed AV valves. Retrograde VA conduction complicates the problem and produces pacemaker syndrome. Programmable VVI units may partly overcome this by being programmed to a lower rate or with hysteresis. VVI pacing in sinus rhythm may also induce AF by retrograde atrial contraction.
- *DVI (AV sequential pacing):* Both atrium and ventricles are paced, but only spontaneous ventricular activity is sensed **(Fig. 16.7)**. Spontaneous atrial

activity is ignored. After a spontaneous ventricular impulse is sensed, the unit resets to one V-A interval and fires an atrial impulse followed by a ventricular impulse. Spontaneous P wave occurring within this V-A interval is ignored.

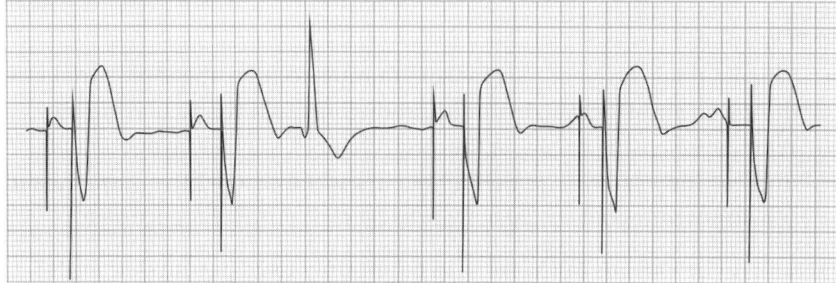

Fig. 16.7: ECG recording in DVI mode.

It can be used in complete AV block, pacemaker syndrome (atrial pacing prior to ventricular pacing prevents retrograde conduction), and sinus bradycardia. It cannot be used in AF.

- *VDD (P-synchronous pacing):* Single ventricular lead but also has sensing electrodes in RA to allow tracking atrial rhythm. Implantation is simpler than dual-chamber devices. P wave sensing results in ventricular pacing after an appropriate AV delay. If the atrial rate becomes very rapid, a specific pacemaker protects the ventricle from a rapid-paced rate. If a spontaneous P wave does not appear, the generator paces the ventricles on demand at its programmed rate. Spontaneous ventricular impulses inhibit the pacemaker, when it is reset to fire after a standby period **(Fig. 16.8)**.

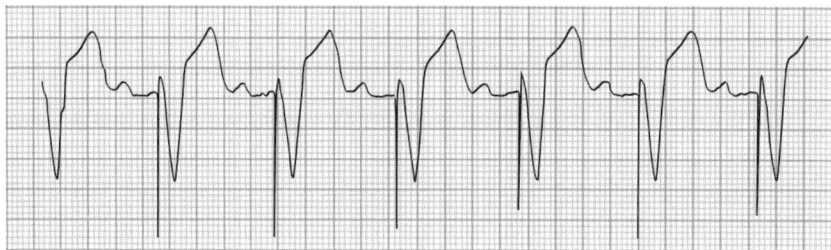

Fig. 16.8: ECG tracing in VDD mode: Atrial rhythm is sinus. After AV delay (programmed), a ventricular stimulus is delivered. Thus, the ventricular paced rate is the same as the sinus rate.

VDD is excellent for CHB in the presence of normal sinus node function. If AF develops, the pacemaker reverts to VVI mode (also occurs if the spontaneous atrial rate falls before the escape rate).

Disadvantage: Absence of atrial backup pacing in the event of sinus bradycardia. PMT may occur in the presence of retrograde conduction.
- *DDD:* Fully automated unit that paces and senses both the atrial and ventricular on demand. During sinus bradycardia, atrial (and, if necessary, ventricular) pacing occurs. During AV block, ventricular pacing occurs following either a spontaneous or a paced atrial impulse. Thus, ventricular pacing can occur in sequence with sinus activity (tracking), and normal rate response to exercise is maintained despite AV block **(Fig. 16.9)**.

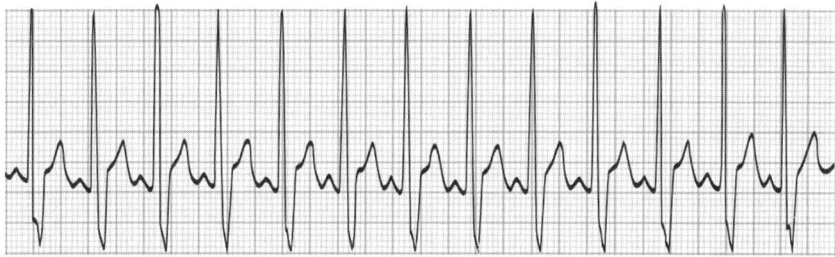

Fig. 16.9: DDD mode (ventricular pacing is triggered by sensed atrial activity).

DDDR devices are available for patients with chronotropic incompetence. It can be used in AV block with intact sinus node function and in sick sinus syndrome with additional AV node disease (an advance on the VDD). If AF develops, it also reverts to VVI mode (mode switching).

Q14. What is the difference between inhibited and triggered pacing?
Ans. Inhibition and triggering are the modes of response of the pacemaker unit to the sensed impulse. Inhibited mode is the demand pacing system. Pacing is inhibited by the sensed spontaneous cardiac impulse (atrial or ventricular). The pacemaker fires a stimulus only after a preset interval if no further impulse is sensed **(Figs. 16.10A and B)**.

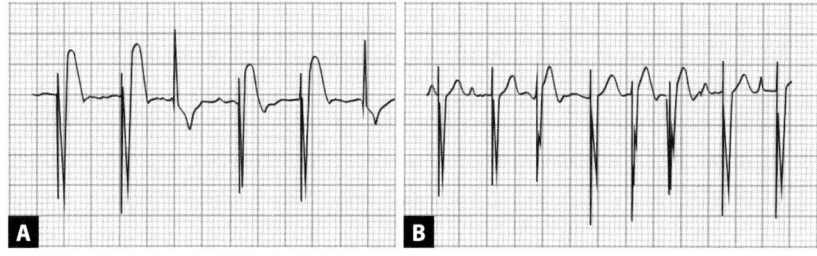

Figs. 16.10A and B: Ventricular inhibited pacing (A) and ventricular triggered pacing (B).

In triggered mode, a sensed spontaneous R wave results in an immediate pacing stimulus fired into the R wave (the heart is refractory and obviously not paced).

Ventricular triggered pacing may be used:
- To avoid electromyography (EMG) inhibition
- When a temporary wire is inserted to cover a failing permanent

Q15. What do you mean by physiological pacing? How is it achieved?
Ans. Utilization of atrial systole to increase left ventricle (LV) end-diastolic volume and COP by either sensing and pacing in synchrony with ventricular pacing is called physiological pacing. Such pacing may improve COP in patients with borderline LV function. In sick sinus syndrome, it may prevent stagnation of blood in a flaccid left atrium, thus avoiding systemic embolism.

It may be achieved by establishing cardiac synchrony in the following ways:
- Atrioventricular sequential pacing—pacing of the atrium followed at a preset interval by pacing of the ventricle. This allows physiologic atrial transport into the LV as in DVI pacing.
- Rate-responsive pacing—via sinus node conduction, i.e., depends on the sinus node as the physiological sensor. Sinus rate is altered according to hemodynamic requirement, and because of AV synchrony, ventricular pacing rate alters accordingly. Example: VDD and DDD.

Physiological pacing system has limitations and cannot be strictly physiological at high heart rates. Some of the limitations are: More expense, shorter battery life, complexity of the unit and programming equipment, occasional pacemaker-medicated tachycardia, and limitations of pacemaker potential on disease progression, e.g., development of sick sinus syndrome in VDD and AF in DDD (should be converted to VVI by programming or automatic mode switching).

Q16. How do environmental factors influence pacemaker function?
Ans.
- *Cellular telephones:* These may interfere with cardiac pacemakers while transmitting or receiving calls. Patients with pacemakers are advised not to carry cellular telephones near the pacemaker site (e.g., shirt pocket) and to hold the telephone to the contralateral arm during use.
- *Electronic article surveillance:* The electromagnetic field may cause pacemaker interference, primarily inhibition of pacemaker output. Patients with unipolar dual-chamber pacemakers are particularly susceptible.
- *High-voltage power lines and electric substations:* These may cause inhibition or asynchronous pacing in a unipolar pacemaker if the patient is quite close to the electric field.
- Metal detectors may be set off because of the detection of a pacemaker; there is generally no appreciable interference with pacemaker function.
- *Magnetic resonance imaging (MRI):* The magnetic force may close the pacemaker and cause asynchronous pacing. One radiofrequency signal

of MRI may inhibit pacing, cause rapid pacing, or cause reversion to reset mode. Unipolar pacemakers are more susceptible to interference from MRI. In general, MRI is avoided in patients with pacemakers.
- *Cardioversion or defibrillation:* The shock may damage the pulse generator or cause the device to be reset. If necessary, the patch electrodes are positioned as far from the pulse generator as possible. A pacemaker evaluation is performed after the procedure.
- *Diathermy:* It may cause pacemaker interference or damage if applied to the region near the pulse generator.
- *Dental equipment:* Some types may cause pacemaker inhibition, particularly for unipolar pacemakers. Vibrations may increase the pacing rate of activity-sensing, rate-adaptive pacemakers.
- *Transcutaneous electric nerve stimulation (TENS):* It is safe for patients with bipolar pacemakers. Patients with a unipolar pacemaker may need a reduction in sensitivity.
- *Electrocautery:* It may cause temporary inhibition of pacemaker output because of oversensing of EMI; electrocautery is used sparingly and in short bursts. The cautery electrode is placed at a distance from the pacemaker site.
- *Extracorporeal shock wave lithotripsy (ESWL):* The shock waves can interfere with or damage a pacemaker. Hence, the pulse generator must be as far as possible from the focal point of the lithotripsy shock waves. Activity-based rate-responsive pacemakers with piezoelectric crystals may be damaged, and the shock wave may cause oversensing and subsequent nonphysiologic rapid pacing rates. Such pacemakers are reprogrammed with the rate-adaptive features deactivated before the procedure. Shock waves may be misinterpreted as atrial activity; therefore, dual-chamber pacemakers are programmed to VVI mode to avoid rapid ventricular pacing.

Q17. What are the indications of pacemaker battery failure? How can battery life be increased?
Ans. The end of life of most pacemaker batteries is indicated by:
- Slowing of the basic pacing rate
- Increasing pulse width/pulse duration
- Decreasing output voltage

Battery life may be increased by: Avoiding low lead impedance with a large electrode tip, avoiding wide pulse width*, avoiding fast pacing rate and constant pacemaker use, and avoiding complex circuitry. Generally, the more complex the pacemaker, the shorter the expected battery life. If a pacemaker with hysteresis mode is available, the takeover rate may be set lower than the basic pacing rate, conserving battery life. A pacemaker may have its battery life prolonged by reducing rate, pulse width, and output. However, reducing pulse width, and/or output voltage should not be performed until enough time has elapsed from implantation to allow for the establishment of the chronic threshold (e.g., 3 months).

Q18. How does a magnet help?
Ans.
- *Diagnostic:* Placing a magnet over the pacemaker units converts them to a faster fixed-rate mode (VOO). This is done to test battery life and satisfactory pacing if there is competition at a slower demand rate. Failure pacemaker stimulus output may produce a pause during a paced rhythm. If the pause resolves with the application of the magnet, the diagnosis of oversensing is most likely. If the pause does not resolve, one of the other causes is considered.
- *Therapeutic:* If a patient is at frequent risk from external interference, he or she may use a magnet to switch the pacemaker to fixed-rate mode, during which it is immune to external signals.

ICD, CRT, EP STUDY

These are special pacing devices used for the management of life-threatening arrhythmias and heart failure. Because of the inability of antiarrhythmic agents to control life-threatening arrhythmias, ICD is being introduced. CRT is designed to bring synchrony in cardiac contraction in heart failure by pacing both ventricles. Often ICD and CRT are combined, i.e., combo device.

Q1. What are the electrotherapies for cardiac arrhythmias?
Ans.
- Direct current electrical cardioversion
- Implantable electrical device, i.e., ICD—monitor rhythm, deliver pacing stimuli, and low- and high-energy shock
- Ablation therapy—destroy myocardial tissue by delivering electrical energy through electrodes on a catheter placed next to an area of the myocardium integrally related to the onset or maintenance of arrhythmia or both.

Q2. What is an ICD? What are the components?
Ans. It is an implantable device that detects life-threatening arrhythmias as well as delivers defibrillating shock to combat that arrhythmia, thus preventing SCD. In light of the evidence for inefficiency and hazards of antiarrhythmic agents for the prevention of SCD, ICD is now a preferred therapeutic option.

Components of ICD are **(Fig. 16.11)**:
- Implantable cardioverter defibrillator box containing a battery and capacitors to store energy to deliver a defibrillation shock

- Ventricular lead and atrial paced-sense lead contain shocking coil and a bipolar pacing electrode at the tip. These sense electrogram and deliver low voltage pulses to pace the heart if the rate is too low(anti-bradycardia pacing) or overdrive, if the rate is too fast, e.g., VT (antitachycardia pacing)
- Microprocessors—contains an algorithm to interpret the sensed electrograms to: (1) Detect tachycardia, (2) discriminate VT/ventricular fibrillation (VF) from nonlife-threatening arrhythmias, e.g., AF, and (3) deliver energy. Some of these are programmable.

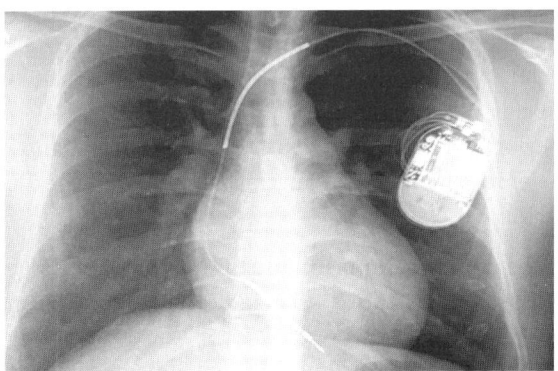

Fig. 16.11: ICD with shocking coil and generator in situ.

Q3. How does an ICD device work?
Ans. An ICD device works by:
- Delivering a defibrillating shock
- Bradycardia pacing (single and dual chamber) and rate-adaptive option
- Antitachycardia pacing (ATP)—terminates a rhythm disturbance without the delivery of a shock
- Incorporating resynchronization therapy, i.e., cardiac resynchronization therapy with defibrillator (CRT-D).

Q4. Enumerate some cardiac conditions where an ICD is beneficial.
Ans.
- Survivors of SCD secondary to VT or VF, where all reversible factors are excluded (secondary prevention)
- Sustained VT and significant structural heart disease, e.g., ischemic cardiomyopathy and dilated cardiomyopathy
- Syncope of undetermined origin and VT or VF inducible on EP study (secondary prevention)
- Sustained VT with reasonable LV function (primary prevention)
- Previous MI with poor LV function [ejection fraction (EF ≤35%)] and inducible VT on EP study (primary prevention)
- Long QT syndrome and Brugada syndrome with history of VT or syncope

- Hypertrophic cardiomyopathy (HCM) or arrhythmogenic right ventricular cardiomyopathy with one or more risk factors for SCD.

Q5. What are the indications of ICD?
Ans. Implantable cardioverter defibrillator is indicated for patients with heart failure with reduced ejection fraction (HFrEF) who are at increased risk of ventricular arrhythmia and SCD. It is indicated for both primary and secondary prevention of SCD.
- *Primary prevention:* (1) Both ischemic and nonischemic cardiomyopathy and EF ≤35% with New York Heart Association (NYHA) class II or III symptoms on guideline-recommended therapy (GRT) for at least 3 months. (2) Patients who are at least 40 days post-MI and with EF ≤35% and NYHA class II symptoms or more while on GRT.
- *Secondary prevention:* For survivors of cardiac arrest and patients with sustained ventricular arrhythmia, irrespective of left ventricular ejection fraction (LVEF)

Q6. What are the complications unique to ICDs?
Ans. Besides the complications associated with the placement of PPM, complications unique to ICD are:
- Failure to deliver appropriate energy when indicated
- Delivery of inappropriate therapy

Q7. What are the limitations of ICD implantation?
Ans.
- Implantable cardioverter defibrillator is only offered to patients who have a reasonable expectation of survival beyond a year in the absence of frailty and/or advanced comorbid conditions.
- ICD shocks (appropriate or not) can lead to anxiety and even post-traumatic stress disorder. Hence, the decision of ICD implantation should be judiciously taken.
- ICD is not a disease-modifying therapy; heart failure progresses even with ICD in situ. Deactivation may be needed at a point when it becomes harmful rather than beneficial.
- ICD should not be implanted in patients with NYHA class IV symptoms who are candidates for LVAD or cardiac transplantation.

Q8. What are CRT, CRT-P, and CRT-D?
Ans. Cardiac resynchronization therapy is a biventricular pacing device for heart failure patients to bring the contraction and relaxation of ventricles into a coordinated manner, thus increasing COP and reducing heart failure symptoms. Patients with heart failure and LBBB exhibit dyssynchrony, i.e., uncoordinated contraction and relaxation of ventricles, because of delayed and heterogeneous depolarization of the LV. By pacing LV and RV simultaneously **(Fig. 16.12)**, CRT improves LVEF and reduces ventricular

dimensions (reverse remodeling). CRT has been shown to improve quality of life, exercise capacity, and EF in patients with advanced congestive heart failure (CHF). As this is achieved by biventricular pacing, it is also called CRT-P. When defibrillation facilities, such as ICD, are incorporated into CRT, it is called CRT-D (often leveled as a combo device).

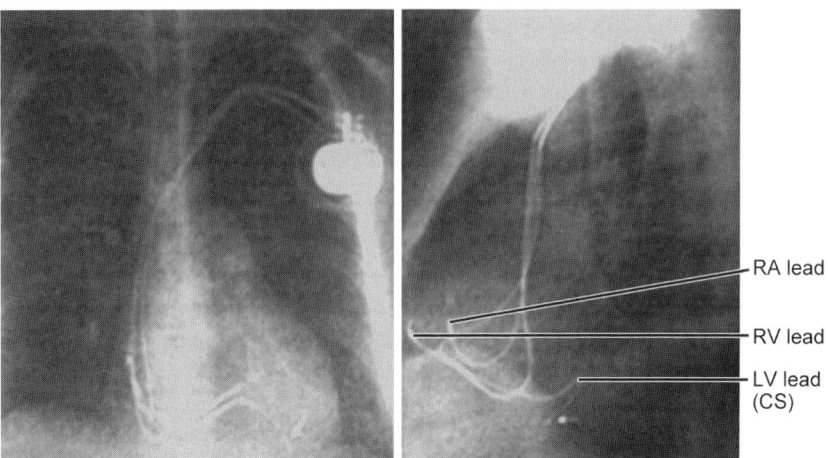

Fig. 16.12: CRT-D chest radiograph showing leads in RA, RV, and LV (the LV lead is placed in the posterolateral branch of the coronary sinus). (CRT-D: cardiac resynchronization therapy defibrillator; CS: coronary sinus; LV: left ventricle; RA: right atrium; RV: right ventricle)

Q9. How does CRT work?
Ans. The device paces the LV and the RV simultaneously, thus improving LVEF and reducing death and hospital admissions in heart failure.

Q10. What are the indications of CRT?
Ans. It is recommended for patients in normal sinus rhythm with LVEF ≤35% and an LBBB with QRS of ≥120 ms. American Heart Association, American College of Cardiology, and Heart Rhythm Society (AHA/ACC/HRS) guidelines (2008) recommend that CRT is indicated in patients with NYHA class III–IV heart failure established on optimal medical therapy, QRS duration >120 ms, LVEF ≤35%, and those in sinus rhythm.

It may also be beneficial in heart failure patients with NYHA class III–IV established on optimal medical therapy, AF with QRS duration >120 ms, and LVEF ≤35%. Also NYHA class III–IV patients and LVEF ≤35% who require frequent RV pacing.

Q11. What is EP study? Give its importance.
Ans. It is the method of recording and/or stimulating cardiac electrical activities by introducing multipolar catheter electrodes and positioning them at various intracardiac sites. An EP study is often combined with catheter ablation to treat the identified arrhythmia.

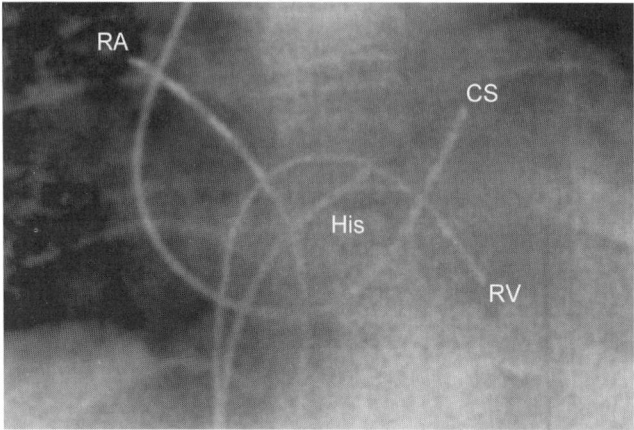

Fig. 16.13: EP study and SVT ablation—fluoroscopic image showing quadripolar catheters in high RA, RV, His bundle, and a decapolar catheter in high RA, RV, His bundle and a decapolar catheter in coronary sinus.

The importance of EP studies is:
- Diagnostic—type of clinical rhythm disturbances and its electrophysiologic mechanism
- Therapeutic—to terminate a tachycardia by electrical stimulation or electroshock, to evaluate the effect of therapy by determining whether a particular intervention modifies or prevents electrical induction of a tachycardia or an induced tachyarrhythmia, and to allocate myocardium involved in the tachycardia to prevent further episodes.
- Prognostic—to identify patients at risk of SCD

Q12. What is catheter ablation? When is it indicated?
Ans. It is the catheter-based antiarrhythmic therapy achieved by ablating or damaging the tissue responsible for arrhythmia by application of radiofrequency energy. Catheter placed in RA, RV, near His bundle, and in coronary sinus via femoral vein **(Fig. 16.13)**. The radio frequency (RF) energy creates a burn by resistively heating the tissue. A cryocatheter that freezes the tissues can also be used for ablation. Acoustic and laser-based ablation systems are also evaluated. For a successful ablation, accurate diagnosis of arrhythmia, mapping to determine the precise location of tissue causing arrhythmia, placement of ablation catheter on site, and application of effective RF energy are needed. Ablation lesion heals by fibrosis. For many arrhythmias, the risks are sufficiently low, and catheter ablation has become an important common therapy.

Indications of catheter ablation:
- Supraventricular tachycardias (SVTs)—AV nodal re-entrant tachycardia (AVNRT), AV reciprocating tachycardias using an accessory pathway,

focal atrial tachycardia, inappropriate sinus tachycardia (modifying S.A. node function), atrial flutter, etc.
- Atrial fibrillation—AV junction ablation (for rate control) and atrial ablation (for maintaining sinus rhythm)
- Ventricular tachycardia—idiopathic focal VT, idiopathic interfascicular re-entrant tachycardia, VT after MI, and bundle branch reentrant VT

Q13. What is myocardial mapping?
Ans. It is the method of recording potentials directly from the heart that is spatially depicted as a function of time in an integrated manner. The mapping system displays the location of the catheter and a three-dimensional representation of the anatomic as well as electrophysiologic character of the tissue. It can display continuous catheter position without the need for fluoroscopy, thus reducing radiation exposure. Integration of cardiac MRI, computed tomography (CT), and echocardiography is needed when extensive ablation is required over complex anatomy, e.g., extensive left atrial ablation in AF. Direct cardiac mapping by catheter electrodes can be used to identify and localize the areas responsible for rhythm disturbances in patients with SVT and VT for catheter or surgical ablation or resection.

Indications are: Wolff–Parkinson–White (WPW) syndrome with accessory pathways, AV node and His bundle ablation in AV node re-entry, and the site of origin of VTs

Q14. What are the indications of an EP study?
Ans.
- Atrioventricular block—to determine the site of block (which cannot be determined by routine ECG), patients with PPMs having symptoms
- Intraventricular conduction disturbances—an HV interval >35 ms raises the possibility of trifascicular block, and an HV interval >80–90 ms indicates an increased risk of AV block.
- Sinus node dysfunction—symptoms attributable to bradycardia or asystole (presyncope or syncope) for whom noninvasive tests provide no explanation.
- Tachycardia—to differentiate aberrant supraventricular conduction from VT
- Unexplained syncope
- Palpitation.

■ SUGGESTED READING

1. Epstein AE, DiMarco JP, Ellenbogen KA, Estes NA 3rd, Freedman RA, Gettes LS, et al. ACC/AHA/HRS 2008 guidelines for device-based therapy of cardiac rhythm abnormalities: a report of the American College of Cardiology/American Heart Association Task Force on Practice Guidelines (Writing Committee to Revise

the ACC/AHA/NASPE 2002 Guideline Update for Implantation of Cardiac Pacemakers and Antiarrhythmic Devices). Circulation. 2008;117:e350-e408.
2. Goldschlager N, Goldman MJ. Cardiac pacing. In: Principles of Clinical Electrocardiography. Appleton & Lange; 1989.
3. Mann DL. Management of heart failure patients with reduced ejection fraction. In: Libby P, Bonow R, Mann D (Eds). Braunwald's Heart Disease: A Textbook of Cardiovascular Medicine, 8th edition. Philadelphia, PA: Saunders; 2008.
4. Ramrakha P, Hill J (Eds). Invasive electrophysiology. In: Oxford Handbook of Cardiology, 2nd edition. Oxford, UK; 2012.
5. Swanton RH. Disturbance in cardiac rhythm. In: Cardiology, 4th edition. Blackwell Science; 1998.

CHAPTER 17

Cardiac Pharmacology

> *"Increasing incidence of CAD and it`s risk factors, more and more use of coronary interventions pharmacological agents are utelized more and more."*
> —Author of the book

■ INTRODUCTION

With an increasing incidence of coronary artery disease (CAD) and more and more use of mechanical intervention, i.e., percutaneous coronary intervention (PCI) and stenting, pharmacological intervention is also utilized more and more. A growing array of drugs is available that are safer and more efficacious to treat as well as to prevent cardiovascular diseases. In this chapter, nitrates, β-blockers, calcium channel blockers (CCBs), antiplatelets, anticoagulants, fibrinolytics, angiotensin-converting enzyme inhibitor (ACEI), diuretics, lipid-lowering agents, antiarrhythmics, and digoxin are discussed. Other cardiac drugs are also discussed in relevant chapters.

■ NITRATES

Q1. How do nitrates achieve their antianginal effect?
Ans.
- Nitrates are an effective vasodilator for angina.
  It increases oxygen (O_2) delivery to ischemic myocardium by:
  - Dilatation of epicardial coronary arteries and coronary resistance vessels. Atherosclerotic coronary arteries with significant stenosis also respond to nitrate
  - Dilatation of collateral vessels
  - Relieving coronary spasm
- Nitrates decrease O_2 consumption by ischemic myocardium by:
  - Dilatation of systemic arteries and a decrease in afterload
  - Dilatation of systemic veins and reduction of preload

Q2. What forms of nitrate therapy are available?
Ans.
- *Nitroglycerine:* It is available as a sublingual tablet or spray. When angina starts, 1 tablet is used sublingually every 3 minutes until the pain goes or a maximum of 4–5 tablets have been given. Also, long-acting oral tablets, intravenous (IV) preparations, and topical preparations (ointment or patch) are available.

- Isosorbide dinitrate—as oral tablets
- Isosorbide-5-mononitrate—available for oral administration; can be used sublingually.

Q3. What are the indications of IV nitrates?

Ans. Nitrates are used IV in the following situations:

- Unstable angina (UA)—not responding to medical treatment orally. An upward dose titration, starting with 5-10 µg/min, titrated up to 200 µg/min, may be needed, depending on clinical course, to overcome tolerance and relieve pain
- *Left ventricular failure (LVF) and pulmonary edema:* These may be secondary to acute mitral regurgitation (MR), acute aortic regurgitation (AR), and hypertension
- Malignant hypertension.

Acute myocardial infarction (AMI) patients with ongoing anginal pain, those with LVF, severe hypertension, or when the differential diagnosis between early transmural AMI and Prinzmetal's angina is not clear. The starting dose is 5 µg/min, increased by 5-20 µg/min every 5 minutes in the first 30 minutes until the mean blood pressure (BP) is reduced to 10% in normotensive patients or 80% in hypertensive patients.

- During and after coronary artery bypass surgery, hypertensive episodes following cardiac surgery
- During cardiac catheterization—intracoronary injection may be needed if chest pain is associated with ST elevation, suggesting coronary spasm and impending infarction.
- During percutaneous transluminal coronary angioplasty (PTCA)—as a prophylactic agent to prevent coronary spasm

Q4. What are the causes of failure of nitrate therapy?

Ans. These are:

- *Development of nitrate tolerance:* During prophylactic therapy with long-acting nitrates, it is a frequent cause of apparent failure. It is treated by interval dosing.
- *Loss of potency of tablets:* Nitrate tablets should be kept in air-tight containers and stored in the cold. Glyceryl trinitrates are sensitive to sunlight (the container should be amber-colored).
- *Incorrect route of administration*: Some sublingual preparations should not be taken orally and vice versa.
- Arterial hypoxemia, especially in chronic obstructive pulmonary disease (COPD).
- Noncompliance, usually caused by headache.
- Increasing severity of angina—worsening of the disease process; it is treated by combination therapy, e.g., when nitrates are less effective than expected owing to tachycardia, combination with β-blocker gives better

result, while excluding aggravating factors such as hypertension, atrial fibrillation (AF), or anemia and considering interventional therapy.
- Others—dry mucosal membrane impairs oral absorption of nitrates.

Q5. What are the nitrate preparations? Give their pharmacokinetics.

Ans. Depending on its route of application, various nitrate preparations are in use with differing pharmacokinetic properties **(Table 17.1)**.

TABLE 17.1: Pharmacokinetic properties of various nitrate preparations.

Drug	Route of administration	Dose	Frequency	Duration of effect and comment
Nitroglycerine	Sublingual	0.5–1.3 mg tablet (maximum 2.5 mg)	As needed for pain relief	1½ minutes–1 hour
	Spray	0.4 mg/dose	As needed	Effect apparent within 5 minutes
	Oral, sustained release	2.6–6.4 mg	b.d. or t.d.s.	4–8 hours
	Intravenous	5–400 µg/min	Continuous	In UA, increasing dose are needed (during intra coronary infusion)
	Topical:			
	• Ointment (2%)	12.5–40 mg	Every 4–6 hours	Duration of effect 3–4 hours
	• Patch	2.5–15 mg	Every 24 hours	Effect start within 1–2 hours, last 8–12 hours during intermittent therapy
Isosorbide dinitrate	Oral tablet	10–40 mg	Every 6 hours	
	Sublingual tablet	2.5–10 mg	Every 2–3 hours	
Isosorbide-5-mononitrate	Oral tablet	10–40 mg	12 hourly	6–10 hours (eccentric dosage needed to avoid tolerance)
	Sustained release-tablet	40–100 mg	Once daily	9 hours

(b.d.: twice daily; t.d.s.: three times daily; UA: unstable angina)

BETA ADRENERGIC RECEPTOR BLOCKERS

Q1. What is the role of β-blocker therapy in treating patients with IHD?

Ans. Beta blockers are the first-line drugs to treat ischemic heart disease (IHD). Use of β-blockers early in the course of acute infarction [both Q and non-ST-elevation myocardial infarction (NSTEMI)], in the absence of contraindications, decreases the risk of death by about 20%. There is a reduction of both sudden and nonsudden cardiovascular mortality. Administration of β-blockers within hours after infarction provides the additional benefit of limiting infarct size and reducing the risk of recurrent ischemia and reinfarction.

Beta blocker therapy is also beneficial in postinfarct survivors, who are at high risk, including those with:
- Large infarction, especially anterior
- Persistent ischemia (angina, positive stress test suggesting significant coronary lesion supplying viable myocardium)
- Complex ventricular ectopy
- Coexisting illness treatable with β-blockers—hypertension, supraventricular tachycardia (SVT), etc.

Q2. How to choose a β-blocker?

Ans. Properties of the agent, availability, personal preference, and experience dictate the choice:
- Hypertensive patients may be best managed with a single-dose schedule taken in the morning. More frequent dose schedules are usually required for angina.
  - Patients with cool peripheries, peripheral vascular disease, diabetes mellitus, or mild bronchospasm should start with a cardioselective drug. In patients with airway obstruction, start on a small dose and monitor peak flows at least twice daily.
- Patients complaining of bad dreams (e.g., on propranolol) should receive a nonfat-soluble drug (e.g., atenolol).
- Renal failure—a β-blocker with hepatic excretion (e.g., propranolol and carvedilol) but at a lower dose than in patients with normal function. Reduction in cardiac output lowers renal plasma flow and may cause a deterioration in renal function.
- Liver disease—first-pass metabolism occurs with fat-soluble drugs (e.g., propranolol and labetalol). Dose of fat-soluble drugs is reduced or switched to a nonfat-soluble drug (e.g., pindolol and nadolol), which is excreted only by the kidneys.
- Heart failure—in mild-to-moderate heart failure, nonselective β-blockers with additional α_1-blocking activity, e.g., carvedilol, at low dose, have been shown to improve left ventricular (LV) function.

- Diabetes mellitus—cardioselective drug is preferable. β-blockade prevents the sympathetic reaction to hypoglycemia; muscle glycogenolysis is mediated via β_2 receptors.
- Pregnancy—labetalol, as a treatment for hypertension in pregnancy.

Q3. How to adjust the dose of β-blockers to get an adequate antianginal effect?

Ans. β-blockers decrease myocardial oxygen demand by decreasing the heart rate (HR) and myocardial contractility both at rest and during exercise. In treating stable angina, it is essential that the dose of β-blockers be adjusted to lower the resting HR to 55–60 beats/min; rates <50 beats/min may be accepted provided that heart block is avoided and there are no symptoms. Reduction in exercise-induced tachycardia during β-blockade therapy is an important determinant of the response to therapy of effort angina with β-blockers, and the aim should be an exercise HR of <100–110 beats/min.

Q4. What is the role of β-blockers in the prevention of IHD?

Ans. In postmyocardial infarction (MI) patients, β-blockers are recommended. Mortality is reduced by 25–35%. Post-MI patients with arrhythmias, inducible ischemia, and high-risk patients with large (usually anterior) MI and compensated LV dysfunction are mostly benefited. The beneficial effects in low-risk patients are less clear, but because of the relatively favorable side effect profile, these patients should also be included. It is commonly recommended that β-blocker therapy be continued indefinitely as long as side effects are not present.

Q5. What is the role of β-blockers in preventing sudden cardiac death (SCD)?

Ans. Beta blockers are the only antiarrhythmic drug found clearly effective in preventing SCD in patients with prior MI. It reduces total cardiac mortality by >40%. This effect is most pronounced in patients who are at high risk for SCD, such as those with congestive heart failure (CHF), atrial and ventricular arrhythmias, post-MI, and diabetes.

Q6. What are the antiarrhythmic effects of β-blockers?

Ans. Both supraventricular and ventricular arrhythmias may respond to β-blockers.
- *Ventricular:*
  - *Acute myocardial infarction:* β-blockers prevent ventricular fibrillation, reduce infarct size. In post-infarction period, it prevents SCD, which may reflect an antifibrillatory mechanism.
  - Ventricular arrhythmias are provoked by high sympathetic tone, increased circulating catecholamine, suppressing torsade de pointes in the long QT syndrome, exercise-induced ventricular tachycardia (VT), CHF, anxiety, anesthesia, and postoperative states.

- Digitalis-induced ventricular arrhythmias
- Arrhythmias of mitral valve prolapse, thyrotoxicosis, etc.
- *Supraventricular:*
  - *In chronic AF without LV failure:* β-blockers may be used to reduce the ventricular response.
  - In acute onset AF, IV esmolol may be useful.

Q7. How to withdraw β-blockers in IHD?
Ans. All patients with IHD must be warned not to stop β-blockers therapy abruptly. Sudden withdrawal may exacerbate angina, sometimes resulting in MI. The β-receptors are upregulated owing to prolonged β-blockade. Circulating catecholamines act on the β-receptors to produce this adverse effect. During discontinuation, β-blockers should be tapered over 3–10 days when possible to avoid rebound worsening of angina. A sudden stop with the patient resting in bed seems to be safe if at all needed. In case of poorly compliant patients, the use of β-blockers with added intrinsic sympathomimetic activity, such as pindolol, appears to lessen withdrawal effects.

Treatment of the withdrawal syndrome is by reintroduction of β-blockade.

Q8. What are the cardiovascular conditions when β-blockers are contraindicated?
Ans.
- Absolute—severe bradycardia (HR <50 beats/min), hypotension (BP <100 mm Hg), high degree atrioventricular (AV) block (2° or 3°), PR interval >240 ms, overt LVF
- Relative—Prinzmetal's angina (unopposed α-spasm), patients receiving high doses of other agents depressing the sinoatrial node (SA) or AV nodes (verapamil, diltiazem, digitalis, and antiarrhythmic agents).

ANTIPLATELETS, ANTICOAGULANT, AND FIBRINOLYTIC AGENTS

Q1. What are the antithrombotic agents?
Ans. Three main types of agents act at different stages of the thrombotic process.
a. *Antiplatelets:* Act on arterial thrombogenesis where endothelial injury and platelet activation are the inciting factors, e.g., AMI, PCI with or without stent deployment. It is also helpful for the primary prevention of MI.
b. *Anticoagulants:* Given acutely (e.g., heparin) limit further thrombus formation, thus preventing ST-elevation myocardial infarction (STEMI) in UA and NSTEMI. Given chronically (e.g., warfarin), act where stasis is dominant factor, e.g., prevention and treatment of deep vein thrombosis

and pulmonary embolism, prevent systemic thromboembolism in AF (from dilated left atrium). Both antiplatelets and anticoagulants are required to inhibit thrombotic complications of PCI.
c. *Fibrinolytic agents:* Acts where thrombus has already formed but recent and still subject to lysis, e.g., STEMI and peripheral arterial thrombosis, especially when prompt mechanical revascularization (primary PCI) is not feasible. Also, these may be beneficial in pulmonary embolism, thrombotic cardiovascular disease (CVD).

The different sites of action of three types of agents mean that combination therapy can be beneficial. For example, fibrinolytic agents are used with antiplatelets and anticoagulants in the management of AMI.

Q2. What antiplatelets and anticoagulants are commonly used in cardiology?
Ans.
- Anticoagulants—heparin [given intravenously or subcutaneously)], warfarin (given orally)
- Antiplatelets—aspirin, thienopyridines [inhibit adenosine diphosphate (ADP)-mediated platelet activation], e.g., clopidogrel, prasugrel, ticagrelor, etc., and glycoprotein IIb/IIIa receptor inhibitors abciximab (Fab fragment of monoclonal antibody directed against platelet GP IIb/IIIa receptor) and eptifibatide. IIb/IIIa receptor inhibitors block platelet aggregation in response to all potential agonists and are approved for clinical use in patients with acute coronary syndrome (ACS) and patients undergoing coronary angioplasty.

Q3. What are the unique features of platelets?
Ans.
- Platelets (platelet, i.e., small plate-shaped) are remnant of cell, i.e., megakaryocytes. These are anucleated, hence unable to synthesize proteins. Aspirin blocks the function of platelets exposed to it for their remaining lifetime (7–10 days) in circulation. This accounts for the lengthy therapeutic effect of aspirin despite a t½ of only 20 minutes.
- Although enucleated platelets are highly active metabolically with adhesion, activation, release reaction, and aggregation in the hemostatic process. It has several receptors, such as ADP receptor, thromboxane (TxA) receptor, von Willebrand factor (VwF) receptor, collagen (COL) receptor, epinephrine (EP) receptor, thrombin (TH) receptor, and fibrin (FIB) receptor. The surface glycoproteins are glycoprotein IIb/IIIa. Platelet aggregation is mediated by fibrinogen through FIB receptors on adjoining platelets, forming a bridge. FIB receptors are formed by the complexing of glycoprotein IIb/IIIa in the membrane of activated platelets. Only some of the many receptors can be blocked by aspirin, clopidogrel, and glycoprotein IIb/IIIa antagonists. Antagonists to several

major receptors, such as those to which COL, the VwF, and TxA_2 bind, have yet to be developed.
- Platelets play a pivotal role in the pathogenesis of AMI. Besides initiation of clot formation after plaque fissuring or rupture, it produces propagation of clot. Secretion of plasminogen activator inhibitor causes clots to become resistant to lysis, and secretion of thromboxane A_2 cause vasoconstriction. They may embolize to cause plugging of the microvasculature. Platelet aggregates are resistant to fibrinolytic therapy.

Q4. What is dual antiplatelet therapy? Give its indications.
Ans. As aspirin and clopidogrel act on different sites on the platelet, a combination of both, i.e., dual therapy, may provide better results in patients with higher risk. It is indicated in the setting of acute vascular injury, whether procedure induced as in stenting, or spontaneous as in ACS (UA, NSTEMI, and STEMI). For AMI, the American College of Cardiology/American Heart Association (ACC/AHA) guidelines recommend (2008) clopidogrel 75 mg daily added to aspirin for at least 7 days. In PCI, clopidogrel (300-mg loading dose, than 75 mg daily) is added to aspirin and continued for at least 12 months after a drug-eluting stent (DES).

Q5. What are the doses and duration of aspirin in various situations?
Ans. Prophylactic aspirin is indicated for all stages of symptomatic IHD, including chronic effort angina, UA, AMI, postinfarction state, after coronary artery bypass grafting (CABG), and during PCI.
- In ACS-STEMI treated with fibrinolytic therapy or primary PCI, and UA/NSTEMI treated with either conservative or invasive strategies, aspirin should be given in both acute and follow-up phases. At the start of AMI therapy, the initial dose should be 162–325 mg of chewable (nonenteric) aspirin, with maintenance of 75–162 mg.
- Secondary prevention—all patients with stable angina, patients with a prior cardiovascular event, such as UA, prior MI, PCI, prior stroke or transient ischemic attack (TIA), and peripheral arterial disease should receive aspirin 75 mg daily. In stable angina, it reduces AMI or sudden death.
- Primary prevention—considered only for high-risk otherwise healthy patients. Even in moderate-risk patients, there are almost as many disabling strokes and major bleeds as MIs prevented, so that aspirin is not recommended.
- Percutaneous coronary intervention with bare metal stent (BMS)—aspirin 325 mg daily for 1 month
- Percutaneous coronary intervention with DES—aspirin 325 mg daily for at least 1-year

Q6. How long to continue dual antiplatelet therapy in patients with DES and BMS?

Ans. Adenosine diphosphate receptor antagonists, clopidogrel, prasugrel help to prevent acute thrombotic closure after coronary artery stenting. For elective PCI, high-dose clopidogrel is sufficient without glycoprotein IIb/IIIa receptor inhibitors.

Drug-eluting stents inhibit vascular smooth muscle cell proliferation and prevent in-stent restenosis. They also delay regrowth of proliferative vascular endothelium, resulting in a longer time period during which patients are at risk for stent thrombosis. Because stent thrombosis has been observed up to and even beyond 1-year following placement of a DES, current guidelines recommend at least 1-year of dual antiplatelet therapy (with aspirin 325 mg and clopidogrel 75 mg/day) after placement of a DES. Patients who, for any reason are poor candidates for long-term clopidogrel, including those who are planned for major surgery in the near future (in the next few months after PCI) should not receive DES.

In patients with BMS placement dual antiplatelet therapy is continued for 30 days, with aspirin 325 mg and clopidogrel 75 mg daily.

Q7. What are the characteristic features of different ADP receptor antagonists?

Ans. Of the ADP receptor antagonists clopidogrel, prasugrel are indirect acting and ticagrelor is direct acting agent.
- Onset of action in clopidogrel is slow (must be converted to an active form). Pretreatment with 300–600 mg loading 12–15 hours prior to PCI produces rapid platelet inhibition (in 2–6 hours). If patients are not pretreated with clopidogrel, a loading dose of 600 mg should be given on the catheterization table if a PCI is to be carried out immediately.
- Prasugrel is 5–9 times more potent than clopidogrel (60 mg loading dose, then 10 mg daily compared with 300-mg loading dose, and then 75 mg daily for clopidogrel) with an onset of action within 1 hour.
- Cangrelor, a reversible ADP-receptor blocker given intravenously acts within 20 minutes and achieves 85% platelet inhibition with less prolongation of bleeding time (compared with GP IIb/IIIa). It is used in ACS and PCI.

Q8. How to achieve maximal platelet inhibition?

Ans. Maximum platelet inhibition logically consists of three types of agents acting at three different sites: Aspirin, clopidogrel, and GP IIb/IIIa. High doses of all three combined with anticoagulant therapy should be reserved for patients with ACS at high risk undergoing PCI. For low-risk patients, acute high-dose clopidogrel is given upstream. Clopidogrel should be added to aspirin to obtain better platelet inhibition in acute vascular injury, but not for stable coronary disease. In patients with prior TIAs or minor stroke, a dual therapy increases life-threatening bleeding without improving cardiovascular (CV) outcome.

ANTICOAGULANTS

Q1. What are the commonly used parenteral anticoagulants?
Ans.
- *Unfractionated heparin (UFH):* It binds to antithrombin for its major antithrombin activity (IIa); also inhibits factor Xa and to a lesser extent XIa and others. Thus, it has a wider spectrum of antithrombotic activity. Monitoring is done with activated partial thromboplastin time (APTT), using IV or subcutaneous (SC) following a bolus. It is indicated in ACS, primary PCI, prevention, and treatment of deep vein thrombosis (DVT). Its anticoagulant effect can be promptly withdrawn by stopping infusion and the action reversed by protamine. In clinical doses, it is not cleared by the kidneys, hence safe in renal failure.
- *Low-molecular-weight heparin (LMWH):* Molecular weight is one third of UFH; has greater bioavailability and a longer half-life than UFH. It binds to antithrombin effectively to inhibit factor Xa, with some direct TH inhibition. Monitoring is not needed; dose reduction is needed in renal impairment and in the elderly.
- *Fondaparinux:* It indirectly inhibits TH by inactivating factor Xa, resulting in reduced generation. Specific anti-Xa activity is about sevenfold higher than LMWH. It has a longer half-life compared to UFH and LMWH, and given SC once daily; needs no monitoring. Dose reduction in renal impairment and in the elderly is needed.
- *Bivalirudin:* It directly inhibits soluble and clot-bound TH (without depending on antithrombin); it is given in IV infusion in UA undergoing PCI; monitoring with APTT needed.

Q2. How to achieve and monitor the therapeutic level of heparin?
Ans.
- Continuous injection—heparin is given IV or subcutaneously. The standard IV schedule is usually a 5,000 unit IV loading dose, followed by a continuous infusion of 1,000 units/h (given by infusion pump). The APTT is checked at 4–6 hours. If it is not within the goal of 1.5–2.5 times baseline, the rate is adjusted up or down (100–200 units/h). Minimally prolonged APTT may require a re-bolus of 5,000 U and if APTT is markedly prolonged, the infusion is held for 1 hour and then a reduced rate resumed. The APTT is rechecked at 4–6 hours. Once an adequate rate is achieved, the APTT should be checked each day.

- Intermittent injections with 10,000 units given as an initial dose, followed by 5,000–10,000 units every 4–6 hours may be preferable in AMI to avoid fluid overload.
- Subcutaneous heparin—after the initial IV loading dose, heparin may be given as a deep SC injection 10,000 units 8 hourly or 15,000 units 12 hourly, using a different site at each time. SC heparin, used prophylactically, is started at 5,000 units every 8–12 hours. It is not monitored, because therapeutic goals are achieved at levels that may not prolong the APTT.

Q3. How to combine heparin with warfarin for long-term anticoagulation?
Ans. Warfarin is started on day 1 of heparin therapy. This allows depletion of vitamin-K dependent factors (which needs 3–4 days), while the patient is fully anticoagulated with heparin. After 5–6 days of heparin and with at least 2 days of a therapeutic prothrombin time/international normalized ratio (PT/INR), heparin can be discontinued.

A minor decrease in PT/INR may be seen as the heparin effect wanes.

Q4. What baseline tests are needed before starting heparin?
Ans. Hematocrit, platelet count, APTT, and (PT with INR).

The APTT serves as a baseline value to gauge the therapeutic dose of heparin.

Prothrombin time/international normalized ratio is the baseline for anticipated warfarin therapy.

The hematocrit and platelet count provide pretreatment values if complications like bleeding and thrombocytopenia arise.

Q5. How to start and follow up warfarin therapy?
Ans. A reasonable guideline for chronic anticoagulation with warfarin is:
- Start with 5 mg orally each day. Large loading doses are not recommended. Use 10 mg for 1–2 days if there is some urgency.
- Check INR daily until a therapeutic level is reached for that clinical setting.
- After 4–6 days, the dosage may need to be adjusted as the individual's sensitivity to warfarin is established.
- Monitor INR twice weekly for 2 weeks, then weekly for 2 months.
- Once the dose is stable, check INR every 1–2 months.
- Never go >2 months for INR check with therapeutic doses. Many factors can influence the anticoagulant intensity and increase the risk of bleeding unpredictably.

Q6. What is INR?
Ans. Measurement of INR is recommended by the World Health Organization (WHO) for monitoring the oral anticoagulant effect of warfarin. The laboratory determined INR is the PT ratio that reflects the result that has been obtained

if the WHO reference thromboplastin has been used to perform the test in the laboratory.

$$INR = \left(\frac{\text{Patient PT}}{\text{Control PT}}\right) \times ISI$$

The INR is based, therefore, on two contributing factors: the PT ratio and the international sensitivity index (ISI). The ISI is a measure of the responsiveness of a given thromboplastin to the reduction in the vitamin-K dependent coagulation factors. Reagent manufacturers assign each lot an ISI, which relates the preparation's activity to that of an international reference thromboplastin.

Results are reported with both the PT and INR values. Problems with standardization of anticoagulant intensity arose in the past with the use of PT, because the thromboplastin used varied among batches in the ability to facilitate coagulation.

Q7. What is the frequency of INR monitoring in warfarin therapy?
Ans. The optimal frequency of INR monitoring is unknown. A reasonable recommendation is to determine the INR every month on an average, but one should wait up to 2 months to recheck the INR in stable patients.

Q8. What are the recommended INR ranges?
Ans. For most conditions of anticoagulation, an INR of 2–3 is adequate.
- High-risk situations may call for greater intensity. i.e., INR 3.0–4.5:
  - Mechanical mitral valve prosthesis
  - Caged ball valve (rather than bileaflet or tilting disc valve)
  - Systemic embolization at a less intense level of anticoagulation
- INR 2.5–3.5: Mechanical valve other than mitral. If aspirin can be used at 100 mg/day, an INR of 2.0–3.0 may be as effective as the higher intensities.

Q9. How does aspirin interact with warfarin therapy?
Ans. Aspirin, by inhibiting platelet function, may increase the risk of bleeding when cotreatment with warfarin is done. Although it does not change warfarin level. This combination must be used carefully and usually requires the INR to be slightly lower than usually indicated.

High doses of aspirin (6–8 tablets/day) may act by a different mechanism to potentiate the anticoagulant effect because the synthesis of clotting factors are impaired.

Q10. List some drugs that alter the PT.
Ans. Warfarin may be subject to approximately 80 drug interactions that alter PT **(Table 17.2)**.

TABLE 17.2: Drugs interacting with warfarin.

Pharmacokinetic (drugs changing warfarin levels)	Pharmacodynamics (drugs not changing warfarin levels)	Mechanism unknown (drugs whose effect on warfarin level is unknown)
Prolongs PT: Metronidazole, trimethoprim-sulfamethoxazole, omeprazole, amiodarone, phenylbutazone, sulfinpyrazone, cimetidine, and disulfiram	Prolongs PT: Second and third generation Cephalosporins, thyroxine, and clofibrates	Prolongs PT: Erythromycin, anabolic steroids, flu and ketoconazole, isoniazid, quinidine, phenytoin, piroxicam, and tamoxifen
Reduces PT: Reduce absorption—Cholestyramine, increases clearance—Barbiturates, rifampicin, carbamazepine, and griseofulvin	• Inhibits platelet function: Aspirin, other NSAIDs, ticlopidine, and clopidogrel • Inhibits blood coagulation: Heparin	Reduce PT: Penicillin

(NSAIDs: nonsteroidal anti-inflammatory drugs; PT: prothrombin time)

Q11. What are the prerequisites for a successful prolonged anticoagulation?
Ans. Successful anticoagulation therapy requires:
- A cooperative patient
- Meticulous medical supervision
- An excellent laboratory
- A constant guard against the use of additional drugs and their interactions.

The safest rule is to tell patients on oral anticoagulants not to take any over-the-counter drugs without consultation, and for the physicians to check any new drug used. If in doubt, more frequent measurements of the PT/INR are required.

Q12. What factors increase the risk of bleeding during warfarin therapy?
Ans.
- Intensity of therapy—INR >3.0 have increased risk
- Age—risk rises with increased age
- Duration of therapy—risk is highest at the start of therapy. The risk of major bleeding during the first month of warfarin therapy is approximately 10 times the risk after the first year of therapy.
- Comorbid conditions—cerebrovascular, renal, heart, and liver diseases are associated with more bleeding complications
- Concurrent medications—some drugs prolong PT/INR and increase the risk of bleeding
- Compliance—regular monitoring and systematic dose adjustment needed for safe and effective warfarin therapy.

Q13. How does NOAC differ from vitamin-K antagonist (VKA)?
Ans. These novel oral anticoagulants (NOAC) differ from VKA, like warfarin in the following aspects:
- Rapid onset of action. Bridging with parenteral anticoagulants is not needed.
- Monitoring is not needed.
- Drug interaction is much less compared to warfarin.
- No excess bleeding; preferred in Asians in terms of both efficacy and safety.
- More effective in the elderly, in preventing stroke and systemic embolism.
- All are excreted by the kidneys; dose modification required in chronic kidney disease (CKD). Rivaroxaban 15 mg b.d.; apixaban 2.5 mg b.d.; and edoxaban 30 mg b.d. dabigatran avoided.
- Warfarin is preferred for patients with creatinine clearance <30 mL/min and patients on hemodialysis.

Q14. What are the NOACs currently recommended for use?
Ans. Currently, four NOACs are approved by the USFDA:
- Dabigatran—a direct TH inhibitor
- Rivaroxaban, edoxaban, and apixaban—factor xa inhibitor

■ FIBRINOLYTIC AGENTS

Q1. What are the advantages and disadvantages of tenecteplase as a thrombolytic agent?
Ans. Tenecteplase is fibrin-specific, has faster lytic action with bolus administration, achieves greater thrombolysis in myocardial infarction (TIMI) 3 flow, and avoids systemic lytic state and antigen–antibody reaction. If available, TNK should be the preferred agent in most patients. High cost, higher risk of intracranial hemorrhage, and less availability are the disadvantages.

Q2. What are the advantages of streotokinase over TNK?
Ans. Streptokinase is cheap and remains the most frequently used agent in the world. SK is highly immunogenic, and neutralizing antibody formation generally precludes readministration. It is preferred over t-PA in patients with low-mortality risk, e.g., inferior MI, and those in whom the risk of intracranial hemorrhage is high, e.g., in the elderly.

Low cost, easy availability, greater familiarity among physicians, and lesser hemorrhagic stroke.

It should be the agent of choice in patients at high risk for intracranial hemorrhage (age >65, female sex, low body weight <70 kg), hypertension at presentation, and prior cerebrovascular disease. Considering the scenario in South Asian countries, SK is still and will remain to be a major thrombolytic agent in STEMI. For providing timely thrombolytic for the highest number of patients, SK will be continued to be the agent of choice.

Q3. What are the benefits of fibrinolytic therapy in STEMI?
Ans. Benefits are:
- Tissue reperfusion and decreased myonecrosis
- Restoration of flow in infarct-related artery; keep it patient
- Prevention of ventricular remodeling
- Minimizing ventricular dysfunction
- Increased survival in the long term.

Q4. Compare different fibrinolytic agents?
Ans. First-generation fibrinolytics (SK and urokinase) are not FIB specific. Second-generation fibrinolytics (alteplase, prourokinase) are FIB specific and act at the thrombus site. Third-generation fibrinolytic agents (reteplase and tenecteplase) are newer, engineered versions of plasminogen activators designed to improve thrombolysis with advantages like longer half-lives and greater FIB specificity. Difference among them are in **Table 17.3**.

TABLE 17.3: Comparison of commonly used fibrinolytic agents.

Point	SK[‡]	Alteplase[†]	Reteplase*	Tenecteplase*
Fib. Specificity	–	+	+	+
Syst, fibrin dep.	+++	+	++	±
Antigenicity	+	–	–	–
Allergic reaction	+	–	–	–
Bolus adm.	–	–	+	+ (single)
TIMI 3 flow	+	++	++	++
Patency (in 90 m)	50%	75%	75%	75%
Cost	Less	More	More	More

*Third-generation fibrinolytic by modification of basic t-PA structure; common feature is prolonged plasma clearance, allowing bolus administration, enhanced potency, and PAI-1 resistance to enhance the efficacy of reperfusion
[†]The very short half-life of alteplase mandates cotherapy with IV heparin to avoid reocclusion.
[‡]SK is not FIB-specific, and treatment with SK leads to proteolysis of fibrinogen, factor V and III, and clotting factor depletion may result in increased bleeding.
(adm.: administration; dep.: deposition; Fib.: fibrin; IV: intravenous; SK: streptokinase; Syst: system; ; PAI-1: plasminogen activator inhibitor-1; TIMI: thrombolysis in myocardial infarction; t-PA: tissue-type plasminogen activator)

Q5. How early administration of fibrinolytics are beneficial?
Ans. Fibrinolytics are most commonly used as reperfusion therapy internationally. Benefit of fibrinolytic therapy is greatest when the agent is administered as early as possible, with the most dramatic result when given within 2 hours of symptom onset.

- Early reperfusion during the golden first hour—can resolve ST elevation without development of Q wave and with very prompt reperfusion, there may be no elevation in biomarkers of necrosis—"aborted MI."
- Between 7 and 12 hours, mortality is still reduced with fibrinolysis, perhaps related more to the benefit of a patent infarct-related artery than to myocardial salvage.
- Fibrinolytic therapy may be the treatment of choice in the first 2 hours and PCI the treatment of choice both in patients with contraindications against fibrinolytic therapy and in those presenting after 3 hours, provided that the procedure can be performed with <60 minutes of PCI-related time delay. For patients within the first 3 hours of symptom onset, more prompt reperfusion with lysis may balance the delayed but more complete and sustained reperfusion with PCI.

Patients with a higher baseline risk of mortality (e.g., anterior wall MI vs. inferior wall MI) are more likely to benefit from fibrinolytic therapy. Second- and third-generation fibrinolytics are superior drugs. Although in cardiogenic shock fibrinolytics are not beneficial (PCI preferred).

Q6. What are reperfusion injuries?
Ans.
- Cellular death of cells
- Vascular—progressive damage to microvasculature-area of no-flow and loss of coronary vasodilatation.
- Stunned myocardium—salvaged myocytes display a prolonged period of contractile dysfunction following restoration of blood flow due to decreased intracellular energy production.
- Reperfusion arrhythmia—bursts of VT, sometimes ventricular failure (VF) within seconds of reperfusion.

Q7. What is the present and future of reperfusion strategy in low middle-income countries?
Ans.
- In many LMICs, many STEMI patients still fail to get any form of reperfusion therapy.
- Thrombolysis is still the reperfusion strategy of choice here.
- Percutaneous coronary intervention capable centers providing round-the-clock service is merger and limited to few major centers.
- Timely reperfusion with thrombolytics should be focused, especially in nonurban and rural areas, if not contraindicated and who cannot get primary PCI within stipulated time frames.
- Early thrombolysis, within 1–3 hours of symptom onset may have mortality benefit equivalent to that of primary PCI. Thus, a health setup capable of providing timely thrombolytics in STEMI is a necessary.

- Urgent referral for unstable, high-risk patients and those with failed thrombolysis for urgent angiography and referral of those with successful thrombolysis for coronary angiography (CAG) after 3–24 hours for PCI, if needed (i.e., PI strategy) may be undertaken to prevent possible reocclusion.

VASODILATORS—INCLUDING ANGIOTENSIN-CONVERTING ENZYME INHIBITORS

Q1. How vasodilators are classified?

Ans. Vasodilators are classified in two ways:
1. According to the site of action in the circulation:
   a. Predominant venodilators (preload reducer): Nitrates and frusemide
   b. Predominant arterial dilators (afterload reducer): Hydralazine, diazoxide, phentolamine, trimethaphan, minoxidil, nifedipines, and other CCB
   c. Balanced dilators (both pre and afterload reducers): Captopril and nitroprusside
2. According to the cellular mechanism of action:
   a. Angiotensin-converting enzyme (ACE) inhibitors—captopril, enalapril, and lisinopril
   b. Nitrate-like agents (stimulate guanyl cyclase and increase cGMP): Nitrates and nitroprusside
   c. Direct smooth muscle relaxants: Hydralazine and diazoxide
   d. Calcium antagonists: Nifedipine, verapamil, and diltiazem
   e. Alpha-adrenergic blockers: Prazosin, terazosin, and doxazocin

Q2. How do ACEI vasodilators differ from non-ACEI vasodilators in their action?

Ans. Angiotensin-converting enzyme inhibitor exerts a direct effect on the renin–angiotensin–aldosterone system (RAAS) by blocking the conversion of angiotensin I to angiotensin II. Circulating aldosterone is reduced as angiotensin II stimulates aldosterone production. Diminished aldosterone levels decrease sodium resorption and potassium secretion in the distal renal tubule. Thus, increased intravascular volume and edema are not the side effects of ACE inhibition; however, hyperkalemia can occur. On the other hand, non-ACEI vasodilators are potent stimulators of the RAAS. This results from lowering of the mean systemic BP and decreased renal perfusion. Activation of RAAS increase aldosterone levels which, in turn, cause sodium and water retention at the distal tubule. The result of this process is increased intravascular volume and edema. Hence, ankle edema is a side effect of most non-ACEI vasodilators. Also the added neurohumoral benefit of ACE inhibitors merits its use as the vasodilator of choice in CHF.

Q3. What are the clinical uses of vasodilators?
Ans. These are:
- Congestive heart failure—ACE inhibitors are the drug of choice. Nitrates combined with hydralazine are also tested to be helpful.
  - Nitrates, being the predominant venous dilator, produce a pharmacologic phlebotomy. This reduces pulmonary congestion in LVF and CHF. Frusemide IV rapidly improves acute pulmonary edema, by venodilatation (even before there is an increased urine output).

  In severe acute MR (also AR), sodium nitroprusside produces acute vasodilatation. Thus, it, by favoring forward ejection of LV volume and lowering regurgitant volume, reduces pulmonary venous pressure and edema.
- *Hypertension:* Balanced dilators and predominantly arterial dilators are agents used as antihypertensives. Calcium antagonists and ACE-inhibitors are first-line antihypertensive agents. Fast-acting IV vasodilators, like nitroprusside, are the agent of choice for rapid lowering of BP in hypertensive crisis.
- *Ischemic heart disease:* Nitrates and calcium antagonists are used as antianginal agents. After MI, ACE inhibitors prevent ventricular remodeling, thus decrease LV size, and improve LV ejection fraction.
- Others—aortic dissection (IV nitroprusside).

Q4. What are the beneficial effects of ACE inhibitors?
Ans.
- Angiotensin-converting enzyme inhibitor may be more effective than other antihypertensive agents for reducing ventricular mass and improving diastolic dysfunction in patients with LVH due to hypertension.
- Angiotensin-converting enzyme inhibitor with sulfhydryl (SH) group, such as captopril prevent nitrate tolerance.
- Angiotensin-converting enzyme inhibitor with SH group, may have a mild antiplatelet effect and may increase insulin receptor sensitivity (insulin resistance is an important component of hypertension).
- Captopril provides more protection against decline in renal function in insulin-dependent patients than other antihypertensives provide. Captopril improves proteinuria in diabetic nephropathy.

CALCIUM CHANNEL BLOCKERS

Q1. How do CCBs differ in their pharmacologic properties?
Ans. Although all act by blocking slow calcium channels, they differ structurally as well as functionally.
- Verapamil is a papaverine derivative, nifedipine is a dihydropyridine and diltiazem is a benzothiazine.

- They have differing binding sites despite clinical similarities. Verapamil and diltiazem interact with different binding sites; both depress nodal tissue as well as vascular tissue (verapamil has more action on AV node and diltiazem on SA node). Whereas, dihydropyridines such as nifedipine bind to a third site and have little clinical effect on nodal tissue.
- Clinically, verapamil, nifedipine, and diltiazem has different spectrum of actions. Vasodilator effect is common to all; hence, they are virtually exchangeable when used for coronary artery spasm. All may be used for mild-to-moderate hypertension and for effort angina.

Q2. What are the important pharmacologic properties of CCB?

Ans. There is structural as well as functional difference among three class of CCBs **(Table 17.4)**.

TABLE 17.4: Calcium channel blockers—pharmacologic properties. There are the important pharmacologic differences in their action.

Parameters	Verapamil	Nifedipine* (and other DHP)	Diltiazem
Arterial vasodilatation	+++	++++	++
SA node inhibition	++++	+	++++
AV node inhibition	++++	–	+++
Negative inotropism	+++	+	++

–, No activity; ++++, most potent effect; intermediate numbers suggest intermediate potency of action.
*Increase in HR due to reflex tachycardia, which is decreased by verapamil and diltiazem (verapamil > diltiazem).
(AV: atrioventricular; DHP: dihydropyridine; SA: sinoatrial)

Q3. Compare the therapeutic uses of various CCB.

Ans. Calcium channel blockers, being a heterogeneous group of drugs, vary in their pharmacologic properties and therapeutic use **(Table 17.5)**.

TABLE 17.5: Calcium channel blockers—therapeutic uses.

	Conditions	Verapamil	Diltiazem	Nifedipine
Angina	Chronic stable	++	++	+/++
	Vasospastic	++	++	++
	Unstable angina	+	+	0
	Angina with hypertension	++	++	++
	Unstable angina (already treated with β-blocker)	+	+	++
	Angina with heart failure	+/–	+	++
	Postinfarction (no LVF)	++	+	0

Contd...

Contd...

	Conditions	Verapamil	Diltiazem	Nifedipine
Hypertension	Severe hypertension	+	+	++
	As first-line monotherapy	++	+	++
	Combination with β-blocker	+	+	++
	As second- or third-line therapy	+	+	++
Arrhythmias	SVT-acute IV use	++	+	0
	SVT-oral prophylaxis	++	+	0
	Ch. AF or flutter (+ digitalis)	++	++	0
Others	Raynaud's phenomenon	0/+	++	+++
	Hypertrophic obstructive cardiomyopathy	++	+	0
	NSTEMI	0/+	+	0

(AF: atrial fibrillation; LVF: left ventricular failure; NSTEMI: non-ST-elevation myocardial infarction; SVT: supraventricular tachycardia)
(+++: strongly indicated; ++: indicated; +: marginal positive effect; 0: no effect; –: negative effect)

Q4. Why are calcium channel antagonists used in patients with PCIs?
Ans. Calcium channel antagonists prevent coronary spasm, which is frequently seen during and shortly after PTCA and other PCIs. They have not been shown; however, to reduce the incidence of restenosis, which usually occurs within the first 6 months after PTCA.

Q5. What is the role of nifedipine in patients with AR?
Ans. Asymptomatic patients with severe AR and normal LV systolic function should be treated with a long-acting nifidipine unless there is a contraindication to its use. It decreases regurgitation by dilation of arteries, thus improving more forward flow.

■ DIURETICS

Q1. When is frusemide preferred over thiazide as a diuretic in cardiovascular conditions?
Ans.
- Frusemide is the diuretic of choice in severe heart failure, because it is more powerful and acts more rapidly. Frusemide promotes venodilatation and preload reduction and is effective (in high dose) in promoting diuresis even in the presence of a low glomerular filtration rate (GFR). These make frusemide the diuretic of choice in acute pulmonary edema. As heart failure ameliorates, frusemide may be replaced by thiazides.

- Hypertension complicated by renal failure-frusemide increases GFR. Low-dose frusemide can be effective even as monotherapy or combined with other agents such as β-blocker and ACEI.

Standard oral dose of frusemide (40–80 mg daily), as used for chronic therapy of heart failure and hypertension, probably causes less hypokalemia than do some thiazides. Short duration of action of frusemide allows postdiuresis correction of potassium. Addition of potassium supplements to frusemide is neither needed nor very effective; addition of potassium-sparing diuretics is probably better.

Q2. When are thiazides preferred over frusemide?
Ans. Thiazide diuretics remain the most widely used first-line therapy for mild hypertension. Longer duration of action and relatively low ceiling (i.e., maximal response is reached at a relatively low dosage) of thiazides compared to furosemides make it a better antihypertensive agent. It may be the initial agent of choice in the elderly, in blacks, and in obese, and when cost and compliance are important. Thiazide diuretics are the best-proven drugs for the treatment of isolated systolic hypertension (ISH). Also, these are often required in controlling severe hypertension when multiple classes of drugs at maximal doses are being used without complete success.

In chronic CHF, thiazides are standard therapy when edema is modest.

Q3. What are the causes of resistance to diuretic therapy in heart failure?
Ans.
- *Incorrect use of diuretics:* (1) Repetitive diuretic administration leads to a reduced diuresis, because the part of the tubular system not affected reacts by reabsorbing more sodium in the face of shrunken intravascular volume. This occurs when diuretics of the same class are combined instead of different classes (sequential nephron block) and (2) the use of thiazide in renal failure (serum creatinine >2.0 mg/dL, GFR <15–20 mL/min).
- Poor renal perfusion—in the face of low cardiac output in CHF or excess hypotension induced by ACEI; diuretic-induced hypovolemia decreases diuresis
- Neurohumoral change in CHF—excess circulating catecholamines, activation of renin-angiotensin-aldosterone system—both produce vasoconstriction and limit renal blood flow
- Eletrolyte imbalance—hyponatremia, hypokalemia, and hypomagnesemia
- Interfering drugs—indomethacin and other nonsteroidal anti-inflammatory drugs (NSAIDs), probenecid and lithium
- Miscellaneous—poor compliance, not restricting dietary salt.

Q4. What are metabolic side effects of diuretics?
Ans.
- *Hyperglycemia:* It is caused by hypokalemia-induced decreased insulin secretion. Patients with a familial tendency to diabetes are prone to a diabetogenic tendency.
- *Dyslipidemia:* Total cholesterol increases in a dose-related fashion (up to 15–20 mg/dL). Also, the low-density lipoprotein (LDL)—cholesterol and triglyceride (TG) increase. During prolonged thiazide therapy a lipid-lowering diet is advisable.
- *Hyperuricemia:* Urate excretion is decreased with the risk of increasing blood uric acid and causing gout in predisposed persons.
- *Hypercalcemia:* Calcium is retained, and hypercalcemia may be precipitated, especially in hyperthyroid patients.

Whether frusemide causes fewer metabolic side effects than conventional thiazides is not clear.

LIPID-LOWERING AGENTS

Q1. What are the advantages of 4-hydroxyl-3-methoxy glutaryl coenzyme A (HMG-CoA) reductase inhibitors (statins) over other lipid-lowering agents?
Ans.
- They directly inhibit hepatic cholesterol synthesis effectively: LDL cholesterol is decreased (18–55%), high-density lipoprotein (HDL) cholesterol is increased (5–15%), and TGs are reduced slightly (7–30%). It is the first-line drug (according to ATP III and IV guidelines of NCEP).
- A single dose at night can be effective, perhaps because cholesterol synthesis occurs at night
- Well tolerated and are by far the most palatable in hypercholesterolemia
- Safe in renal disease (hepatic excretion only)
- Can also be combined with other lipid-lowering agents, e.g., fibrates, etc.
- Since the publication of the 4S study (with simvastatin) and CARE study (with pravastatin) demonstrating regression or cessation of progression of angiographic coronary atherosclerosis, a statin drug is a must therapy for a patient with an ischemic syndrome and a cholesterol level >200 mg/dL or an LDL cholesterol level >100 mg/dL.

Q2. How to monitor therapy with statins?
Ans.
- *Monitoring for side effects:* Monitoring of hepatic aminotransferase levels is recommended during therapy. Therapy should be discontinued when greater than threefold elevation occurs. Enzyme levels typically return to normal within 2 weeks. Either lower doses of the same medication can be reinstituted, or a different agent can be used.

Levels should be measured 6 weeks and 3 months after initiation of therapy and every 6 months thereafter. Creatinine kinase (CK) measurements are not needed unless symptoms of myopathy occur. CK level of >10 times the upper limit of normal may occur with myopathy (a rare complication).

- *Monitoring benefit of therapy:* Serial blood lipid profiles are required to confirm the benefit of therapy. Failure to achieve target lipoprotein levels merits an increase in dose or institution of combination therapy. The target LDL cholesterol level of 100 mg/dL or less may be difficult to attain. Addition of low-dose bile acid resins to the ongoing statin regimen usually results in greater LDL lowering than doubling the statin dose.

Q3. How are lipid-lowering drugs used in combination?
Ans. As each type of lipid-lowering agent has a different mechanism of action, combination therapy may be needed in appropriate cases. For example, an excellent combination with colestipol–niacin–lovastatin in familial hypercholesterolemia decreases total cholesterol by 55%, LDL cholesterol by 66%, TG by 42%, and increases HDL cholesterol by 35% (risk of myositis is increased by lovastatin and niacin). In general, the combination of reductase inhibitors and fibrates or nicotinic acid should not be used to avoid the risk of myositis.

Q4. How dyslipidemia of DM managed with lipid-lowering agents?
Ans.
- *4-Hydroxyl-3-methoxy glutaryl coenzyme A reductase inhibitors (statins):* Lowers cholesterol without any adverse effect on glycemic control. Simvastatin was found more efficacious in secondary prevention of IHD in diabetic patients than nondiabetics in a study.
- *Fibric acid derivatives:* Hypertriglyceridemia of diabetes can be effectively treated. Gemfibrozil may cause a 5–15% drop in LDL levels in patients with normal TG levels, but in patients with hypertriglyceridemia, LDL levels go up.
- *Bile acid-binding resins:* These can decrease levels of LDL in diabetic patients, but they can also cause a significant rise in TG levels, especially if the very low-density lipoprotein (VLDL) level is already high or if diabetes is poorly controlled.
- *Nicotinic acids:* These acids Lower both cholesterol and TG levels while raising HDL levels. It has an adverse effect on glycemic control due to its induction of insulin resistance; hence not generally indicated.

Q5. What are the effects of different lipid-lowering agents on lipid profile?
Ans. Different classes of lipid-lowering agent vary in their lipid-lowering properties **(Table 17.6)**.

TABLE 17.6: Lipid-lowering agents—effect on lipid profile.

Drugs	Effect on lipid profile
• Drugs: – HMG-CoA reductase inhibitors (statins, simvastatin, atorvastatin, fluvastatin, rosuvastatin, lovastatin, etc.)	LDL-C ↓ 18–55% HDL-C ↑ 5–15% TG ↓ 7–30%
Fibric acids (gemfibrozil, fenofibrate, and clofibrate)	TG ↓ 20–50% HDL-C ↑ 10–20% LDL-C ↓ 5–20% (may increase in patients with high TG)
Bile acid sequestrates (cholestyramine and colestipol)	LDL-C ↓ 15–30% HDL-C ↑ 3–5% TG-no change or increase
Nicotinic acid	TG ↓ 20–50% HDL-C ↑ 15–35% LDL-C ↓ 5–25%

(HDL: high-density lipoprotein; HMG-CoA: 4-hydroxyl-3-methoxy glutaryl coenzyme A; LDL: low-density lipoprotein; TG: triglyceride)

Q6. How to treat hypertriglyceridemia?
Ans.
- Borderline-raised TG (200–400 mg/dL)—lifestyle modification (LSM):
    - Diet (limit sugar and carbohydrate, fat, limit alcohol completely eliminate if the level is very high), include fish in diet
    - Exercise—maintain regular aerobic exercise: 30 minutes on most of the days of a week
    - Body weight—obtain and maintain ideal weight
    - Smoking cessation
- Level above 400 mg/dL—LSMs continued for 6 months. Pharmacotherapy (if the level remains above 500 mg/dL)
- Level above 1,000 mg/dL (high risk for acute pancreatitis)—combination of aggressive LSM and drugs

Q7. How are lipid-lowering agents chosen for various dyslipidemic conditions?
Ans. The lipid profile can determine which drug to be used here.
- Patients with CAD—a treatment strategy to further reduce LDL-C is appropriate, as it causes the greatest risk reduction. Statins are potent LDL-C lowering agents; they also increase HDL-C levels slightly and can lower TG up to 30%.
- Patients with low LDL-C, low HDL-C, and high TG-fibric acid derivations (clofibrate, fenofibrate, and gemfibrozil) are a reasonable choice. Here, HDL-C increases by 10–20% (LDL-C may increase slightly).
- Patients with isolated hypertriglyceridemia—fibric and derivatives are the drug of choice. Combination therapy can be used, but patients must be monitored carefully because of the risk of liver toxicity.

INOTROPIC AGENTS

Q1. What are the inotropic agents?
Ans. These are the class of drugs that increase the availability of Ca^{2+} to the contractile elements of cardiac muscle at the time of excitation–contraction coupling.

There are two classes of inotropic agents:
1. Glycosides include digoxin and digoxin-like agents
2. Nonglycosides:
   a. Sympathomimetic amines include EP, norepinephrine, isoproterenol, dopamine, dobutamine, and methoxamine
   b. Phosphodiesterase inhibitors—amrinone, milrinone, etc.

Q2. What are the basic differences between glycosides and nonglycosides?
Ans.
- Cardiac glycosides, e.g., digitalis, have, besides a positive inotropic effect, negative chronotropic, (especially in AF) and a sympatholytic effect. The bradycardic effect is universally beneficial unless there is digitalis toxicity. The combined inotropic-bradycardic action of digitalis is unique when compared to many nonglycosides, which all tend to cause tachycardia.
- Most nonglycosides have vasodilator action along with positive inotropic effect, hence called inodilators. Although vasodilatory action is variable (marked with phosphodiesterase inhibitors and low dose dopamine), it is beneficial in afterload reduction in CHF, cardiogenic shock, etc. Digitalis has no such action.
- Nonglycosides are not available for oral use. Digitalis is available as oral as well as IV preparation. It remains as the basic inotrope for oral use.
- Digitalis acts by inhibition of Na/K ATP-ase pump with an increase in intracellular sodium, which, in turn, enhances calcium influx by sodium–calcium exchange mechanism. By virtue of the vagal effect, it causes sinus slowing and AV nodal inhibition. It exerts a sympatholytic effect on muscles in CHF.
- Nonglycosides act by increasing myocardial and vascular cyclic adenosine monophosphate (AMP). β-receptor stimulation occurs in sympathomimetic amines [phosphodiesterase inhibitors (PDIs) act directly].

Q3. Mention the pharmacologic properties of inodilators.
Ans. Sympathomimetic agents such as EP, norepinephrine, and dopamine and their synthetic analogs such as isoproterenol, dobutamine, and PDI are inodilators that have vasodilatory as well as inotropic action **(Table 17.7).**

TABLE 17.7: Inodilators: Pharmacologic properties.

Drugs	Receptor involved	Inotropic effect	Arteriolar vasodilatation	Vasoconstriction	Chronotropic effect	Effect on BP	Direct diuretic effect	Arrhythmic risk	Use in CHF	Use in resuscitation
Epinephrine	Mixed β_1, β_2 (also some α)	++	+	+	++	0/+	0	+++	0	+/0
NE	$\alpha > \beta$	+	0	++	+	+	+	+	+	+
Isoproterenol	$\beta_1 > \beta_2$	+++	+	0	+++	+SBP	0	+++	0	+/0
Dopamine	Dopaminergic DA_1, DA_2	++	++	+	0/+	0/+ (high dose)	++	0/+ (high dose)	++	++
Dobutamine	β_1 (also β_2)	++	+	0	0/+	0/+	0	+/++	++	++
PDI (amrinone, milrinone)	0	+	++	0	++	0/–	0	+/++	++	0

(+: increase; 0: no effect; –: negative effect; BP: blood pressure; CHF: congestive heart failure; NE: norepinephrine; PDI: phosphodiesterase inhibitors; SBP: systolic blood pressure)

Q4. How does the action of dopamine varies?
Ans. Dopamine is a flexible molecule. It can fit into different receptors at different doses. Besides action on dopaminergic receptors, it can cause direct β_1 and β_2 stimulation, as well as α-stimulation.
- *In doses <2 µg/kg/min:* It stimulates the dopaminergic receptors (DA_1); promotes renal perfusion and improves cerebral, coronary, and mesenteric circulation.
- *In 2-5 µg/kg/min*: It has predominantly inotropic effect, increase cardiac contractility; cardiac output increases with little change in HR.
- *In 5-10 µg/kg/min*: It increases BP, HR, and peripheral vascular resistance, and a decrease in renal blood flow.
  In refractory heart failure, the dose started at 0.5-1 µg/kg/min and is raised until an acceptable urinary flow, BP, or HR is achieved.
- In cardiogenic shock or AMI, 5 µg/kg/min of dopamine is enough to give a maximum increase in stroke volume; arrhythmia may appear at 10 µg/kg/min

■ DIGITALIS

Q1. What is the mechanism of action of digitalis?
Ans.
- *Positive inotropic effect:* It inhibits membrane-bound Na-K ATP-ase (sodium pump). This results in an enhanced transient increase in the intracellular sodium which, in turn, enhances calcium intracellularly by the sodium calcium exchange mechanism. An increased cytosolic calcium concentration results in enhanced myocardial contractility.
- Slowing of AV conduction—by increasing vagal activity via an action on the central nervous system. It causes prolongation of AV refractory period. The beneficial effect in rapid AF is mediated by its action on AV conduction. The inhibitory effect on the AV node is usually preceded by the inotropic effect.
- *Other effects:* Sympathetic inhibition may play an important role in the control of CHF. It inhibits muscle sympathetic nerve activity (it cannot be achieved by dobutamine infusion). In contrast, part of the toxic effect is by the sympathomimetic effect (site of action is on the floor of the fourth ventricle), which probably acts together with intracellular calcium overload to cause arrhythmias.
- Digitalis produces alterations in electrical properties of both contractile cells and the specialized cells, particularly evident with higher does. It occurs by inhibition of Na K ATP-ase causing hypokalemia within cells and predisposing to arrhythmia. With lowering of the resting potential, the rate of rise of action potential is reduced with slowing of conduction of

impulse, which is conducive to the development of re-entry. Increase in cytoplasmic calcium causes delayed after depolarization, thus, triggered impulse may be initiated producing arrhythmia.

Q2. How does the inotropic effect of digitalis differ from that of sympathomimetic amines?

Ans. Digitalis differs from sympathomimetic amines (dopamine and dobutamine) regarding inotropic action as follows:

- Digitalis decreases HR (by the vagal effect), whereas sympathomimetic amines increase it.
- The inotropic effect of digitalis is much weaker than that of sympathomimetics.
- In CHF, digitalis has a sympatholytic effect—inhibiting muscle sympathetic nerve activity.
- Digitalis is effective with oral administration even in patients with gut congestion (in CHF).

Q3. What are the indications of digitalis?

Ans.

- Congestive heart failure with AF—classic indication
- *Congestive heart failure and sinus rhythm:* CHF with dilated left ventricle, imparted systolic function, and a S_3 gallop are prime candidates.
- *Heart failure in children*: It is the mainstay of therapy
- Atrial fibrillation—control of chronic AF (e.g., in paroxysmal AF; if episodes are frequent and prolonged).
- *Acute SVTs*: It is sometimes used alone or in combination with verapamil, diltiazem, or β-blockers.
- Atrial flutter may not respond to digitalis, except in high doses. It may be converted to AF.

Q4. What are the contraindications of digitalis?

Ans.

- *Hypertrophic obstructive cardiomyopathy:* The inotropic effect worsen the obstruction.
- Significant AV nodal block—second-degree AV block (Mobitz type II), intermittent CHB with history of Stokes Adam's attack, or in the setting of AMI, or acute myocarditis
- Diastolic dysfunction (as in severe LVH)—does not respond to digitalis
- Some cases of Wolff-Parkinson-White (WPW) syndrome: It may accelerate antegrade conduction through the bypass tract to precipitate VT of VF.
- Severe renal failure
- Digitalis toxicity—should be confirmed by the measurement of serum digoxin

- *Relative contraindications are:* Chronic cor pulmonale, AF due to thyrotoxicosis hypokalemic states, renal failure, early AMI and postinfarct, severe myocarditis, prior to DC cardioversion, concomitant treatment with drugs causing bradycardia (β-blocker, verapamil, diltiazem, etc.)

Q5. How is the dose of digoxin determined?
Ans.
- *Slow digitalization:* It can be done by using multiple doses over a long period unless urgent indications exist. Thus, a steady-state plasma and tissue concentration may be achieved in 5–7 days. For example, oral digoxin 0.5 mg two times daily for 2 days or 0.5 mg three times daily for 1 day.
- *Rapid digitalization:* In urgent situation, a loading dose may be required, because a certain amount of digoxin is required to saturate the skeletal muscle receptors throughout the body and for tissue penetration until equilibrium is reached. Loading dose of digoxin: 0.75–1 mg IV. Alternatively, a combination of digoxin 0.5 mg IV followed by oral digoxin 0.25 mg, one or two doses to a total of 0.75–1.0 mg.

The usual maintained dose remains 0.25 mg daily. In patients with severe renal insufficiency, a maintenance dose of 0.125 mg/day is recommended. Subsequent dose adjustment may be done from serum digoxin levels.

Weight governs the loading dose, because a low skeletal mass means less binding to skeletal muscle receptors, so that the blood level for any given loading dose is higher in a thin old man.

Q6. What factors influence digoxin dose?
Ans.
- Renal function is the most important determinant of daily digoxin dosage in all groups. A major portion of digoxin is excreted by the kidney unchanged. Renal failure reduces the volume of distribution.
- *Body weight:* A decrease in skeletal muscle and lean body mass causes increased blood digoxin levels, because digoxin binds to cardiac and skeletal muscles.
- Electrolyte imbalance—hypokalemia, hypocalcemia, and hypomagnesemia increase sensitivity to digoxin.
- Chronic pulmonary diseases—increase sensitivity to the toxic action of digitalis.
- Cardiac diseases—AMI, myocarditis (viral or rheumatic), thyrotoxic heart disease—increase sensitivity.
- Concomitant drug—diuretics induce hypokalemia, quinidine causes approximately double blood digoxin levels, amiodarone also elevates serum digoxin levels. Drugs with added effect on the SA or AV node, e.g., verapamil and diltiazem β-blockers, increase sensitivity to digoxin.

Q7. How do electrolyte disturbances influence the effect of digitalis?
Ans. *Potassium interacts with digoxin in two ways:* (1) They inhibit each other's binding to Na-K ATP-ase, thereby hyperkalemia reduces the enzyme-inhibiting action of digoxin, whereas hypokalemia facilitates these action; (2) abnormal cardiac automaticity is inhibited by hyperkalemia, thus moderately increased extracellular K⁺ reduces the effect of digoxin. Calcium facilitates the toxic effect of digoxin by accelerating the overloading of intracellular Ca⁺ stores that appear to be responsible for digitalis-induced abnormal automaticity. Hypercalcemia increases the risk of digoxin-induced arrhythmia. Magnesium effect appears to be opposite to Ca⁺.

Q8. How does digitalis action vary in failing and nonfailing heart?
Ans.
- The positive inotropic effect is exhibited in normal nonfailing, hypertrophied, as well as in failing hearts. However, in the absence of heart failure, it does not increase cardiac output, as it is not limited by cardiac contractility here.
- In patients with sinus rhythm, digitalis slows HR by withdrawing sympathetic activity. It is negligible in a nonfailing heart. Hence, it should not be used for the treatment of sinus tachycardia unless heart failure is present.

Q9. What are the toxic manifestations of digitalis? How does it occur?
Ans. Intoxication due to digitalis excess is common. The typical patient with digitalis toxify is usually elderly with advanced heart disease and AF, often associated with abnormal renal function and pulmonary disease. However, it should be considered in any patient receiving digitalis who presents with new gastrointestinal (GI) (anorexia, nausea, vomiting, and diarrhea) or neurologic (confusion, vertigo, colored vision, etc.) manifestations, or in whom a new arrhythmia or AV conduction disturbance develops.

Mechanism of digitalis toxicity: (1) Intracellular calcium overload predisposing to calcium-dependent delayed after depolarization, which in turn, may develop increased automaticity, (2) excessive vagal stimulation predisposing to AV block, (3) direct depressive effect on nodal tissue, and (4) sympathetic stimulation.

Digitalis induced arrhythmias: A slow pulse is a useful alerting signal.

The most frequent disturbance of cardiac rhythm is premature ventricular beats, which may take the form of bigeminy. AV block of varying degrees of severity may occur. Accelerated junctional or ventricular arrhythmias, when combined with AV nodal block, are highly suggestive of digitalis toxicity. Sinus arrest, sinoatrial exit block, and multifocal PVC may also occur.

Electrocardiographic manifestations depend in part upon the age of the patient and the state of the myocardium. Acceleration of vagal effect with AV block is more common in young healthy individuals whereas, digitalis-intoxicated patients with advanced cardiac disease develop ventricular ectopy.

Q10. What are the electrocardiogram (ECG) changes of digitalis use?
Ans. *Digitalis effect:* ST segment manifests a slight downward slope with a sharp terminal rise, i.e., mirror image of check or correction mark. It is unrelated to serum levels of the drug. This characteristic change develops in leads with the tallest R waves. As a result of the shortening of the electrical systole QT interval shortens.

Digitation toxicity: Ventricular extrasystole are most common, often bigeminy, VT may occur with advanced heart disease. Sinus bradycardia (due to sinus arrest or SA exit block) may occur in patients with high vagal tone. First-degree heart block is common. Second-degree (Mobitz type I) and third-degree AV block may also manifest occasionally (although bundle branch block is not expected).

Q11. How do you manage digoxin toxicity?
Ans. These include:
- Discontinuing digoxin
- Potassium—if hypokalemia is present. Tachyarrhythmia's, particularly multifocal ventricular premature beats or VT, should be treated with lidocaine. Lidocaine should be given only after correction of K^+.
- Digibind (digoxin antibody)—if digoxin toxicity, e.g., second- or third-degree AV block or VT (digibind) should be administered.

Q12. How to monitor digoxin therapy?
Ans. The optimal maintenance dose varies from 0.1 to 0.75 mg daily (depending on renal function). Each patient's dose must be individually adjusted.
- *Clinical:* In AF, the aim is to achieve a resting HR (apical rate) <90 beats/min and a mild postexercise rise. Verapamil or β-blockers may be added if CHF is absent. Here, a test of digoxin level is not usually needed.
- *Laboratory:* Normal level for laboratory therapeutic response is 0.8–2 mg/mL. A level of 3 mg/mL should be avoided, because it is always associated with clinically serious toxicity. Serum digoxin level estimation is advisable only when digoxin toxicity is suspected.

■ ANTIARRHYTHMIC AGENTS

Q1. What are the treatment options for arrhythmia management?
Ans.
- No therapy—if arrhythmia is not significant symptomatically, prophylactic treatment of arrhythmias has been severely questioned by the results of the Cardiac Arrhythmia Suppression Trial (CAST) study.

- Pharmacologic therapy—antiarrhythmic drug selection is often empirical. The side effect profile of available drugs are very different and are often the determining factors in drug selection. Pharmacologic therapy is undertaken when the benefit of treatment clearly outweigh the risk involved.
- *Electrical therapy:* (1) Direct current conversion—it is done if an arrhythmia cause angina, hypotension, or heart failure. (2) Automatic implantable cardioverter defibrillator (AICD)—these sense lethal ventricular arrhythmias and deliver an internal electric shock within 10-15 seconds of arrhythmia onset. They can effectively protect against both tachycardia and bradycardic SCD. Regardless of the underlying heart disease or conditions triggering the arrhythmias. (3) Radiofrequency ablation—by percutaneous catheter; used for ablating accessory pathway in patients with WPW syndrome, ablating His-bundle in some SVT when symptoms are impossible to control with drugs. It may also be applied in some refractory VTs.
- *Surgical therapy:* Aneurysmectomy, CABG, etc.

Q2. What antiarrhythmic agents are effective in preventing SCD?
Ans.
- β-blockers—class II agents are the only antiarrhythmic drugs found clearly effective in preventing sudden cardiac death in patients with prior MI.
- Amiodarone—a class III antiarrhythmic agent (with additional class I, II, and IV properties) has been shown to reduce SCD rates significantly following MI. In patients with CHF who are at high risk for SCD prophylactic therapy with amiodarone has been shown to decrease mortality.
- Sotalol—a potent class III antiarrhythmic agent with nonselective β-blocking effect has been shown to suppress inducible VT in patients presenting with sustained ventricular arrhythmias.

Q3. What is the role of lignocaine in the control of arrhythmia?
Ans. It is effective for the acute suppression of sustained ventricular arrhythmias, especially in the presence of acute myocardial ischemia or infarction. It has no role in the control of chronic recurrent ventricular arrhythmias. Lignocaine has become the standard IV agent for suppression of ventricular arrhythmias with AMI and cardiac surgery.

Use in AMI is recommended in: (1) Frequent, multiform ventricular ectopy, especially R on T-phenomenon, or short runs of nonsustained VT, (2) ventricular ectopics, so frequent or so timed that it significantly impairs hemodynamics, and (3) after an episode of VT or VF requiring electrical conversion or after cardiopulmonary resuscitation (CPR).

Although some data suggest that lignocaine decreases VF in patients admitted within 6 hours of the onset of symptoms in AMI, no evidence shows a beneficial effect in its routine or prophylactic use.

Q4. Classify antiarrhythmic drugs with their indications.

Ans. Antiarrhythmic agents have different sites of action in action potential of cardiac tissues. Thus indications of the four classes of antiarrhythmic vary. Also, digoxin and adenosine are antiarrhythmic agents having their own indications **(Table 17.8)**.

TABLE 17.8: Antiarrhythmic agents—indications.

Drug	Mechanism of action	Primary site of action	Indications
Class IA Disopyramide, procainamide, quinidine	Block fast Na channel, (1a↑ APD, 1b↓ APD Ic no effect)	Ia-atrium, ventricle, bypass tract; Ib-ventricles Ic-His-Purkinje, ventricle, bypass	Extrasystole and tachyarrhythmia (atrial and ventricular) SVT (all types), pre-excitation with AF, and flutter (control ventricular rate)
Class IB Lidocaine, mexiletine, and phenytoin	"	"	Lignocaine-VT and VF especially during acute ischemia and MI. Mexiletine-ventricular tachyarrhythmia's Phenytoin-digitalis induced tachyarrhythmias, polymorphic VT (c̄ ↑QT)
Class IC Flecainide Encainide	"	"	Refractory atrial and ventricular tachyarrhythmia's; SVT due to AV node re-entry and AV bypass tracts
Class II Propranolol and other adrenoceptor blockers	β-receptor blockade	Sinus and AV nodes	Slowing of ventricular rate during AF, atrial flutter, and other atrial tachycardia's (in the absence of pre-excitation); SVT-due to AV nodal re-entry and re-entry utilizing bypass tracts, arrhythmia due to sympathetic over activity (e.g., exercise, hyperthyroidism, VT with congenital long QT syndrome)
Class III Amiodarone	Potassium channel blockade (↑APD)	Atrium, ventricle, AV node, His-Purkinje accessory pathway	Refractory atrial and ventricular tachyarrhythmia's; refractory SVT due to AV nodal re-entry and AV re-entry utilizing bypass tract

Contd...

Contd...

Drug	Mechanism of action	Primary site of action	Indications
Bretylium	"	"	"
Sotalol	(Has combined Class II and Class III activity)	"	Refractory VT and VF, especially due to acute ischemia
Class IV Verapamil and diltiazem	Slow calcium channel blocker	AV node	Slowing of ventricular rate during AF and other atrial tachycardia's in the absence of preexcitation, SVT due to AV nodal re-entry, and AV reciprocating tachycardia
Others: Digoxin	Block Na^+–K^+ ATPase pump, activation of parasympathetic (vagal) system	Sinus and AV node	Slowing of ventricular rate during AF, flutter, and other atrial tachycardia's in the absence of pre-excitation, SVT due to AV nodal re-entry and AV reciprocating tachycardias
Adenosine		AV node predominantly; also, sinus node	PSVT (AV nodal reentrant tachycardia, AV tachycardia, AV re-entrant tachycardia in WPW). In broad complex tachycardia's (to differentiate VT from SVT)

(AF: atrial fibrillation; ATP: adenosine triphosphate; AV: atrioventricular; MI: myocardial infarction; PSVT: paroxysmal supraventricular tachycardia; SVT: supraventricular tachycardia; VF: ventricular fibrillation; VT: ventricular tachycardia; WPW: Wolff–Parkinson–White syndrome)

Q5. What precautions are needed in using amiodarone?
Ans. Thyroid function should be measured every 3 months in all patients receiving amiodarone. The effect on thyroid function is not dose dependent and can occur at any time after initiating treatment. Because of high lipid solubility and long half-life of amiodarone, this effect can persist up to 1-year after discontinuing therapy.

Q6. What is proarrhythmic effect of antiarrhythmic agents?
Ans. Proarrhythmia is defined as a new higher form of arrhythmia, especially with hemodynamically important symptoms, occurring early after the drug use (<30 days) and is not due to other obvious reasons. A tenfold increase in nonsustained VT or frequency of PVC per hour when the baseline PVC frequency is <100/hour on Holter monitoring and threefold increase when PVC frequency is >100/hour is adequate to identify proarrhythmia. Proarrhythmic sudden death was responsible for increased mortality in the CAST study.

This can be overcome by (1) avoiding the use of class I, and especially class IC agent, (2) not treating unless the overall effect will clearly be beneficial, (3) defining subjects at high risk for proarrhythmias and arrhythmic death, and (4) potentially reversing proarrhythmic effect of class IC agents by β-blockers.

SUGGESTED READING

1. Opie LH, Gersh LH. Drugs for the Heart, 7th edition. Philadelphia, PA: Saunders; 2009.
2. Swanton RH. Cardiology, 4th edition. UK: Blackwell Science; 1998.
3. Ramrakha P, Hill J (Eds). Drugs for the heart. In: Oxford Handbook of Cardiology, 2nd edition. UK: Oxford; 2012.

18. Interventional Cardiology

"Percutaneous coronary intervention has evolved dramatically over the past 2 decades fundamentally altering the management of ischemic cardiovascular disease."
—Eric J Topol

■ INTRODUCTION

Catheter-based interventional treatments for patients with coronary, valvular, congenital, and peripheral vascular diseases are effective in many cases. In the absence of diffuse multivessel coronary artery disease (CAD) and left ventricular (LV) dysfunction, percutaneous coronary intervention (PCI) is often the preferred method of revascularization for most patients. Percutaneous mitral valvuloplasty, aortic valve intervention, and percutaneous device implantation for structural heart diseases and some cases of heart failure are widely practiced treatment option nowadays.

Q1. What is interventional cardiology?
Ans. These are catheter-based therapies for the treatment of cardiovascular diseases that provide an effective nonsurgical alternative for patients with coronary, valvular, congenital, and peripheral vascular diseases.

It includes:
- *Intervention for CAD:* Percutaneous transluminal coronary angioplasty (PTCA), stents, atherectomy, and lesser
- *Noncoronary angioplasty:* For renal artery stenosis, peripheral vascular diseases (femoral, popliteal, subclavian, and mesenteric), and aortic (coarctation of aorta, aortitis, etc.)
- *Valvular stenosis:* Pulmonary balloon valvuloplasty, mitral balloon valvuloplasty, and aortic balloon valvuloplasty
- *Congenital:* Atrial septotomy in transposition of the great arteries (TGAs), device closure of atrial septal defect (ASD), ventricular septal defect (VSD), patent ductus arteriosus (PDA), coil closure of collaterals, and tumor feeding vessels
- *Arrhythmia:* Electrophysiological study (EPS) and radiofrequency ablation, automatic implantable cardioverter defibrillator (AICD)
- *Heart failure:* Cardiac resynchronization therapy (CRT)
- *Others:* Percutaneous trans-septal myocardial ablation (PTSMA) for hypertrophic obstructive cardiomyopathy (HOCM), renal denervation therapy (RNT) for resistant hypertension, etc.

Q2. What are PCIs?

Ans. These are coronary revascularization procedures done percutaneously. It comprises a broad array of balloon, stent, and adjunctive devices (e.g., embolic protection, atherectomy devices, and aspiration devices) required to perform the procedure safely and effectively. PCI is generally reserved for patients in whom there is objective evidence of ischemia or symptoms, as well as angiographic evidence of obstructive CAD.

Percutaneous coronary intervention includes:
- PTCA
- Implantation of intracoronary stents
- Atherectomy (i.e., removal of atheromatous material from a heavily diseased segment), which includes directional coronary atherectomy (DCA), laser atherectomy, rotational atherectomy, and extraction atherectomy

Q3. What are the sequential advances in PTCA technology?

Ans.
- *Implantation of stents:* To overcome the problems of elastic recoil and negative remodeling following PTCA.
- *Drug-eluting stent (DES):* To prevent neointimal proliferation and in-stent restenosis (ISR).
- *Advances in stent platform:* Design, material, and strut thickness, thus reducing the quantity of metals with less wall injury and restenosis.
- *Bioabsorbable stents:* These will be completely absorbed over time, while maintaining vessel patency by altering arterial geometry at the time of implantation. Besides, successful absorption vasomotion is restored, i.e., the ability of the coronary artery to contract and expand with normal prestent flexibility.

Q4. What factors favor PCI as a treatment option?

Ans. The ideal candidate for PCI should have the following characteristics:
- Symptomatic with viable myocardium; symptoms not fully controlled by drugs
- Anticipated high likelihood of myocardial infarction (MI), death, if left untreated
- Low procedure-related risk for adverse events: MI, death, and peripheral vascular complications

For those who do not fulfil these criteria, careful judgement must be exercised in reassessing the benefit-risk ratio in conjunction with the patient and his or her family.

Q5. What is percutaneous old balloon angioplasty (POBA)? Give its indications.

Ans. Percutaneous old balloon angioplasty is the procedure where only balloon dilatation of the stenotic coronary artery is done (without deploying a stent).

Indications are:
- Very small vessel (<2.25 mm)
- Predilatation before stent placement
- Postdilatation following stent deployment

Q6. What is a stent?

Ans. These are flexible, balloon-mounted, and expandable stainless steel tubes that scaffold the dilated coronary lesions. Stents are effective in treating dissections, reducing abrupt closure and late restenosis. Two varieties of stents are bare metal stent (BMS) and DES.

Q7. What are the steps in stent deployment?

Ans.
- Guide catheter (size: 6–9 Fr) is placed; standard Judkin's right and left guide catheters are usually used. Sometimes, Amplatz and extra backup (for supporting guidewire and balloon) interventional catheters are used.
- Coronary guidewire is fed into the catheter through an adjustable hemostatic valve using an introducer needle. Wire is threaded into the coronary artery until the tip is positioned as distally as possible in the target vessel (small contrast injections are usually needed to assist the wire position).
- The target lesion is predilated with a balloon (to give the stent space to straddle the lesion).
- Balloon sizing is done with reference to an adjacent nonstenosed vessel segment. Balloon catheter is prepared by flushing the central lumen with heparinized saline, and then emptied under negative pressure and replaced with a diluted contrast agent.
- Stent-mounted balloon is fed over the wire and advanced into the artery (without advancing or retracting wire).
- The balloon is carefully positioned over the stenosed segment (with the help of radio-opaque markers in it).
- The balloon is gradually inflated with a diluted contrast agent (with continued screening so that the balloon does not slip forward or backward). Inflation pressure is increased up to 10–14 atm until either the waist at the stenosed segment disappears or a maximum pressure is reached. The balloon is usually kept inflated for 10–60 seconds **(Fig. 18.1)**.

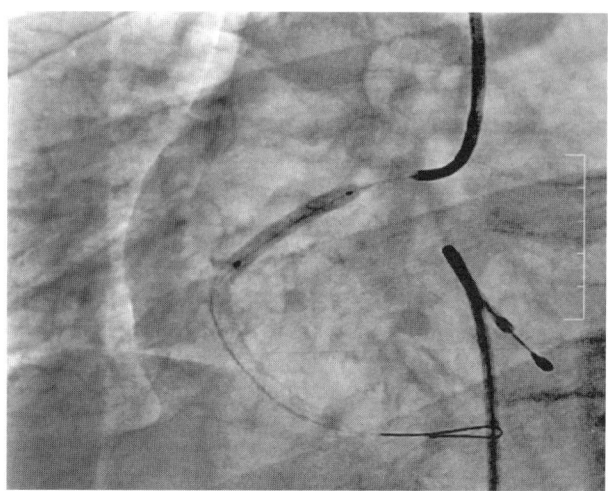

Fig. 18.1: PCI of RCA lesion (guidewire in situ; balloon inflation and stent deployment in progress); also seen TPM lead.

- The balloon is deflated completely and withdrawn from the artery.
- Angiogram is done to assess result.

Q8. What precautions are needed in stent deployment during PCI?
Ans.
- Avoid damage to stent while passing balloon through hemostatic valve (open the valve wide). Stent may not pass easily through the tortuous segment or into side branches (SBs). The vessel may be traumatized, and stent deformed or dislodged from the balloon if the balloon catheter is forced.
- Position of the wire to be maintained always. In severe dissection or acute vessel closure, it may not be possible to revive the vessel if the wire slips back. Hydrophilic and stiff wire increase the likelihood of crossing severe, tortuous stenosis but the stiff wire may traumatize or perforate the vessel.
- For very tight, stenosed lesions, predilatation with a small diameter low-profile balloon may subsequently allow a larger balloon to cross the lesion. An extra backup guide catheter is needed for traversing complex lesions, tortuous vessels, or right angle bends or where the risk of procedural complication (e.g., dissection) is high.
- Very proximal or ostial lesions require catheter with side holes because of occluding the vessel with the catheter. It may also be helpful in PTCA to right coronary artery (RCA) (prone to spasm).
- To preserve SBs, flexible stents, coil stents (instead of mesh or slotted tube stents), and stents with low cell density (i.e., less amount of metal) are recommended.

Q9. What are the various types of balloons?
Ans.
- *Monorail balloon:* Most balloons operate on a "monorail" system, only the distal few centimeters of the balloon catheter ride on the guidewire.
- Over-the-wire balloons require a very long guidewire and are sometimes used in peripheral vascular interventions.
- *Compliant balloon:* Most often used for PCI. As inflation pressure is increased, the balloon diameter also increases; a balloon with 3-mm diameter at the nominal pressure may increase to 3.5 mm at high pressure.
- *Noncompliant (NC) balloon:* Expand relatively little beyond nominal pressure and is useful for hard, calcified lesions and localized areas of underexpansion within stents (require high inflation pressure).
- *Cutting balloon:* Three or four sharp metal microtome blades mounted on a noncompliant balloon, used for atherectomy, i.e., incise coronary atheroma during balloon dilatation.
- *Drug-coated balloon (DCB):* Balloon impregnated with antiproliferative drugs (as in DES)

Q10. When is DCB indicated?
Ans. The effectiveness and safety of DCBs with balloon delivery of a short burst of an antiproliferative agent to a targeted vessel segment are promising. RCTs have shown the safety and efficacy of DCB in the treatment of coronary ISR and treatment of de novo and nonstented restenotic lesions in the superficial femoral artery (SFA). Its role in coronary de novo disease needs further evaluation.

Q11. How to classify stents?
Ans. Stents may be classified as follows:
- Based on composition: Metallic or polymeric
- Mode of expansion: Self-expandable or balloon expandable
- Bioabsorption: Degradable (bioabsorbable) or biostable (durable)
- Configuration: Slotted tube, coiled wire, etc.
- Coatings: None or passive coating as heparin or polytetrafluoroethylene (PTFE) or bioactive coatings such as DES

Q12. What are the components of DES?
Ans. Drug-eluted stent consists of three principal components: (1) The stent backbone itself, (2) the pharmacologic agents intended to reduce neointimal hyperplasia and sometimes other adverse effects, and (3) a polymer design to slow the release of the pharmacologic agent, such that it remains at a sufficient concentration for long enough to interdict relevant biologic processes.

Q13. What are the situations where BMS is preferred over DES?
Ans. The BMS is favored in patients receiving PCI before major surgery or in situations that possess a significant contraindication to long-term antiplatelet therapy.

These are:
- Bleeding diathesis
- Need for chronic warfarin therapy
- Impending noncardiac surgery, which needs discontinuation of dual antiplatelet therapy, predisposing to stent thrombosis

Q14. How to classify DES?
Ans. With the rapid evolution of DES technologies, DESs are classified into several generations of development.
- *First-generation:* Used early BMS platform thick strut stainless steel platform with durable polymer to deliver either sirolimus (Cypher) or paclitaxel (TAXUS) (manufacturing discontinued in 2011 and 2016, respectively).
- *Second-generation:* Currently used; use more deliverable thinner-strut made from cobalt chromium or platinum alloy with more biocompatible polymers eluting (in most cases) rapamycin-analogs, such as zotarolimus (Endeavor, Resolute, and Resolute Onyx) and everolimus (Xience Prime, Xience Expedition, Promus Element, and Promus Premier).

Points to ponder:
- Polymer-free DES is underway, which can be used with a short period of dual antiplatelet therapy (DAPT) in patients with high bleeding risk.
- A variety of bioabsorbable polymer (BP)-based DES has been developed and widely used in Europe and Asia, and approved for use in the USA.

Q15. What are the drugs used in DES?
Ans. The DES provides sustained local delivery of antiproliferative agents at the site of injury. Depending on the agents used, two types of DES are: (1) Sirolimus-eluting stent (Cypher) and (2) paclitaxel eluting stent (TAXUS). Sirolimus is a naturally occurring immunoproliferative agent that produces cytostatic inhibition of cell proliferation. Paclitaxil is a microtubular stabilizing agent having anti-inflammatory effect and inhibits cell migration and division. The release of these agents is completed within 30 days, but they remain in polymer coating indefinitely.

Q16. What are the indications of stents? What are the advantages and limitations?
Ans.
- *Elective (primary stenting):* Primary treatment of complex lesions, restenotic lesions, total occlusions, and lesions with a high restenosis rate [proximal left anterior descending artery (LAD) and saphenous vein grafts]
- As a "bail out" procedure: If coronary dissection occurs, or the vessel occludes

Limitations:
- It is expensive. In some countries, coronary artery bypass grafting (CABG) is the cheaper alternative when more than two stents are required for a procedure.
- A substantial proportion of lesions are either inaccessible (severely tortuous or calcified vessels) or not recommendable for stenting (small and diffusely diseased vessels).

Q17. Why is PCI not preferred as a treatment option?
Ans. The PCI is generally reserved for patients in whom there is an objective demonstration of ischemic symptoms as well as an angiographic demonstration of obstructive CAD.

It is not generally indicated in:
- Asymptomatic or mildly symptomatic patients who have only a small area of jeopardized myocardium
- Have no objective evidence of ischemia
- Have other life-threatening diseases
- Have a low likelihood of success

Q18. When is PCI said to be successful?
Ans. The PCI is said to be successful clinically when there is relief of signs and symptoms of ischemia, plus there is angiographic improvement of coronary obstruction, i.e., residual stenosis of <50% (or <20% with stent) without major in-hospital complications (i.e., death, CABG, and MI).

Q19. What are the current expectations of PCI?
Ans. These are:
- Success rate of 90%
- Mortality rate <1%
- ST-elevation myocardial infarction (STEMI) <1.5%
- Emergency CABG 1–2%.

Q20. Compare BMS with DES.
Ans. The DESs are now widely used because of their lower rate of restenosis. The BMS have a limited use. They differ from each other in the aspects mentioned **Table 18.1**.

TABLE 18.1: Bare metal stent (BMS) and drug-eluting stent (DES).

Points	BMS	DES
Endothelization	2–4 weeks	Delayed; strut-platelet contact for years
In-stent restenosis	More	Less
In-stent thrombosis	Less	More
Dual antiplatelet	Needed (for 1 month)	Needed for 1 year (at least)

Q21. How to assess the results of PCI symptomatically?
Ans.
- Patients should expect to have no anginal symptoms early after discharge.
- Ongoing angina suggests persistent untreated disease or poor result at the treatment site.
- Initial symptomatic relief followed by the recurrence of symptoms after 2-6 months suggests restenosis of the dilated segment.
- Symptom recurrence one or more years after successful angioplasty suggests progression of disease at another site.

Q22. How to classify coronary lesions for PCI?
Ans. The American Heart Association-American College of Cardiology (AHA-ACC) classification of coronary lesion is as follows:
- *Type A lesion:* Discrete lesion (<10 mm length), concentric lesion, lesions easily accessible, nonangulated, smooth contour without calcification, not involving major branches, not ostial, and no thrombus present. These lesions generally have a high success rate (>85%) and are of low risk **(Fig. 18.2)**.

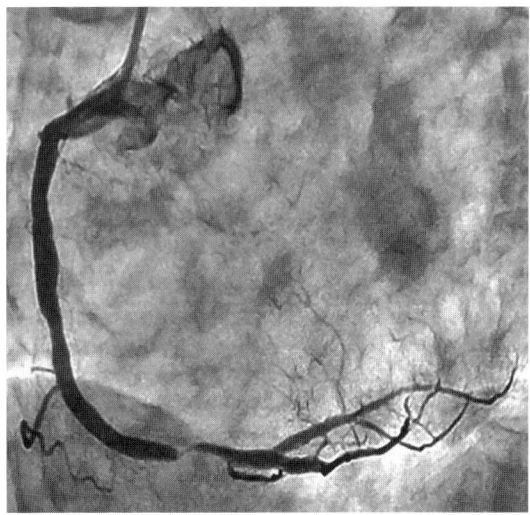

Fig. 18.2: Type A lesion in distal RCA.

- *Type B lesions:* Tubular lesions (10-12 mm long), eccentric, moderately angulated, irregular contour, moderate tortuosity of proximal segment to the lesion, ostial lesions, recent total occlusion (<3 months), at point of bifurcation (often requiring two wires), moderately heavy calcification, and some thrombus present. The success rate is moderate (60-85%) and is of moderate risk **(Fig. 18.3)**.

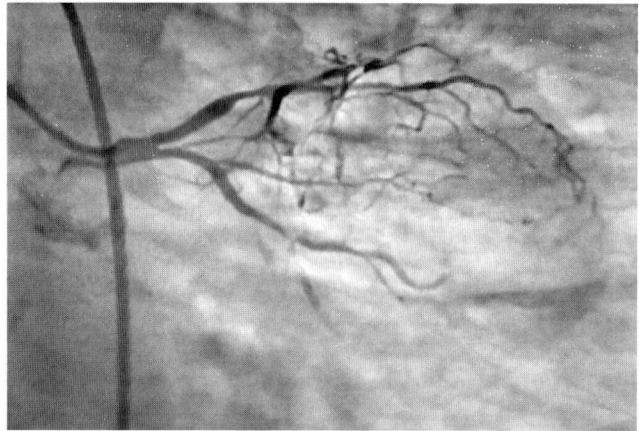

Fig. 18.3: Type B lesion (bifurcation lesion involving LAD and LCx).

- *Type C lesion:* Diffuse lesion (>2 cm long), chronic total occlusion (CTO) (>3 months), excess tortuosity of proximal segment, inability to protect major branches, extremely angulated, and vein graft with friable lesion. The success rate is low (<60%) and is of high risk **(Fig. 18.4)**.

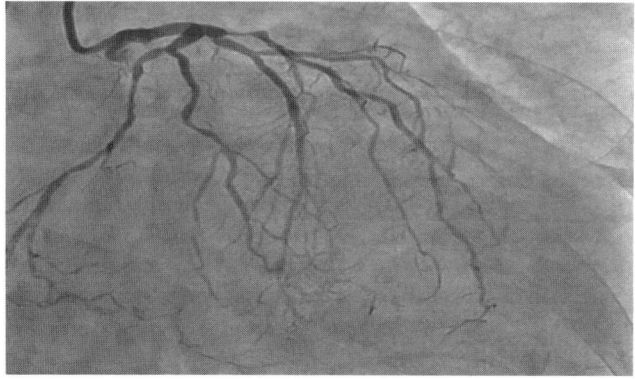

Fig. 18.4: Type C lesion (diffuse lesion in LAD and LCx).

Q23. What are the characteristic features of PCI in type B lesion?
Ans.
- Osteal lesion may be aorto-osteal (taken as a possible bifurcate lesion) and branch osteal lesion.
- Side branch protection is done by placing wire in the bifurcate lesion.
- The two-stent strategy for the main and SB is an accepted approach.
- Dilatation of the main branch (MB) is done first if the wiring SB is difficult.
- Final kissing inflation is proceeded by high-pressure inflation on the SB.
- Glycoprotein IIb IIIa is to be used routinely.

Q24. What are the special features of type C lesion intervention?
Ans.
- The incidence of acute complications and restenosis is high.
- It is often associated with diabetes mellitus (DM) and multivessel disease.
- Rotational atherectomy may be a rational approach to the long-calcified lesion and may render it responsive to balloon dilatation.
- May not be a suitable candidate for conventional bypass grafting due to the involvement of the distal vascular territory

Q25. What is coronary revascularization? Who should get it?
Ans. Coronary revascularization means restoration of vascular supply in the coronary bed. It is done by PCI or CABG. Candidates for coronary revascularization should have the following features: (1) The presence of symptoms that are not acceptable to patients either because of restriction of physical activity or lifestyle or because of side effects from medications or (2) the presence of findings that indicate clearly that patients would have a better prognosis with revascularization than with medical therapy. Anatomic consideration for revascularization is based on the assessment of the grade and class of angina experienced by the patient, presence and severity of evidence of myocardial ischemia on noninvasive stress testing, the distribution and severity of CAD, and the degree of LV function on CAG.

In young patients, revascularization is usually done for both prognostic and symptomatic reasons. In elderly patients, the risk of interventions increases and symptom control may be the main indication for therapy.

Q26. What are the things to consider in determining the mode of revascularization procedures?
Ans. When revascularization is indicated, the choice between PCI and CABG is determined by the factors listed in **Table18.2**.

TABLE 18.2: Revascularization-PCI vs. CABG.

Favor PCI	Favor CABG
Single vessel disease	Left main stem disease
Two-vessel disease without sig. proximal LAD lesion, especially if the LV function is normal	• Two-vessel disease with proximal LAD lesion • Three-vessel disease characteristics that are unfavorable for PCI • Multivessel disease with severe LV dysfunction
Unstable angina (high-risk patients) and acute MI with or without cardiogenic shock	Concomitant valvular, aortic root, or congenital heart disease that will require surgery
Severe comorbidity (e.g., COPD) that makes risk for surgery prohibitive	Long-standing diabetes mellitus with diffuse multivessel disease, especially if with LV dysfunction

Contd...

Contd...

Favor PCI	Favor CABG
Limited life expectancy but requires palliative therapy for symptomatic CAD	Multivessel restenosis (especially diffuse in-stent) or repeated restenosis of proximal single vessel
No more available bypass conduits (in patients with prior CABG)	Strong patient preference to avoid repeat revascularization

(CABG: coronary artery bypass grafting; CAD: coronary artery disease; COPD: chronic obstructive pulmonary disease; LAD: left anterior descending artery; LV: left ventricle; MI: myocardial infarction; PCI: percutaneous coronary intervention)
Note: Improved hardware, technology, and newer drugs allow the use of PCI for a wider range of coronary lesions.

Q27. What are the limitations of PCI?
Ans.
- Although PCI attenuates symptoms, it has not yet been shown to improve survival or attenuate the incidence of MI.
- The PCI should be done only in setting where there is ready-on site access to emergency cardiac surgery, e.g., emergency CABG may be needed in persistent coronary occlusion with ongoing ischemia and hemodynamic instability.
- Expert interventionist is mandatory for PCI assurance that the operator can treat the lesion with a high probability of success.
- The incidence of restenosis is considerable, ranging from 16% to 74%, depending on a variety of factors including clinical presentation and lesion characteristics. Typically, 80% of restenosis will be declared within 3 months of PTCA and almost all by 6 months post-PTCA.
- Outcome is poor in thrombotic, ostial, and calcified lesions.

Q28. How often does restenosis occur following PTCA? What are the predictors for restenosis?
Ans. In general, the restenosis rate is approximately 20–30% within 3–6 months, and it can be even greater in complex lesions. Typically, 80% of restenosis will be declared within 3 months of PTCA, and almost all cases by 6 months post-PTCA.

Predictors of restenosis:
- *esion-related factors:* Total occlusion, vessel size <3 mm, location in ostium, proximal LAD or vein graft, previous angioplasty to the same site, and bifurcation lesion or bend lesion
- *Patient-related factors:* Male, recent symptom onset, and unstable or variant angina
- *Procedure-related factors:* Incomplete dilatation with residual stenosis and dilatation without evident intimal tear

Points to ponder: Not all symptoms after PCI are attributable to restenosis. Symptom persistence/recurrence within the first month is more typical for incomplete revascularization, and those after 6 months are almost always secondary to new lesions.

Q29. What are the indications for PTCA in chronic stable angina?
Ans. PTCA is indicated in following patients with single- and multivessel diseas **(Box 18.1)**.

> **BOX 18.1:** PTCA in chronic stable angina—indications.
>
> - *In single-vessel disease:*
>   - Symptomatic patients with a significant lesion in a major vessel supplying a large area of viable myocardium, PTCA is indicated if any of the following exists:
>   - Intolerance to medical therapy
>   - Continued anginal symptoms despite medical therapy
>   - Inducible ischemia on stress testing done on medical therapy
>   - In asymptomatic patients, PTCA is indicated for single-vessel disease affecting a large area of myocardium if any of the following are present:
>   - Significant inducible ischemia on stress testing
>   - Survivors of a "near death episode" without an MI
>   - History of MI with an ischemic stress test
>   - Planned high-risk noncardiac surgery with objective evidence of ischemia
> - *Multivessel disease:*
>   - For symptomatic patients, significant lesions should involve each of the two major arteries, both supplying a moderate area of viable myocardium. Furthermore, there should be objective evidence for ischemia on stress testing, angina unresponsive to maximal medical therapy, and/or intolerance to medications. Lesion characteristics should suggest a moderate to high success rate, and patients should be in a low-risk group for morbidity and mortality for PTCA
>   - Asymptomatic patients depend on the presence of the same conditions as for single-vessel disease, provided that a large area of myocardium must be supplied by the diseased vessel. Additional lesions supply small or nonviable regions
>
> (MI: myocardial infarction; PTCA: percutaneous transluminal coronary angioplasty)

Q30. What are the antiplatelet agents currently used for PTCA?
Ans.
- *Aspirin:* Most widely used therapy. Dose 75–300 mg daily. Prior treatment with aspirin is associated with a 50% reduction in the rate of vessel occlusion after PTCA.
- *Thienopyridine:* They block adenosine diphosphate (ADP)-mediated platelet aggregation without affecting the cyclo-oxygenase pathway. These are ticlopidine and clopidogrel. Clopidogrel, 300–525 mg loading dose, unless pretreatment for several days has been performed, followed by 75 mg daily (for 2 weeks). It is used in combination with aspirin, especially when stenting is planned. This combination reduces cardiac events and vascular complications.

- *Glycoprotein IIb/IIIa receptor antagonists:* They inhibit the final common pathway of platelet aggregation and are potent antiplatelet agents. These have been proven to have a mitigating role for periprocedural adverse events.

    Abciximab is a monoclonal antibody fragment that blocks the GP IIb IIIa receptor and is most widely used. Evidences show its efficacy in high-risk coronary interventions, especially in patients with unstable angina.

    The recommended dose is 0.25 mg/kg bolus, 10-minute preprocedure, and then 10 μg/min for 12–24 hours afterward.

    Synthetic oral analogs (tirofiban and integrilin) are also becoming available and may be useful in the future.

Q31. How are postprocedural PCI complications defined?
Ans.
- *Abrupt closure:* Obstruction of contrast flow [thrombolysis in myocardial infarction (TIMI) 0 or 1] in a dilated segment with previously antegrade flow.
- *Dissection:* Persistence of contrast after washout of contrast material from the remaining portion of the vessel or an intimal flap as evident by a discrete filling defect in apparent continuity with the arterial wall.
- *Perforation:* Extravasation of the contrast material confined to the pericardial space immediately surrounding the artery, not associated with tamponade (localized) or a jet with tamponade (nonlocalized).
- *Distal embolization:* Migration of a filling defect or thrombus to distally occlude the target vessel or one of its branches.
- *Coronary spasm:* Transient or permanent narrowing >50%, when a <25% stenosis has been previously noted.

Q32. What is multilesion and multivessel PCI?
Ans.
- *Multilesion PCI:* PCI in multiple arterial segments in a patient with single-vessel disease or in a patient with multivessel disease.
- *Multivessel PCI:* It means PCI in more than two or all three major coronary arteries [LAD, left circumflex artery (LCx), and RCA]. The presence of multivessel disease increases the complexity of PCI. Most PCI patients with multivessel disease have two-vessel disease, whereas most patients undergoing CABG with multivessel disease have three-vessel involvement, and they have more severe LV dysfunction.

Q33. What are the types of revascularization undertaken in multivessel diseases?
Ans.
- *Complete revascularization:* Successful treatment of all lesions with 70% or more lesions. In patients with extensive disease, PCI is less likely to achieve complete revascularization than CABG.

- *Incomplete revascularization:* When a significant residual lesion remains, usually in a distal segment or a distal lesion too small to treat may account for incomplete revascularization.
- *Incomplete but adequate revascularization:* When the unrevascularized artery supplies the nonviable myocardium. It is more common in PCI than in CABG.
- *Culprit lesion revascularization:* A strategy of dilating only the lesion thought to be principally responsible for the patient's ischemia and leaving other lesions untreated. It is usually associated with good clinical outcome.

Q34. How does abrupt closure occur in PCI?
Ans.
- Formation of obstructive intimal dissection flap and intramural hematoma by extensive disruption of intima
- *Thrombus:* Most common after stent implantation (more with DES), especially when stents are inadequately deployed by traditional inflation pressure (6–8 atm) with poor apposition of stent struts to the arterial wall. Stent thrombosis arises primarily at the site of poorly apposed atherosclerotic plaque or stent struts protruding into the arterial lumen.
- *Propagation of pre-existing mural thrombus at the treatment site:* In acute coronary syndrome (ACS) patients
- *Local coronary vasoconstriction:* From platelet and endothelial derived vasoconstrictor factors and loss of endothelium-derived relaxing factor (EDRF)

BIFURCATION LESIONS

Bifurcation lesion intervention is an enigma. It is one of the most complex and controversial procedures with a high risk of stent thrombosis and restenosis. There is still no consensus about the strategy for bifurcation intervention. The bifurcation lesion consists of the MB and the SB. The optimal expansion of MB stent without compromising SB is the ultimate goal. Most cases can be treated with a provisional approach, but there are some cases that need two-stent strategies from the beginning.

When dedicated DESs for bifurcate lesions become available, the use of a two-stent strategy may become more liberal. It may facilitate conquest of one of the most challenging areas in interventional cardiology.

Q1. What is a bifurcation lesion?
Ans. A bifurcation lesion is one that occurs at, or adjacent to, a significant division of the major epicardial coronary artery. In true bifurcation lesion, the MB and the SB are both significantly narrowed (>50% diameter stenosis). All other lesions involving bifurcation site are non-true bifurcations.

Q2. How to classify bifurcation lesions?

Ans. Among the various classifications, the "Medina" classification is still the most simplified and widely used approach to classify the distribution of atherosclerotic plaque at the bifurcation site. The presence of "1" means >50% diameter stenosis and "0" means the absence of stenosis, in each of the three bifurcation segments, starting with proximal MB, distal MB, and proximal SB: 1, 1, 1 is a critical stenosis in all three segments and 1, 1, 0 where only the proximal and distal MB are affected.

Q3. What are the strategies of bifurcation lesion stenting?

Ans.

- *Provisional stenting:* Stenting the MB only with provisional stenting of the SB. Provisional T-stenting with SB stenting remains the gold standard, and the most frequently used technique for most bifurcate lesions. Here, after stenting of the MB, proximal optimization technique (POT), FKBI in the SB, and a final POT, a second stent is placed in the SB when the result is unsatisfactory [>75% residual stenosis, dissection, TIMI flow <3 in >2.5 mm, or fractional flow reserve (FFR) <0.80]. SB stenting is performed with T-stenting or T-stenting and small protrusion of 1–2 mm into the MB (TAP), reverse internal crush, or provisional culotte technique, followed by kissing balloon inflation. FFR or optical coherence tomography (OCT) can evaluate SB results after balloon dilation.

- *Two-stent strategy:* Stenting both the MB and the SB. Routine two-vessel stenting does not improve either angiographic or clinical outcomes for most cases of bifurcate lesions. It is reserved only for selected "true" bifurcations. The size and territory of distribution of SB, length of lesion at ostium of SB (e.g., a large SB with ostial disease extending >5 mm from carina), angle MB and SB, and narrowing at SB ostium are to be considered in decision-making.

Techniques are (1) Culotte technique (second stent advanced and expanded into the MB after rewiring through the stent struts in SB and optimization by POT). It gives the best coverage of the carina. As struts toward SB need dilation, open-cell design stents are recommended here. (2) The mini-crush technique (the SB stent crushed by the MB stent). (3) Double kissing (DK) crush where the protruding SB stent crushed by the MB balloon, followed by a second crush by the second stent advanced in MB. (4) The V and simultaneous kissing stent (SKS) technique, where two stents are implanted in MB and SB together; a new carina is created by pull back of both stents and kissing inflation is performed. (5) In T-stenting, a second stent is advanced into the SB following adequate dilatation of the MB stent struts. The stent is positioned at the SB ostium, trying to minimize any possible gap, and a second kissing balloon inflation is done.

Kissing balloon inflation for carina reconstruction is optional in provisional stenting but mandatory in two-stent techniques.

Q4. What is the inter-relationship between MB and SB?
Ans.
- The angle between MB and SB may be acute, close to 90°, or obtuse. The narrower the angle between MB and SB, the higher the risk of plaque shift and compromise of the ostium of SB.
- The term SB may be misleading sometimes. In some anatomical conditions, SB is as important as MB, regarding size and territory of distribution. Left main coronary artery (LMCA) bifurcating into LAD and LCx, an RCA bifurcating into PDA, a number of posterolateral branches, a dominant LCx bifurcating into distal circumflex, and a large OM are situations in which SBs are important vessels that may generate a large ischemia if left untreated.
- In bifurcation stenting, SB should be protected by inserting the wire and leaving it until MB stenting is completed. During jailed wire retrieval, trauma to coronary ostium should be avoided.

Q5. What is POT?
Ans. The POT is carried out after MB stenting by inflation of a short larger-diameter balloon just proximal to carina; it should be performed before SB rewiring to facilitate access. Also, the procedure should be finalized by POT after kissing to correct the proximal MB stent distortion.

CHRONIC TOTAL OCCLUSION

The CTO PCI should be considered in patients with angina resistant to optimal medical therapy and those with large ischemic burden. It is shown to provide relief angina and dyspnea and improve exercise capacity and LV function. It has been shown to be cost-effective in highly symptomatic patients. Successful CTO PCI improves symptoms, ejection fraction (EF), and long-term clinical survival. Complications are higher with CTO PCI compared with non-CTO PCI.

Q1. Define CTO.
Ans. The CTO is defined as a coronary occlusion known to be present for 3 months or a newly documented occlusion not attributable to a similarly recent ischemic event. Here, occlusion means stenosis within which there is neither a continuous visible lumen nor any visible antegrade flow, i.e., TIMI grade 0. Clinically, a CTO imitates a lesion with an FFR of 0.8 or less.

Coronary occlusion must be detected by catheter-based angiography. Computed tomography (CT) angiography cannot be used to reliably distinguish CTO from high-grade stenosis with preserved flow. When a long tortuous microchannel exists within a previous occlusion, it is a recanalized CTO.

A lesion with TIMI grade 1 flow, i.e., trace antegrade flow is a subtotal occlusion.

Lesion with a residual lumen but without an antegrade flow because of competing collateral flow is referred to as pseudo-occlusion.

Q2. What are the challenges in CTO PCI?
Ans. Chronic total occlusion is a frequent reason for not proceeding with PCI. CTO PCI is a major technical challenge for intervention cardiologists. Factors contributing are (1) initial traversing of lesion with a guidewire, (2) length of occlusion, (3) presence of calcification, and (4) fibrosis at the suture line after graft failure.

Q3. What are the unique features of CTO lesions?
Ans.
- Chronic total occlusion connotes more advanced atherosclerosis. Patients are on average 1–2 years older, more likely to be male, and more likely to have diabetes and hypertension. Multivessel CAD is more commonly present, as is PAD and cerebrovascular disease.
- Viability of myocardium distal to a CTO is dependent upon collateral circulation. Both ischemia- and flow-mediated shear stress stimulate collateral development.
- Diagnosed incidentally, despite long-standing CTO, an ACS arising in other coronary segments is a common trigger for cardiac catheterization that leads to CTO detection.
- CTO PCI is a complex procedure that demands experienced operators at centers with specialized CTO equipment and access to circulatory support and cardiac surgery. Ad hoc CTO PCI (coincident with diagnostic catheterization) is discouraged.
- Primary indication in the setting of single-vessel CAD is a relief of ischemic symptoms that persist despite drug therapy. The frequency of CTO PCI is much lower than for obstructive nonocclusive CAD in practice and varies widely among physicians and centers.
- Some unique complications are related to retrograde techniques.

▪ PRIMARY PERCUTANEOUS CORONARY INTERVENTION

Primary PCI is now the mainstay of reperfusion therapy in patients with STEMI. It is superior to thrombolytic therapy in reducing death, reinfarction, reocclusion of infarct-related artery, ischemia, and intracranial hemorrhage (ICH) in patients with STEMI irrespective of patient's risk or whether interhospital transfer for PCI is required. High efficacy and low contraindications in patients presenting early or late after symptom onset are its advantages.

Interventional Cardiology

Q1. What is primary PCI?

Ans. It is the strategy of emergent coronary angiography followed by coronary angioplasty with or without stenting of the infarct-related artery and without prior administration of fibrinolytic therapy. It has become the standard of care for STEMI. The current guidelines recommend primary percutaneous coronary intervention (PPCI) as the default reperfusion strategy for patients with STEMI presenting within the first hours from the symptom onset. PPCI improves survival even in patients with STEMI who have contraindications to fibrinolysis or in patients presenting outside the therapeutic window of fibrinolysis.

Q2. What is the current status of primary PCI?

Ans. The PCI has revolutionized care of ACS; 80% of PCI done in ACS in the USA is primary PCI.

- Initially introduced as an alternative to fibrinolytic therapy in STEMI, now recognized as the reperfusion therapy of choice.
- The current guidelines recommend PPCI as the default reperfusion strategy for patients with STEMI.
- Restores coronary flow promptly in >90% cases.
- Superior to thrombolytic therapy in reducing death rate, reinfarction, intracranial bleeding, reocclusion of infarct-related artery, and recurrent ischemia.

Q3. Mention the time targets in reperfusion of STEMI.

Ans. The target interval of time recommended for STEMI cases is shown in **Table 18.3**.

TABLE 18.3: Target time in STEMI.

Time intervals	Targets
FMC to ECG and diagnosis*	≤10 minutes
STEMI diagnosis to PPCI (wire crossing)†	≤120 minutes
STEMI diagnosis to wire crossing (at PPCI hospitals)	≤60 minutes
STEMI diagnosis to wire crossing in transferred patients	≤90 minutes
STEMI diagnosis to start of fibrinolysis‡	≤10 minutes
Start of fibrinolysis to evaluation of its efficacy	60–90 hours
Start of fibrinolysis to evaluation angiography	2–24 hours

*ECG should be interpreted immediately.
†To choose PPCI strategy over fibrinolysis (if the target time cannot be met, consider fibrinolysis).
‡in patients unable to meet PPCI target times.
(ECG: electrocardiogram; FMC: first medical contact; PPCI: primary percutaneous coronary intervention; STEMI: ST-elevation myocardial infarction)

Q4. What are the indications of PPCI in STEMI patients?
Ans. Class I indications of PPCI according to the ACC/AHA guidelines are: (1) Patients with STEMI with ischemic symptoms <12 hours (level of evidence A); (2) patients with STEMI with ischemic symptoms <12 hours who have contraindications to fibrinolysis irrespective of time delay from first medical contact (level of evidence B), and (3) patients with STEMI and cardiogenic shock or severe heart failure irrespective of the time delay from STEMI onset (level of evidence B).

■ INTERVENTION OF STRUCTURAL HEART DISEASE

Structural heart disease interventions include various interventions for valvular and congenital heart diseases, as well as interventions undertaken in heart failure. Commonly done interventions for structural diseases are balloon mitral valvuloplasty (BMV) for severe mitral stenosis, device closure of secundum ASD, device closure of PDA, transcatheter aortic valve replacement (TAVR), etc. BMV and heart failure interventions are discussed here. The rest of the things are discussed elsewhere.

Q1. What is percutaneous balloon valvuloplasty?
Ans. These are cardiac interventions involving the dilatation of stenotic cardiac valves with large diameter balloon catheters introduced percutaneously.

Q2. What are the major steps in BMV?
Ans. The BMV is commonly done by the Inoue balloon technique **(Figs. 18.5A and B)**. The Inoue balloon is self-positioning and pressure extensible, low profile (4.5 mm), and size (24–30 mm in diameter). Its three parts have differing elasticity, enabling them to be inflated sequentially, thus minimizing the risk of mitral leaflet injury and mitral regurgitation (MR). Serial hemodynamic measurements, alone or in combination with echocardiography, evaluate the result of BMV. The major steps are:

- Trans-septal puncture is done with the Brockenbrough needle via the right femoral vein.
- 8F Mullins sheath with a dilator is introduced through the septal puncture.
- After entry into the left atrium (LA), the needle and dilator are removed, and a stiff wire is introduced into the LA.
- Inoue balloon is introduced into the LA.

Distal portion of the balloon dilated first with 1–2 mL of diluted contrast medium, thereafter pulled back and anchored at MV. Subsequently, inflation of the proximal and middle portion is done. At full inflation, the waist of the balloon in its mid portion disappears.

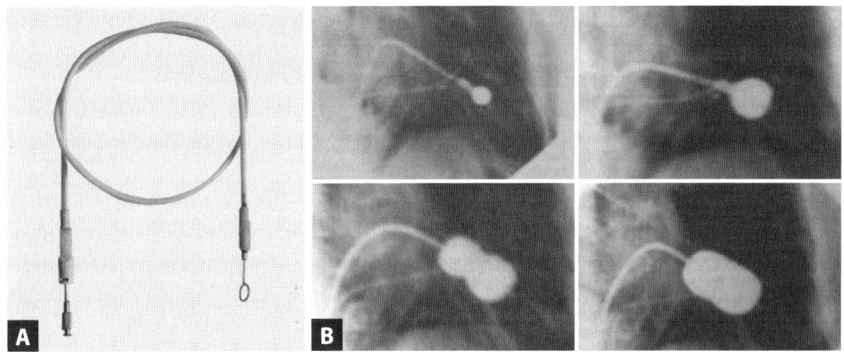

Figs. 18.5A and B: (A) BMV-Inoue balloon; (B) Inflation in progress.

Q3. What are the desired endpoints in BMV? What are its contraindications?

Ans. Desired endpoints of BMV are mitral valve area (MVA) >1.5 cm^2, complete opening of at least one commissure, and appearance or increment of MR >1/4.

The BMV contraindicated in the presence of LA thrombus, MR >2/4, massive or bicommissural calcification, severe aortic valve disease, or severe tricuspid stenosis plus regurgitation, and severe concomitant coronary heart disease (requiring CABG).

Q4. Besides BMV, what are the other indications of trans-septal puncture?

Ans. Besides BMV, other situations needing trans-septal puncture are percutaneous mitral valve (MV) repair, left atrial appendage (LAA) closure, some cases of PFO closure, and atrial fibrillation (AF) ablation.

Interatrial septum (IAS) is crossed through fossa ovalis below limbus fossa ovalis (an area of 2 cm in diameter). It is located posterior and inferior to the aortic root in the mid portion of IAS. The procedure is performed using the Brockenbrough needle introduced through an 8 Fr. Mullins sheath and dilator combination.

Q5. What are interventions for heart failure?

Ans. These include interventions for primary and secondary valve disease, e.g., TAVR in aortic stenosis, percutaneous MV repair (MitraClip system) in functional MR, repair of severe functional tricuspid regurgitation in right heart failure, and implantable hemodynamic monitors such as PAP monitoring and interatrial shunt device.

■ SUGGESTED READING

1. Antman EM, Anbe DT, Armstrong PW, Bates ER, Green LA, Hand M, et al. American College of Cardiology/American Heart Association. ACC/AHA guidelines for the management of patients with ST-elevation myocardial infarction--executive summary: a report of the American College of Cardiology/

American Heart Association Task Force on Practice Guidelines (Writing Committee to Revise the 1999 Guidelines for the Management of Patients With Acute Myocardial Infarction).Circulation. 2004;110(5):588-636.
2. Khanna NN, Henry M (Eds). Handbook of Interventions for Structural Heart and Peripheral Vascular Disease, 1st edition. New Delhi: Jaypee Brothers Medical Publishers (P) Ltd; 2016.
3. Levine GN, Bates ER, Blankenship JC, Bailey SR, Bittl JA, Cercek B, et al. 2011 ACCF/AHA/SCAI guideline for percutaneous coronary intervention: a report of the American College of Cardiology Foundation/American Heart Association Task Force on Practice Guidelines and the Society for Cardiovascular Angiography and Interventions. Circulation. 2011;124(23):2574-609.
4. Thach N, Dayi H, Shao L, Moo-Hyun K, Shigeru S, Cindy G, et al. Practical Handbook of Advanced Interventional Cardiology, 4th edition. Willey-Blackwell; 2013.
5. Topol EJ, Teirstein PS (Eds). Textbook of Interventional Cardiology, 8th edition. Elsevier; 2019.

CHAPTER 19

Diseases of the Aorta

"Palpation as well as auscultation is usually unrevealing. Chest radiography, echocardiography, CT, MRI, and aortography are imaging modalities for diagnostic examination of the aorta."

—EM Isselbacher

■ INTRODUCTION

Aorta, the largest and strongest artery of the body, is both tensile and elastically distensible. It is commonly involved by aneurysm, dissection, and autoimmune process (e.g., Takayasu arteritis).

Q1. What are the diseases of the aorta?
Ans.
- *Congenital:* Coarctation—preductal (infantile) and postductal (adult type), and aneurysm of sinus of Valsalva
- *Acquired:* Atherosclerosis, aortitis, infection, e.g., syphilitic, extension of atrioventricular (AV) endocarditis, autoimmune (Takayasu's aortitis), trauma (may produce false aneurysm), dissecting aneurysm—type A (involve ascending aorta with or without extension into descending aorta) and type B (involve descending aorta with or without involvement of ascending aorta).

Q2. What is coarctation of the aorta? What are the types?
Ans. Coarctation is a localized narrowing of aortic lumen due to deformity of aortic media. If the defect is predominantly in the intima, it is called stenosis, e.g., stenosis of abdominal aorta, etc.

Types:
- Adult type: Coarctation at or below the insertion of ductus arteriosus (i.e., distal to origin of left subclavian artery)
- Infantile type: Diffuse involvement of preductal aorta with cyanosis and patent ductus arteriosus
- Reversed coarctation—acquired in Takayasu aortitis

Q3. What are the associations and complications of coarctation of the aorta?
Ans.
- *Associations:* Bicuspid aortic valve (46%), patent ductus arteriosus (PDA), isolated ventricular septal defect (VSD), hypoplastic aortic arch, and berry aneurysm

- *Complications:* Left ventricular failure, aneurysm formation and dissection of ascending aorta, subarachnoid hemorrhage from ruptured berry aneurysm, infection of coarctation or bicuspid AV, and persistent hypertension despite repair of coarctation.

Q4. How does hypertension occur in coarctation? What are the special features?

Ans. Coarctation of aorta is a cause of secondary hypertension. Here, both the systolic and diastolic pressures above the coarctation are elevated; systolic pressure in legs is lower than that in arms, and diastolic pressure is usually normal or slightly lower below the coarctation. Mechanisms are: (1) Increased resistance to aortic flow by the coarctation; (2) decreased capacity and distensibility of vessels into which LV ejects, and (3) humoral factors, such as activation of renin–angiotensin system by diminished flow into the kidneys.

Special features are:
- Hypertension presents only in upper extremities
- It usually increases during first several months of life and then tend to diminish again as collateral circulation improve.
- Some patients with severe coarctation and well-developed collaterals around the coarctation may be normotensive at rest, but have inappropriate hypertension with exercise.
- Timely surgical repair cures the hypertension.
- If repair delayed or hypertension is long-standing prior to repair, it may persist even after repair. It is due to renal involvement.

Q5. What murmurs are found in coarctation?

Ans.
- *Murmur due to coarctation itself:* An ejection systolic murmur at level of fourth intercostal space posteriorly and left second intercostal space anteriorly close to the sternum.
- *Murmur (bruit) of collateral circulation:* Low-pitched, continuous, bilateral; heard over the chest, particularly posteriorly; and seldom before adolescence.
- Due to associations, e.g., bicuspid AV produces ejection sound with short mid systolic [in aortic stenosis (AS)] and early diastolic murmur [in aortic regurgitation (AR)], murmur of VSD or PDA, etc.

Q6. What collaterals develop in coarctation? What are their diagnostic importance?

Ans. Several collaterals develop in the anterior and posterior systems.
- *Anterior system:* This system originates from internal mammary artery and makes use of epigastric artery in abdominal wall to supply lower extremities.

- *Posterior system:* This system involves parascapular arteries that connects to posterior intercostal arteries (branch of descending thoracic aorta) and carries blood to distal aorta, principally for supply to abdominal viscera. These dilated posterior intercostal arteries produce rib notching.
- *Anterior spinal arteries:* Receiving branch from proximal and distal segments of coarctation are also dilated and tortuous.

Rib notching produced by posterior system occurs from the age of 6 to 8 years. It does not occur in first and second ribs (first two posterior intercostal arteries do not arise from aorta but from costocervical branch of subclavian arteries). Presence of rib notching on X-ray chest examination are suggestive of coarctation.

Q7. What are the radiologic features of coarctation of aorta?
Ans.
- *Rib notching:* Notching in lower margins from third rib in their posterior aspect
- Typical aortic knuckle is absent and is replaced by a double knuckle in a figure of "3" manner. Upper part is the dilated subclavian artery, and lower part is poststenotic dilatation of descending aorta. Left ventricle (LV) is normal or variably enlarged.
- Left ventricular hypertrophy **(Fig. 19.1).**

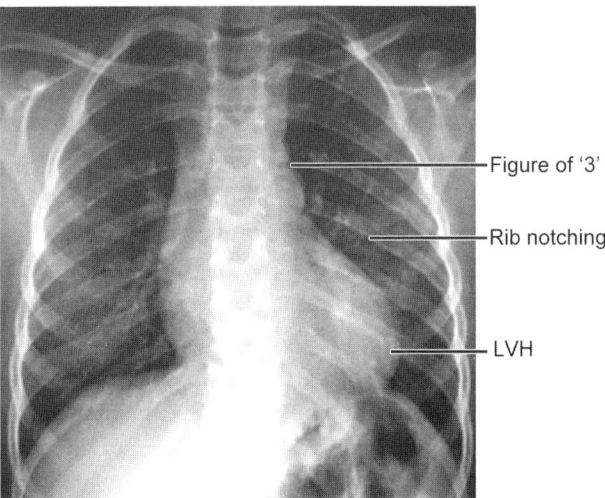

Fig. 19.1: Chest X-ray showing coarctation of aorta.

Q8. How MRI helps in diagnosis of coarctation?
Ans. MRI is the ideal investigation for demonstrating coarctation. It shows the coarctated segment, collaterals developed as well as intercostals arteries **(Fig. 19.2).**

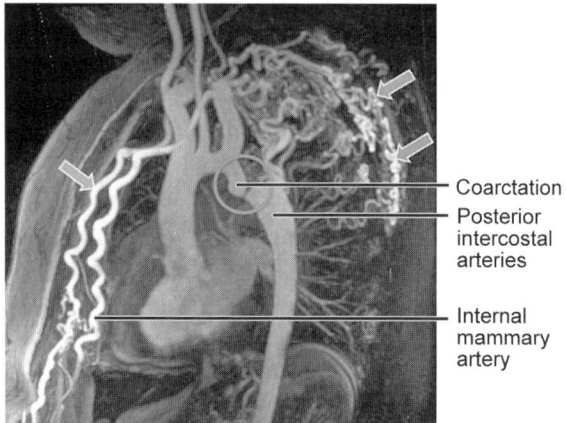

Fig. 19.2: MRI in coarctation of the aorta with extensive collaterals.

Q9. What is the treatment of coarctation?
Ans.
- Surgical resection and end-to-end anastomosis or if necessary, by graft insertion are the treatment options. Elective correction is recommended between 1 and 4 years or at time of diagnosis (which may be late). If corrected before 1 year, recoarctation occurs and if done after 6 years, hypertension may persist.
- Balloon angioplasty—particularly effective in cases of recoarctations, stent placement may be considered as primary measure for selected older patients.

Q10. What are the presentations of aortic dissection?
Ans. Severe chest and/or back pain is the typical presenting symptom. Pain is of sudden onset. Its severity is maximum at onset, in contrast to the pain of myocardial infarction (MI), which is more gradual in onset. The pain is described as tearing or stabbing; often follows the course of dissection, i.e., anteriorly in proximal dissection and to the back or interscapular area, with distal (i.e., type B) dissection.

Less common presentations include: Congestive heart failure (CHF) (due to severe, acute AR in proximal dissection), syncope (cardiac tamponade due to rupture into pericardial cavity), neurologic features, such as paraplegia (in distal type), CVD (proximal dissection), etc.

Q11. What are the BP findings in aortic dissection?
Ans.
- *Hypertension:* Often seen in dissection, frequently as the cause and occasionally as a complication (distal dissection involving renal artery producing ischemia)

- *Hypotension:* It may be found in proximal dissection, with involvement of aortic root, producing hemopericardium and cardiac tamponade.
- *Pseudohypertension:* When subclavian artery is involved with resultant compression, hence underestimation of BP.

Q12. How to differentiate aortic dissection from acute MI?

Ans. Aortic dissection and acute MI are cardiac emergencies, needing urgent attention and management. They differ from each other in the aspects mentioned in **Table 19.1**.

TABLE 19.1: Difference between aortic dissection and acute MI.

Points	Dissection	Acute MI
Risk factors	Hypertension, sometimes CT disease	Hypercholesterolemia, smoking, DM, and hypertension
Chest pain	Tearing pain maximum at onset; usually radiate to interscapular area	Compressing pain, gradually increasing in severity; radiates to left arm
BP (at presentation)	Often increased, rarely decreased	Hypertension unusual; may be hypotensive in cardiogenic shock
ECG	LVH common, no ST elevation or Q (very rarely occur if coronary ostia involved in dissection producing MI)	St elevation and Q wave are typical
Cardiac enzymes	Normal	Elevated
Treatment: Intravenous beta blockers	Used to prevent further dissection in all patient (to↓ cardiac ejection velocity)	May be used to relieve uncontrollable chest pain, prevent cardiac rupture and arrhythmia, especially in anterior MI
Intravenous nitroprusside	To decrease afterload; used in all patients	To reduce afterload in some patients with heart failure
Streptokinase	Contraindicated (even if MI occur as complication)	Indicated
Surgery	Repair generally needed in proximal type (type A)	CABG in some patients with complications

(CABG: coronary artery bypass grafting; CT: computed tomography; DM: diabetes mellitus; MI: myocardial infarction; LVH: left ventricular hypertrophy)

Q13. How will you manage a suspected case of aortic dissection?

Ans. The patient should be admitted to the intensive care unit for close monitoring. Intravenous β-blockers should be started immediately. Then intravenous nitroprusside should be started to maintain mean arterial pressure of 60–70 mm Hg.

Diagnosis is confirmed by several investigations such as echocardiography [transthoracic echocardiography (TTE) and transesophageal echocardiography (TEE)], MRI, and CT. Aortic dissection cases are managed according to the steps shown in **Flowchart 1**.

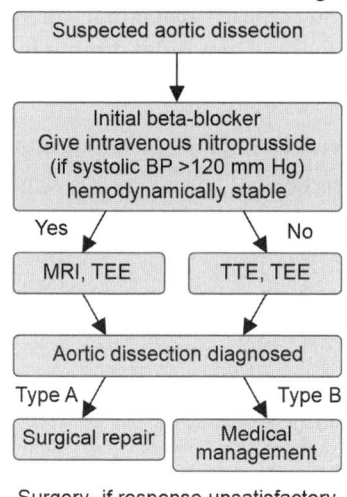

Flowchart 1: Aortic dissection-management.

(TEE: transesophageal echocardiography; TTE: transthoracic echocardiography)

SUGGESTED READING

1. Isselbacher EM. Diseases of the aorta. In: Libby P, Bonow RO, Mann DL, Zipes DP (Eds). Braunwald's Heart disease: A Textbook of Cardiovascular Medicine, 8th edition. Saunders: Philadelphia, PA; 2008.
2. Singh B. Diseases of vessels. In: Manchanda O (Eds). Oram's Clinical heart Disease, 3rd edition. CBSP: New Delhi; 1999.

CHAPTER 20

Pulmonary Heart Diseases (Pulmonary Embolism, Cor Pulmonale, and Sleep Disordered Breathing)

"Three main factors associated with deep vein thrombosis are stasis, hypercoagulability of blood and injury to the vessel wall."
—Rudolf Ludwig Carl Virchow

INTRODUCTION

Pulmonary circulation has large cross-sectional surface area with thin-walled distensible vessels along with large recruitable vascular reserve. The pulmonary vascular resistance is approximately one-eighth of systemic vascular resistance. When total cross-sectional area is decreased by destruction or obliteration of lung tissue, as in chronic obstructive airway disease or occlusion of pulmonary vasculature, and in pulmonary embolism (PEm), the end result is pulmonary hypertension (PH). When PH involves the right heart, cor pulmonale results.

Q1. What are the peculiarities of pulmonary circulation?
Ans.

- In adults lying flat, normal pulmonary arterial pressure (PAP) is 15–25 mm Hg systolic and 5–10 mm Hg diastolic. Compared to the systemic circulation, it is a short circuit but high flow zone. Cardiac output (CO) here is same to that in systemic circulation (in absence of a systemic or pulmonary communication).
- Pulmonary vascular resistance is approximately one-eighth of systemic vascular resistance. Pulmonary circulation has a large capacity, great distensibility, and a low resistance to flow owing to the presence of modest amount of smooth muscles in small arteries and arterioles. Hence, pulmonary circulation is not predisposed to become hypertensive.
- Large cross-sectional surface area coupled with distensibility of thin-walled vessels and large recruitable vascular reserve allows a fourfold increase in flow during exercise without any change in PAP and concomitant PVR.
- Pulmonary arteries (PAs) carry deoxygenated blood. Bronchial arteries provide nutrition to the airways, which amounts to 1% of CO. Some bronchial veins empty into pulmonary veins (remainder into systemic). The bronchial circulation constitutes a physiological right-to-left (R-L) shunt.

Q2. What are the diseases of PA?
Ans.
Pulmonary stenosis: It is usually congenital and rarely acquired (e.g., carcinoid and rheumatic). Congenital stenosis may also involve PA and its branches (coarctation of PA).
- *Pulmonary regurgitation:* It is acquired, functional (secondary hypertension to PH), most common, secondary to surgery, infective endocarditis, trauma, rheumatic carditis, etc., and congenital-idiopathic dilatation of pulmonary trunk.
- *Pulmonary hypertension:*
  - Primary pulmonary hypertension (PPH)
  - Secondary:
    - Acquired disorders of left heart, e.g., mitral and aortic valvular disease, myocardial disease
    - Congenital heart diseases, e.g., atrial septal defect (ASD), ventricular septal defect (VSD), patent ductus arteriosus (PDA)
    - *Respiratory disorders:* Chronic obstructive pulmonary disease (COPD), interstitial fibrosis (idiopathic, or due to connective tissue diseases)
    - *Occlusive pulmonary vascular disease:* Thromboembolism.

Q3. What do you mean by venous thromboembolism (VTE)?
Ans. Venous thrombosis occurs when there is stasis. The platelet-rich red thrombus thus formed easily embolizes to lung, leading to PE. Many of these are microemboli, and resolve automatically. Thus, venous thrombosis and PE occur almost simultaneously. Hence, the term venous thromboembolism.

Q4. What are the risk factors for VTE?
Ans. Factors leading to development of venous thrombosis include stasis, vascular damage, and hypercoagulability—*the Virchow's triad* (described by *Rudolf Ludwig Carl Virchow* in 1856). Following clinical conditions predispose development of VTE **(Box 20.1)**:

BOX 20.1: Venous thromboembolism risk factors.

- *Surgery:* Orthopedic, thoracic, abdominal, and genitourinary
- *Neoplasm:* Pancreatic, lung, ovary, testes, urinary tract, breast, and stomach
- *Trauma:* Fracture of spine, pelvis, femur, tibia, and spinal cord injury
- *Immobilization:* Acute myocardial infarction (AMI), congestive heart failure (CHF), stroke, postoperative convalescence, and long air halt travel
- *Pregnancy:* Particularly third trimester and first month postpartum
- *Estrogen:* Use oral pills, hormone replacement therapy (HRT)
- *Hypercoagulable states:* Deficiency of protein C, protein S, and antithrombin III, antiphospholipid antibody, myeloproliferative diseases, dysfibrinogenemia, disseminated intravascular coagulation (DIC)
- Venulitis—thromboangiitis obliterans, Behçet's disease, and homocystinuria
- History of previous deep vein thrombosis (DVT)

Q5. When the diagnosis of PEm should be considered?
Ans. Pulmonary embolism should be considered in a hypotensive patient when:
- There is evidence of venous thrombosis or its precipitating factors.
- There is evidence of acute cor pulmonale, such as acute right ventricular failure (RVF), increased jugular venous pressure (JVP), S_3 gallop, right ventricular (RV) heave, tachycardia, and tachypnea.
- There is echocardiographic findings of RV dilatation and hypokinesia, or electrocardiogram (ECG), evidences of acute cor pulmonale such as $S_1Q_3T_3$, new incomplete right bundle branch block (RBBB), and RV ischemia.

Q6. How to classify PEM?
Ans. Depending on the hemodynamic embarrassment produced, PE may be massive, submassive, and small **(Box 20.2)**.

BOX 20.2: Classification of PEm.
- *Massive PE:* Systolic blood pressure (BP) <90 mm Hg, poor tissue perfusion, multiorgan failure plus high clot burden
- *Submassive PE:* Hemodynamically stable, moderate to severe RV dysfunction or enlargement
- *Small to moderate PE:* Normal hemodynamics and normal RV size

---

Q7. How will you differentiate acute PEm from AMI?
Ans. Both are present with acute severe chest pain. The differentiating points are listed in **Table 20.1**.

TABLE 20.1: Acute pulmonary embolism and acute myocardial infarction—difference.

Points	Acute pulmonary embolism (PEm)	Acute myocardial infarction (AMI)
Risk factors	Stasis (bed rest, pregnancy, CHF), endothelial damage (trauma and inflammation), and hypercoagulable state (in cancer, genetic)	That of CAD [hypercholesterolemia, smoking, DM, and hypertension]
Symptoms	Chest pain—severe, dyspnea, hemoptysis, and faintness	Chest pain, sweating, and vomiting
Signs	Cyanosis (central)	Nil
	↑ JVP (early), tachycardia (invariable)	JVP-N (↑ in heart failure), tachycardia common (if anterior MI)

Contd...

Contd...

Points	Acute pulmonary embolism (PEm)	Acute myocardial infarction (AMI)
	Hypotension (common)	Only in complicated MI, i.e., shock, heart failure
	S_2—widely split, may be loud	S_1, S_2—soft
Investigation: ECG	No ST elevation, Q and $\downarrow$T in lead III (but not in II), in association with $\downarrow$T in V_1–V_4—strongly suggestive	ST elevation, followed by Q and $\downarrow$T waves in respective leads
Chest x-ray	Oligemic lung field; linear or wedge-shaped opacity, pleural effusion, raised hemidiaphragm, etc.	Usually normal, pulmonary edema in LVF
Blood exam: Cardiac enzymes-	Normal	Raised
Plasma D-dimer	Usually +ve	–ve
PaO_2 and $PaCO_2$	$\downarrow$	Normal
Pulmonary angiography	+ve	– ve
Coronary angiography	–ve	+ve
Treatment L: Heparin	Anticoagulation with heparin—always	±
Thrombolytics	If there is hemodynamic compromise, a lobe or multiple segments are obstructed. Heparin is withheld until the thrombolytic infusion is completed	Always (if no contraindication)

(CHF: congestive heart failure; CAD: coronary artery disease; DM: diabetes mellitus; JVP-N: normal jugular venous pressure; LVF: left ventricular failure)

Q8. How heparin helps patients with PEm?
Ans.

- *Prevention of DVT and subsequent development of pulmonary embolism:* Subcutaneous heparin 5000 U, every 8–12 hours, treatment continued till immobilization or till precipitating factors persist. Activated partial thromboplastin time (APTT) is maintained 1.5–2 times to prevent thromboembolism. Low-molecular-weight heparin (LMWH) is being increasingly used, particularly in high-risk patients (e.g., those undergoing total knee and hip replacement). Dose: Enoxaparin 40 mg SC (daily).
- *Treatment of PE:* Heparin administered IV 5,000 units bolus followed by a maintenance dose of 30,000–40,000 units/24 h by continuous infusion.

- Lower dose is administered if patient is considered at high risk for bleeding. APTT, followed at 6 hours intervals until it is consistently in the therapeutic range of 1.5–2.0 times to prevent thromboembolism. Documented PE should be treated for 3 months. Longer treatment may be needed when significant risk factors persist.
- Warfarin is initiated as soon as APTT is therapeutic, and heparin should be maintained until a therapeutic international normalized ratio (INR) of 2.0–3.0 has been overlapped with a therapeutic APTT for three consecutive days.

When LMWH is used, then enoxaparin 1 mg/kg SC is initiated every 12 hours. Warfarin is initiated within 24 hours after. At least 5 days of therapy with LMWH is appropriate; INR should be 2.0 or greater for two consecutive mornings prior to discontinuing LMWH.

Q9. How long to continue anticoagulant therapy in PEm?
Ans. Etiology of the condition determines the duration **(Box 20.3)**.

> **BOX 20.3:** Duration of anticoagulant therapy in pulmonary embolism.
> - *First provoked PE/proximal leg DVT:* 6 months
> - *Second provoked PE:* 12 months or indefinitely
> - *Third VTE:* Indefinitely
> - *Cancer patients:* 6 months or indefinitely
> - *Unprovoked VTE:* Indefinitely
>
> (PEm: pulmonary embolism; DVT: deep vein thrombosis; VTE: venous thromboembolism)

Q10. What is PH?
Ans. Pulmonary hypertension is defined as an increase in mean pulmonary arterial pressure (mPAP) of 25 mm Hg at rest, as assessed by right heart catheterization.

Q11. How to classify PH?
Ans. It is classified into five groups, which are as follows:
- *Pulmonary arterial hypertension (PAH):* Idiopathic PH or PPH, in coronary heart disease (CHD), connective tissue (CT) disease. In PAH, the distal PAs are mainly affected, and pulmonary veins are classically unaffected. Bronchial arteries undergo significant remodeling that may cause episodic hemoptysis.
- *Pulmonary hypertension due to left heart disease:* Left ventricular (LV) dysfunction, valvular disease
- *PH due to lung disease, and/or hypoxia:* COPD, interstitial lung disease (ILD), sleep-disordered breathing (SDB)
- Chronic thromboembolic PH, and other PA obstructions
- PH with unclear and/or multifactorial mechanisms—chronic hemolytic anemia, myeloproliferative diseases, sarcoidosis, etc. In absence of other potential causes of PH, such as left-sided heart disease, COPD, an

estimated right ventricular systolic pressure (RVSP) > 40 mm Hg warrants further evaluation of a patient with unexplained dyspnea.

Q12. What are the forms of PH?
Ans. Pulmonary hypertension may be acute or chronic. The acute form is due to PE or adult respiratory distress syndrome. Chronic PH is due to long standing structural changes in the pulmonary vasculature.

Q13. What are the causes of PH?
Ans. Causes of PH are as follows:
- *Primary or idiopathic*
- *Secondary:*
  - *Passive:* It is due to increased resistance to left ventricular filling, e.g., in mitral stenosis and left ventricular failure (LVF).
  - *Active or vasoconstrictive:* It is due to alveolar hypoxia, e.g., in COPD and high altitude.
  - *Obstructive or obliterative:* It is due to decrease in cross-sectional areas of pulmonary vascular bed, e.g., in emphysema, thromboembolic diseases of PAs, extensive pulmonary fibrosis.
  - *Hyperkinetic:* It is due to a significant increase in pulmonary arterial flow, e.g., in left-to-right shunts (ASD, VSD, PDA, PAPVD, etc.).

  Common causes of PH: Mitral valvular diseases, COPD, and LVF:

Q14. What is pre- and postcapillary PH?
Ans. Precapillary PH is defined as a mPAP of 25 mm Hg or more, a pulmonary capillary wedge pressure (PCWP) of 15 mm Hg or less, and a PVR of more than 3 Wood units. It may be group 1, group 3, group 4, or group 5 in origin. Postcapillary PH is present when mPAP or more, and the PCWP is 15 mm Hg or more. It is most common in group-2 patients; it may also occur in group-5 patients.

Q15. How PAH in CHD differs from primary PAH, prognostically?
Ans. Pulmonary arterial hypertension in CHD—with early onset in life—right ventricular adaptive response and marked RV hypertrophy as well as preservation of a fetal-type phenotype allows the patient to sustain an increased afterload with better RV function for many years or decades than those in whom PAH develops later in life. Hence, survival time for patients with Eisenmenger syndrome is better than those with IPPH. Currently approved PAH-specific therapies have demonstrated benefit in patients with Eisenmenger syndrome.

Q16. What are the echocardiographic features of PAH?
Ans. Common echocardiographic features of PAH include right atrial (RA) enlargement, RV enlargement and dysfunction, small underfilled left-sided heart chambers, flat interventricular septum, tricuspid

regurgitation (TR) with reduced tricuspid annular plane systolic excursion (TAPSE). Echocardiography overestimates RVSP, and a diagnosis of PH should not be made without confirmatory right heart catheterization. However, it is useful in disease follow up and assessing therapeutic interventions.

Q17. How to select drug therapies for patients with PH?
Ans.
- *Calcium-channel blockers:* Long-acting nifedipine, diltiazem, and amlodipine are used. A positive response is defined as a fall in mPAP of at least 10–40 mm Hg or less with no change in CO.
- *Endothelin receptor antagonists:* Endothelin-1 is a potent vasoconstrictor and smooth muscle mitogen that contributes to the pathogenesis of PAH. Three drugs—bosentan, ambrisentan, and macitentan are currently available.
Phosphodiesterase (PDE) inhibitors: They inhibit hydrolysis of cyclic guanosine monophosphate (cGMP) and have proved to be an effective therapy for PAH. Sildenafil 20 mg t.d.s and tadalafil 40 mg once daily are the approved drugs.
- *Other agents:* Parenteral prostanoids such as epoprostenol and treprostinil are used at special centers. Soluble guanylate cyclase stimulators like Riociguat directly stimulate soluble guanylate cyclase independent of nitric oxide (NO) and increase sensitivity of soluble guanylate cyclase to NO.

Q18. Justify the use of PDE5 inhibitors for other cardiac conditions.
Ans.
- Besides their proven application in PH, PDE5 inhibitors need to be used in patients with coronary artery disease (CAD) with erectile dysfunction (ED). These are useful for treatment of ED in patients with stable ischemic heart disease (SIHD), but they should not be used in patients receiving nitrate. Nitrates should not be administered to patients within 24 hours of tadalafil administration. Switching from nitrate to ranolazine in patients with CAD, receiving PDE5 inhibitors for ED is an alternative.
- Sildenafil is safe as PDE3 receptors dominantly present in cardiac myocyte are not affected by PDE5 inhibitors. Sildenafil reduces BP by 3–5 mm Hg, hence no chance of orthostatic hypotension.

Q19. What is PPH? How to treat it?
Ans. It is an intrinsic disorder of pulmonary vascular bed, characterized by sustained elevation in pulmonary vascular resistance and PA pressure that generally leads to RVF and death. PPH is a rare disease, hence requires clinical exclusion of other conditions that can produce PH (i.e., secondary PH).

Treatment include:
- *Long-term oral vasodilator:* Oral calcium-channel blockers (nifedipine or diltiazem). Other agents like IV prostacyclin (PGI_2), epoprostenol, and adenosine may also be helpful.

Surgery: Atrial septostomy (to decompress the overloaded right heart and improve systemic output of under filled LV), and lung transplantation when PH has progressed to the stage of RVF.

Q20. What is cor pulmonale?
Ans. Cor—heart and pulmonale—lung, i.e., heart disease due to pulmonary cause. Thus, cor pulmonale is defined as involvement of right ventricle (by dilatation or hypertrophy), with or without failure resulting from diseases affecting the function and/or structure of the lung.

It is due to PH resulting from lung disorders.

Classification is as follows:
- *Acute cor pulmonale:* Occurs in acute massive PEm
- *Chronic cor pulmonale:* Chronic obstructive pulmonary disease, pulmonary fibrosis (diffuse), recurrent pulmonary thromboembolism, hypoventilation syndrome, obstructive sleep apnea, chest wall diseases, and PPH.

Q21. How does cor pulmonale occur in COPD?
Ans. Chronic bronchitis leads to hypoxic vasoconstriction of pulmonary vasculature and secondary polycythemia. On the other hand, emphysema leads to loss of pulmonary vasculature. Vasoconstriction and vascular loss lead to an increase in total peripheral resistance. Polycythemia increases CO. An increase in CO and peripheral resistance leads to development of PH, and in due course of time, cor pulmonale **(Flowchart 20.1)**.

Flowchart 20.1: Mechanism of development of cor pulmonale.

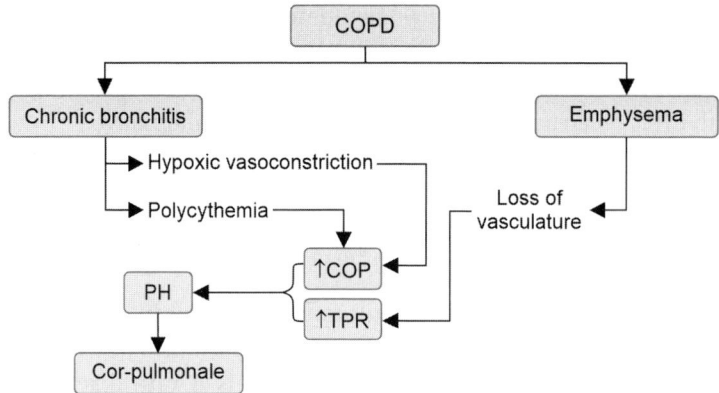

(COPD: chronic obstructive pulmonary disease; CO: cardiac output; TPR: total peripheral resistance, PH: pulmonary hypertension)

Q22. What are the echocardiographic findings of cor pulmonale?
Ans.
- M-mode findings are absent or diminished A wave. In RVF, absent A wave may reappear (atrial component of RV diastole increased); thus, a normal A wave does not exclude PH. Midsystolic closure or notching remains a valuable sign for PH.
- 2-DE findings include RV dilatation and/or hypertrophy and diminished RV function. RV enlargement with flattening of IVS produces a small D-shaped LV **(Fig. 20.1)**.

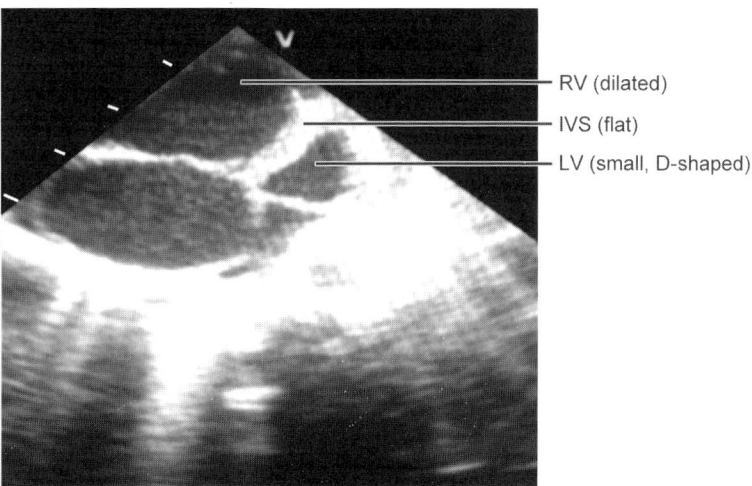

Fig. 20.1: 2DE showing features of cor pulmonale. (RV: right ventricular; IVS: interventricular septum, LV: left ventricle)

- *Doppler study:* Right ventricular, and thus PA systolic pressure may be measured from tricuspid regurgitation. PA diastolic pressure may be measured if pulmonary regurgitation is present.
    Echocardiography can exclude mitral valve disease, congenital heart diseases, and cardiomyopathies, etc.

Q23. How to treat heart failure in chronic cor pulmonale? How it differs from RVF secondary to left heart disease?
Ans.
- Correction of hypoxemia and CO_2 retention by low flow O_2 therapy (high flow O_2 may remove hypoxic drive). Arterial P_aO_2 to be restored more than 60 mm Hg. Some patients may benefit from long-term domiciliary O_2.
- Bronchodilators to improve oxygenation and relieve bronchospasm
- Antibiotics for acute exacerbation of bronchitis (may precipitate failure)
- Corticosteroids may help patients with reversible airway obstruction.

Diuretic is the mainstay of therapy for RVF. Therapy is carefully monitored by measurement of electrolytes as well as P_aO_2 and P_aCO_2.

- *Vasodilators:* Pulmonary vasodilators are efficacious in some patient with PPH. Otherwise, vasodilators are of limited benefit, as peripheral vessels are already dilated by hypoxia (in contrast to RVF due to left heart disease).
- *Digoxin:* It may be harmful as myocardium is hypoxic and right-sided muscle mass is only one third (compared to LV). It should be used extremely cautiously in following situations:
  - Certain digitalis responsive supraventricular arrhythmia, e.g. atrial fibrillation (AF)
  - Treating coexistent LV dysfunction
  - For patients who are refractory to other measures.

Q24. What are pulmonary vasodilators?
Ans. These are drugs that selectively dilate the pulmonary vasculature.

These are as follows:
- *Endothelin receptor antagonists:* Bosentan (in NYHA class III–IV)
- *Phosphodiesterase-5 inhibitors:* Sildenafil and tadalafil (longer acting)
- Prostacyclin and its analogs (epoprostenol).

They produce symptomatic and functional improvement in patients with PH.

Q25. What is SDB and its cardiovascular consequences?
Ans. Sleep-disordered breathing is characterized by repetitive episodes of partial or complete upper airway occlusion occurring during sleep with resultant intermittent hypoxemia and sleep disturbances.

Sleep-disordered breathing-related cardiovascular consequences are: Hypertension, heart failure, stroke, arrhythmia, ischemic heart disease, PAH, etc.

Q26. What is the mechanism of SDB?
Ans. Sleep-disordered breathing causes chronic episodic hypoxemia, sympathetic activation, intrathoracic pressure swings, and sleep fragmentation that result in oxidative stress, vascular inflammation, hypercoagulability that influence cardiac and vascular functions. These may contribute to development of hypertension, atherosclerosis, arrhythmia, and heart failure. Growing evidence implicates SDB as an independent risk factor for hypertension, CAD, cardiovascular disease (CVD), stroke, AF, and mortality.

■ SUGGESTED READING

1. Das PK, Rahman F, Shetty PK, Shetty DP. Pulmonary embolism: An observational study at Narayana Hrudayalaya Institute of Cardiac Sciences, Bangalore, India. Mymensingh Med J. 2010;19(3):399-404.

2. Gami AS, Somers VK. Sleep apnea and cardiovascular disease. In: Libby P, Bonow RO, Mann DL, Zipes DP (Eds). Braunwald's Heart Disease: A Textbook of Cardiovascular Medicine, 8th edition. Philadelphia: Saunders; 2008.
3. Goldhaber SZ. Pulmonary embolism. In: Libby P, Bonow RO, Mann DL, Zipes DP (Eds). Braunwald's Heart Disease: A Textbook of Cardiovascular Medicine, 8th edition. Philadelphia: Saunders; 2008.
4. Miller MA, Sweeny JM, Lawrence C, Brighton KL. Chronic cor pulmonale. In: Fuster V, Walsh RA, Harrington RA (Eds). Hurst's The Heart Manual of Cardiology, 13th edition. USA: McGraw-Hill; 2011.
5. Veasey SC, Guilleminault C, Strohl KP, Sanders MH, Ballard RD, Magalang UJ. Medical therapy for obstructive sleep apnea: a review by the Medical Therapy for Obstructive Sleep Apnea Task Force of the Standards of Practice Committee of the American Academy of Sleep Medicine. Sleep. 2006;29(8):1036-44.

CHAPTER 21

Peripheral Vascular Diseases

"Concomiitant CAD present in 30 to 50% of patients with peripheral arterial disease and thus it is considered a risk equivalent."
—EJ Topol

■ INTRODUCTION

Peripheral arterial diseases (PADs) are frequently associated with coronary and cerebral atherosclerosis but are commonly underdiagnosed and undertreated. Issues relating to diagnosis and management of PAD are discussed in this chapter. Also, diseases involving veins and lymphatics are highlighted in brief.

Q1. What are PAD and peripheral vascular diseases (PVD)?
Ans. Peripheral arterial diseases are diseases obstructing flow to upper and lower limbs due to atherosclerosis, thrombosis, embolism, vasculitides, fibromuscular dysplasia, entrapment, etc. Conventionally, all arterial involvements, besides coronary and cerebral atherosclerosis, are designated as PAD. Thus, renal artery stenosis and mesenteric vascular occlusion are also examples of PAD.

Peripheral vascular diseases encompasses a group of diseases afflicting blood vessels, including PAD, as well as atherosclerotic renal and carotid arterial diseases, vasculitides, vasospasm, venous thrombosis, venous insufficiency, and lymphatic disorders.

Q2. How the risk factors for PAD differ from that of coronary artery disease (CAD)?
Ans. All four major risk factors of atherosclerosis, such as dyslipidemia, smoking, diabetes mellitus (DM), and hypertension, act as risk factors for the development of PAD with the following differences:
- *Smoking:* It is more linked to PAD than CAD.
- *DM:* It produces severe and extensive PAD with more calcified distal arterial bed.
- *Low-density lipoprotein (LDL):* Some but not all studies show it as a risk factor for PAD, but for CAD it is a universal risk factor.
- *Hypertension:* The link between hypertension and PAD is found in some but not in other studies.

Q3. How to classify PAD?
Ans. Fontain classification for staging of PAD are listed in **Box 21.1**:

> **BOX 21.1:** Stages of PAD.
> - *Stage I:* Asymptomatic
> - *Stage II:* Intermittent claudication
>   - *Stage IIa:* Pain free, claudication walking >200 meters
>   - *Stage IIb:* Pain free, claudication walking <200 meters
> - *Stage III:* Rest and nocturnal pain
> - *Stage IV:* Necrosis, gangrene

Q4. What is the ankle–brachial index (ABI)?
Ans. It is the ratio of systolic blood pressure (BP) measured at the ankle by Doppler ultrasound to systolic BP measured at the brachial artery by stethoscope (or Doppler).

Normal ABI is 1 or more. ABI correlates inversely with walking distance and speed.

In patients with leg claudication, ABI is 0.5–0.8, in critical limb ischemia it is <0.5.

Q5. What is the importance of exercise treadmill test (ETT) in patients with PAD?
Ans. Exercise treadmill test helps in patients with PAD in two ways:
1. *Clinical significance of PAD:* Detection of initial claudication distance (point at which claudication first appears), and absolute claudication distance (point at which patient can no longer continue walking because of severe leg claudication).
2. *Objective evidence of PAD:* Normally, increase in BP during exercise shall be same in upper and lower limbs with ABI >1. In PAD, ABI decreases because of peripheral arterial stenosis, because the increased BP observed in arm is not matched by a comparable increase in ankle BP. A 25% or greater decrease in ABI after exercise is diagnosed.

Q6. What is acute limb ischemia (ALI)? What are its causes?
Ans. Acute limb ischemia is the arterial occlusion that suddenly reduces blood flow to arms or legs. It presents with 5 *P*s: *P*ain, *p*ulselessness, *p*allor, *p*aresthesia, and *p*aralysis.

Causes of ALI are: Arterial embolism, thrombosis in situ, dissection, and trauma.

Q7. How to classify ALI ? State its treatment.
Ans. Categories of ALI are listed in **Box 21.2**.

BOX 21.2: Acute limb ischemia classification.

- *Category I:* Viable, not immediately threatened, no sensory or motor abnormality, blood flow detected on Doppler
- *Category II:* Threatened
  - *IIa:* Marginally threatened, minimal or no sensory loss, no motor weakness, Doppler signal audible: Salvageable, if promptly treated
  - *IIb:* Immediately threatened, rest, pain, mild to moderate muscle weakness, Doppler signal inaudible: Salvageable with immediate revascularization
- *Category III:* Irreversible loss of sensation, paralysis, and absence of blood flow, as detected by Doppler, in both arteries and veins distal to occlusion.

Treatment of ALI includes: Analgesics, IV heparin, intra-arterial thrombolytics, percutaneous mechanical thrombectomy, and surgical revascularization.

Q8. How to differentiate embolic ALI from thrombotic ALI?
Ans. Acute limb ischemia may result from thrombosis of the vessel involved, or from distal embolization from a remote source. The two differ in the aspects mentioned in **Table 21.1**.

TABLE 21.1: Acute limb ischemia—embolic and thrombotic.

Points	Embolic	Thrombotic
Severity	Complete (no collateral)	Incomplete (collateral)
Onset	Seconds to minutes	Hours to days
Leg–arm involvement	3:1	10:1
Multiple sites	Common	Rare
Source	Heart (usually AF)	In situ
H/o claudication	Absent	Present
Artery on palpation	Soft, tender	Hard, calcified
Bruit	Absent	Present
Contralateral leg pulse	Present	May be absent
Diagnosis	Clinical	Angiography
Treatment	Thrombolytics, embolectomy	Thrombolytics, bypass, angioplasty
Prognosis	Loss of life >loss of limb	Loss of limb >loss of life

(AF: atrial fibrillation; H/o: history of)

Q9. What are the diseases of veins?
Ans.
- Varicose vein
- Deep vein thrombosis (DVT) and venous thromboembolism (VTE)
- Phlebitis and superficial venous thrombosis
- Chronic venous insufficiency.

Q10. What are the differences between arterial and venous thrombus?
Ans. Thrombus may develop in arteries by endothelial injury or in veins by stasis. They have distinct features **(Table 21.2)**.

TABLE 21.2: Difference between arterial and venous thrombus.

Arterial thrombus	Venous thrombus
Endothelial injury is the initiating factor	Stasis is the initiating factor
Thrombus is fibrin-rich white	Thrombus is platelet-rich red
May obstruct lumen producing infarction	Usually nonobstructive
Propagation is less	Propagates along direction of flow
Distal embolism is less	Embolism more, producing PE
Thrombolytics are more beneficial	Thrombolytics are less beneficial
Antiplatelets are more useful in prevention	Anticoagulants are more useful in prevention

Q11. What are phlegmasia cerulea dolens and phlegmasia alba dolens?
Ans. In some patients with DVT, deoxygenated hemoglobin in stagnant veins imparts a cyanotic hue to the limb called phlegmasia cerulea dolens. In markedly edematous legs, the interstitial tissue pressure may exceed the capillary perfusion pressure, causing pallor, a condition designated as phlegmasia alba dolens.

Q12. What are the imaging modalities for PAD?
Ans. The imaging modalities for PAD are:
- Duplex ultrasound imaging
- Magnetic resonance angiography (MRA)
- Computed tomography angiography (CT angiography)
- Contrast angiography

Q13. How does duplex ultrasound imaging help in diagnosis of PAD?
Ans. Duplex ultrasound examination provides a direct, noninvasive means of assessing both the anatomical and functional significance of PAD. It incorporates ultrasound imaging for direct visualization of arterial walls, atherosclerotic plaques, pulsed-wave Doppler to determine blood flow within the arterial lumen, and color-flow mapping to localize the stenotic site.

Q14. What are the utilities of CT angiography and MRA in diagnosis of PAD?
Ans.
- *Computed tomography angiography:* It is commonly used to detect peripheral arterial obstruction. It requires radiocontrast and ionizing radiation, but can be used in patients with metallic clips, stents, pacemakers **(Fig. 21.1)**.

- *Magnetic resonance angiography:* Gadolinium-enhanced MRA produces resolution of arteries like that of contrast digital subtraction angiography (DSA). It is done in patients at risk for renal, allergic, or other complications of conventional angiography.

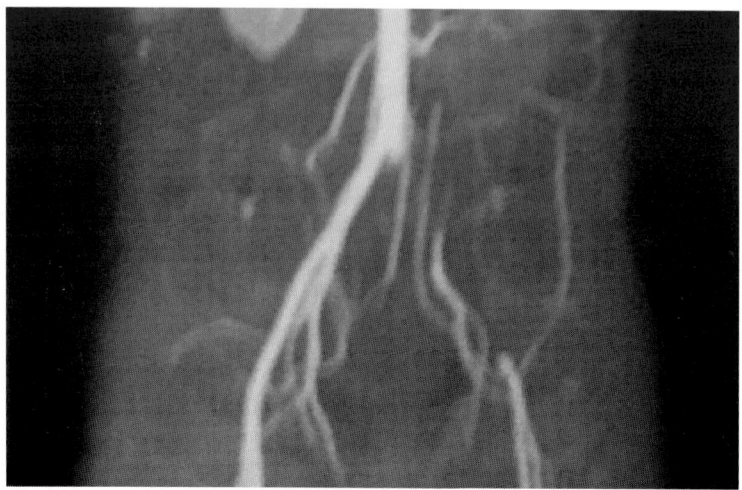

Fig. 21.1: CT angiography of lower limb showing totally occluded left iliac artery.

Q15. How does peripheral angiography (PAG) help in the diagnosis of PAD?

Ans. Peripheral angiography by DSA technology directly visualizes peripheral arteries and detects the lesions. It allows intervention to be undertaken (**Fig. 21.2**).

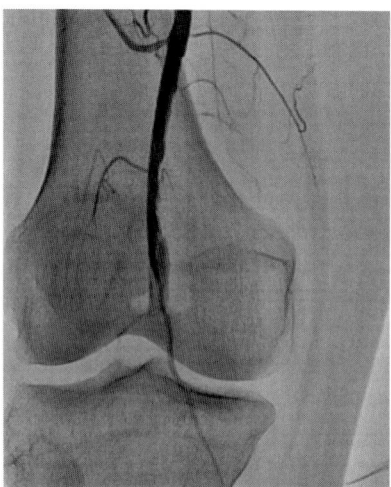

Fig. 21.2: PAG showing completely occluded right popliteal artery.

Q16. What are the interventions for PAD?
Ans.
- Endovascular interventions for iliac artery stenosis are initial therapy of choice, because success rate and medium- and long-term patency are comparable to those of surgical revascularization. It is the preferred strategy for patients with anatomically appropriate lesions. It may be repeated if needed, but repeat surgery is more challenging.
- Surgery is preferred for patients with common femoral and proximal profunda femoris obstructive PAD.

SUGGESTED READING

1. Creager MA, Libby P. Peripheral arterial diseases. In: Libby P, Bonow RO, Mann DL, Zipes DP (Eds). Braunwald's Heart Disease: A Textbook of Cardiovascular Medicine, 8th edition. Philadelphia: Saunders; 2008.
2. Hirsch AT, Haskal ZJ, Hertzer NR, Bakal CW, Creager MA, Halperin JL, et al. ACC/AHA 2005 guidelines for the management of patients with peripheral arterial disease (lower extremity, renal, mesenteric, and abdominal aortic): executive summary a collaborative report from the American Association for Vascular Surgery/Society for Vascular Surgery, Society for Cardiovascular Angiography and Interventions, Society for Vascular Medicine and Biology, Society of Interventional Radiology, and the ACC/AHA Task Force on Practice Guidelines (Writing Committee to Develop Guidelines for the Management of Patients With Peripheral Arterial Disease) endorsed by the American Association of Cardiovascular and Pulmonary Rehabilitation; National Heart, Lung, and Blood Institute; Society for Vascular Nursing; Transatlantic Inter-Society Consensus; and Vascular Disease Foundation. J Am Coll Cardiol. 2006;47(6):1239-312.
3. Khanna NN, Ashish G, Suparna R. Critical Limb Ischemia. In: Khanna NN, Henry M (Eds). Handbook of Interventions for Structural Heart and Peripheral Vascular Disease, 1st edition. New Delhi: Jaypee Brothers Medical Publishers (P) Ltd; 2016.

22 Diabetes and Heart Diseases

"All diabetics should be considered to be at high risk of CVD; those with additional CV risk factors are at very high risk."
—Eric Jeffrey Topol

▇ INTRODUCTION

Diabetes accelerates atherosclerosis and coronary heart disease. 80% of all deaths among diabetics are due to atherosclerosis. Conventional coronary artery disease (CAD) risk factors such as hypertension, dyslipidemia, and obesity cluster in patients with impaired glucose tolerance or diabetes. Diabetic patients have lipid-rich atheromatous plaques that are more vulnerable to rupture than plaques found in nondiabetic patients. Diabetes is also a strong and independent risk factor for congestive heart failure (CHF).

Q1. What are the diagnostic criteria for diabetes mellitus (DM)?
Ans. The American Diabetic Association (ADA) criteria for diagnosis of DM are listed in **Box 22.1**.

> **BOX 22.1:** The American Diabetes Association (ADA) diagnostic criteria.
> - *Fasting plasma glucose (FPG):* 126 mg/dL or more
> - *2-hours postprandial glucose:* 200 mg/dL or more during an oral glucose tolerance test (OGTT)
> - Symptoms of DM (polyuria, polydipsia, and unexplained weight loss)
> - Random plasma glucose of 200 mg/dL or more

Q2. What are impaired fasting glucose (IFG), impaired glucose tolerance (IGT), and metabolic syndrome (MetS)?
Ans. Impaired fasting glucose is a fasting plasma glucose of 110–125 mg/dL and IGT is a 2-hours postprandial glucose of 140–199 mg/dL during OGTT.

These two metabolic disturbances predispose diabetes and *cardiovascular disease* (CVD) and are leveled as prediabetes. Before the development of diabetes, subjects passed through a stage of impaired glucose metabolism characterized by IFG and IGT.

Metabolic syndrome is a cluster of lipid and nonlipid risk factors of metabolic origin, mediated by insulin resistance, such as pathologic glucose metabolism, obesity, hypertension, and dyslipidemia.

Q3. What is normal blood glucose?

Ans. Fasting blood glucose (FBG) of <110 mg/dL and a 2-hours post-prandial plasma glucose of <140 mg/dL are considered as normal. The threshold above which hyperglycemia becomes atherogenic is not known but may be in the range defined as IGT (i.e., FBG >126 mg/dL with 30-, 60-, or 90-minutes blood glucose concentration of >200 mg/dL, and a 2-hours plasma glucose level of 140–200 mg/dL during an OGTT).

Q4. How DM acts as a risk factor for atherosclerosis?

Ans. In addition to metabolic disturbances, diabetes alters the function of multiple cell lines, including endothelial cells, smooth muscle cells, and platelets.

- *Hyperglycemia:* The degree and duration of hyperglycemia are strong risk factors. Even IGT increases cardiovascular (CV) risk.
- *Dyslipidemia:* Increased triglyceride (TG), decreased high-density lipoprotein (HDL), more small, dense low-density lipoprotein (LDL)
- Insulin resistance and hyperinsulinemia start 15–20 years before the onset of clinical diabetes. It induces inflammation and causes endothelial dysfunction, dysfunction of smooth muscle cells leading to restenosis [after percutaneous coronary intervention (PCI)], and platelet dysfunction leading to a prothrombotic state.
- Associated conditions, such as obesity and renal dysfunction also contribute to diabetes-associated CAD.

Q5. Diabetes is a CAD-risk equivalent—explain.

Ans. In 2001, Adult Treatment Panel III (ATP III) of National Cholesterol Education Program (NCEP) recommended that diabetes be considered a CAD-risk equivalent, thus mandating aggressive CV-risk prevention. The reasons for this are as follows:

- Diabetic patients without known CAD have the same likelihood of experiencing a myocardial infarction (MI) as nondiabetic counterparts with a previous history of MI.
- Diabetic persons without prior evidence of CVD [i.e., MI, angina, or ischemic-electrocardiogram (ECG) changes] have the same long-term mortality as nondiabetic patients with established CVD.

Q6. What are the patterns of coronary lesions in diabetic patients with CAD?

Ans. Angiographic studies show that the greater the impairment of glucose metabolism (i.e., normal, IGT, newly diagnosed diabetes, or known diabetes), the smaller the average vessel diameter, and longer the coronary lesions. Patients with diabetes, more frequently, have left main coronary artery lesions, multivessel disease, diffuse CAD, and unstable plaques. Diabetics are likely to have an impaired ability to develop coronary collaterals compared with nondiabetic counterparts. They are less likely to undergo favorable remodeling—an early compensatory enlargement at atherosclerotic sites in response to atherosclerosis (negative remodeling).

Q7. What are the stages of development of diabetes? How are they related with the development of CAD?

Ans.

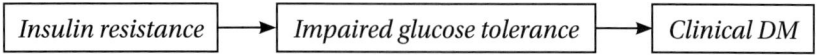

Insulin resistance may be present as long as 15–25 years before the onset of clinical diabetes. Several atherogenic factors are associated with insulin resistance, which can start the atherosclerotic process years before clinical hyperglycemia ensures. Conversely, hyperglycemia plays an important role in enhancing the atherosclerotic process in type 2 DM (T2DM). The threshold above which hyperglycemia becomes atherogenic is not known but may be in the range defined as IGT (i.e., FPG level <126 mg/dL with 30-, 60-, or 90-minutes plasma glucose concentrations >200 mg/dL, and a 2-hours plasma glucose level of 140–200 mg/dL during an OGTT).

Q8. What is insulin resistance?

Ans. It is the reduced sensitivity of body tissues to the action of insulin that affects both glucose disposal in muscle and fat, and insulin suppression of hepatic glucose output. As a consequence, higher concentration of insulin is needed to stimulate peripheral glucose disposal and to suppress hepatic glucose production in patients with type 2 diabetes than those without diabetes. On a biological basis, insulin resistance has been associated with increased coagulation, proinflammation, and endothelial dysfunction (reduced endothelial dependent vasodilatation). Insulin resistance is the first measurable metabolic disturbance among individuals who will subsequently develop type 2 diabetes, and is a key feature of MetS.

Insulin resistance and hyperinsulinemia starts 15–20 years before the onset of clinical diabetes. It induces inflammation and causes endothelial and smooth muscle dysfunction. It may produce alteration of coagulation pathway and platelet dysfunction leading to hypertension, alteration of coagulation, and a prothrombotic state. Associated conditions, such as obesity, hypertension, and renal dysfunction also contribute to atherosclerosis.

Q9. How does diabetes lead to atherosclerosis?

Ans.
- Hyperglycemia leads to endothelial vasomotor dysfunction, systemic inflammation, and a prothrombotic state.
- Systemic inflammation leads to increased oxidative stress and lipid-rich atherosclerotic plaque.
- Diabetic dyslipidemia increases atherosclerotic risk-high TG, low HDL-cholesterol (C), and increased small, dense LDL.

- Altered coagulation, fibrinolytic pathway, and platelet function produce a prothrombotic state.
- Altered functioning of multiple cell lines, including endothelial cells, smooth muscle cells, and platelets contributes.

Q10. What are the indications of cardiac testing in diabetic patients?

Ans. The American Diabetes Association recommendations for cardiac testing in diabetic patients are listed in **Box 22.2**.

> **BOX 22.2:** Indications of cardiac testing.
> - In patients with ≥1 of the following:
>   - Typical or atypical cardiac symptoms
>   - Resting ECG—suggestive of ischemia or infarction
>   - Peripheral or carotid occlusive arterial disease
>   - Sedentary lifestyle, age ≥35 years, and plan to begin a vigorous exercise program
> - In patients with ≥1 of the following risk factors in addition to DM: Dyslipidemia, hypertension, smoking, family history of premature CAD, and positive microalbuminuria test

Q11. What are the things to consider while selecting antidiabetic agents in cardiac patients?

Ans.

- *Metformin:* It lowers hemoglobin A1c (HbA1c) by 1–2%. It can be used to treat MetS, it lowers TG, body weight, and plasminogen activator inhibitor-1 (PAI-1) activity. It should not be used in renal failure (serum creatinine >1.5 mg/dL in male, >1.4 mg/dL in female), potential hypoxic states, such as CHF and severe pulmonary disease (risk of lactic acidosis). It should be discontinued on the day patients receive iodinated contrast media prior to a surgical procedure. Dose is resumed 48 hours later if serum creatinine is normal.
- *Pioglitazone:* It is cardioprotective, improves LDL concentration, LDL particle size, TG, and HDL concentration. It should not be used in CHF.
- *Rosiglitazone:* It is not cardioprotective, also it should not be used in CHF.
- *Repaglinide:* It is particularly useful for elderly patients with CHF, patients who are erotic eaters.
- *Nateglinide:* It is effective in lowering postprandial glucose. Just like in repaglinide, its dose should be omitted if a meal is skipped.
- *Incretins—dipeptidyl peptidase-4 (DPP-4) inhibitor:* DPP is the enzyme degrading glucagon-like peptide-1 (GLP-1) and gastric inhibitory polypeptide (GIP). GLP-1 agonists decrease BP, body weight, and reduce inflammation. There are GLP-1 receptors in cardiac muscles, and treatment with GLP-1 improves myocardial function.

- *Acarbose (alpha-glycosidase inhibitors):* It is not absorbed, delays absorption of complex carbohydrates in brush border of gut and acts as an adjunctive therapy.
- *Insulin:* Its use offers smooth control of hyperglycemia during acute MI. In long-term use, caution to avoid weight gain is needed.

Q12. How does metformin help cardiac patients? What caution to be taken in its use?

Ans. Metformin controls hyperglycemia by decreasing hepatic glucose output and stimulating glucose uptake by skeletal muscle and adipocytes. It lowers HbA1c by 1–2%. It lowers serum TG, PAI-1 activity and body weight, and is used in MetS.

Metformin should be discontinued on the day patients receive iodinated contrast material for radiographic studies as well as before any surgical procedures. The metformin dose may be resumed 48 hours later if serum creatinine is in normal range.

Q13. What are the indications of sodium–glucose cotransporter 2 (SGLT2) inhibitors in various heart diseases?

Ans.
- *Patients with T2DM and heart failure with reduced ejection fraction (HFrEF):* To reduce hospitalization and CV death
- *Heart failure:* Empagliflozin and dapagliflozin are recommended for patients with HFrEF regardless of diabetic status [in addition to optimal medical therapy with an angiotensin-converting enzyme inhibitor (ACEI)/angiotensin receptor–neprilysin inhibitor (ARNI), beta-blocker, and mineralocorticoid receptor antagonist (MRA)].
- Prevention of heart failure in patients with T2DM [European Society of Cardiology (ESC) guidelines 2021]
- To reduce CV death due to MI, unstable angina (UA), stroke, irrespective of the diabetic status
- *Patients with heart failure with preserved ejection fraction (HFpEF):* Recent trials have shown benefits.

Q14. What is diabetic heart disease?

Ans. Diabetic patients may develop CHF in the absence of hypertension, CAD, or other evident source of cardiac disease—the entity known as diabetic heart disease. Accumulation of matrix protein induced by hypoglycemia, collagen deposition followed by fibrosis induced by angiotensin II (AT II) receptor, and high level of AT II appear to be responsible in its pathogenesis.

Q15. What are the treatment goals for diabetic patients?

Ans. The American Diabetes Association recommendations for treatment goal in diabetes are listed in **Box 22.3**.

BOX 22.3: Treatment goals in diabetic patients.

- *Glycemic control:***
  - *Hemoglobin A1c (HbA1c):* <7%
  - *Preprandial capillary plasma glucose:* 90–130 mg/dL (5.0–7.2 mmol/L)
  - *Peak postprandial capillary plasma glucose:* <180 mg/dL (<10.0 mmol/L)
- *Blood pressure (BP)**: <130/80 mm Hg
- *Lipids:*
  - *Low-density lipoprotein (LDL):* <100 mg/dL (<2.6 mol/L)
  - *Triglyceride (TG):* <150 mg/dL (<1.7 mmol/L)
  - *High-density lipoprotein (HDL):* >40 mg/dL (>1.1 mol/L)

*Tight BP control may be more beneficial than tight glycemic control in terms of cardiovascular (CV)-risk reduction [United Kingdom Prospective Diabetes Study (UKPDS) trial].
**Improved glycemic control mainly lowers TG and has a modest effect on raising HDL.

SUGGESTED READING

1. American Diabetes Association—The Expert Committee on the Diagnosis and Classification of Diabetes Mellitus. Report of the Expert Committee on the Diagnosis and Classification of Diabetes Mellitus. Diabetes Care. 1997;20(7):1183-97.
2. American Diabetes Association. Executive Summary: Standards of Medical Care in Diabetes-2010. Diabetes Care. 2010;33(Suppl 1):S4-10.
3. Expert Panel on Detection, Evaluation, and Treatment of High Blood Cholesterol in Adults. Executive Summary of The Third Report of The National Cholesterol Education Program (NCEP) Expert Panel on Detection, Evaluation, and Treatment of High Blood Cholesterol in Adults (Adult Treatment Panel III). JAMA. 2001;285(19):2486-97.

23 Pregnancy and Heart Disease

"Heart disease in pregnancy is a high-risk condition for mother, baby, or both."
—Author of the book

■ INTRODUCTION

Hemodynamic changes of pregnancy can influence both maternal and fetal wellbeing. Heart disease may manifest for the first time in pregnancy. Management and prognosis of the cardiac ailment are influenced by hemodynamic load of pregnancy. Also, heart disease may influence course and outcome, and hence, management of a pregnancy. Drugs used for maternal cardiac condition may affect fetal growth and development.

Q1. What are the physical signs in pregnancy that may mimic heart disease?

Ans. Hemodynamic changes of normal pregnancy lead to an increase in cardiac output and a decrease in peripheral resistance. These lead to changes that may mimic heart disease.

Heart rate: It increases, pulse may be bounding.
- *Blood pressure (BP):* Despite the significant increase in blood volume and cardiac output, BP decreases due to peripheral vasodilatation and mechanical pressure by the gravid uterus on inferior vena cava in supine position (supine hypotension of pregnancy).
- *Jugular venous pressure (JVP):* It rises (with brisk descents) due to volume overload and decreased peripheral resistance.

Edema: It is common as pregnancy advances.
- S_1, S_2 may be loud, S_3 is common. Ejection systolic murmur in pulmonary areas is common, which may mimic atrial septal defect or pulmonary hypertension. A continuous murmur at the base of the heart may be due to cervical venous hum or mammary souffle.

Q2. What cautions are needed in using cardiac drugs during pregnancy?
Ans.
- *Drugs contraindicated:*
  - *Warfarin:* In the first trimester, it crosses the placenta, and causes embryopathy (bone stippling, nasal hypoplasia, optic atrophy, mental retardation), fetal loss, and abortion. It causes more bleeding in

fetus in the third trimester if normal delivery is allowed (fetal liver cannot produce vitamin K and revert warfarin action quickly). Hence, switching to heparin before labor is needed.
- *Angiotensin-converting enzyme inhibitor (ACEI) and angiotensin receptor blocker (ARB):* They cause oligohydramnios and intrauterine growth retardation (IUGR), renal failure, and abnormal bone ossification.
- *Amiodarone:* It causes goiter, hypothyroidism, and hyperthyroidism in fetus.

- *Relatively safe:* Unfractionated heparin intravenous (IV) or subcutaneous (SC) does not cross the placenta, and no fetal abnormality occurs. It should be started as soon as pregnancy is diagnosed in mothers needing anticoagulants (in place of warfarin) and continued up to 13 or 14 weeks (when embryogenesis completes), then warfarin is reinstituted, and then switch to heparin from 36 weeks till delivery. Some continue heparin throughout pregnancy. Low-molecular weight-heparin with low dose aspirin may also be used instead.
  - Low-dose aspirin (in high dose, it may cause closure of the ductus arteriosus)
  - Betablockers (with small risk of fetal bradycardia and IUGR)
  - *Others:* Quinidine, calcium channel blockers (CCBs), and procainamide can be used.

Drugs that are safe to use: Alpha-methyldopa, digoxin, hydralazine, furosemide, and lignocaine.

Q3. What are the types of heart diseases in pregnancy?
Ans. Heart diseases in pregnancy may be classified into two categories:
1. *Preexisting heart diseases:* Valvular, congenital, coronary artery diseases, etc.
2. *Pregnancy-induced heart diseases,* e.g., peripartum cardiomyopathy and gestational hypertension.

Q4. What is the effect of pregnancy in mother and fetus?
Ans.
- *Effect on mother:* Increase in blood volume (50% by 32 weeks), cardiac output, and heart rate impose a hemodynamic burden on the maternal cardiovascular system. Estrogen causes vasodilatation, dilatation of aorta and left atrium. All these aggravate preexisting heart disease symptoms, or symptoms manifest for the first time during pregnancy.
- *Effect on fetus:* Decreased placental flow and IUGR, abortion.

Q5. What are the predictors of maternal cardiac risk during pregnancy?
Ans. Some conditions increase maternal cardiac risk during pregnancy **(Box 23.1)**.

BOX 23.1: Predictors of maternal cardiac risk in pregnancy.
- *Prior cardiovascular events before pregnancy:* Myocardial infarction (MI), arrhythmia, heart failure (HF), cardiovascular disease (CVD), transient ischemic attack (TIA)
- Baseline New York Heart Association (NYHA)-class higher than II
- Cyanosis
- *Left heart obstruction:* Mitral valve area (MVA) <2 cm^2, aortic valve area (AVA) <1.5 cm^2, peak pressure gradient (PPG) in left ventricular outflow tract (LVOT) >30 mm Hg [on echocardiography (echo)]
- *Decreased left ventricular (LV) function:* Ejection fraction (EF) <40%

Q6. What are the cardiac conditions where pregnancy is well tolerated?
Ans.
- *Valvular regurgitations:* Mitral and aortic regurgitations, where patients are asymptomatic or mildly symptomatic.
- Atrial septal defect (ASD), ventricular septal defect, patent ductus arteriosus without evidence of large left-to-right (L-R) shunt, and pulmonary hypertension. ASD patients carry small risk of paradoxical embolism during pregnancy.
- Tricuspid and pulmonary valve diseases
- *Congenitally corrected transposition of the great arteries (TGA):* As long as EF of systemic ventricle is preserved.
- *Ebstein's anomaly:* Risk of paradoxical embolism, if ASD present (in 50% cases)

Q7. What are the cardiac conditions in which pregnancy should be avoided?
Ans. Some maternal cardiac conditions need avoidance of pregnancy, at least before their correction or treatment **(Box 23.2)**.

BOX 23.2: Cardiac conditions where pregnancy needs to be avoided.
- Cyanotic congenital heart diseases, e.g., uncorrected tetralogy of Fallot (TOF) and Eisenmenger syndrome. Cyanosis poses risk to mother and fetus. Decreased peripheral resistance increases L-R shunt and aggravates maternal cyanosis. Erythrocytosis in pregnancy increases the risk of thrombosis, paradoxical embolism, and stroke.
- *Pulmonary hypertension:* When pulmonary arterial pressure is more than 60% of systemic pressure.
- Hypertrophic obstructive cardiomyopathy
- Marfan syndrome with aortic diameter >4.5 cm (aorta dilates by estrogen effect)
- Coronary artery disease, especially in women with diabetes
- Dilated cardiomyopathy with EF <40%.

Q8. What is the risk of mitral stenosis during pregnancy?
Ans. As blood volume, cardiac output, and heart rate increase during pregnancy, pressure gradient across the mitral orifice increases that further

increases pulmonary venous pressure, leading to pulmonary edema. Thus, even moderate mitral stenosis may become symptomatic during pregnancy. Atrial fibrillation (AF) may develop or preexist. AF may aggravate due to pregnancy-induced left atrial dilatation.

During delivery, maternal circulation receives an additional 500 mL of blood from placenta (autotransfusion), which may cause pulmonary edema.

Q9. How does pregnancy induce cardiomyopathy?
Ans. A dilated cardiomyopathy presents itself during the peripartum period (i.e., last month of pregnancy, or first 6 months postpartum). The condition is pregnancy induced, but etiology is idiopathic. Hence, valvular, ischemic, hypertensive, congenital, or any other known etiologies should be excluded.

Q10. What are the risk factors for the development of peripartum cardiomyopathy?
Ans. Common risk factors are as follows:
- Peripartum cardiomyopathy in previous pregnancy
- Twin pregnancy
- Preeclampsia
- Advanced maternal age
- Multiparity

Q11. What is the prognosis of peripartum cardiomyopathy?
Ans.
- About 50% recover their left ventricular ejection fraction (LVEF) within 6 months after the diagnosis.
- 20% deteriorate, and either die or develop refractory HF.

The risk during subsequent pregnancy is not uniform—LVEF may decline in next pregnancy in both who recover from LV dysfunction and in those with persistent impairment of LVEF.

Q12. What are the types of hypertension in pregnancy?
Ans.
- *Chronic hypertension:* Raised BP present before pregnancy, or before 20 weeks of gestation. 25% of chronic hypertension develops preeclampsia.
- *Gestational hypertension:* Raised BP develops after 20 weeks; BP normalizes by 12 weeks postpartum. No proteinuria. 50% of gestational hypertension develops preeclampsia.
- *Preeclampsia and eclampsia on chronic hypertension:* Raised BP above patient baseline with proteinuria or end-organ dysfunction
- *Preeclampsia and eclampsia:* Proteinuria (0.3 g over 24 hours) with new hypertension.

Q13. What are the antihypertensives used in pregnancy?
Ans.
- Women with preexisting hypertension are advised to continue their current medication, except for ACEI, ARB, and aliskiren.
- *Methyldopa:* Drug of choice
- *Labetalol:* It has comparable efficacy with methyldopa. In case of severe hypertension, it could be given intravenously.
- *Calcium channel blockers:* Oral nifedipine or IV isradipine could be given in hypertensive emergencies.
- *Antihypertensives contraindicated in pregnancy:* ACEI/ARB, direct renin inhibitors, and atenolol. Diuretics are contraindicated in preeclampsia.
- *Antihypertensives used with caution:* Metoprolol is safe in late pregnancy, avoided in early pregnancy. Diuretics can be used in chronic hypertension before gestation in patients who are salt sensitive. Hydralazine causes perinatal adverse effects; hence, it is no longer a drug of choice.

Q14. How to manage patients with prosthetic valves in pregnancy?
Ans. Maternal risk in pregnancy with prosthetic valves increases due to thromboembolic complications and hemorrhagic complications from anticoagulation. Prophylaxis against valve thrombosis must be maintained with adjusted dose of regular heparin [activated partial thromboplastin time (APTT): 1.5–2 times of control]. If pregnancy is contemplated, a bioprosthetic tissue valve may be used to avoid anticoagulation. Metallic prosthesis is often needed subsequently after completion of reproductive life as it degenerates.

Q15. What are the principles of drug use in pregnancy?
Ans. Drugs may have harmful effects on embryo or fetus at any time during pregnancy. During the first trimester, congenital malformation may develop; risk is greatest during 3rd–11th week of gestation. Even during second or third trimester, drugs may affect growth and functional development.

Principles of drug use:
- Use drugs only if benefits outweigh potential risks to fetus.
  Use drugs with longest safety record, in lowest dose for shortest duration.
- Avoid multidrug regimen, if possible.
  - *Antihypertensives:*
    - A methyldopa drug of choice which is the most trusted.
    - *Angiotensin-converting enzyme inhibitor/angiotensin receptor blocker:* Contraindicated; cause oligohydramnios, IUGR, and malformation
    - *Betablockers:* Cross placenta; cause growth retardation, bradycardia, hypoglycemia
    - *Calcium channel blockers:* Safe

- *Diuretics:* Aggressive dose may decrease placental flow and cause growth retardation
- *Hydralazine:* Safe
- *Warfarin:* Contraindicated in the first trimester; crosses placenta, may cause fetal embryopathy; vaginal delivery contraindicated, switching to heparin needed.
    - *Antiplatelet low-dose aspirin:* Safe; high dose may cause ductal closure.
- *Antiarrhythmics:*
    - *Lignocaine:* Safe
    - *Amiodarone:* Crosses placenta; may cause neonatal goiter
    - *Digoxin:* Safe

SUGGESTED READING

1. Elkay am U, Bitar F. Valvular heart disease and pregnancy; part I: native valves and part II: prosthetic valves. J Am Coll Cardiol. 2005;46(2):223-30; 46(3):403-10.
2. Hirsh J, Fuster V, Ansell J, Halperin JL. American Heart Association/American College of Cardiology Foundation guide to warfarin therapy. J Am Coll Cardiol. 2003;41(9):1633-52.
3. Oakley C, Child A, Lung B, Presbitero P, Tornos P, Klein W, et al. The Expert consensus document on management of cardiovascular diseases during pregnancy: The Task Force on the Management of Cardiovascular Diseases During Pregnancy of the European Society of Cardiology. Eur Heart J. 2003;24(8):761-81.

CHAPTER 24

Renal Diseases and the Heart

"The heart and the kidneys act in synchronization to control BP, diuresis, intravascular volume homeostasis, and oxygenation-if heart fails kidney also starts to fail."
—Author of the book

■ INTRODUCTION

Patients with heart disease have a high prevalence of chronic kidney disease (CKD), which itself also increases risk of coronary artery disease (CAD), hypertension, heart failure (HF), peripheral vascular disease, arrhythmias and sudden death, pericarditis, etc. Assessment of renal function is essential for patients with heart disease to reduce the risk of acute kidney injury (AKI) associated with diagnostic procedures, such as coronary angiography, and therapeutic interventions, such as percutaneous coronary intervention (PCI).

Q1. What are AKI and CKDs?

Ans. Acute kidney injury is a sudden decrease in kidney function that develops within 7 days, as shown by an increase in serum creatinine, or a decrease in urine output, or both. Cause of AKI may be prerenal, intrinsic renal, or postrenal.

Chronic kidney disease is a long-term kidney disease, in which there is a gradual loss of kidney function occurring over a period of months or years.

Diagnostic criteria for CKD are listed in **Box 24.1**.
The stages of CKD are mentioned in **Box 24.2**.

> **BOX 24.1:** Chronic kidney disease—diagnostic criteria.
>
> *Chronic kidney disease is defined as:*
> - Kidney damage ≥3 months (pathological abnormality, or markers of kidney damage, e.g., urine sediments, renal imaging abnormalities, abnormalities in blood or urine composition)
> - Estimated glomerular filtration rate (eGFR) <60 mL/min/1.7 m^2 for ≥3 months without kidney damage

> **BOX 24.2:** Stages of chronic kidney disease (CKD).
>
> - *Stage I:* Only risk factors of CKD; glomerular filtration rate (GFR) is preserved in the presence of damage to the kidney
> - *Stage II:* GFR: 80–70 mL/min/1.73 m^2; mild decrease in kidney function
> - *Stage III:* GFR: 50–40 mL/min/1.73 m^2; moderate decrease in kidney function
> - *Stage IV:* GFR: 15–29 mL/min/1.73 m^2; severe decrease in kidney function
> - *Stage V:* End-stage renal disease (ESRD); GFR: <15 mL/min/1.73 m^2
> - Increased rates of adverse events are generally seen below an eGFR of 60 mL/min/1.73 m^2

Q2. How does CKD increase the risk of CAD?

Ans. Chronic kidney disease acts as a risk factor for CAD in the following ways as listed in **Box 24.3**:

> **BOX 24.3:** Risk of coronary artery disease (CAD) in chronic kidney disease (CKD)—contributing factors.
> - *Dyslipidemia:* Increased triglyceride (TG), lipoprotein(a) [Lp(a)], low-density lipoprotein (LDL), and decreased high-density lipoprotein (HDL)
> - Renin–angiotensin aldosterone (RAS) hyperactivation
> - Sympathetic nervous system hyperactivation
> - *Chronic volume overload:* Decreased response to natriuretic peptide
> - Anemia
> - *Hyperhomocysteinemia:* Increase in homocysteine
> - Coagulopathy and platelet dysfunction
> - Inflammation and endothelial dysfunction
> - Oxidative stress (increased oxidation of LDL)
> - Imbalance between endothelin and nitric oxide (NO)—increases BP
> - Stress of dialysis

Q3. What are the cardiac drugs that need dose adjustment in CKD?

Ans.
- Low-molecular-weight heparin (30% dose reduction is needed if creatinine clearance is <30 mL/min; Xa monitoring is needed) and bivalirudin
- Glycoprotein (GP) IIb/IIIa inhibitors (abciximab, eptifibatide, and tirofiban)
- *Methyldopa:* Reduce to t.i.d. dose if creatinine clearance is <30 mL/min
- *Digoxin:* Reduce dose by 50%
- *Milrinone:* Reduce dose by 25%
- *Angiotensin-converting enzyme inhibitors (ACEIs):* All except captopril and enalapril
- *Betablockers:* Atenolol and sotalol

Others: Antiarrhythmics (disopyramide, flecainide, mexiletine, procainamide, and dofetilide), gemfibrozil, nicotinic acid, and hydralazine

Q4. How does CKD contribute to HF?

Ans. Contributors of HF in CKD are as follows:
- Pressure overload due to raised BP
- Volume overload due to fluid retention
- Anemia due to decreased erythropoiesis
- Cardiomyopathy, especially in diabetes
- Electrolyte imbalance
- Metabolic acidosis
- *Coronary artery disease:* CKD acts as a predisposing factor for CAD
- *Arteriovenous (AV) fistula:* In patients receiving hemodialysis

Q5. How does HF contribute to renal failure?
Ans.
- Decreased renal blood flow in systolic dysfunction leading to AKI on top of CKD.
- *Drugs*: ACEI and angiotensin receptor blocker (ARB) may increase serum creatinine level.

Angiotensin-converting enzyme inhibitor and ARB decrease mortality and development of ESRD, hence should be continued down to GFR: 15 mL/min/1.7 m^2, below this level hyperkalemia rate is high.

Q6. What is cardiorenal syndrome (CRS)?
Ans. It is defined as the disorders of heart and kidneys where acute or chronic dysfunction in one organ may induce acute or chronic dysfunction of the other. As both heart and kidney play a prominent role in BP regulation as well as intravascular homeostasis disorder of one organ may affect other.

Types of CRS are as follows:
- *Type I (acute CRS):* Acute worsening of cardiac function leading to renal dysfunction as in cardiogenic shock and acute decompensated HF.
- *Type II (chronic CRS):* Chronic abnormality of cardiac function leading to renal dysfunction, as in congestive heart failure (CHF).
- *Type III (acute renocardiac syndrome):* Acute worsening of kidney function causing acute cardiac dysfunction, e.g., in AKI and glomerulonephritis
- *Type IV (chronic renocardiac syndrome):* CKD causing decline in cardiac function as in chronic glomerulonephritis (CGN) and interstitial nephritis.
- *Type V (secondary CRS):* Systemic conditions causing kidney and cardiac dysfunction, e.g., sepsis, diabetes mellitus (DM).

Q7. What is cardiorenal failure?
Ans. Heart failure may lead to renal impairment, and renal impairment may in turn precipitate HF—the entity leveled as cardiorenal failure.

Q8. How does CKD precipitate acute coronary syndrome (ACS)?
Ans. Renal dysfunction is a highly inflammatory state that induces plaque rupture leading to ACS. It carries a poor outcome because of the following:
- Presence of comorbidities, e.g., DM and HF
- Drug toxicity
- Therapeutic inertia
- *Special biologic and pathophysiologic factors:* Vascular pathology, dyslipidemia (increased TG, Lp(a), LDL, and decreased HDL), more oxidized LDL, and homocystinemia

Q9. What coronary intervention is preferred in patients with CKD—PCI or CABG?
Ans. Patients with CAD with CKD (especially ESRD) have worse prognosis in medical therapy. Coronary artery bypass grafting (CABG) is superior to

multivessel PCI. If CABG is not possible, PCI with drug-eluting stent (DES) is done.

Q10. What are the predictors of cardiovascular (CV) risk in CKD?
Ans.
- *Glomerular filtration rate:* In early stage of CKD, a major reduction of GFR is still compatible with serum creatinine within normal limit, because it depends also on nonrenal factors (particularly muscle mass).
- *Albuminuria:* It occurs as a result of endothelial dysfunction in glomerular capillary. In the absence of albuminuria, CV risk conferred by reduced renal function is markedly less.

Q11. What is microalbuminuria? How does it act as a risk factor for CAD?
Ans. It is defined as a random urine albumin to creatinine ratio (ACR) of 30–300 mg/g. An ACR >300 mg/g is gross proteinuria. A spot urine ACR offer test for microalbuminuria.

Q12. What is contrast-induced nephropathy (CIN)? How can it be prevented?
Ans. Acute kidney injury with serum creatinine >25% or >0.5 mg/dL above baseline after intravenous (IV) contrast administration. Factors contributing are toxicity of contrast, dehydration, and vasoconstriction.

Prevention: Choosing low osmolar agent, such as iodixanol; maintaining proper hydration and maintaining urine output of 15 mL/h.

■ SUGGESTED READING

1. Brosius FC 3rd, Hostetter TH, Kelepouris E, Mitsnefes MM, Moe SM, Moore MA, et al. Detection of chronic kidney disease in patients with or at increased risk of cardiovascular disease: a science advisory from the American Heart Association Kidney and Cardiovascular Disease Council; the Councils on High Blood Pressure Research, Cardiovascular Disease in the Young, and Epidemiology and Prevention; and the Quality of Care and Outcomes Research Interdisciplinary Working Group: developed on collaboration with the National Kidney Foundation. Circulation. 2006;114(10):1083-7.
2. Chobanian AV, Bakris GL, Black HR, Cushman WC, Green LA, Izzo JL Jr, et al. The Seventh Report of the Joint National Committee on Prevention, Detection, Evaluation, and Treatment of High Blood Pressure: the JNC 7 report. JAMA. 2003;289(19):2560-72.
3. McCullough PA. Interface between renal disease and cardiovascular illness. In: Libby P, Bonow RO, Mann DL, Zipes DP (Eds). Braunwald's Heart Disease: A Textbook of Cardiovascular Medicine, 8th edition. Philadelphia: Saunders; 2008.

Chapter 25: Cerebrovascular Diseases and the Heart

"Risk factors for stroke overlap with those for CAD; majority of stroke patients die of their cardiac ailment rather than stroke."
—Author of the book

■ INTRODUCTION

Risk factors for stroke overlap with those for coronary artery disease (CAD). Atherosclerosis and other vascular diseases affect both the heart and the brain. The most frequent cause of death in stroke patients is CAD. Again, heart diseases often lead to cerebral dysfunction, and conversely, cerebrovascular diseases can influence the heart and its function. The inter-relationship between cerebrovascular and cardiac disease is discussed in this chapter.

Q1. Compare and contrast between heart attack and stroke.
Ans. Heart attack or acute myocardial infarction (AMI) and stroke are both two grave manifestations of cardiovascular disease (CVD). They have some common etiology but differ in several aspects regarding pathogenesis and management **(Table 25.1)**.

TABLE 25.1: Heart attack and stroke—comparison.

Points	Heart attack	Stroke
Cause	Coronary thrombosis with myocardial infarction (MI)	Both cerebral thrombosis with infarction and hemorrhage
Risk factor	Dyslipidemia appears to be universal	Smoking and hypertension appear to be more important
Hemorrhagic transformation	±	May occur
Antiplatelets	Always indicated in AMI and as secondary prevention	Indicated for ischemic
Heparin	NSTEMI, STEMI with ongoing pain and after rt-PA	Not indicated in infarct infarction
Thrombolytics	In STEMI within 12 hours	Indicated in some cases of infarction within 3 hours
Interventional	Primary PCI (with stent)	Endovascular therapy in proximal MCA occlusion (using rt-PA)

(MCA: middle cerebral artery; rt-PA: recombinant tissue plasminogen activator)

Q2. What are the causes of cardiogenic stroke?
Ans. Cardiogenic stroke can occur when:
- Embolus from the heart, as in atrial fibrillation (AF)
- Cerebral hypoperfusion in cardiogenic shock and pump failure
- Drug-induced–drugs used for heart disease having neurologic adverse effects, e.g., digitalis-induced hallucination, confusion, etc.

Q3. What is paradoxical embolism? How is the diagnosis made?
Ans. Paradoxical embolism is the emboli entering the systemic arterial circulation from thrombus arising in the venous side through a right to left shunt. The most common potential intracardiac shunt is a residual patent foramen ovale (PFO).

Four out of the following five criteria establish the diagnosis:
1. A situation that promotes thrombosis in leg or pelvic veins
2. Increased coagulability
3. Sudden onset of stroke during sexual intercourse, straining at stool, or other activities that include a Valsalva maneuver.
4. Pulmonary embolism within a short time before or after the neurological event.
5. Absence of other putative cause of stroke

Q4. What are the risk factors of cerebral embolism in AF? How to prevent it?
Ans.
- Age >65 years
- Mitral valvular disease
- Dilated left atrium
- Mitral annular calcification (on echocardiography)

Q5. What are the cardiac effects of cerebral lesions?
Ans.
- *Arrhythmias:* Sinus bradycardia, sinus tachycardia, premature ventricular contraction (PVC), atrioventricular (AV) block, ventricular tachycardia (VT), AF, etc.
- Neurogenic pulmonary edema—in subarachnoid hemorrhage (SAH), subdural hemorrhage, and may develop despite normal cardiac function.
- *Electrocardiogram (ECG) changes:* Prolonged QT interval with giant, wide, roller coaster-inverted T waves, and U waves, especially in SAH
- *Echocardiographic changes:* Takotsubo cardiomyopathy (also called broken-heart syndrome) is transient left ventricular apical ballooning. It has been found after severe emotional stress, especially in postmenopausal women. Cerebral lesions causing it are ischemic stroke and SAH, causing marked sympathetic activation. On echocardiography,

left ventricular (LV) end-systolic shape resembles an octopus catcher (takotsubo) used in Japan.
- *Sudden death:* Voodoo death is sudden death occurring in stressful situations that involves central nervous system (CNS). It may occur in SAH, intracranial hemorrhage (ICH), and ischemic stroke. Cardiac arrhythmias may be the mechanism.
- *Cardiac changes:* Patchy myocardial necrosis, subendocardial hemorrhage, found in hearts of patients dying of acute CNS lesions.

Q6. What are the cerebral complications of cardiac interventional procedures?
Ans.
- *Cardiac catheterization:* Stroke, transient ischemic attack (TIA) due to embolic phenomena
- *Percutaneous coronary intervention (PCI) and stenting:* Stroke: 0–4%
- *Electrophysiology (EP) procedures and cardioversion:* Thromboembolic stroke
- *Percutaneous closure of left atrial (LA) appendage:* An alternative to chronic warfarin for stroke prevention in patients with nonvalvular AF
- *Percutaneous valvuloplasty:* Balloon valvuloplasty of aortic and mitral valves has been complicated by stroke.
- *Intra-aortic balloon pump (IABP):* Spinal cord infarct by local thromboembolism or aortic dissection.

Q7. What are the coexistent vascular disorders that affect both the brain and the heart?
Ans.
- Atherosclerotic diseases predominantly involve the origin of internal carotid and vertebral arteries in the neck at site of branching and diversion of blood flow. Patients with internal carotid artery (ICA)-origin disease have a high frequency of hypercholesterolemia, CAD, and peripheral vascular disease (PVD). Although patients with intracranial occlusive disease do not have a high incidence of CAD or PVD.
- *Hypertension:* Acute and chronic high blood pressure (BP) damage deep, penetrating intracranial arteries; accelerate atherosclerosis in extra-cranial and large intracranial arteries, producing lacunar infarct, ICH, and diffuse ischemic degeneration. CVDs are manifested as pure motor hemiplegia, pure sensory stroke, ataxic hemiplegia, and dysarthria-clumsy hand syndrome. An increase in BP can cause ICH by vessel leakage. An abrupt increase in BP can sometimes lead to SAH, although SAH is not directly caused by hypertension in most cases.
- *Coagulopathy:* It can lead to serious ICH, SAH, or subdural and epidural hemorrhage. Hemorrhage develops more insidiously and evolves slowly. Anticoagulants should be stopped immediately, and their effect reversed

by fresh frozen plasma or vitamin K. Anticoagulation resumed after 7–14 days with heparin, if indicated (as in case of mechanical valves).
- *Aortic dissection:* Involving innominate or common carotid arteries causes stroke and TIA.

Q8. What are the cardiac sources of cerebral embolism?
Ans. The three groups are as follows:
1. *Cardiac chamber abnormalities:* Cardiomyopathies, hypokinetic and akinetic ventricular regions after myocardial infarction (MI), ventricular aneurysm, atrial myxoma, atrial septal aneurysm, septal defects, and PFO.
2. *Valvular:* Rheumatic mitral and aortic disease, prosthetic valves, bacterial endocarditis, mitral valve prolapse (MVP), and mitral annular calcification
3. *Arrhythmias:* AF and sick sinus syndrome.

Some cardiac sources are strong, such as prosthetic valves, AF, sick sinus syndrome, ventricular aneurysm, akinetic LV wall, mural thrombus, cardiomyopathy, and diffuse ventricular hypokinesia, and some are weak sources, such as MI >6 months old, aortic and mitral stenosis and regurgitation, congestive heart failure (CHF), MVP, hypokinetic LV segment, and mitral annular calcification.

The incidence of embolism is highest during the period of active thrombus formation (first 1–3 months), but risk remains in patients with AF, CHF, or those with persistent myocardial dysfunction.

Q9. What are the indications of anticoagulants in patients with acute ischemic stroke?
Ans. The American Heart Association/American Academy of Neurology recommendations for use of anticoagulants in acute ischemic stroke are given in **Box 25.1**.

> **BOX 25.1:** Anticoagulation in acute ischemic stroke.
> - Patients with atrial fibrillation (AF)—associated stroke benefit from long-term anticoagulation unless contraindicated [e.g., previous ICH, history of fall, etc.]. Those with large stroke and with uncontrolled hypertension are at higher risk of spontaneous intracranial hemorrhage.
> - Emergent anticoagulation with goal of improving neurological outcome, or preventing early recurrent stroke—not recommended.
> - Urgent anticoagulation for moderate to severe stroke—not recommended as risk of intracranial hemorrhage is high.
> - Anticoagulant initiation within 24 hours of treatment with intravenous (IV) recombinant tissue plasminogen activator (rt-PA)—not recommended.

Q10. What is the role of antiplatelets in acute ischemic stroke and its prevention?
Ans. Aspirin is beneficial if begun within 48 hours of acute ischemic stroke. Aspirin 169–375 mg daily, and not any other antiplatelet alone or

in combination, shown to be beneficial. The combination of aspirin and clopidogrel, in various studies, was associated with a significant increased risk of bleeding complications without any significant reduction of stroke. Aspirin lowered the risk of nonembolic stroke in one study. It reduces risk of recurrent stroke. 15% of stroke survivors will have a second stroke within 1 year, and 30% within 5 years. Risk of developing stroke in TIA is 10% over 90 days (highest risk over first week).

Q11. Hemorrhagic or infarctive stroke—which one is more common among hypertensives? What is the mechanism?

Ans. Infarctive strokes are more common in hypertensives—80% of strokes in hypertensives are due to infarction, and only 20% are due to hemorrhage. Hypertensive intracranial hemorrhage accounts for 10% of all stroke cases.

- *Cerebral infarction:* Hypertension accelerates atherosclerosis in extracranial and large intracranial arteries and produces lacunar infarcts. Besides, it also produces diffuse ischemic changes in white matter and basal grey matter.
- *Intracranial hemorrhage:* High BP (acute or chronic) damages deep penetrating small intracranial arteries, leads to development of microaneurysm with subsequent rupture. Hematoma develops at the same site of lacunae.

An acute elevation of BP and/or blood flow to the brain causes vessel leakage.

Q12. Cerebral hemorrhage is an important cause of stroke, but cardiac hemorrhage seldom occurs—why?

Ans. Penetrating intracranial vessels undergo microaneurysm formation in persons with chronically elevated BP. These not being adequately supported by adjacent brain matter, may undergo rupture with resultant hemorrhagic stroke. On the contrary, intramural coronary arteries are always adequately supported by myocardial tissues and are kept under pressure by cardiac contraction. Hence, aneurysm formation and rupture of intramural coronaries do not happen, and intracardiac hemorrhage does not occur.

Q13. How to reduce elevated BP in stroke patients?
Ans.
- Relatively aggressive treatment of elevated BP is needed in patients receiving IV rt-PA to reduce risk of bleeding.
- In those who are not thrombolized and who do not have malignant hypertension (hypertensive encephalopathy, aortic dissection, acute renal failure, acute pulmonary edema, AMI, or BP >220/120 mm Hg), a controlled reduction of BP is needed. Precipitous drop may further compromise already ischemic brain, potentially increasing the stroke.

- In hemorrhagic stroke with high BP, rapid reduction of BP is needed to prevent more blood leak and increase of intracerebral hematoma.

Q14. What is the reperfusion strategy in ischemic stroke?
Ans. Reperfusion therapy for ischemic stroke is advocated as quickly as possible to minimize further damage and consists of IV thrombolysis with recombinant tissue plasminogen activator (rtPA) with or without catheter-based reperfusion therapy, including intra-arterial thrombolysis, mechanical thrombectomy, or balloon angioplasty with or without stent deployment. The only approved agent for acute ischemic stroke is IV tPA within 3–4.5 hours of onset and without contraindications. Rapid initiation of IV tPA with a door-to-balloon time of less than 60 minutes is important for a good outcome.

Q15. What are the contraindications of thrombolysis in stroke?
Ans.
- *Clinical:* History of ICH, systolic blood pressure (SBP) >185 mm Hg, diastolic blood pressure (DBP) >110 mm Hg, rapid improvement in neurological status, mild neurological impairment, SAH, history of stroke or head trauma within the last 3 months, gastrointestinal or genitourinary tract hemorrhage, or major surgery within 3 weeks, recent MI, seizure with stroke, oral anticoagulant intake, and received heparin within 48 hours.
- *Radiologic:* Evidence of ICH
- *Laboratory findings:* International normalized ratio (INR) >1.7, total platelet count <100,000, elevated activated partial thromboplastin time (APTT), and blood glucose <50 mg/dL.

Q16. What are the pitfalls in using thrombolytic in ischemic stroke?
Ans.
- The risk-to-benefit ratio for tPA in ischemic stroke is narrow. It has limited effectiveness in recanalizing proximal stroke-related arteries with a large clot burden [<10% for ICA occlusion to approximately 10% for middle cerebral artery (MCA) distal branch occlusion].
- The risk of hemorrhage is increased for older adult patients and those with large strokes, diabetes mellitus, a history of stroke, or thrombocytopenia.
- Stroke thrombi usually have an embolic origin, and are larger in volume, making them older, more organized, and more resistant to lysis. Moreover, tortuosity of cerebral vessels can make clot-busting therapy more difficult than the treatment of AMI.

Stroke centers outlined by the Brain Attack Coalition (BAC) in 2000 recommend quick identification and triage of stroke patients to provide the most timely treatment. These include basic acute stroke care, 24-hours access to computed tomography (CT) scans and advanced neuroimaging capabilities, on-demand neurosurgical and endovascular interventional capabilities, etc.

Q17. What is the role of interventional cardiologists in stroke management?

Ans. Many interventional cardiologists are currently performing carotid stent placement and intracerebral angiography. Excellent catheter skills, experience of managing atherosclerotic risk factors for stroke, and management of coexisting cardiac disease, e.g., AF, are their strength. A stroke neurologist, in consultation with the interventional cardiologist and neuroradiologist, is initially called to assess the patient and determine the need for intervention. Stroke patients may be considered eligible for intervention if the delay is less than 8 hours from symptom onset. Lack of on-demand interventional therapy for most stroke patients who are not candidates for lysis is a concern.

SUGGESTED READING

1. Megan CL, Louis RC. Cerebrovascular disease and neurological manifestations of heart disease. In: Fuster V, Walsh RA, Harrington RA (Eds). Hurst's The Heart, 13th edition. New York: McGraw-Hill; 2011.
2. The Cerebral Embolism Task Force. Cardiogenic brain embolism. The second report of the Cerebral Embolism Task Force. Arch Neurol. 1989;46(7):727-43.
3. The Stroke Prevention in Atrial Fibrillation Investigators. Predictors of thromboembolism in atrial fibrillation: II. Echocardiographic features of patients at risk. Ann Intern Med. 1992;116(1):6-12.

26 Anesthesia, Surgery, and Heart Diseases

"Patients with clinically stable heart disease may not need extensive investigation and preoperative interventions are rarely needed for them."
—Eric J Topol

■ INTRODUCTION

Patients with heart disease or cardiac risk factors needing noncardiac surgery, cardiovascular mortality and morbidity increase significantly. High-risk patients with risk of perioperative myocardial injury need to be identified prior to the procedure.

Q1. What are the major clinical predictors of increased perioperative cardiovascular risk?

Ans. Major predictors of increased perioperative cardiovascular risk are shown in **Box 26.1**.

> **BOX 26.1:** Predictors of perioperative MI and cardiac death.
> - Acute myocardial infarction (AMI) (within 7 days) and recent MI (>7 days and up to 1 month), with evidence of ischemia based on symptoms or noninvasive testing
> - Unstable or severe angina (class III or IV)
> - Decompensated heart failure
> - High-grade atrioventricular (AV) block
> - Symptomatic ventricular arrhythmias with underlying heart diseases
> - Supraventricular arrhythmia with uncontrolled ventricular rate
> - Severe valvular heart disease

Q2. How to stratify perioperative cardiovascular risk in noncardiac surgery?

Ans. Cardiovascular risk stratification in noncardiac surgery is shown in **Box 26.2**.

> **BOX 26.2:** The American Heart Association/American College of Cardiology (AHA/ACC) Task Force stratification of surgical procedures.
> - *High risk (cardiac risk >5%):*
>   - Emergency major operations, particularly in elderly
>   - Aortic, major vascular, and peripheral vascular surgery
>   - Extensive operations with large volume shift or blood loss
>   - Intermediate risk (cardiac risk <5%)
>   - Intraperitoneal and intrathoracic

Contd...

Contd...

- Carotid endarterectomy
- Head and neck surgery
- Orthopedic
- Prostate
- Low risk (cardiac risk <1%):
  - Endoscopic procedures
  - Superficial biopsy
  - Cataract
  - Breast surgery

Q3. Patients needing percutaneous coronary intervention (PCI) and a subsequent surgery—how to manage?

Ans. Whenever possible, noncardiac surgery should be delayed 6 weeks after bare metal stent placement, by which time stents are generally endothelialized and a course of antiplatelet therapy to prevent stent thrombosis has been completed.

Drug-eluting stents (DES) should not be implanted before planned noncardiac surgery unless surgery can be safely performed on dual antiplatelet therapy, or elective noncardiac surgery can be delayed for 12 months to allow effective post-DES antiplatelet therapy. If clopidogrel must be discontinued before major surgery, aspirin must be continued and clopidogrel restarted as soon as possible.

Surgery may be undertaken 2–4 weeks after plain old balloon angioplasty (POBA).

Q4. How beta-blockers reduce perioperative cardiac risk in noncardiac surgery?

Ans. Beta-blockers reduce perioperative cardiac mortality. The AHA/ACC recommend treatment with a beta-blocking agent for patients previously receiving these agents, and for patients with positive stress tests undergoing major vascular surgery. Such therapy should be initiated several days or more in advance and titrated to a heart rate of 60–70 beats/min.

Prophylactic use of beta-blockers in patients with major risk factors for coronary artery disease (CAD) is recommended.

Q5. What is a "cardiac anesthetic"?

Ans. There is no best general anesthetic technique for patients with CAD undergoing noncardiac surgery. Hence, the concept of a "cardiac anesthesia" is abandoned. General anesthesia is done by inhalational agents, high-dose narcotics, or by a balanced mechanism (low-dose narcotics with an inhalation agent).

- *Inhalational anesthetics:* They cause reversible myocardial depression and decrease O_2 demand. They also cause ischemic preconditioning of the myocardium.

- *Narcotic anesthetic (high dose):* It lacks myocardial depressant action, it also provides hemodynamic stability.
- *Propofol intravenous (IV):* It is used for both induction and maintenance of general anesthesia. It may produce profound hypotension but clears rapidly. It has been used to assist early extubation after coronary artery bypass grafting (CABG).

Q6. What are the cardiovascular effects of spinal and epidural anesthesia?
Ans. Spinal or epidural techniques can produce sympathetic blockades, which can reduce blood pressure (BP) and slow heart rate. Spinal anesthesia and lumbar, or low thoracic epidural anesthesia can also evoke reflex sympathetic activation above the blockades, which might lead to myocardial ischemia.

Q7. Patients with a mechanical prosthetic valve undergoing noncardiac surgery—how to manage?
Ans. Oral anticoagulants are contraindicated during surgery. They are discontinued several days prior to surgery. Short half-life allows patients to undergo surgery safely within a few hours of discontinuation. Patients should receive heparin postoperatively until oral anticoagulation is fully therapeutic. Re-establishment of therapeutic level usually requires several days after warfarin is started.

SUGGESTED READING

1. Fleisher LA, Beckman JA, Brown KA, Calkins H, Chaikof EL, Fleischmann KE, et al. 2009 ACCF/AHA focused update on perioperative beta blockade incorporated into the ACC/AHA 2007 guidelines on perioperative cardiovascular evaluation and care for noncardiac surgery: a report of the American College of Cardiology Foundation/American Heart Association Task force on Practice Guidelines. Circulation. 2009;120(21):e169-276.
2. Tarakji KG. Assessing and managing cardiac risk in noncardiac surgical procedures. In: Griffin BP, Topol EJ (Eds). Manual of Cardiovascular Medicine, 3rd edition. Philadelphia: Lipincott Williams and Wilkins; 2009.

CHAPTER 27

Neoplastic Heart Disease and Cardio-oncology

> "Population aging and improved cancer survival lead to a convergence of heart disease and cancer."
> —Author of the book

■ INTRODUCTION

Primary tumors of the heart are rare. Myxoma is the most common primary cardiac tumor. Secondary involvement, directly or indirectly by extracardiac tumor is 20–40 times more common. Cardio-oncology refers to diagnosis, treatment, monitoring, and prevention of CV disease in patients with cancer. CVD and cancer being the leading cause of mortality globally cardio-oncology aims to provide optimal oncotherapy with minimal CV mortality and morbidity.

Q1. How do neoplastic diseases involve the heart?
Ans.
- *Directly:* By local invasion, e.g., pericardial involvement in bronchogenic and breast cancer, lymphatic spread causing superior vena cava syndrome in bronchogenic carcinoma.
- *Indirectly:* By producing hyperviscosity syndrome, e.g., myeloproliferative diseases, causing coronary ischemia
- *Drug and radiation induced:* For example, cardiomyopathy by doxorubicin, radiation-induced pericardial effusion, and constrictive pericarditis
- *Coexistence:* Cardiovascular (CV) diseases and cancer share common risk factors, e.g., smoking, causing coronary artery disease (CAD) and bronchogenic carcinoma. Thus, both may coexist in the same patient.

Q2. What is the causal relationship between IHD and cancer?
Ans.
- Both the conditions may have common risk factors, e.g., smoking is a risk factor for both bronchogenic carcinoma and IHD.
- A common biological mechanism may act in both the conditions.
- Patients with CV disease may develop cancer.
- Cancer patients are at risk of developing CV disease secondary to cancer therapy (cardiotoxicity).

Q3. What are the CV effects of anti-cancer drugs?
Ans. Cardiotoxicity may manifest heart failure (HF), arrhythmia, hypertension (HTN), pulmonary HTN, IHD, pericardial disease, peripheral vascular disease, and venous and arterial thrombosis. With improved treatment regimen and increased longevity of cancer patients, chances of cardiotoxicity are increasing. Moreover, cancer therapies are rapidly evolving; "targeted" strategies may affect signaling pathway in cardiomyocytes and endothelial cells, and hemostasis.
- *Anthracyclines:* Doxorubicin, daunorubicin—cardiac arrhythmia, cardiomyopathy, and HF
- *Paclitaxel:* Arrhythmia and ischemia
- *Alkylating agents (cyclophosphamide):* Myocarditis, arrhythmias, cisplatin, carboplatin, etc.—endothelial dysfunction, arterial vasospasm, and HTN
- *Antimetabolites, e.g., 5-fluorouracil (5-FU):* Coronary spasm, ischemia, myocardial infarction (MI), arrhythmia
- *Monoclonal antibody (tyrosine kinase inhibitors):* HF
- *Estrogen receptor modulator, e.g., tamoxifen:* Thrombosis
- *Small molecule tyrosine kinase inhibitors, e.g., sunitinib:* HTN, cardiomyopathy, and HF.
- *Radiation therapy:* Valvular heart disease, pericardial disease—CAD, CM, and HF.

Q4. How to provide CV care for cancer patients?
Ans. Safe and effective delivery of cancer therapy through the identification of patients at high risk of CV disease, optimization of CV-risk factors, such as HTN, diabetes mellitus (DM), dyslipidemia, obesity and smoking, and careful management of CV diseases. American Society of Clinical Oncology (ASCO) recommends screening and optimization of CV disease and its risk factors through history taking, doing physical examination and investigations, including an echocardiographic examination. CV care of cancer patients is taken at three stages: Prior to, during, and after cancer therapy.

Q5. What are the causes of pericardial effusion in a cancer patient?
Ans.
- Malignant invasion
- Radiation induced
- Infective—tuberculosis, fungal, and bacterial
- Iatrogenic
- Idiopathic

Q6. What are the tumors involving the heart?
Ans.
- *Primary:* Uncommon, usually benign. Myxoma most common, others are papillary fibroelastoma, rhabdomyoma, lipoma, and hemangioma. Rarely malignant neoplasm may be sarcoma or lymphoma.

- *Secondary:* Direct invasion of primary lung, breast, and esophageal cancer; hematogenous or retrograde lymphatic spread may occur in lymphoma, melanoma, Kaposi's sarcoma, etc.

Q7. What are the special features of myxoma?
Ans. Myxomas are the most common cardiac neoplasm.
- They arise from multipotent mesenchymal cells.
- Although benign, they may recur at multiple sites.
- They may grow from embolic tumor fragments (maybe called metastases).

Q8. What are the echocardiographic findings of left atrial (LA) myxoma?
Ans.
- *M-mode echocardiography (echo):* Tumor echo completely fills the mitral valve throughout the diastole. With the cursor across LA and aortic valve, the echo producing mass is seen within LA hind the aortic valve.
- *2-dimensional echocardiography (2DE):* A mobile, echogenic mass attached to interatrial septum by a pedicle in the region of fossa ovalis. A myxoma with a long stock is seen to show to-and-fro motion, occupying the mitral orifice during diastole and coming back within LA during systole **(Figs. 27.1A and B)**.

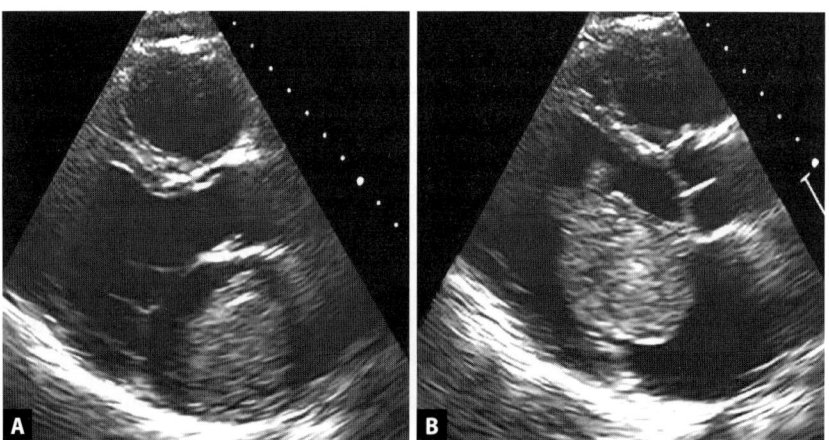

Figs. 27.1A and B: 2DE showing left atrial myxoma (A), prolapsing through mitral orifice (B).

Q9. What is the presentation of myxoma?
Ans. Triad of presentation is as follows:
1. *Obstructive:* Dizziness, dyspnea, cough, pulmonary edema, congestive heart failure (CHF) resulting from mechanical interference of mitral valve.
2. *Embolic:* To any organ or tissue
3. *Systemic:* Fever, weight loss, fatigue, arthralgia, muscle weakness, and Raynaud's phenomenon

Q10. What is Carney syndrome?
Ans. It is an autosomal dominant disorder characterized by myxoma formation in cardiac and several extracardiac sites, spotty skin pigmentation, endocrine hyperactivity, and other tumors, e.g., testicular Sertoli cell tumor, etc.

SUGGESTED READING

1. Armenian SH, Lacchetti C, Barac A, Carver J, Constine LS, Denduluri N, et al. Prevention and Monitoring of Cardiac Dysfunction in Survivors of Adult Cancers: American Society of Clinical Oncology Clinical Practice Guideline. J Clin Oncol. 2017;35(8):893-911.
2. Lyon AR, López-Fernández T, Couch LS, Asteggiano R, Aznar MC, Bergler-Klein J, et al. ESC Guidelines on cardio-oncology developed in collaboration with the European Hematology Society for Therapeutic Radiology and Oncology (ESTRO) and the International Cardio-oncology Society (IC-OS): Developed by the task force on Cardio-Oncology of the European Society of Cardiology (ESC). 2022;43:4229-361.
3. McManus M, Lee, CH. Primary tumors of the heart. In: Libby P, Bonow RO, Mann DL (Eds). Braunwald's Heart Disease: A Textbook of Cardiovascular Medicine, 8th edition. Philadelphia, PA: Saunders; 2008.

28. Air Pollution, Toxins and the Heart

"Exposure to ambient and household air pollution is a leading cause of death worldwide with seven million premature deaths globally."
—Global Burden of Disease Study

■ INTRODUCTION

Air pollution has been an inevitable consequence of civilization; the level of pollution has increased most significantly since the industrial revolution. Long-term exposure to particulate matter <2.5 µm (PM2.5) is associated with increased risk of atherosclerosis, hypertension, myocardial infarction (MI), and stroke. A staggering 80% of cardiovascular disease (CVD) deaths are linked to air pollution, and over 60% of these deaths are attributed to indoor air pollution.

Many toxins affect cardiovascular system (CVS) adversely. These include alcohol, illicit drugs, and commonly used pharmacological agents, etc.

Q1. How is air pollution related to CVD?
Ans. Air pollution with particulate matter, nitrous oxide (N_2O), and ozone (O_3) all have similar effects on CVS. It causes CVD directly by oxidative stress, inflammation, autonomic imbalance, endothelial dysfunction, and thrombosis, and indirectly by triggering arrhythmia, hypertension, respiratory infection, and exacerbation of chronic obstructive pulmonary disease (COPD). Direct consequences lead to atherosclerosis and its complications like ischemic heart disease (IHD), cardiac arrest, heart failure, stroke, etc. Type of pollutant, dose, duration of exposure, and individual health status are factors determining the net result. Fine PM2.5 air pollution is the most important environmental risk factor contributing to global cardiovascular (CV) mortality and disability.

Q2. What are the various types of air pollution?
Ans.
- *Aerosols:* Most pollution consist of aerosols containing a mixture of both particles and gases. Of these, PM2.5 suspended in air has received the most attention, because it is easily measured and readily related to the adverse health effects of polluted air.

- *Gaseous pollutants:* Carbon monoxide, sulfur dioxide, nitrogen oxide, ozone, etc. are greenhouse gases (GHGs). There emission results from fossil-fuel use, deforestation, expansion of human habitats, changing pattern of land-use, and change in lifestyles.
- *Outdoor pollution:* From industry, traffic, and agriculture.
- *Indoor pollution:* Unclean cooking and using kerosene and biomass for cooking purpose.

Q3. What are the mitigation strategies for air pollution?

Ans. Achieving a zero-carbon emission economy is essential. Mitigation strategies that may help are as follows:
- Shifting to clean cooking fuel and transport options.
- Using face masks and air purifiers among vulnerable communities.
- Awareness about adverse effects of air pollution by using air quality index (AQI); creating country-wide air quality monitoring network and generating citizen awareness.
- Establishing a national clean air program to implement mitigation strategies.
- Lifestyle adjustments like avoiding use of incense or candles indoor.
- Wearing N95 masks which can filter PM2.5, particularly if we need to go outside.

Q4. How is alcohol cardioprotective?

Ans. Moderate intake of alcohol (ethanol), e.g., 2–7 drinks in a week decreases CV mortality in both males and females. All alcoholic beverages exert such an effect although it is the strongest with wine **(Box 28.1)**. Consumption of excessive amounts has the opposite effect.

> **BOX 28.1:** Beneficial effects of ethanol.
> - Increases high-density lipoprotein-cholesterol (HDL-C) and apoprotein A1
> - Decreases platelet aggregation
> - Decreases serum fibrinogen
> - Increases antioxidant activity—by phenolic compounds and flavonoids contained in red wine
> - Increases fibrinolysis

These cardioprotection may be more among those with increased risk [older, high low-density lipoprotein-cholesterol (LDL-C), female with multiple risk factors].

Q5. What are the toxic effects of alcohol on the CVS?

Ans. Consumption of alcohol in excess amount exerts toxic effects on the CVS as listed in **Box 28.2**.

> **BOX 28.2:** Alcohol—toxic effects on the cardiovascular system (CVS).
>
> - *Nonischemic cardiomyopathy:* By direct toxic effect on myocardium
> - *Systemic hypertension:* Excessive intake raises blood pressure (BP) instantaneously
> - *Arrhythmias:* Most commonly atrial fibrillation (AF); may also cause ventricular ectopic, supraventricular tachycardia, and atrial flutter. New-onset AF among youth after binge drinking in weekends is called "holiday heart syndrome". Hypertension, sleep apnea, and electrolyte imbalance contribute besides direct toxicity
> - *Accelerating atherosclerosis:* Heavy ethanol use increases triglyceride (TG), elevates BP, increases left ventricular (LV) mass and thus augments atherosclerosis. It is also seen in heavy smokers
> - *Sudden cardiac death:* Due to coronary artery disease (CAD) and arrhythmias

Q6. What is the mechanism of myocardial toxicity of alcohol?
Ans.
- Direct toxicity
- Deficiency of thiamine and K^+
- Additives—lead and cobalt that are toxic to myocardium
- Decreases oxidation of free fatty acids by liver—increases TG, LDL-C, and total cholesterol

Q7. How does cocaine cause CAD?
Ans. Cocaine causes vasoconstriction of epicardial coronaries and decreases oxygen (O_2) supply by its sympathomimetic (α-agonist) action. It also increases heart rate, LV wall tension, and LV contractility, thus increasing all three determinants of myocardial O_2 consumption.

Q8. What are the cardiovascular complications of cocaine?
Ans. Cocaine, by dint of its sympathomimetic action leads to following CVS features when consumed in excessive dose **(Box 28.3)**.

> **BOX 28.3:** Cardiovascular effects of cocaine.
>
> - Coronary artery disease (CAD)—myocardial infarction (MI) in young
> - Arrhythmias
> - Sudden cardiac death
> - Pulmonary edema
> - Acute aortic dissection
> - Cardiomyopathy
> - Endocarditis

Q9. When to suspect cocaine abuse as a cause of MI?
Ans. When subjects with no or few risk factors for atherosclerosis, particularly those who are young, or have a history of substance abuse present with AMI, cocaine abuse should be suspected. Urine and blood samples should be analyzed for cocaine and its metabolites.

Q10. What are the cardiac manifestations of organophosphorus compound (OPC) poisoning?
Ans. Cardiac manifestations of acute OPC poisoning are: Bradycardia, ST-segment elevation, and atrioventricular conduction disturbances. Long-term changes include QT prolongation, polymorphic ventricular tachycardia (VT), and sudden cardiac death.

SUGGESTED READING

1. Costanzo S, Di Castelnuovo A, Donati MB, Iacoviello L, de Gaetano G, et al. Alcohol consumption and mortality in patients with cardiovascular disease: a meta-analysis. J Am Coll Cardiol. 2010;55(13):1339-47.
2. Particulate matter air pollution and cardiovascular disease: An update to the scientific statement from the American Heart Association. Circulation. 2010;121(21):2331-78.
3. Richard AL, Hills LD. Toxins and the heart. In: Libby P, Bonow RO, Mann DL (Eds). Braunwald's Heart disease A Textbook of Cardiovascular Medicine, 8th edition. Philadelphia, PA: Saunders; 2008.

29 Traumatic Heart Disease

"The heart is subject to lifetime biological and psychological trauma but accidental physical trauma may occur."

—Anonymous

■ INTRODUCTION

Accidental or iatrogenic cardiac trauma may occur, although the heart has a protective surrounding by the chest case and adjacent lungs. Cardiac trauma can easily be overlooked in the presence of distressing injuries, as it can occur in the absence of chest pain or visible trauma.

Q1. What are the causes of traumatic heart diseases?
Ans.
- Iatrogenic—catheterization and pericardiocentesis
- Physical injury—penetrating and nonpenetrating
- Metabolic cardiac injury (MCI)—in response to burn, sepsis, electrical injury, and systemic inflammation
- Others—burn, electrocution, etc.

Q2. What are the cardiac complications of electrical injury?
Ans. Electrocution, lightning, and strikes may cause immediate cardiac arrest, acute myocardial necrosis and ventricular failure, pseudoinfarction, myocardial ischemia, dysrhythmias, conduction abnormalities, and acute hypertension with peripheral vasospasm.

This is by direct effect on excitable tissues, heat generated from electrical currents, and associated injuries (fall, explosion, fire, etc.)

Q3. What are the cardiac complications of burn?
Ans.
- Capillary leakage is caused by endothelial injury due to burn resulting in a profound decrease in cardiac output.
- *Myocardial depression:* When surface burn is 20–25%; caused by release of myocardial depressant factor, tumor necrosis factor (TNF), vasopressin, O_2-free radical, interleukin, etc.

Q4. What is MCI?

Ans. Metabolic cardiac injury refers to cardiac dysfunction in response to traumatic injury associated with burn, electric injury, sepsis, and other systemic inflammation and multisystem trauma. It produces decreased myocardial contractility and various conduction disturbances.

SUGGESTED READING

1. Matthews JW Jr, Danny C, Kenneth LM. Traumatic heart disease. In: Libby P, Bonow RO, Mann DL, Zipes DP (Eds). Braunwald's Heart Disease: A Textbook of Cardiovascular Medicine, 8th edition. Philadelphia, PA: Saunders; 2008.

CHAPTER 30

Genetics and Heart Diseases

"Cardiovascular genomics is the advanced frontier of modern CVD management."
—Anonymous

■ INTRODUCTION

Hypertrophic cardiomyopathy is the first inherited cardiovascular (CV) disorder to be successfully genotyped. There is a familial clustering of CV diseases. A family history of premature coronary artery disease leads to a threefold increase in risk of CHD in offsprings. Understanding the mechanisms by which single genes cause CV disease and understanding the genetic susceptibility to common CV diseases and trials of CV gene therapy are emerging matters in CV medicine. With the advancement of molecular genetics, number of diseases resulting from mutations in different genes are increasing.

Q1. What is genetics, genomics, and epigenetics?

Ans. Genes are the region of deoxyribonucleic acid (DNA), which codes for a specific protein. DNA is the functional building block of life and contains four bases: (1) Alanine, (2) tyrosine, (3) guanine, and (4) cytosine. These are packed into 22 pairs of autosomes and two sex chromosomes. The human body is composed of billions of cells (derived from zygote). The nuclei of these cells contain chromosome composed of DNA that codes for proteins. The study of genes is genetics, and the study of all genes together is genomics.

Epigenetics is the phenotypic changes caused by external factors in addition to altered DNA sequences that influence process of gene transcription.

Q2. What are the genetic CV diseases?

Ans. The following CV disorders are solely genetic in origin **(Box 30.1)**:

BOX 30.1: Genetic cardiovascular diseases.

- *Familial hypercholesterolemia (AD) and raised LP(a)*
- *Connective tissue diseases—Marfan syndrome, Ehlers–Danlos syndrome, and Loeys–Dietz syndrome*
- *Cardiomyopathies—HCM, DCM (50% cases), arrhythmogenic RV cardiomyopathy, and LV noncompaction*
- *Arrhythmogenic disorders—Brugada syndrome and long QT syndrome*
- *Valvular diseases—MVP, bicuspid AV, and Noonan's syndrome with PS*
- *Inborn errors of metabolism—hemochromatosis, mucopolysaccharidosis, Gaucher's disease, and L-carnitine deficiency*
- *Chromosomal abnormalities—Down syndrome (MVP and TOF), Turner syndrome (coarctation of aorta), and Edward's syndrome (ASD and VSD)*

Q3. What are the common genetic CV diseases?
Ans. These are hypertrophic cardiomyopathy (most common), Marfan syndrome, familial hypercholesterolemia (FH), dilated cardiomyopathy, long QT syndrome, Brugada syndrome, raised lipoprotein (a) [LP(a)], etc.

Q4. How is familial hypercholesterolemia diagnosed?
Ans. A very high serum low-density lipoprotein-cholesterol (LDL-C) level, early-onset myocardial infarction (MI), and a family history of premature MI suggest FH. An extremely high LDL-C (above 400 mg/dL) and MI result from defects in the LDL receptor genes. A history of premature CHD, family history, presence of tendinous xanthoma **(see Fig. 2.1)**, corneal arcus, very high serum LDL-C, and DNA analysis detecting mutation in LDL receptor, apolipoprotein B (ApoB), or proprotein convertase subtilisin/kexin type 9 (PCSK9) establish the diagnosis.

Q5. What is the pharmacological treatment of FH?
Ans. The pharmacological treatment is as follows:
- Bempedoic acid—inhibitor of adenosine triphosphate (ATP) citrate lyase
- PCSK9 inhibitors, such as alirocumab and evolocumab
- Inclisiran—a small interfering RNA (siRNA) molecule.

Q6. What are the CV manifestations of Marfan syndrome?
Ans. Marfan syndrome is a connective tissue disease inherited as autosomal dominant involving the CV, skeletal, and ocular systems. Classic features are tall stature, arachnodactyly **(Fig. 30.1)**, dolichostenomelia, pectus excavatum, and ectopia lentis. CV manifestations are aortic aneurysm, aortic dissection, MVP, tricuspid valve prolapse, and arrhythmias. Aortic dissection is the most common cause of death.

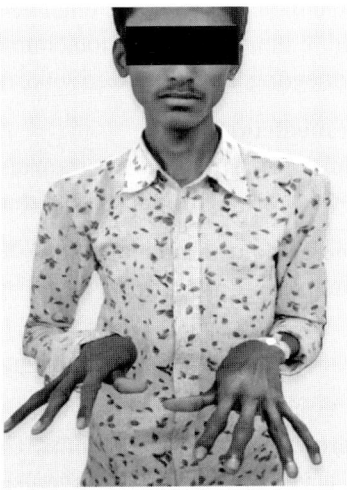

Fig. 30.1: Arachnodactyly in Marfan syndrome.

Q7. What are the magnetic resonance imaging (MRI) features in Marfan syndrome?

Ans. In patients with Marfan syndrome, MRI can detect aortic dissection. It can show the tear of inner aortic wall, and allows visualization of a false lumen, indicating dissection **(Fig. 30.2)**.

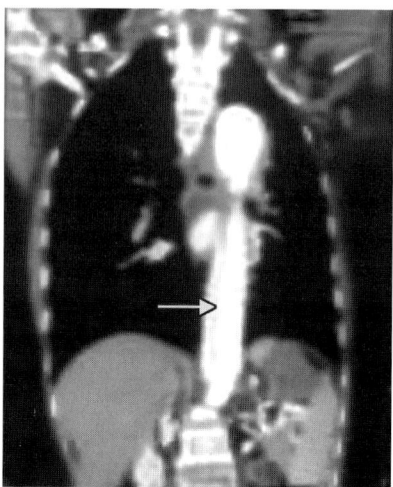

Fig. 30.2: Cardiac MRI showing aortic dissection in the same patient.

Q8. What are genetic engineering and biotechnology?

Ans. Genetic engineering (genetic modification or manipulation) is a specific set of techniques used to alter an organism's genetic makeup. It involves manipulating DNA, RNA, or protein to introduce new traits or characteristics.

Biotechnology uses biological systems, living organisms, or parts of them to create products or technologies. Genetic engineering is a powerful tool within the broader field of biotechnology. Biotechnology is the overarching field, while genetic engineering is a specialized set of techniques within it.

Q9. What is molecular medicine?

Ans. It is the understanding of the molecular basis of disease from the genome and gene regulation to the proteins produced from the genome.

Q10. Enumerate the molecular therapies available for CV diseases.

Ans. The molecular therapies are as follows:
- Gene therapy
- Stem cell therapy

Gene therapy: It is an experimental technique that uses genes to treat or prevent disease by correcting genetic problems. Genome editing is the technique that allows scientists to alter an organism's DNA by addition, removal, or modification of genetic material at specific locations in the genome. CRISPR-Cas9 is a prominent gene editing technology. It can correct faulty genes or introduce protective genes.

Stem cell therapy: It involves transferring cells into a patient to treat or prevent disease; maybe autogenic or allogenic. Stem cells are primitive cells with the possibility of both self-renewal and differentiation. Totipotent (embryonic) stem cells can form any tissue types.

Q11. How is PCSK9 related to CHD?

Ans. Proprotein convertase subtilisin/kexin type 9 mutation causes FH. Thus, a genetically raised level of PCSK9 is a risk factor for CHD. Individuals with loss of function of PCSK9 mutation are genetically protected from CHD without suffering any known adverse effects.

Thus, antibody-based drugs targeting PCSK 9 protein such as alirocumab and evolocumab may reduce risk of CHD. There is a large reduction in blood LDL-C level with these agents. Anti-PCSK9 monoclonal antibodies bind to the LDL receptors and direct it to lysosomal degradation, and are now available for clinical use.

Q12. How is screening done for genetic cardiac diseases?

Ans. After the recognition of a potential genetic cause for a cardiac aliment, a systemic family screening can identify it precisely. Family history and phenotyping patients and their relatives may contribute in characterizing a correlation between genetic and overall risk and outcome.

Q13. What is gene silencing or RNA interference? How is it utilized clinically?

Ans. It is the method to silence, suppress, or reduce the expression of certain genes of interest by genetic engineering techniques. It aims to reduce or eliminate the production of a protein from its corresponding gene. Gene silencing is switching off a gene by a mechanism other than genetic modification. Some gene silencing occurs naturally in utero.

It is done by RNA interference using small interference RNA (siRNA) or microRNA (miRNA). SiRNA binds to messenger RNA (mRNA) to cleave it and make it unavailable to form protein. miRNA binds to the target mRNA transcript and blocks the translation process. It is utilized in making LDL-lowering agent inclisiran, in preparing anticancer agents, and in controlling infectious diseases. The technique is also widely used in the agriculture sector.

■ SUGGESTED READING

1. Farnier M. PCSK9: From discovery to therapeutic applications. Arch Cardiovasc Dis. 2014;107(1):58-66.
2. Li C, Pan Y, Zhang R, Huang Z, Li D, Han Y, et al. Genomic Innovation in Early Life Cardiovascular Disease Prevention and Treatment. Circ Res. 2023;132:1628-47.
3. O'Donnell CJ, Nabel EG. Genomics of cardiovascular disease. N Engl J Med. 2011;365(22):2098-109.

CHAPTER 31

Heart Diseases in the Elderly: Geriatric Cardiology

"The heart never grows better by age; I fear rather worse, always harder."
—Lord Chesterfield

■ INTRODUCTION

There is a marked increase in longevity in Western countries as well as in Bangladesh. The number of people over the age of 65 years is expected to double, and individuals over 75 years are one of the fastest growing segments of the population in our country. Concurrently, with this shift there will be an increased prevalence of geriatric disorders including cognitive dysfunction, mobility limitations, frailty, and auditory and visual impairment. Cardiovascular disease (CVD) being a disease of aging, coronary artery disease (CAD), hypertension, valvular diseases, heart failure (HF), stroke, and arrhythmias become more common with each passing decade. Older adults are likely to develop CVD as a result of pathophysiological changes of aging, even without prior risk factors of CVD. Besides the fundamental biological changes, cumulative effects of lifestyles and comorbidities are causative factors.

Q1. Why is geriatric cardiology necessary?
Ans. Geriatric cardiology is an evolving field. It will continue to advance in coming years as demographics continue to shift towards older patients with CVD. Geriatric cardiologists aim to provide coordinated care with other clinicians including medical and surgical subspecialists, physical therapists, and palliative care specialists, wherever appropriate. It is likely that a group of cardiovascular subspecialists will develop specific expertise in aging-related issues in order to become "geriatric cardiologists".

Q2. What are the special attributes of CVDs in geriatric population?
Ans. An increase in left ventricular (LV) mass, left atrial (LA) size, myocardial deposition, calcium deposition in valvular structures and coronary arteries and stiffness of large elastic arteries due to more collagen deposition, calcification and endothelial dysfunction are documented in geriatric population. As a result of these changes, certain diseases are seen almost exclusively in older adults. These are: Isolated systolic hypertension, calcific aortic stenosis, senile cardiac amyloidosis, etc. Also, a high prevalence of coronary atherosclerosis, atrial fibrillation (AF), and HF is encountered with advancing age.

Q3. What is geriatric syndrome? How is it related to CVD?
Ans. It refers to multifactorial problems of old age that do not fit into classical disease categories. These include frailty, cognitive impairment, delirium, falls, incontinence, and functional decline, etc. The inter-relationship of CVD with geriatric syndrome are as follows:
- CVD is a risk factor for geriatric syndrome. Geriatric syndrome in turn contributes to the new onset or progression of CVD.
- When both coexist, the risk of adverse health outcomes is higher than the risk associated with either condition alone.
- Medications used for one may worsen another or increase the risk of drug-related adverse events.
- Presence of geriatric syndrome is a poor prognostic marker for mortality, functional decline, and lack of treatment benefit in older adults with CVD.

Q4. What are the unique features of various CVDs in older adults?
Ans.
- *Ischemic heart disease (IHD):* Increasing age is the strongest predictor of IHD. The structural and functional changes that occur with increasing age along with the increasing prevalence of most atherosclerotic risk factors and a progressively sedentary lifestyle, all contribute to higher likelihood of developing IHD with increasing age. Furthermore, subclinical, cardiovascular, and other medical diseases are highly prevalent among older patients. As a result, older patients with IHD often present later and with more severe diseases, resulting in substantially higher risk of adverse outcomes. In old age, atherosclerosis is more severe and diffuses with a higher prevalence of left main stenosis, multivessel disease, and impaired LV function. Presentation may be atypical with exertional fatigue and dyspnea, lack of energy, epigastric discomfort, etc. Postprandial and emotional stress symptoms are common. Silent ischemia may occur.

  Acute coronary syndrome (ACS): Although ACS is predominantly a disease of middle-aged males, number of women with ACS increase in old age. Among adults above 75 years, the number of men and women with ACS are similar, and in the population of over 80 years of age, more women are affected than men. Mortality rates are generally higher in older women than men with ACS. Non-ST-segment elevation (NSTE)-ACS is far more prevalent than ST-segment elevation myocardial infarction (STEMI) in the older population. Typical chest pain is less; autonomic symptoms like dyspnea, diaphoresis, nausea and vomiting, syncope, weakness, altered mentation or confusion are more. Early and correct diagnosis is reduced, leading to delay in management. ACS is precipitated more by hemodynamic stressors like infection and dehydration.

- *Heart failure:* Incidence and prevalence rise exponentially with age. Whereas HF is more frequent in men than women at younger age, women

predominate at older age. More than half of older HF patients have HF with preserved ejection fraction (HFpEF).
- *Valvular heart disease:* With aging left heart valves undergo myxomatous degeneration and collagen infiltration. In aortic valves, these lead to aortic sclerosis, calcific aortic stenosis (AS), aortic regurgitation (AR), etc. Mitral annular calcification occurs, particularly in older women. Mitral regurgitation (MR) due to myxomatous degeneration may occur; functional MR may also develop.
- *Cardiac arrhythmias:* Bradyarrhythmia due to sinus node dysfunction and AV block increases with age. Less than 10% of pacemaker cells are functional by the age of 75 years. Medications (e.g., betablockers for IHD) may increase incidence of bradyarrhythmia. AF occurs in about 12% of patients of age 75 years or older. It depends on age-related changes in atrial tissue, hypertension, and structural heart disease common in older age.
- *Venous thromboembolism (VTE):* Deep vein thrombosis (DVT) and pulmonary embolism increase with advancing age; hypercoagulability, decreased mobility, and laxity of large venous valves contribute.
- *Syncope:* Prevalence increases with age
- *Peripheral arterial disease (PAD):* Abdominal aortic aneurysm, aortic dissection, and lower extremity PAD increase in incidence with aging.
- *Cerebrovascular disease and stroke:* Older patients have increased mortality and morbidity, increased hemorrhagic transformation, reduced neurologic recovery, and are more susceptible to iatrogenic effects of stroke therapy.

Q5. What are the complications of acute myocardial infarction (AMI) in old age?
Ans. Acute myocardial infarction in older adults is attended with more mechanical as well as electrical complications. These are related to pathophysiological changes of aging, greater severity of CAD and LV dysfunction at diagnosis, comorbidities, and frailty. Aging is also associated with diminished collateral circulation and lower number and lesser function of endothelial progenitor cells to facilitate myocardial recovery after myocardial infarction (MI).

Q6. How does AS in old age differ from that in younger patients?
Ans.
- Symptoms may not be as prominent in elderly with sedentary lifestyles, resulting in delayed presentation or incidental diagnosis of severe AS at time of presentation for other medical problems.
- Older individuals with severe AS are less likely to exhibit delayed upstroke of carotid pulse wave (pulsus parvus et tardus) as a result of increased arterial stiffness.

- As older patients are more likely to have LV dysfunction, the prevalence of low flow, low gradient AS producing "pseudo" severe AS increases with age.
- Paradoxical low flow, low gradient AS with normal systolic function is more common in older individuals and produces a similar pseudo severe AS.

Assessing the response to dobutamine infusion may be helpful in distinguishing severe AS from such pseudo severe AS, i.e., low calculated aortic valve area in absence of severe obstruction to flow.

Q7. What are the interventional treatments for older patients with AS?
Ans.
- Surgical aortic valve replacement (SAVR)
- Transcatheter aortic valve replacement (TAVR)—for elderly, frail AS patients who are not considered suitable candidates for SAVR. It is also indicated for intermediate- and high-risk older patients, or inoperable patients with severe AS. TAVR showed comparable or superior benefit compared to medical or surgical therapy.

Q8. What perioperative CV management are advised for older adults?
Ans.
- *Hypertension:* Treat very high blood pressure (BP) (>180/110 mm Hg); avoid aggressive lowering that may increase risk of intraoperative hypotension.
- *Myocardial infarction:* Pain may be masked by narcotics; ST elevation warrants biomarker estimation. Management is similar to that for nonsurgical patients.
- *Arrhythmia:* It may be due to infection, hypotension, hypokalemia or hypomagnesemia, hypothermia, pulmonary embolism, ischemia, hypoxemia, and pain. AF is the most common arrhythmia. Heart rate (HR) control and unfractionated heparin (UH) or low-molecular-weight heparin (LMWH) are used.
- *Heart failure:* It may occur with fluid overload on reduced cardiac reserve of aging. Management includes early ambulation, compression stockings, or boots and anticoagulation.
- *Deep vein thrombosis:* Venous stasis, hypercoagulable state, and high-risk orthopedic, and pelvic operations increase the risk.

Q9. How are perioperative medications advocated for older adults?
Ans.
- *Drugs to be discontinued:* Aspirin, nonsteroidal anti-inflammatory drugs (NSAIDs) 5-7 days before surgery to decrease bleeding, anticoagulants 1-4 days before surgery, diuretics to be held for 24 hours, hypoglycemic to be held.

- *Drugs to be continued:* CV and antihypertensives, insulin in half dose, steroid in stress dose, betablockers started several days before and continued for at least one month following surgery (HR goal: 55–60 beats/min)
- *Drugs to be avoided:* Prophylactic nitroglycerine

Q10. Compare HF in old age with that in young.
Ans. Incidence of HF increases with increasing age. Older patients with HF differ from that in younger in some respects as listed in **Table 31.1**.

TABLE 31.1: Heart failure (HF) in older and younger patients—difference.

Characteristics	Older	Younger
Prevalence	More	Less
Gender	F > M	M > F
Type of HF	HFpEF more	HFrEF more
Etiology	HTN more	CAD more
Comorbidities	Multiple	Few

(CAD: coronary artery disease; F: female; HTN: hypertension; M: male; HFpEF: heart failure with preserved ejection fraction; HFrEF: heart failure with reduced ejection fraction)

Q11. How to provide palliative care?
Ans. Palliative care is a holistic approach for patients facing a life-threatening illness. It focuses on symptomatic standard care as well as psychosocial and spiritual care. In some respects, geriatric cardiology and palliative care overlap. Palliative care improves overall survival time. For example, for an older, frail patient TAVR may mitigate symptoms and increase survival, which initially seems to be an end-stage disease. Hospice care is given to patients with an expected survival rate of <6 months, and who have agreed to forgo more aggressive treatment.

Geriatric cardiologists can play a role in making end-of-life decisions including decision regarding resuscitation. Genoscience is an emerging field that aims to understand the relationship between aging and age-related diseases to prevent it.

■ SUGGESTED READING

1. Bell SP, Orr NM, Dodson JA, Rich MW, Wenger NK, Blum K, et al. What to Expect From the Evolving Field of Geriatric Cardiology. J Am Coll Cardiol. 2015;66(11):1286-99.
2. Forman DE, Rich MW, Alexander KP, Zieman S, Maurer MS, Najjar SS, et al. Cardiac care for older adults. Time for a new paradigm. J Am Coll Cardiol. 2011;57(18):1801-10.

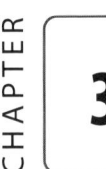

32 Heart Diseases in Women

"Because women don't expect to have heart disease, a lot of times they don't seek help if they have the early symptoms of a heart attack."
—Laura Bush

■ INTRODUCTION

Cardiovascular disease (CVD) is the leading cause of death in women as in men. However, women receive less recognition and treatment than men, as the female pattern of ischemic heart disease (IHD) is characterized by lower obstructive coronary artery disease (CAD). About one third of women over the age of 65 years will have some form of CVD. There are both biological and sociocultural differences in CVD in women. These result in a difference in pathophysiologic mechanisms, risk factors, presentation, diagnosis, and management of CVD among women. Women with IHD differ from men in terms of epidemiology, diagnostic test accuracy, and treatment. The female pattern IHD is characterized by lower obstructive CAD and preserved left ventricular ejection fraction (LVEF). Special attributes of CAD in women are discussed. Other heart diseases in women are discussed in respective chapters.

Q1. What are the characteristics of coronary heart disease (CHD) in women?
Ans.
- Coronary arteries are smaller than those in men, but myocardial perfusion is higher in women. Average endothelial shear stress is higher that inhibits atheroma formation.
- Atherosclerosis is diffuse in epicardial coronary arteries.
- Long "latent" period of developing diffuse coronary atherosclerosis
- Microvascular dysfunction is more. Chest pain may be atypical; angina equivalent may be more prevalent.
- The acute coronary syndrome (ACS) presentation is delayed or late and is associated with high mortality.
- Inaccurate diagnostic test results including electrocardiogram (ECG) may show nonspecific ST-T changes; exercise tolerance test (ETT) results may be false positive; coronary angiography (CAG) may be normal after an attack of myocardial infarction (MI), and the entity called myocardial infarction with nonobstructive coronary arteries (MINOCA).
- Response to medical treatment and invasive procedures differs.

Q2. What is the implication of a "normal" coronary in women with ACS?
Ans. In the setting of an ACS, "normal" coronary arteries do not have a benign prognosis. Despite less obstructive CAD, women have a poorer prognosis after ACS, particularly in younger women.

Q3. What are the risk factors for CVD in women?
Ans.
- *Age:* Lags at least 10 years compared with men; increase after the age of 60 years, with one in three women having evidence of CHD after the age of 65 years.
- *Family history:* More potent than in men
- *Hypertension (HTN):* Have a higher overall prevalence compared with men, especially after the age of 60 years. HTN rises two to threefold in women taking oral contraceptives. The risk of congestive heart failure (CHF) and stroke is more in women related to their greater life expectancy.
- *Diabetes mellitus (DM):* Risk is greater in women; also risk of fatal CHD is 3.5 times that in nondiabetic women and is higher than in diabetic men.
- *Dyslipidemia:* High-density lipoprotein cholesterol (HDL-C) is around 10 mg/dL higher than in men throughout their lives. Adverse changes in lipid profile accompany menopause and include increased levels of total cholesterol, low-density lipoprotein cholesterol (LDL-C), and triglycerides (TG), and decreased HDL-C.
- *Smoking:* More detrimental in women than men. Female smokers die 14.5 years earlier than nonsmoker women. The use of oral contraceptives and smoking imparts an even greater risk of MI.
- *Sedentary behavior:* More common in women; inactivity increases with age, physical inactivity is associated with higher blood pressure (BP), poor glucose metabolism, worse cholesterol levels, obesity, and poor mental health.
- *Metabolic syndrome and obesity:* More prevalent
- *Nontraditional risk factors:* Depression, menopause, polycystic ovary syndrome (PCOS), pregnancy-induced conditions like gestational HTN, gestational diabetes, etc.

Q4. What is MINOCA?
Ans. Myocardial infarction without obstructive CAD is referred to as MI with non-obstructive coronary arteries (MINOCA). It is more frequent in women, particularly younger women. All traditional risk factors, except dyslipidemia, are frequently present. Factors contributing to MINOCA are coronary microvascular disease, myocarditis, coronary vasospasm, takotsubo cardiomyopathy, hypertrophic cardiomyopathy (HCM), and spontaneous coronary artery dissection (SCAD). All-cause mortality appears to be lower in MINOCA. Diagnosis requires additional investigations and imaging to determine the cause.

Q5. What is ischemia with nonobstructive coronary arteries (INOCA)?

Ans. The Women's Ischemia Syndrome Evaluation (WISE) study showed that 57% of women with ischemic symptoms had no obstructive CAD by CAG. Majority of them continue to have symptoms and signs of myocardial ischemia and undergo repeated hospitalizations and angiographic evaluation. They have higher mortality when compared with asymptomatic women. Thus, the prognosis in women with INOCA is not benign.

Women with microvascular angina (formerly called "cardiac syndrome X") also have nonobstructive CAD resulting from microvascular coronary reactivity and dysfunction occurring in the setting of underlying atheroma. This is also more prevalent in women, possibly because of risk factor clustering and hormonal alterations. It is associated with atypical symptoms and adverse outcomes in women.

Q6. Ischemic heart disease or CAD—which terminology is more appropriate for women?

Ans. Women have less anatomical obstructive CAD and relatively more preserved left ventricular (LV) function. Adverse coronary reactivity, microvascular dysfunction, and distal microembolization from plaque may contribute. Thus, the term IHD is more useful than CAD for women.

Q7. What is Yentl syndrome?

Ans. It is the different course of action that MI usually follows for women than men. Yentl was the heroine of Issac B. Singer's short story in the 19th century who had to disguise herself as a man in order to receive the education she desired. The phrase was coined in an academic paper in the year 1991 by Dr Bernadine Healy titled "The Yentl Syndrome" (published in N Engl J Med). Most of the medical research has focused primarily on MI in men and MI in women is often misdiagnosed as their symptoms present differently. Decades of sex-exclusive research have reinforced the myth that CHD is a disease of men. As CHD afflicts older people, at a time in life, men and women are affected with equal frequency. Moreover, women live longer than men, by as much as 7 years on average. Major commitment is to conduct research on women's health and illness needed and make women's health a priority, not just in the interest of women but for the well-being of the people in general. It is expected that Yentl syndrome will slip back into history, but the bold, charming heroine Yentl will survive.

Q8. What is Variation in Recovery: Role of Gender on Outcome of young AMI patients (VIRGO) classification system in MI patients?

Ans. The VIRGO study researchers showed that one in eight young women (<55 years) presenting with acute MI (AMI) fall in an unclassified category when using the current established classification system for AMI. So, they proposed a new classification system for AMI **(Table 32.1)**.

TABLE 32.1: VIRGO classification for young MI.

Class	
Class I	Plaque mediated culprit lesion—with obstruction (or near obstruction) of a major epicardial vessel
Class IIa	Obstructive CAD with evidence for supply-demand mismatch. Epicardial vessel stenosis >50% but no culprit lesion identified; an additional insult implicated
Class IIb	Obstructive CAD (stenosis >50%); no evidence for supply-demand mismatch
Class IIIa	Nonobstructive CAD (stenosis <50%); no culprit lesion with evidence of supply-demand mismatch; an additional insult implicated
Class IIIb	Nonobstructive CAD; no culprit lesion; no supply-demand mismatch
Class IV	Nonatherosclerotic pathophysiologic mechanism, including vasospasm, dissection, and embolism
Class V	Indeterminate; presentation fits into two or more of the above classes

(AMI: acute myocardial infarction; CAD: coronary artery disease; MI: myocardial infarction; VIRGO: Variation in Recovery: Role of Gender on Outcome of young AMI patients)

Q9. What is SCAD?

Ans. The SCAD is a sudden separation of coronary artery layers creating an intimal flap, intraluminal hematoma that obstructs coronary flow resulting in AMI. It is a rare cause of AMI in women during the peripartum period. Left anterior descending (LAD) artery dissection is more common. It is diagnosed with computed tomography (CT) angiography or magnetic resonance imaging (MRI). The typical presentation is a sudden onset of ACS in young healthy women without traditional atherosclerotic cardiovascular disease (ASCVD) risk factors.

Q10. How is risk stratification for IHD done in women?

Ans. The IHD risk classification in women is done as follows:
- *Low risk:* Premenopausal women with symptoms
- *Low to intermediate risk:* Symptomatic women in the fifth decade and capable of performing routine activities of daily living (ADLs)
- *Intermediate risk:* If the performance of ADLs compromised; also women in their 60s
- *High risk:* Women 70 years of age and older

Q11. How to investigate IHD in women?

Ans.
- Women at low IHD risk are not candidates for a diagnostic evaluation. Starting at puberty, women have higher resting heart rates compared with men.

- In low-intermediate or intermediate risk cases, an exercise ECG if she has a functional capacity estimate of five metabolic equivalent of tasks (METs) or higher.
- Women at intermediate-high IHD risk with an abnormal 12-lead ECG—noninvasive imaging including echocardiography, cardiac magnetic resonance (CMR), or coronary computed tomography angiography (CCTA).
- Women with high IHD risk with stable symptom—functional assessment of ischemic burden and guidance for post-test anti-ischemic therapy done by stress imaging, e.g., myocardial perfusion imaging (MPI), stress echo, etc.

Q12. What is the importance of ETT in women?

Ans. The American Heart Association (AHA) consensus statement emphasizes the usefulness of ETT as the initial test of choice for women with a normal ECG who are able to exercise. Although it has been considered less useful in women because of a high false-positive test result, a negative ETT has a significant diagnostic value. The negative predictive value of ST segment depression in symptomatic women is similar to that in men. A woman with a negative ETT and normal exercise abilities has an excellent event-free survival rate and a low risk of obstructive CAD. A markedly abnormal ETT with ≥2 mm ST depression, in particular occurring at low workload (<5 METS) or persisting for >5 minutes into recovery, is associated with a high likelihood of obstructive CAD for both women and men. The WOMEN (What is the Optimal Method for Ischemia Evaluation in Women) trial showed that the prognostic value of ETT is no different than an exercise MPI test. It also reduces radiation exposure.

Q13. What are the characteristic features of percutaneous coronary intervention (PCI) in women?

Ans. Although sex difference in procedural and clinical success is narrow, the number of women receiving PCI is much less compared to men. The following features are observed among women:
- They tend to be older with more comorbidities.
- They have more high-risk characteristics, such as older age, DM, HTN, heart failure (HF), dyslipidemia, and unstable angina (UA).
- More bleeding risk, transfusion requirements, and more vascular complications (reduced by using a radial route)
- More residual angina, more 1-year mortality following PCI compared with men

Q14. How to prevent CHD in women?

Ans. The INTERHEART study has shown that conventional CVD risk factors are similar in men and women, but the impact of preventive measures is greater in women. Women often receive less intensive medical therapy or lifestyle counseling and less revascularization, which influences the outcome adversely.

Primary and secondary preventive measures advocated are as follows:
- No smoking
- Weight reduction/maintenance
- Regular exercise
  Control high BP; optimal BP <120/80 mm Hg
- Reduce high cholesterol; optimal LDL <100 mg/dL, HDL >50 mm Hg, TG <150 mg/dL
- Control blood sugar

SUGGESTED READING

1. Enas EA, Senthilkumar A, Juturu V, Gupta R. Coronary artery disease in women. Indian Heart J. 2001;53(3):282-92.
2. Herz CN. The Yentl syndrome is alive and well. Eur Heart J. 2011;32:1313-5.
3. Spartz ES, Curry LA, Masudi FA, Zhou S, Strait KM, Gross CP, et al. The variation in recovery: role of gender on outcome of young AMI patients(VIRGO) classification system: a taxonomy for young women with acute myocardial infarction. Circulation. 2015;132:1710-8.

CHAPTER 33

Systemic Diseases Involving the Heart

"The heart nourishes and charishes all other systems of the body and their diseases may affect the heart in turn."

—Anonymous

■ INTRODUCTION

Diseases affecting multiple organ systems may also impact the cardiovascular system. This chapter aims to familiarize the readers with the clinical features of systemic diseases that affect the heart and blood vessels.

Q1. What are the common systemic diseases involving the heart?

Ans. Many systemic diseases affect the heart. Some are minor, but some others are life-threatening manifestations **(Table 33.1)**.

TABLE 33.1: Systemic disease involving the heart.

Systemic disease	Cardiac manifestations
Hyperthyroidism	Palpitation, AF, SVT, and systolic hypertension
Hypothyroidism	Bradycardia, hypotension, PE, DCM, and CHF
Acromegaly	HF (systolic and diastolic)
Pheochromocytoma	Hypertension, palpitation, and CHF
Carcinoid	Tricuspid and pulmonary valve disease and RHF
SLE	Pericarditis, Libman-Sacks endocarditis, myocarditis, and arterial and venous thrombosis
Rheumatoid arthritis	Pericarditis, PE, myocarditis, valvulitis, and coronary arteritis
Systemic sclerosis	PE, CHF, myocarditis, microvascular angina, and tachyarrhythmia
Ankylosing spondylitis and other sero negative arthritis	Aortitis, AR, MR, and conduction abnormalities
Ehler–Danlos syndrome	Aortic and coronary aneurysm, MVP, and TV prolapse
Marfan syndrome	Aortic aneurysm and dissection, AR, and MVP
Amyloidosis	CHF, restrictive CM, valvular regurgitation, and PE
Sarcoidosis	CHF, CM (dilated or restrictive), ventricular arrhythmia, and heart block
Hemochromatosis	CHF, arrhythmia, and heart block

Contd...

Contd...

Systemic disease	Cardiac manifestations
Tuberculosis	Pericarditis, pericardial effusion, and myocarditis (rare)
COVID-19	Acute cardiac injury, ACS, myocarditis, TCM, HF, and arrhythmia
HIV	Myocarditis, DCM, and PE

(ACS: acute coronary syndrome; AF: atrial fibrillation; AR: aortic regurgitation; CHF: congestive heart failure; CM: cardiomyopathy; COVID-19: coronavirus disease 2019; DCM: dilated cardiomyopathy; HF: heart failure; HIV: human immunodeficiency virus; MR: mitral regurgitation; MVP: mitral valve prolapse; PE: pulmonary embolism; RHF: right heart failure; SLE: systemic lupus erythematosus; TCM: Takotsubo cardiomyopathy; TV: tricuspid valve)

Q2. How to manage atrial fibrillation (AF) in hyperthyroid patients?
Ans.
- Atrial fibrillation may be the first symptom of thyroid hormone excess in the elderly.
- Treatment of hyperthyroidism with beta-blockers followed by antithyroid drugs or radioiodine should be the first-line therapy in patients with overt hyperthyroidism and AF to obtain conversion to sinus rhythm and to improve hemodynamics.
- Patients usually require a higher dose of digitalis in hyperthyroidism because of the decreased vagal tone, increased rate of clearance, and decreased drug sensitivity due to the high level of sodium-potassium adenosine triphosphatase (Na^+, K^+-ATPase).
- In younger patients with hyperthyroidism with AF in the absence of other heart disease, hypertension, or other independent risk factors for thromboembolism (CHAD VASC score = 0), the benefit of anticoagulation is not established.
- Hyperthyroid patients who do not regain sinus rhythm spontaneously within 4 months of normalization of thyroid function, pharmacologic, or electrical cardioversion should be considered after evaluation of the age of the patient and underlying cardiac status. Many such patients need anticoagulants.

Q3. How to treat hypothyroidism in patients with known or suspected coronary artery disease (CAD)?
Ans.
- In case of stable ischemic heart disease patients in whom revascularization is not indicated, treatment with low-dose levothyroxine (12.5 µg/day) started with stepwise increment (12.5–25 µg/day) every 6–8 weeks until the serum thyroid-stimulating hormone (TSH) level normalizes.

The ability of thyroxin to decrease afterload and improve myocardial efficacy can decrease signs of myocardial ischemia.
- In patients potentially at risk for CAD but without any signs or symptoms, thyroid hormone replacement can be started at a low dose (25–50 µg) and then increased by 25 µg/day every 6–8 weeks until the serum TSH level normalizes. If signs or symptoms of ischemic heart disease (IHD) develop, the same recommendations as for patients with known IHD apply here.
- If patients are not candidates for percutaneous coronary intervention (PCI) and have unstable angina, left main (LM) disease, or TVD with impaired left ventricular (LV) function, even in the setting of overt hypothyroidism, CABG can be performed. Thyroid hormone replacement can be delayed until the postoperative period, when it can be administered in full doses parentally or orally.
- Patients younger than 50 years with no history of IHD tolerate full replacement dose of thyroxin (1.5 µg/kg/day without untoward cardiac side effect).

Q4. What are the cardiovascular manifestations of coronavirus disease 2019 (COVID-19)?

Ans. Severe acute respiratory syndrome coronavirus-2 (SARS-CoV2) causes COVID-19, which has become a pandemic affecting every country of the world. Cardiac involvement appears to be a prominent feature of the disease occurring in 20–30% of hospitalized patients and is an important cause of mortality. Cardiovascular manifestations of COVID-19 are as follows:
- *Acute cardiac injury:* Most common, incidence 8–12%, and elevation of troponin I above 99th percentile of the upper reference limit
- *Acute coronary syndrome (ACS):* Type II myocardial infarction (MI); uncommonly Type I
- Myocarditis and myopericarditis
- *Heart failure (HF):* Manifestation of myocarditis, acute cardiac injury, and myocarditis
- *Arrhythmias:* Both tachy- and bradyarrhythmia

Q5. What are the commonly elevated biomarkers in COVID-19? How to interpret elevated troponin I?

Ans. Commonly elevated biomarkers are troponin I, natriuretic peptide (NT pro-BNP/BNP), D-dimer, ferritin, interleukin-6 (IL-6), and lactate dehydrogenase (LDH).

The most documented biomarker is troponin I.
- A mildly elevated troponin I below the 99th percentile carries a good prognosis.
- A progressively elevated troponin I carries a worse prognosis.

- An elevated troponin I, along with the rise of other biomarkers, indicates cytokine storm, myocarditis, or ACS.

Q6. How does COVID-19 interact with heart diseases?
Ans. Although the lung is the primary target for the SARS-CoV-2 virus, the heart may also be involved. It binds to the angiotensin-converting enzyme 2 (ACE2) receptor, which is abundant in the lung and heart. Severe COVID-19 is a systemic illness characterized by a hyperinflammatory response and cytokine storm. Preexisting heart disease and its risk factors increase vulnerability to COVID-19. Conversely, COVID-19 can worsen underlying heart disease and even precipitate new cardiac malfunction.

Q7. How does HF occur in COVID-19?
Ans. Recognition of signs and symptoms of HF in patients with COVID-19 pneumonia is a challenging clinical scenario. One may mask the other, and HF may be exaggerated by COVID-19.

Both left and right HF may occur, although left HF is uncommon.
- *Left HF:* Acute cardiac injury, ACS, and myocarditis may cause myocardial dysfunction and features of acute left HF.
- *Right HF:* Venous thromboembolism (VTE) occurs in 20–30% of severe COVID-19 cases that may lead to pulmonary thromboembolism. Also, inflammatory damage incurred by the virus causes pulmonary endothelial damage and formation of microthrombi. D-dimer splits into blood as a result of fibrinolysis. These together lead to the development of pulmonary hypertension and right HF.

Q8. How does COVID-19 mimic heart diseases?
Ans.
- The COVID-19 patients present with respiratory distress, which is also a presenting symptom of heart disease, especially acute left ventricular failure (LVF).
- Chest pain of myopericarditis or pneumonic involvement in COVID-19 may mimic ischemic pain.
- Right HF in pulmonary hypertension resulting from pulmonary thromboembolism mimics congestive heart failure (CHF).
- Electrocardiogram (ECG) findings of ST elevation in Takotsubo syndrome of COVID-19 mimic ST-elevation myocardial infarction (STEMI).
- A raised troponin due to acute cardiac injury or myocarditis in COVID-19 mimics ACS.
- Radiological findings of ground glass pulmonary opacity in COVID-19 may mimic pulmonary edema of acute LVF. Opacities in COVID-19 are mostly peripheral, whereas these are mostly perihilar in acute LVF.

Q9. What is the differential diagnosis of ST elevation in a COVID-19 patient?
Ans.
- The ST elevated MI—type II, sometimes type I
- Takotsubo cardiomyopathy
- Pericarditis or myopericarditis

Q10. Compare and contrast the respiratory distress of acute LVF and COVID-19 pneumonia.
Ans. Both conditions produce respiratory distress as their main feature. The two may be differentiated clinically **(Table 33.2)**.

TABLE 33.2: Respiratory distress in LVF and COVID-19 pneumonia—difference.

Points	Acute LVF	COVID-19 pneumonia
Background	Underlying heart disease	Systemic viral illness during the pandemic
Cough	Productive of pinkish frothy sputum	Mostly dry cough
Wheeze	May be present	More
Decubitus	The propped-up position gives relief	Awake prone position gives relief

(COVID-19: coronavirus disease 2019; LVF: left ventricular failure)

Q11. Why is anticoagulation recommended in COVID-19 patients?
Ans. In COVID-19, there is pulmonary vascular thromboembolic formation with increased dead space ventilation. Autopsy studies also demonstrated VTE in deceased patients. Early anticoagulation may prevent the propagation of microthrombi at presentation and thus decrease mortality.

In acutely hospitalized patients, heparin should be started. Heparin binds tightly to COVID-19 spike proteins. It also downregulates IL-6 and dampens the immune activation. Directly acting oral anticoagulants (DOACs) do not appear to have these anti-inflammatory properties. However, these are recommended after the acute stage is over.

Q12. How to use anticoagulants in COVID-19 patients with heart disease?
Ans. Thromboembolism prevention and treatment guidelines for COVID-19 patients include:
- In the absence of contraindications, all acutely hospitalized patients with COVID-19 should receive thromboprophylaxis therapy. D-dimers, prothrombin time, and platelet count should be measured in hospitalized patients. The possibility of thromboembolism should be evaluated when rapid deterioration of pulmonary, cardiac, or neurological function occurs.

- Low-molecular-weight heparin (LMWH) or fondaparinux should be used for thromboprophylaxis over unfractionated heparin (UH) and DOACs, e.g., rivaroxaban.
- COVID-19 patients should receive prophylaxis with anticoagulants for at least 6 weeks in high-risk patients as recommended by the International Society on Thrombosis and Haemostasis.
- Patients on anticoagulant or antiplatelet therapies for underlying conditions should continue these medications if a diagnosis of COVID-19 is made.

SUGGESTED READING

1. Das PK, Rahman F. Heart disease and COVID-19. Univ Heart J. 2020;31(2):1-156.
2. Hendren NS, Drazner MH, Bozkurt B, Cooper Jr LT. Description and proposed management of the acute COVID-19 cardiovascular syndrome. Circulation. 2020;141(23):1903-14.
3. Remick J, Georgiopoulou V, Marti C, Ofotokun I, Kalogeropoulos A, Lewis W, et al. Heart failure in patients with human immunodeficiency virus infection: epidemiology, pathophysiology, treatment and future research. Circulation. 2014;129(17):1781-9.

CHAPTER 34

Heart Diseases in South Asians

"While the burden of CVD is on the decline globally, it is on the rise among South Asians."
—Current Atherosclerosis Rep. 2018

■ INTRODUCTION

South Asians have demonstrated a higher burden of premature coronary artery disease (CAD) compared with other ethnicities. This has been found among both immigrant South Asians and nonimmigrants. South Asians have some unique features in their heart diseases, especially CAD. Ethnicity as well as environmental factors resulting from nutritional transition are involved. Although epidemiological data are insufficient, various aspects of heart diseases in South Asians are discussed here with data obtained from research conducted in India, Bangladesh, and other South Asian countries.

Q1. What are the cardinal features of CAD in South Asians?
Ans. South Asian populations demonstrate some unique features regarding the prevalence and mode of occurrence of CAD **(Box 34.1)**.

> **BOX 34.1:** Cardinal features of CAD among South Asians.
>
> - Premature atherosclerosis and CAD—onset of first MI occurs 5–10 years earlier compared with other populations. More young people develop MI here; the incidence of MI among people <40 years of age is 5–10-fold higher here
> - The incidence of CAD and its mortality is 2–4-fold higher
> - Greater severity—more triple vessel disease, larger MI with more complications
> - Higher prevalence of emerging risk factors—lipoprotein(a), low HDL, small dense LDL, homocysteine, triglycerides, fibrinogen, and PAI-1
> - Lower prevalence of conventional risk factors, except DM
> - Higher prevalence of insulin resistance—DM and metabolic syndrome
> - Higher CAD rates at a given level of conventional risk factors
> - Higher proportion of vulnerable plaques; clinical events are higher for a given degree of atherosclerosis
>
> (CAD: coronary artery disease; DM: diabetes mellitus; HDL: high-density lipoprotein; LDL: high-density lipoprotein; MI: myocardial infarction; PAI-1: plasminogen activator inhibitor-1)

Q2. What are the factors contributing to increasing CAD in South Asian countries?
Ans. Various sociodemographic and lifestyle factors are responsible for the increasing CAD **(Box 34.2)**.

BOX 34.2: Increasing CAD in South Asian countries—factors contributing.

- Urbanization of rural areas and large-scale migration of the rural population to urban areas
- Increased sedentary lifestyle
- Increased obesity, particularly abdominal
- Nutritional transition increased the use of atherogenic diets, including fried food, processed food, and fast food that are high in calories, saturated fat, and trans-fat. Also, there is an increased consumption of food with a high glycemic index and inadequate consumption of fruits, vegetables, and fibers
- Tobacco abuse
- Poor awareness and control of CAD risk factors, such as hypertension, diabetes, and dyslipidemia

(CAD: coronary artery disease)

Q3. What are the desirable levels of various CAD risk factors among South Asians?

Ans. Since the risk of development of CAD in people of South Asia is double for any level of risk factor compared with the Western population, lower desirable levels are suggested for these people **(Table 34.1)**.

TABLE 34.1: Goal of CAD risk factors—desirable for South Asians.

Risk factor	Desirable levels
Total cholesterol	<160 mg/dL
LDL-cholesterol	<100 mg/dL (<70 for CAD and DM)
Triglyceride	<150 mg/dL
HDL-cholesterol	>40 mg/dL (men); >50 mg/dL (women)
Non-HDL-cholesterol	>130 mg/dL (<100 mg/dL for CAD and DM)
Lipoprotein(a)	<20 mg/dL
Blood pressure	<130/80 mm Hg (<120/80 mm Hg for DM and HF)
Hemoglobin A1c	<6.5%
Waist circumference	<90 cm (men); <80 cm (women)
BMI	<23 (men and women)

(BMI: body mass index; CAD: coronary artery disease; DM: diabetes mellitus; HDL: high-density lipoprotein; HF: heart failure; LDL: low-density lipoprotein)

Q4. What are the CAD risk levels for South Asians?

Ans. According to the Indo-US Healthcare Summit recommendation, three risk levels for South Asians are listed in **Table 34.2**.

TABLE 34.2: CAD risk levels for South Asians.

Risk status	Criteria
High risk	- Established CAD - Cerebrovascular disease - Peripheral arterial disease - Abdominal aortic aneurysm - End-stage or chronic renal disease - DM - Metabolic syndrome - 10-year Framingham global risk ≥10%
At risk	- One major CAD risk factor includes cigarette smoking, poor diet, physical inactivity, central obesity, F/H of premature CVD (<55 years in males, <65 years in females, hypertension, and dyslipidemia) - Evidence of subclinical vascular disease, e.g., coronary calcification - Poor exercise capacity on TMT and/or - Abnormal heart rate recovery after stopping exercise
Optimal risk	- A healthy lifestyle, with no risk factors (Framingham global risk <5%) - Control of blood glucose, diabetes, and metabolic syndrome through intense lifestyle modification and medications if necessary - Complete smoking cessation (cigarette smoking, beedis, and chewing tobacco)

(CAD: coronary artery disease; CVD: cardiovascular disease; DM: diabetes mellitus; F/H: family history; TMT: treadmill test)

Q5. What are the unique risk factors of CAD in South Asians?
Ans.
- Smoking and tobacco use—alarming
- Type 2 diabetes mellitus (DM) and insulin resistance
- *Hypertension:* Liberal use of salt aggravates it
- *Lipid abnormalities:* The most common pattern seen is borderline elevated low-density lipoprotein (LDL), low high-density lipoprotein (HDL), high triglyceride (TG), high lipoprotein(a) LP(a), high apolipoprotein B (apo-B), and low apolipoprotein A1 (apo-A1)
- Abdominal obesity and ectopic fat deposition
- Sedentariness and lack of physical exercise
- Inadequate consumption of fruit and vegetables

Q6. What are the special features of rheumatic heart disease (RHD) in South Asians?
Ans. In South Asians, RHD has a malignant course with an accelerated natural history. The following features are noticeable:
- More young patients are afflicted here.

- The initial attack of rheumatic fever (RF) occurs at a younger age.
- The interval between the initial attack of RF and the onset of symptomatic RHD is shorter—as short as 2 years.
- Pulmonary hypertension develops rapidly.

Q7. What are the unique features of obesity in South Asians? How is it related to CAD?
Ans. South Asians have:
- More central deposition of fat and a tendency to abdominal obesity; these fats are metabolically more active
- More visceral fat deposition
- More ectopic fat deposition, fatty liver, etc.

Also, lower cutoff values for body mass index (BMI) and waist circumference defining overweight and obesity are recommended for South Asians (Table 34.3):

TABLE 34.3: Revised cutoffs of BMI defining overweight and obesity for South Asians

Parameter	Optimum	Overweight	Obese
BMI	<23 kg/m²	23–25 kg/m²	>25 kg/m²
WC (optimum): <90 cm (men), <80 cm (women)			

(BMI: body mass index; WC: waist circumference)

Q8. What weight management is appropriate for South Asians?
Ans. Achievement and maintenance of a healthy weight and waist size by balancing caloric intake and expenditure is recommended. Here, the specific BMI cutpoint for overweight is >23 kg/m², and for obesity is >25 kg/m², which are lower than that for the Western population. Also, the waist circumference cutpoint for males is >90 cm and for females is >80 cm (10 cm lower than that for the Western population).

Q9. How to prevent CAD in South Asians?
Ans. Primordial prevention (population-based)—prevention of the development of risk factors, such as high cholesterol, high blood pressure (BP), tobacco use, obesity, and DM, through healthy lifestyle changes.
- Primary prevention (also called high-risk, individual-based prevention): It aims at identifying individuals with markedly elevated risk factors (conventional and emerging) who have not yet suffered a coronary event and targeting them for interventions. Maximum lifestyle changes, as in primordial prevention, as well as drug therapy, are used.
- Secondary prevention—prevention of mortality and morbidity among those having myocardial infarction (MI) or other forms of CAD, by aggressive medical treatment

- Bangladesh needs a balanced combination of population-based and high-risk, individual-based strategies for effective control of CAD. An enlightened public health policy, a trained medical professional, and a motivated public are needed for it.

Q10. What secondary prevention of CAD should ideally be undertaken for South Asians?

Ans. Here, secondary prevention measures need to be aggressively implemented with optimal use of cardiac rehabilitation and medications.

- *Aspirin and clopidogrel*
  - Aspirin 75–150 mg/day started and continued indefinitely in all patients unless contraindicated.
  - Clopidogrel 75 mg/day in combination with aspirin continued for up to 12 months in patients after acute coronary syndrome, ≥12 months for percutaneous coronary intervention (PCI) patients receiving drug-eluting stents, and ≥1 month for bare metal stents.
  - Patients undergoing PCI with stent placement should initially receive high-dose aspirin at 325 mg/day for 1 month for bare metal stents (BMS) and 6 months for drug-eluting stents (DES).
- Beta-blockers—start and continue indefinitely in all patients with MI, uric acid (UA), or left ventricular (LV) dysfunction with or without heart failure (HF) symptoms, unless contraindicated. In all other patients with coronary or other vascular diseases or diabetes, chronic therapy is considered, unless contraindicated.
- Statins—for all (unless otherwise contraindicated), low-density lipoprotein cholesterol (LDL-C) should be ≤100 mg/dL; a further reduction to ≤70 mg/dL is reasonable, especially if baseline LDL-C is 70–100 mg/dL. If on treatment LDL-C is ≥100 mg/dL, therapy is intensified (may require combinations).

    If TG is 200–499 mg/dL, non-HDL cholesterol (HDL-C) is measured and lowered to ≤130 mg/dL (further reduction to ≤100 mg/dL is reasonable). Option to reduce non-HDL-C: More intense LDL-C lowering therapy, and addition of fibrates or niacin. If TG ≥500 mg/dL, fibrates or niacin is given to prevent pancreatitis before LDL-lowering therapy and treat LDL-C to goal after TG lowering therapy; non-HDL-C goal of ≤130 mg/dL achieved, if possible.
- Angiotensin-converting enzyme inhibitor (ACEI)/angiotensin receptor blocker (ARB)—start and continue indefinitely in all patients with left ventricular ejection fraction (LVEF) ≤40%, in those with hypertension, DM, or chronic kidney disease (CKD) (unless contraindicated). Its use is optional in patients with normal LVEF. ARB is used in patients who are intolerant to ACEI. In severe HF, ACEI may be combined with ARB.

- Aldosterone blockers—in post-MI patients with LVEF ≤40%, who are already receiving therapeutic doses of ACEI and or ARB without significant renal dysfunction or hyperkalemia.
- Poly pills—combining antihypertensive, statin, and aspirin under consideration

Q11. What should be an ideal heart-healthy diet for South Asians?
Ans.
- Reduce glycemic load by limiting carbohydrates, especially refined carbohydrates (e.g., high-calorie soft drinks), particularly for those with high TG levels, metabolic syndrome, prediabetes, and diabetes.
- Limit daily intake of total fat to 25–35% of calories and saturated fat <7% of the calories, by limiting butter, ghee, full-fat dairy products, tropical oils (palm oil and coconut oil), fried foods, and other sources of trans-fat (all crispy foods, e.g., cheeps, etc.).
- Reduce salt intake to <2.3 g Na (1 TSF of salt) per day.
- Increase intake of monounsaturated fats to 20%.
- Increase the intake of fruit and vegetables (at least 500 g/day), legumes, and whole grain foods [Prudent diet or dietary approaches to stop hypertension (DASH) diet].
- Moderation in the use of lean meat and nuts
- Avoid alcohol by those with a family history of alcoholism, or personal history of inability to control the intake, high TG, or high BP. Those who are habituated should limit to an amount not >1 drink/day for women and not >2 drinks/day for men (1 drink = 45 mL of spirit or 12 oz of beer).
- Encourage modification of the school tiffin to a healthier type.

SUGGESTED READING

1. Ahmed ST, Rehman H, Akeroyd JM, Alam M, Shah T, Kalra A, et al. Premature coronary heart disease in South Asians: burden and determinants. Curr Atheroscler Rep. 2018;20(1):6.
2. Enas EA, Senthilkumar A. Coronary artery disease in Asian Indians: an update and review. Internet J Cardiol. 2002;1(2):10-24.
3. Ghaffer A, Reddy KS, Singh M. Burden of non-communicable diseases in South Asia. BMJ. 2004;328(7443):807-10.
4. Misra A. Revisions of cutoffs of body mass index to define overweight and obesity are needed for the Asian-ethnic groups. Int J Obes Relat Metab Disord. 2003;27:1294-6.
5. Yousuf S, Howkan S, Ounpue S, Dans T, Avezum A, Lanas F, et al.; INTERHEART Study Investigators. Effect of potentially modifiable risk factors associated with myocardial infarction in 52 countries (the INTERHEART study): case-control study. Lancet. 2004;364(9438):937-52.

CHAPTER 35

Artificial Intelligence in Cardiology

"Instinct is the domain of animals and intelligence is the domain of human. The scope of instinct is within a narrow limit but the ultimate goal of intellect has not yet been discovered."
—Rabindra Nath Tagore

■ INTRODUCTION

Artificial intelligence (AI) is a computing paradigm to replicate human intelligence. It is the science of making intelligent machines that execute tasks comparable to, or beyond, the capability of a human brain. It may allow faster, more accurate, less cumbersome, and easily reproducible results. AI is utilized for the screening, detection, and classification of diseases, risk stratification, proper selection of therapy, and prognostication in cardiology.

Q1. What is AI?

Ans. Artificial intelligence is the area of computer science where machines are trained to perform tasks that require human-like intelligence. AI is a novel data analytics tool that is capable of analyzing enormous databases encompassing demographic, clinical, genetic, and epigenetic data.

Q2. What are machine learning (ML) and deep learning (DL)?

Ans. Machine learning is a division of AI that uses a multilayer convolutional neural network (CNN) algorithm, typically containing three layers or less. Computers are made to work like a human brain with interconnected nodes called neurons, arranged in a network called CNN.

Deep learning is a subdivision of ML that uses CNN with more than three layers and typically several hundred hidden nodes to process input. It can handle more data than ML and enhance the accuracy of the generated model even more. Basically, there are three steps in DL:
1. Training
2. Internal validation
3. Testing

For example, lacs of electrocardiograms (ECGs) of males are being fed into the machine, so that machine learns to identify the ECG of males. Similarly, lacs of ECGs of females are fed, so that the machine learns to identify the ECG of females. Then, a set of ECGs, again in lacs, are being fed, and the machine identifies whether the ECG is of a male or female, and the accuracy is estimated. This process is known as internal validation. If the accuracy is acceptable, then the machine is subjected to test the data given, i.e., testing.

Q3. What is the difference between ML and DL?

Ans. Both ML and DL are AI tools with the following differences **(Table 35.1)**.

TABLE 35.1: Machine learning versus deep learning.

Machine learning	Deep learning
Able to complete tasks with lesser amounts of data	Usually benefits from a large volume of data
Shorter time required for training	Longer time required for training
An expert is usually needed	Determined by neural networks; an expert is not needed
Improve with experience	Imitate neural networks
Reliant on certain functions in drawing conclusions	Can learn extremely complicated functions

Q4. What are artificial neural networks (ANN) and CNNs?

Ans. Artificial neural networks are complex networks of nodes, similar to the communication of neurons in the human brain. It has the capability to modify its own algorithms, gaining new knowledge by handling fresh data.

A CNN is a specific type of ANN used mostly in AI applications and is a highly efficient DL approach for evaluating visual input. Here, connections are made similar to the way neurons arranged in the human brain.

Q5. How can AI be applied for ECG interpretation?

Ans. Artificial intelligence may change the total outlook of ECG interpretation. AI/ML algorithms learn and derive important clinical information besides those found in the paper version of ECGs, such as the age of the subject, gender, any evidence of left ventricular (LV) dysfunction, prior episodes of atrial fibrillation (AF), significant aortic stenosis (AS), etc. Thus, it is used for ECG interpretation, diagnosis of arrhythmia and its management, clinical decision-making in AF and ventricular arrhythmias, etc. AI algorithms may aid in the diagnosis of infectious diseases like coronavirus disease 2019 (COVID-19). It has been shown that a completely normal ECG practically excludes the presence of COVID-19 infection and possibly other acute infectious diseases.

Q6. How does AI aid in echocardiographic examination?

Ans. Automatic echocardiographic assessment of left ventricular ejection fraction (LVEF) using AI/ML has been shown to be noninferior to experienced echocardiographers. It will allow speedy, unbiased, and precise estimation of echo parameters. Robotic arms are in development that automatically search for the optimal probe position to enhance image quality, thereby further improving AI/ML-guided echocardiography. High patient load, lack of ample time, and inadequate experience may be mitigated by the recent introduction of AI, which provides a much-needed solution to these problems. AI is applied to estimate various echo parameters such as LVEF, LV volumes, LV mass, LV longitudinal strain, diastology, stress echo, right ventricular (RV) function, valvular heart diseases [the severity of AS and mitral regurgitation (MR), screening of rheumatic heart disease (RHD), planning for transcatheter aortic valve replacement (TAVR), etc.], intracardiac masses, amyloidosis, and sarcoidosis.

Q7. What is the utility of AI in computed tomography (CT) coronary angiography?

Ans. Analysis of fat attenuation in the perivascular area in epicardial and pericardial locations provides new insights into the inflammatory status of plaques within the coronary circulation. This can be detected by the fat attenuation index (FAI) with the help of AI/ML. This provide new insights into the inflammatory status of plaques within the coronary circulation **(Fig. 35.1)**. Noninvasive detection of coronary inflammation via FAI can lead to timely and aggressive initiation of primary prevention for patients with no visible coronary artery disease (CAD) but unstable atherosclerotic plaques that may potentially lead to myocardial infarction (MI) if untreated. The FAI can also guide future trials in assessing novel but affordable therapeutic agents that target inflammation.

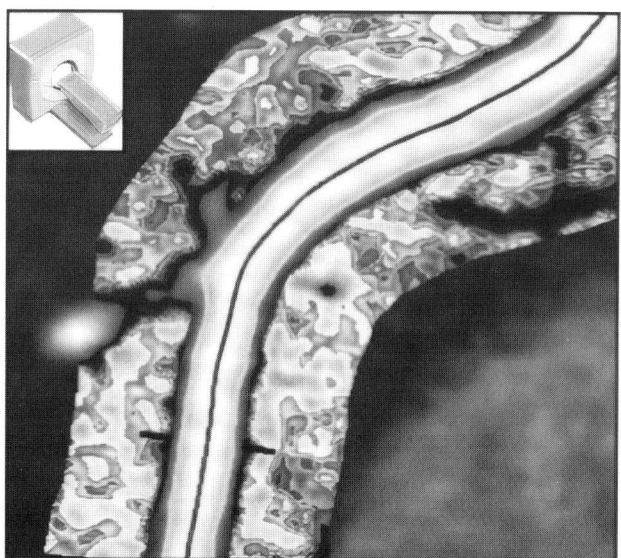

Fig. 35.1: FAI by AI/ML in the perivascular area of the coronary artery.

Q8. How is AI used in cardiovascular magnetic resonance imaging (CMRI)?

Ans. Artificial intelligence/machine learning algorithms allow cardiac volume changes and ejection fraction within seconds, allowing more rapid and highly standardized imaging analysis. While cardiovascular magnetic resonance (CMR) is executed at a high resolution, analysis of the scan by the clinician remains variable, time-consuming, and prone to errors. DL has been used to provide automated information from CMR images. A DL-driven CMR technology named virtual native enhancement (VNE) can generate images without using gadolinium-based contrast.

Q9. How does facial recognition by AI give information on cardiovascular (CV) status?
Ans. Facial photos can detect coronary diseases and predict outcomes precisely. The algorithm analyzes the hair structure and density and wrinkles on the forehead, around the eyes, and the chin and derives a comprehensive analysis. It takes advantage of previous studies, such as baldness, ear lobule crease, and xanthelasma, to predict CV outcomes. AI applications have the future potential to generate results from simple interventions such as taking a selfie

Q10. How does voice change detection by AI give information on CV health?
Ans. Artificial intelligence/machine learning is able to provide information about the health status of a patient based on speech analysis. Acute decompensated heart failure (HF) affects both laryngeal function and respiratory rate and hence the quality of speech. Automated speech analysis technology can identify voice alteration reflecting HF decompensation, thus aiding in outpatient follow-up. Also, AF may be detected from speech signals, and voice-based identification of AF is possible with acceptable accuracy.

Q11. What is the application of AI in HF management?
Ans. Artificial intelligence/machine learning is able to provide information about the health status of HF patients based on speech analysis. Automated speech analysis technology can identify voice alteration reflecting HF decompensation, thus aiding in outpatient follow-up. Acute decompensated HF affects both laryngeal function and respiratory rate and hence the quality of speech.
- *Screening and early diagnosis:* ECG-aided diagnosis of HF, DL-aided echo assessment, identification of novel risk factors of HF
- *Medication management:* Phenogrouping by guideline-directed medical therapy (GDMT) response and identification of GDMT adherence, optimization of device therapy by preprocedural identification of cardiac resynchronization therapy (CRT) responders, prediction of RV failure after left ventricular assist device (LVAD) implantation, and postprocedural identification of high-risk patients, prediction of response to LVAD, prediction of adverse events post-implantable cardioverter-defibrillator (ICD) implantation, etc.

- *Prognostic modeling:* Identification of variables predicting poor outcomes--both in-hospital and in the long term

Q12. How is cardiovascular disease (CVD) risk stratification and prediction done by AI?

Ans. Many established risk models based on conventional statistics, such as the Framingham risk scoring system, modified risk factor test (MRFT) and atherosclerotic cardiovascular disease (ASCVD) risk calculator, provide limited predictive performance. Accurate prediction needs a huge amount of patient data, and such huge amounts of data require modern AI/ML algorithms for efficient analysis. Thus, outcome prediction is higher using ML strategies. AI models can analyze large and complex datasets, including patient demographics, medical history, genetic information, imaging data, and sensor-based measurements, to provide more accurate and personalized risk assessments. Thus, the individual risk of developing CVDs is possible. High-risk patients who may benefit from targeted interventions and life style measurements are thus identified.

Q13. How does AI help in the screening and prediction of outcomes in sudden cardiac death (SCD)?

Ans. Sudden cardiac death is the most common cause of death worldwide, accounting for >50% of CV deaths. AI and ML applications, by using simple measures of heart rate and breathing rate, detect immediate collapse or hypotension within minutes. These methods, with the ability to interpret huge volumes of data, well outside the scope of human interpretation, may predict SCD. These include heart rate variability and indices of other autonomic modalities, indices of abnormal impulse conduction, and indices of abnormal repolarization, such as T-wave alterations.

Q14. How are wearable digital devices utilized in AI?

Ans. The combination of wearable devices and AI enables continuous monitoring, real-time data analysis, personalized interventions, and decision-making.
- Artificial intelligence-powered wearable ECG devices can detect arrhythmias and alert healthcare providers to potential cardiac events. Modern ECG wearables are equipped with wireless communication capability, allowing real-time data transmission to smartphones or cloud-based platforms through Bluetooth automatically. Thus, healthcare providers can track the cardiac status of patients outside traditional healthcare settings, and this is particularly beneficial for patients with chronic CV conditions in remote settings or where hospital visits are challenging.
- Artificial intelligence-powered stethoscope can provide clinicians with information about murmurs, asymptomatic LV dysfunction, and AF,

thereby aiding in the triage of patients and selection of appropriate investigations.
- Wearable Holter monitors, photoplethysmography devices, and implantable cardiac monitors can also be useful in this regard.

Q15. What is a cardiac digital twin (CDT)?
Ans. Cardiac digital twin is the concept of creating a personalized three-dimensional (3D) model of the heart. It is intended for use in planning surgery, personalized therapy, and cardiac rehabilitation. It may provide more accurate and individualized patient care.

Q16. What is ChatGPT? What is its use in cardiology practice?
Ans. *ChatGPT*: *C*hat *G*enerative *P*re-*T*rained *T*ransformer (*G*enerative: creating something new, e.g., poems, articles, short stories; *P*re-training from the domain of ML using a vast pool of data, thus acquiring knowledge about language and sentence formation; *T*ransformer: designing AI models using text data, etc., to generate output).

ChatGPT are large language models (LLMs) in AI systems, which have the ability to interact with human intuition and computer-like intelligence. LLMs have a potential role in cardiology, ranging from medical education, diagnosis, manuscript preparation, and editing. It helps in the automation of various tasks and patient education. Its uses are as follows:
- Aiding in diagnosis and decision support
- Maintaining electronic health records
- Guiding in continuing professional development
- Helping in patient education
- Helping in the automation of administrative tasks

Q17. What are the ethical issues involved in AI?
Ans. The use of AI in medicine may need several ethical aspects to consider. These are informed consent, data privacy and confidentiality, bias mitigation, safety monitoring and oversight, transparency and open communication, beneficence and nonmaleficence, respect for autonomy, compliance with ethical guidelines, public trust and collaboration, social responsibility, etc.

Q18. How to translate AI technology into future clinical practice?
Ans. Despite its huge potential, AI is something new, unfamiliar, and sometimes difficult to comprehend. AI systems can be flawed; generalizability to new settings may produce bad outcomes and lead to poor decision-making. Education of the public regarding AI and the logic behind its applications is vital for understanding the commercialization of AI applications. Medical engineering, computational science, coding, and algorithms need to be addressed in their teaching and training. The Food and Drug Administration (FDA) and the European Union have proposed a regulatory framework with the aim to establish safe and effective AI-based

medical devices. India introduced its National Strategy for AI in 2018. Bangladesh has very recently formulated the National AI Policy 2024 (AI Policy 2024) to effectively address the social, legal, and ethical issues associated with AI, prioritizing health care by the establishment of an independent National Artificial Intelligence Center for Excellence (NAICE).

Q19. What are the present limitations of AI technology?
Ans. Artificial intelligence has its own limitations. Legal considerations are of importance in its application. Many countries have their own guidelines for its application. Bangladesh is going to make its own guidelines for the use of AI. The following are a few of its limitations in the application of AI:

- *"Black box" nature of AI models:* AI algorithms construct complex models directly from raw data, leading to a lack of transparency and understanding. Lack of explicit reasoning in critical medical contexts may pose a challenge.
- Reliance on leveled data in some ML models may introduce potential bias in the leveling process.
- High-quality data is needed for training AI algorithms. Analysis may be compromised if the data is imperfect.
- Scarcity of prospective studies with reliable clinical outcomes: Absence of prospective studies limits our understanding of the true effectiveness and safety of AI applications in clinical practice.
- Using large databases containing sensitive data may raise ethical and legal challenges. Data security and the potential for unauthorized disclosure of information are a concern.
- Artificial intelligence's automated generation of clinical and/or management decisions fails to take into account each patient's unique clinical, physical, environmental, and social situations. Thus, the results may not always correspond to patient care, and this form of intelligence, though helpful, still remains "artificial".

Q20. How AI may prove to be a real intelligence rather than "artificial"?
Ans. The use of AI in cardiology is rapidly developing in our fast-paced world and has the potential to completely transform patient treatment. The identification, classification, and diagnosis of cardiac diseases may be aided by AL algorithms. It will enhance the use of noninvasive diagnostics and reduce the need for costly and complicated invasive tests. By the early identification of subtle changes in cardiac hemodynamics, AI promises to aid clinicians in better predicting, anticipating, and reducing mortality from cardiac ailments. Cardiologists will thus be able to tell an asymptomatic patient whether they will develop a lethal arrhythmia or an MI and what needs to be done to avoid this. Cardiologists should educate themselves in the development of AI, take part in AI innovations, and utilize them in their practice. Short courses and postgraduate degrees on AI in health care may be

undertaken. Overcoming the current limitations and ethical aspects, AI may prove to be a real intelligence rather than "artificial".

SUGGESTED READING

1. Antoniades C, West HW. Coronary CT angiography as a 'one-stop shop' to detect the high-risk plaque and the vulnerable patient. Eur Heart J. 2021;42:3853-5.
2. Davis A, Billick K, Horton K, Jankowski M, Knoll P, Marshall JE, et al. Artificial intelligence in cardiology. J Am Coll Cardiol. 2018;71(23):2668-79.
3. Karakuş G, Degirmencioglu A, Nanda NC. Artificial intelligence in echocardiography: Review and limitations including epistemological concerns. Echocardiography. 2022;39(8):1044-53.
4. Lin S, Li Z, Fu B, Chen S, Li X, Wang Y, et al. Feasibility of using deep learning to detect coronary artery disease based on facial photo. Eur Heart J. 2020;41:4400-11.
5. Oikonomou EK, Williams MC, Kotanidis CP, Desai MY, Marwan M, Antonopoulos AS, et al. A novel machine learning-derived radio transcriptomic signature of perivascular fat improves cardiac risk prediction using coronary CT angiography. Eur Heart J. 2019;40:3529-43.
6. Yasmin F, Shah SMI, Naeem A, Shujauddin SM, Jabeen A, Kazmi S, et al. Artificial intelligence in the diagnosis and detection of heart failure: the past, present, and future. Rev Cardiovasc Med. 2021;22(4):1095-113.

CHAPTER 36: Preventive Cardiology

"Prevention is better than cure; it can create a new generation in whom low risk factor for CAD is the rule and high risk factor is the exception."

—Author of the book

■ INTRODUCTION

Behavioral changes, lifestyle modifications, and drugs are effective in the prevention of heart diseases. As clinical manifestations of atherosclerotic cardiovascular disease (ASCVD) occur late in its course, ample opportunity exists for preventive measures to arrest the disease or stop the progression. Evidences from various trials show that primary and secondary prevention of ASCVD are effective. Risk stratification of individuals in assessing cardiovascular (CV) risk is an essential measure in choosing appropriate preventive measures.

Q1. What are the levels of prevention of coronary artery disease (CAD)?

Ans.

- *Primordial prevention:* Prevention of the development of risk factors of CAD, e.g., preventing the appearance of hypertension, diabetes mellitus (DM), and dyslipidemia, which will prevent the development of CAD in the long term
- *Primary prevention:* Prevention of the development of disease among those with a high prevalence of risk factors by controlling risk factors through lifestyle modification and drugs. This is exemplified by the prevention of CAD among those with hypertension, DM, and dyslipidemia.
- *Secondary prevention:* Prevention of the progression of CAD in those already developing CAD by vigorous lifestyle modification and drugs

Q2. What is a prevention paradox?

Ans. Since the risk associated with most CAD risk factors is a continuum, more people making small changes result in large benefits to society (i.e., primordial prevention) as opposed to a large change in a small number of high-risk patients (i.e., primary prevention). Application of primordial prevention for the total population is called the population-based strategy of prevention. It aims to lower risk factors in the entire population and create a new generation in which low risk is the role and high risk is the exception. Thus, lowering the mean population cholesterol level or mean blood pressure (BP) has a far greater impact than the treatment of those with hypercholesterolemia or hypertension. This is what is called a prevention paradox.

Q3. How to assess ASCVD risk?
Ans. Stratification of ASCVD risk is done as follows:
- *High risk:* 10-year risk: >20%. Risk calculation is done according to the Framingham Risk Score. These are patients with established CAD or evidence of ASCVD in noncoronary beds, e.g., peripheral vascular disease (PVD), abdominal aortic aneurysm, symptomatic carotid disease, DM, or the presence of multiple risk factors. The target low-density lipoprotein-cholesterol (LDL-C) is 100 mg/dL.
- *Moderate risk:* 10-year risk: 10–20%. These are patients with two or more risk factors for cardiovascular disease (CVD) events. The target LDL-C is <130 mg/dL.
- *Low risk:* 10-year risk <10%. These are patients with no or one risk factor. The target LDL-C here is <160 mg/dL.

Q4. What is the importance of waist circumference?
Ans. Waist circumference is an indicator of abdominal or central obesity. However, a mere increase in the waist circumference cannot differentiate subcutaneous fat from visceral fat. Increased waist circumference [for a given body mass index (BMI)] with increased triglycerides (TGs), also known as a hypertriglyceridemic waist, is indicative of ectopic fat and altered cardiometabolic risk profile.

Q5. What is the clinical importance of visceral fat deposition?
Ans. Visceral adiposity and fatty liver is a marker of dysfunctional subcutaneous adipose tissue, which occurs when subcutaneous tissue fails to expand. Individuals lacking subcutaneous fat develop excess visceral fat as well as fat accumulation in normally lean tissue, such as the liver, heart (epicardium and pericardium), blood vessels, kidney, and skeletal muscle, i.e., ectopic fat deposition. Thus, it is a consequence of the inability of subcutaneous adipose tissue to act as a protective "metabolic sink". Ectopic fat is prodiabetogenic, inflammatory, and atherogenic. Visceral adipose tissue acts as an endocrine organ. It is hyperlipolytic, producing free fatty acids and TGs, increasing hepatic glucose production, and reducing insulin extraction, leading to type 2 diabetes mellitus (T2DM). Evidence suggests that excess liver fat is a key abnormality responsible for several cardiometabolic complications found in viscerally obese patients. Susceptibility to visceral fat deposition is greatest in Asians.

Q6. What is sarcopenic adiposity?
Ans. It refers to a condition where there is less muscle mass and more adipose tissue for a given BMI. The smaller body volume of Bangladeshis necessitates a hyperinsulinemic response, which is further intensified by insulin resistance caused by sarcopenic adiposity. This vicious cycle of

intense hyperinsulinemia is a reason for the early onset of all the risk factors at a low BMI among Bangladeshis.

Q7. What is an obesity paradox?

Ans. Despite the established relationship between BMI and CV risk, such as hypertension, dyslipidemia, and T2DM, some studies suggest that obese individuals with these conditions paradoxically may have a better outcome than lean persons, the entity known as an "obesity paradox". Highly functional adipocytes are different from poorly functioning adipocytes found in visceral fat. These poorly functioning fats are rich in macrophages, causing low-grade inflammation. Individuals with a high BMI may be physically fit and have lower mortality compared to those with a low BMI and poorly functioning adipocytes—the "fit and fat" or metabolically healthy obesity.

Q8. What are the therapeutic lifestyle changes (TLCs) recommended to prevent CAD risk?

Ans. Diet is said to be the driver for CAD. A heart-healthy diet, lifestyle changes with regular physical activity, avoiding smoking and psychosocial stress, and maintaining a healthy body weight are recommended **(Box 36.1)**.

> **BOX 36.1:** Prevention of CAD-TLC recommendations.
>
> - *Healthy diet:*
>   – Total fat: 25–35% of total calories; saturated fat: <7% of total calories; cholesterol <200 mg/day; polyunsaturated fat: Up to 10% of total calories; monounsaturated fat: Up to 20% of total calories
>   – Carbohydrates: 50–60% of total calories
>   – Total protein: 15% of total calories
>   – Dietary fibers: 20–30 g/day
>   – Therapeutic options for LDL-C lowering—plant stanols/steroids: 2 g/day, increased viscous soluble fiber (5–10 g/day; 10–25 g/day may have added benefits)
> - Regular physical activity—to expend at least 200 kcal/day
> - Maintaining a healthy weight
> - Avoiding smoking and tobacco use
> - Avoiding psychosocial stress and practicing meditation
>
> (CAD: coronary artery disease; LDL-C: low-density lipoprotein-cholesterol; TLCs: therapeutic lifestyle changes)

Q9. What is a heart-healthy oil?

Ans. The health benefits of oils depend on their fat composition and the ratio between saturated fatty acids (SAFA), monounsaturated fatty acids (MUFA), and polyunsaturated fatty acids (PUFA). A heart-healthy oil should have a ratio of SAFA:MUFA:PUFA = 1:1.5:1, and there should be no trans-unsaturated fatty acids (TUFA). None of the available cooking oils fulfills the criteria of various lipid contents. Thus, it is desirable to blend or rotate different cooking oils such as mustard oil, groundnut oil, canola oil, and rice bran oil with favorable lipid contents. The use of ghee and butter as cooking oil should be limited. Also, the use of oils that solidify at room temperature, e.g., coconut oil and palm oil, is discouraged.

Q10. What is the importance of dietary fat and oils?

Ans. The terms lipids, oils, and fats are used interchangeably. Fats that are liquid at room temperature are called oil (with unsaturated fatty acids). Fats broadly mean solid fats at room temperature. Fat provides energy three times more than carbohydrates and proteins. It increases the taste of food, protects the body from winter, and is an essential component of body cells.

Cholesterol is present in very small amounts in plants. So, plant oils are devoid of cholesterol and are heart healthy.

Q11. What is the role of trans fat in CAD?

Ans. Incomplete hydrogenation of vegetable oils results in the formation of TUFA, and complete hydrogenation produces saturated fat.

It confers texture and structural stability to foods. Even low consumption of 1–3% of the total calorie intake of TUFA leads to an increased risk of CAD. Thus, it is the most harmful fatty acid to CV health. Increased intake increases CVD risk, because it increases LDL, TGs, and lipoprotein(a) [LP(a)] and decreases high-density lipoprotein (HDL). It adversely affects the metabolism of essential fatty acids and prostaglandins, thus promoting thrombogenesis and insulin resistance. The risk of CAD nearly doubles with a 2% increase in the intake of TUFA calories, whereas a 15% increase in SAFA is needed to produce a similar CAD risk. The sources of TUFA are dalda, vanaspati, ghee, margarine, baked foods, ready-made mithais, processed foods, and ready-to-eat snacks.

Q12. What are the various fatty acids?

Ans.
- *Saturated fatty acids*—solid; increase LDL and are present in animal fat, milk products, and coconut and palm oils.
- Monounsaturated fatty acids decrease LDL and increase HDL (through the liver); they are present in olive, mustard, peanut, canola, and rice bran oils.
- Polyunsaturated fatty acids—invisible fat—are present in cereals and sunflower, cotton seed, and groundnut oils.
- *Omega-3 fatty acids:* Essential for the body; cannot be synthesized; decrease TGs, inhibit platelets, and strengthen the endothelium of blood vessels.

Q13. How to implement a smoking cessation program?

Ans.
- Smoking cessation should be considered an important therapeutic intervention for people with heart disease and implemented as part of routine clinical care for these patients.

- Identification of smokers, advise to quit, and educate on the health benefits of quitting that begin to develop soon after quitting.
- Nicotine replacement therapy (NRT) with a nicotine patch, gum, lozenge, inhaler, nasal spray, etc., can be suggested.
- Varenicline, a partial nicotine receptor agonist, can be used.
- Bupropion, an antidepressant, can be prescribed, which may help in combating nicotine dependence.

Q14. How does physical activity reduce ASCVD risk?
Ans. Physical activity has multiple, potentially beneficial effects on atherosclerotic risk factors. It reduces systolic BP, body weight, blood glucose, and TGs and increases high-density lipoprotein-cholesterol (HDL-C) level.

Q15. What preventive measures are advised for athletes with ASCVD?
Ans. Vigorous exercise increases the risk of sudden cardiac death (SCD) and acute myocardial infarction (AMI) in adults with occult ASCVD and those with diagnosed congenital heart disease (CHD). Vigorous exercise acutely increases CV risk by plaque disruption.
- *Take moderate-degree endurance exercise:* A moderate amount of exercise confers as much benefit as more intense exercise.
- A minimum of 2 years of aggressive lipid-lowering therapy should be suggested to reduce lipids to the lowest possible level before returning to competition.
- Continue aspirin and other antiplatelet agents.
- Continue betablockers and discontinue other antihypertensives on the day of the athletic event because exercise acutely reduces BP.

Q16. What is the role of aspirin in the primary prevention of ASCVD?
Ans. The US Preventive Services Task Force recommendations on aspirin for the primary prevention of ASCVD (2016) are as follows:
- Use aspirin for adults aged 50–59 years with a 10-year ASCVD risk of ≥10%, not at increased risk of bleeding, life expectancy of ≥10 years, and willing to take aspirin for ≥10 years.
- For adults aged 60–69 years with a 10-year ASCVD risk of 10%, not at increased risk of bleeding, life expectancy of ≥10 years, and willing to take aspirin for ≥10 years, the decision is individualized.
- There is no recommendation for adults aged <50 or ≥70 years.

Q17. How can yoga prevent heart diseases?
Ans. Yoga (Sanskrit: "yuj") means to join together. It aims at joining the mind with the body. Yoga appears to be especially beneficial for the prevention and control of CVD. This is through controlling stress and improving the neuroendocrine and autonomic nervous system. It may contribute to the control of risk factors such as hypertension, DM, obesity, dyslipidemia, tobacco use, and psychosocial stress. Yoga has been shown to alter the

behavior of an individual that helps them follow a healthy lifestyle. The exercise and dietary components of yoga that encourage taking a vegetarian diet also augment the CV benefits. Benefits have also been reported in the secondary prevention of heart diseases and cardiac rehabilitation. Yoga is very useful in controlling stress, anxiety, and depression, which are frequent accompaniments of CVD and carry a worse prognosis.

> *"He who is regulated in his habit of eating, sleeping, recreation, and work drives away the worldy miseries and sufferings by practicing yoga."*
> —Bhagavad Gita (ch. 6, sloka 17)

■ SUGGESTED READING

1. Dehghan M, Mente A, Zhang X, Swaminathan S, Li W, Mohan V, et al. Associations of fats and carbohydrate intake with cardiovascular disease and mortality in 18 countries from five continents (PURE): a prospective cohort study. Lancet. 2017;390(10107):2050-62.
2. Estruch R, Ros E. Salas-Salvado J, Covas MI, Corella D, Arós F, et al.; PREDIMED Study Investigators. Primary prevention of cardiovascular disease with a Mediterranean diet. N Engl J Med. 2013;368:1279-90 [published correction appears in N Engl J Med. 2014;370:886].
3. Joshipura KJ, Hung HC, Li TY, Hu FB, Rimm EB, Stampfer MJ, et al. Intakes of fruits, vegetables and carbohydrate and the risk of CVD. Public Health Nutr. 2009;12:115-21.
4. Manchanda SC. Yoga—A promising technique to control cardiovascular disease. Indian Heart J. 2014;66(5):487-9.
5. World Health Organization. (2003). Diet, nutrition and prevention of chronic diseases: report of a Joint FAO/WHO Expert Consultation. WHO Technical Report Series 916. Geneva, Switzerland.

Index

Page numbers followed by *b* refer to box, *f* refer to figure, *fc* refer to flowchart, and *t* refer to table.

A

Acarbose 442
Accelerated junctional rhythm 317*f*
Actinobacillus 225
Activated partial thromboplastin time 129
Acute coronary syndrome 106, 129, 239, 245, 264, 452, 479, 490, 491
Acute ischemic stroke 457
    anticoagulation in 457*b*
Acute kidney injury 450
Acute pulmonary
    edema 255, 277
    embolism 423, 423*t*
Acute renal failure 277, 277*f*
    arthritis of 138
    carditis of 138
    diagnosed 137
Acute renocardiac syndrome 452
Adams-Stokes attack 318, 318*t*
Adenosine 309, 392
    triphosphate 392
Adequate revascularization 407
Adrenaline 293, 326
Adrenergic neuron blockers 335
Adrenoceptor blockers 391
Adult coronary heart disease 190
Adult respiratory distress syndrome 277
Advanced life support 320, 322, 322*f*, 323, 333
Aerosols 468
Air pollution 468
    mitigation strategies for 469
    types of 468
Akinesia 57
Albuminuria 453
Alcohol 266, 470, 470*b*
    cardioprotective 469
    toxic effects of 469
Alcoholic cardiomyopathy develop 236
Aldosterone blockers 500
Alkylating agents 465
Allen test, modified 78
Allergic reaction 233
Alpha-glycosidase inhibitors 442
Alpha-methyldopa 445
Ambulatory electrocardiogram
    monitoring 330
    recordings, types of 38
Amiodarone 371, 326, 390, 445, 449
Ampicillin 230
Amyloidosis 234, 236
Analgesics 265
Anemia 274, 451
Anesthesia 461
Aneurysm formation 120
Angina 7*t*, 93, 98, 176, 377
    atypical 95
    causes of 98
    equivalents 95
    implication of 107
    last, episode of 97
    pectoris 7, 95, 237
        chest pain of 7
        limiting 74
    types of 95
Anginal attack, typical 96
Anginal pain 7*t*
    differentiate 7
    location of 97
    radiation of 97
Angiocardiography, indications of selective 71
Angiography 80*t*
    digital subtraction 436
    peripheral 436
Angiotensin receptor
    blocker 288, 445, 448
    neprilysin inhibitor 288
Angiotensin-converting enzyme 330
    inhibitors 4, 114, 146, 285, 288, 359, 375, 445, 448, 451, 499
        beneficial effects of 376
    vasodilators 375
Ankle-brachial index 433
Ankylosing spondylitis 175
Anorexia 388
Anthracyclines 465
Antianginal drugs 103*t*, 124
    uses of 102
Antianginal effect 359
Antiarrhythmic agents 328, 330, 389, 390, 391, 391*t*
    proarrhythmic effect of 392
Antibiotic
    adequate doses of 227
    prophylaxis 204
    selection of 227
    therapy 229
Anti-cancer drugs, effects of 465
Anticoagulant 146, 364, 365, 368, 493
    therapy 425
        duration of 425*b*
        strategies for 185

Antidiabetic agents 441
Antihypertensive agent 266, 269
Antihypertensive drugs 267, 270, 271
   therapy 264
Antimetabolites 465
Antimicrobial agent 231
Antiplatelet 364, 365
   agents 405
      use of 128
      role of 457
Antistreptolysin O titer 140
Antithrombotic agents 364
Anxiety state, pain of 7t
Aorta 415
   ascending 415
   coarctation of 415-417, 417f, 418f
   complications of coarctation of 415
   descending 417
   diseases of 415
Aortic area 18
Aortic dissection 7, 175, 376, 418, 419, 419t, 476f
   differentiate 419
   management 420fc
   presentations of 418
Aortic enlargement 46
Aortic injection 72
Aortic murmur 169
Aortic regurgitation 141, 175, 177-179, 180f, 239, 490
   acute 176
   chronic 176
   classify 175
   diagnosis of severity of 180
   mild 180
   moderate 181f
   murmur of 177t
   peripheral signs in 177, 177t
   semiology in 178t
   severe 180f, 182
      chronic 179f
   stages of chronic 175
   symptomatology in 178t
Aortic sclerosis, classify 169
Aortic stenosis 19, 167, 168, 177, 178, 191, 235, 238t, 305, 336
   different grades of 172
   grades of 172t
   grading severity of 173t
   moderate 174f
   semiology in 178t
   severe 169
   signs of severe 170
   symptomatology in 178t
Aortic valve 2f, 239, 253, 277
   disease, classify 167
   large vegetation on 225f
   replacement 144, 171, 178
      indications of 182
   stenosis 238

Aortic valvotomy, role of 175
Aortic valvuloplasty 190
Aortitis 415
Apical 2-chamber view 57
Apical 4-chamber view 57
Apprehensive facies 9
Arcus lipidicus 10
Arrhythmia 15, 39, 274, 308, 325, 333, 378, 394, 455, 457, 470, 481
   control of 390
   digitalis induced 388
   management, treatment options for 389
Arrhythmic death 393
Arrhythmic syncope, characteristic features of 333
Arrhythmogenic disorders 474
Arterial desaturation 71
Arterial graft 104
Arterial switch 222
Arterial thrombus 435, 435t
Arteriovenous fistula 451
Arthritis comparison 138t
Artificial intelligence 501, 503, 504, 507
   aid 502
   application of 504
   digital devices utilized in 505
   in cardiology 501
   technology 506, 507
Artificial neural networks 502
Artificial valve 185, 186
   function 185
Aspirin 209, 301, 305, 365, 366, 370, 405, 499
   limitations of 103
   role of 513
Asthma
   bronchial 283, 284t
   cardiac 283, 284t
Asymmetric septal hypertrophy 240
Atenolol 362
Atherosclerosis 83, 415, 440
   accelerating 470
   risk factor for 439
Atherosclerotic cardiovascular disease 505, 509
   prevention of 513
   risk 510
      reduce 513
Atherosclerotic cardiovascular risk, reducing 86
Atherosclerotic coronary artery disease 92
Atherosclerotic diseases 456
Atherosclerotic lesions, classification of 92
Athlete's heart 242, 243, 243t
Atrial abnormalities 32
Atrial fibrillation 150, 157, 236, 274, 300, 300f, 308, 308f, 357, 378, 392, 434, 478, 490
   causes of 301
      temporary 306
   chronic 303

classification of 300b
episodes of 502
first episode of 305
hemodynamic consequences of 301
management of 301, 490
types 304
Atrial flutter 33f
Atrial infarction 115
Atrial rhythm 348f
Atrial septal defect 48, 70, 188, 190, 192-196,
    195t, 198, 199, 212, 220f, 305
    anatomical types of 192
    primum 198
    types of 192, 196
Atrial situs 54
Atrial systole, loss of 301
Atrioventricular block 315, 318f
Atrioventricular dissociation 316, 317f, 317t
Atrioventricular sequential pacing 350
Atropine 326
Auscultation 18
Autoimmune 415
    inflammatory disease 261
Automatic external defibrillation 331

B

Bacteremia, induce 230
Balloon
    angioplasty 418
    atrial septostomy 190
    catheter 396
    mitral valvuloplasty 146, 156, 157, 412,
        413, 413f
    types of 398
    valvotomy 155
    valvuloplasty 175
Bare metal stent 366, 400, 400t
Basic life support 320, 322, 323, 333
Batista operation 289
Beck's triad 251
Beriberi 234, 273
Beta adrenergic receptor blockers 362
Beta-blocker 103, 123, 146, 236, 237, 270, 285,
    302, 309, 341, 362, 364, 390, 448,
    451, 462, 499
    antiarrhythmic effects of 363
    dose of 363
    position of 266
    role of 129, 363
    therapy, role of 362
    withdraw 364
Bicuspid aortic valve 415
Bifascicular block 37, 37f
Bifurcation lesion 402f, 407, 408
    stenting, strategies of 408
Bile acid-binding resins 381
Bioabsorbable stents 395

Bioprosthetic prosthesis 184t
Bioprosthetic valves 184
    indications of 184
Bipolar pacemakers 339
Bivalirudin 368
Bjork-Shiley disc valve 184
Blalock-Taussig shunt 219
Bleeding complication occurs 132
Blood cholesterol, treatment of 86
Blood culture 228, 229
    results 223
Blood glucose
    fasting 439
    normal 439
Blood pressure 88, 262, 264, 276, 286, 288,
    322, 346, 384, 418, 443, 444
    categories of 262t
    causes of elevated 270
    diastolic 94, 260, 262, 264
    diurnal variation of 263
    high 498
    lowering 267
    reduce elevated 458
    systolic 131, 260, 262, 264, 384
Body mass index 90t, 496, 498
Bradyarrhythmias 333
    mechanism of 296
Bradycardia 314
    causes of symptomatic 314
    severe 364
    symptomatic 314
Bretylium 392
    tosylate 326
Bruce protocol 42
Brugada syndrome 313, 328
Bundle branch block 27, 32, 34, 119, 308
Burn, cardiac complications of 472

C

Caffeine 266
Calcific aortic
    stenosis 144
    valve 168f
        diseases 167
Calcium 279
    chloride 326
    gluconate 326
Calcium-channel
    antagonists 378
    blocker 103, 302, 309, 359, 376, 377t,
        427, 448
        pharmacologic properties of 377
Cancer 464
Cannon wave 15
Carbomedics valve 183
Cardiac anesthetic 462
Cardiac apex 18

Cardiac arrest 320-322, 322t, 326, 327, 333, 333t
  causes of 321, 325
  classification of 320b
  management of 326
Cardiac arrhythmia 295, 480
  electrotherapies for 352
  suppression trail 314
  treatment of 300
Cardiac catheterization 22, 63, 65, 165, 198, 456
  complications of 69
  contraindications of 69
  during 360
  indications of 68
  role of 174, 181
  routes of 63
Cardiac chamber
  abnormalities 457
  enlargement 46
  normal pressure in 69
Cardiac changes 456
Cardiac cirrhosis 256
Cardiac computed tomography 80t
Cardiac conditions 49, 51, 226, 446, 446b
Cardiac death 461b
Cardiac digital twin 506
Cardiac diseases 47, 387
Cardiac drugs 451
  during pregnancy 444
Cardiac edema 6
  features of 6
Cardiac enzymes 419
Cardiac failure 291
Cardiac glycosides 383
Cardiac hemorrhage 458
Cardiac illness 9
Cardiac index 275, 276
Cardiac injury, acute 491
Cardiac interventional procedures 456
Cardiac lesions 10, 229
Cardiac output 421, 428
  reduced 334
Cardiac pacing 337
Cardiac pharmacology 359
Cardiac physical diagnosis 8
Cardiac radiology 46
Cardiac resynchronization therapy 282, 337
  defibrillator 355f
  indications of 355
Cardiac rhythm disturbances 329
Cardiac risk factors 461
Cardiac surgery, during 341
Cardiac syncope 333, 334t, 335
  causes of 332
Cardiac tamponade 251, 256t
  echocardiographic findings of 253
Cardiac testing, indications of 441, 441b
Cardiac troponin 117
  estimation of 113

Cardiobacterium hominis 225
Cardiocerebral resuscitation 324
Cardiogenic shock 122, 132-134, 272, 290-293, 321, 322t, 332
  mechanism of 290, 291fc
  treatment of 292
Cardiogenic stroke, causes of 455
Cardiology
  practice 506
  preventive 509
Cardiomyopathy 233, 234, 236, 327, 447, 474, 490
  classification of 235b
  infiltrative 245
  nonischemic 470
  terminology of 235
Cardiopulmonary bypass 293
Cardiopulmonary resuscitation 322f
Cardiorenal failure 452
Cardiorenal syndrome 452
  types of 452
Cardiotoxicity 464
Cardiovascular conditions 378
Cardiovascular disease 261, 430, 438, 464, 468, 476, 478, 483, 497, 505
  risk factors for 484
  signs of 4
  symptoms of 4
Cardiovascular effects 463
Cardiovascular imaging techniques 45
Cardiovascular magnetic resonance 52
  principle of 50
Cardiovascular risk, predictors of 453
Cardiovascular system
  anatomy and physiology of 1
  components of 1
  toxic effects on 470b
Cardioversion 324, 351
  contraindications of 304, 325
  indications of 325
Carditis 139
  diagnosis of 141
Carney syndrome 467
Carnitine deficiency 234
Carotid pulsation 16t
Carotid sinus massage 311
Carpentier-Edwards porcine valve 183
Carvedilol 362
Catheter 64
  ablation 300, 356
    indications of 356
  and introducer sheath 68
Catheterization 256
  techniques 68
Cathode 339
Cellular telephones 350
Central nervous system 124
Cephalization 49

Index **519**

Cerebral artery, middle 454
Cerebral complications 456
Cerebral embolism
    cardiac sources of 457
    risk factors of 455
Cerebral hemorrhage 458
Cerebral infarction 458
Cerebral lesions, cardiac effects of 455
Cerebrovascular diseases 88, 454, 480
Chagas disease 234
Channelopathy 313
Characterize plaque composition 91
ChatGPT 506
Chemical cardioversion 304
Chest pain 145
    acute 97, 98
    cardiac causes of 6
    causes of acute 98
Chest X-ray 46, 48, 48t, 182, 199, 202, 212, 239, 251, 252f, 255f, 286
Chlamydia 225
Cholesterol 498
    bad 85
    deadly 85, 86
    good 85
    ugly 85
Chromosomal abnormalities 474
Chronic coronary
    artery disease 95
    syndrome
        clinical presentations of 99
        suspected case of 99
Chronic kidney disease 261, 264, 372, 450, 450b, 451b, 453
    increase 451
    stages of 450b
Chronic obstructive pulmonary
    disease 103, 297, 404, 428, 468
Chronic renocardiac syndrome 452
Chronic total occlusion 409
    lesions 410
Cigarette smoking 89
Cimetidine 371
Circulatory failure 272
Circumflex artery 73f
Clopidogrel 365, 499
Coagulopathy 456
Coarctation
    diagnosis of 417
    treatment of 418
Cocaine 470
    abuse 470
    cardiovascular
        complications of 470
        effects of 470b
Coenzyme Q10 279
Coexistent vascular disorders 456
Collagen disease 255

Collapsing pulse 177
Collateral circulation, murmur of 416
Color Doppler 180
Color flow imaging 186
Colored vision 388
Common genetic cardiovascular diseases 475
Common systemic diseases 489
Commotio cordis 246
Comorbid psychiatric diseases 97
Comorbid somatoform diseases 97
Complete heart block 114, 296, 316, 316f, 317, 317t, 338
    classification 316b
    development of 38
Complete revascularization 406
Compliant balloon 398
Computed tomography 419
    angiography 435
Concurrent diabetes, implications of 93
Congenital heart disease 30, 188, 189, 191, 222, 327, 329, 422
    percutaneous interventions in 190b
    surgical operations in complex 222b
Congenital lesions 144, 308
Congenital ventricular septal defects exist 201
Congestion 272
Congestive heart failure 4, 198, 202, 242, 251, 256, 256t, 272, 299, 363, 376, 384, 386, 438, 490
Connective tissue diseases 248, 474
Constrictive pericarditis 244, 244t, 255, 256t
    causes of 255
    chronic 256t
Continuous wave Doppler 164, 164f, 173, 181, 205, 240
Contrast echo 53, 197
Convolutional neural network 502
Cor bovinum 179
Cor pulmonale 421, 428, 429
    acute 428
    chronic 428, 429
    mechanism of development of 428fc
Coronary angiography 22, 52, 63, 72, 80t, 109, 145, 245, 330, 483, 503
    indications for 74
    limitations of 75
    pitfalls of 76
Coronary artery 3, 72, 73f, 503f
    bypass grafting 61, 104t, 331, 336, 404, 419
        types of 104
    calcium 261
    dissection, spontaneous 484, 486
    imaging 50
    left 3, 73, 73f
        main 59, 409
    nonobstructive 485
    normal 44
    right 3, 73f, 74, 104, 114, 119, 122f, 291

Coronary artery disease 24, 82, 99, 264, 321, 329, 359, 394, 404, 424, 427, 432, 438, 450, 451, 454, 462, 470, 482, 483, 486, 490, 495-497, 497t, 503, 511, 512
    cardinal features of 495, 495b
    diagnosis of 41, 100
    goal of 496t
    increasing 496b
    prevention of 105, 498, 509, 511b
    risk factors of 83, 88, 90, 92, 453, 497
    risk of 85, 451, 451b
    secondary prevention of 499
    syndromic presentation of 99
Coronary circulation 2
Coronary computed tomography angiography 100
Coronary dominance 75
Coronary heart disease 279, 483
    causes of 188
    classify 189
    complex 189
    prevent 487
    secondary prevention of 103
Coronary lesion 439
    degree of 76
Coronary revascularization 403
Coronary risk factors 82
Coronary sinus 355f, 356f
    defect 192
    posterolateral branch of 355f
Coronary spasm 406
Coronary stenosis, severity of 76
Coronavirus disease-2019 490-493, 502
    patients 493
    pneumonia 493, 493t
Corrigan's pulse 177
Cough
    cardiopulmonary resuscitation 324
    cardiovascular causes of 4
Coxiella burnetii 225
C-reactive protein 137
Critically ill patients 59
Culprit lesion revascularization 407
Cutting balloon 398
Cyanosis 8
    causes of 193
    differential 8, 208
Cyanotic spells occur 215
Cyclophosphamide 465

D

Dabigatran 372
DDD mode 349f
De Musset's sign 177
Decapolar catheter 356f
Decubitus angina 95
Deep learning 501, 502, 502t

Deep vein thrombosis 58, 425, 481
    prevention of 424
Defibrillation 324, 351
    contraindications of 325
    indications of 325
Dental equipment 351
Deoxyribonucleic acid 474
Dextrocardia 191
Diabetes 438
    development of 440
    mellitus 84, 234, 363, 419, 424, 484, 495-497, 509
        diagnostic criteria for 438
        noninsulin-dependent 269
        type 2 497, 510
Diabetic dyslipidemia 440
Diabetic heart disease 442
Diabetic patients 441
    ischemia in 93
    treatment goals for 442, 443b
Diarrhea 388
Diathermy 351
Dietary fat and oils 512
Digital echo 54
Digital infarct 227
Digitalis 385
    contraindications of 386
    effect of 388
    indications of 386
    mechanism of action of 385
    toxic manifestations of 388
Digitation toxicity 389
Digoxin 146, 302, 309, 312, 341, 392, 430, 445, 449, 451
    determined 387
    dose, influence 387
    role of 157
    therapy, monitor 389
    toxic dose of 306
    toxicity 389
    use of 285
Dihydropyridine 376, 377
Dilated cardiomyopathy 52, 233, 235, 273, 490
    types 235b
Diltiazem 376, 392
Dipeptidyl peptidase-4 inhibitor 441
Diphtheria 234
Disopyramide 391, 451
Distal embolization 406
Disulfiram 371
Diuretic 132, 378, 449
    advantages of 269
    incorrect use of 379
    low-dose 266
    metabolic side effects of 380
    therapy, causes of resistance to 279
    usefulness of 266

Dobutamine 135, 293
  echo 171
Dofetilide 451
Door-to-needle time 122, 131
Dopamine 134, 135, 293
  varies, action of 385
Doppler echo 53, 153
  criteria 141
  role of 163
  utility of 152
Down syndrome 9
Drug
  in pregnancy, principles of 448
  therapy, target blood pressure for 264*t*
  treatment 146
  use, principles of 448
Drug-coated balloon 398
Drug-eluting stent 367, 395, 399, 400, 400*t*, 462
  components of 398
  classify 399
Dual antiplatelet therapy 366, 367
Dual-chamber pacing 242
Duroziez's sign 177
Dyskinesia 57
Dyslipidemia 84, 87, 88*t*, 380, 381, 439, 451, 484
Dyspnea 5, 145, 237
  cardiac causes of 5
Dysrhythmias, control 238

E

Early advanced cardiac care 322
Ebstein's anomaly 189, 221, 308, 446
  characteristic features of 221
  huge cardiomegaly in 47*f*
Echo aid 59
Echocardiography 52, 138, 182, 186, 205, 213, 216, 229, 330
  changes 455
  modalities 53
  role of 252
  utility of 145
Eclampsia 447
Ectopic beat counter 39
Ectopic fat deposition 510
Edema 444
  cardiovascular causes of 6
Eggshell calcification 49
Ehlers–Danlos syndrome 474
Eikenella 225
Eisenmenger's syndrome 204, 217, 217*t*, 220, 220*f*
Ejection fraction 256
  estimating 50
Electric substations 350

Electrical cardioversion 304
Electrical injury, cardiac
  complications of 472
Electrical therapy 390
Electrocardiogram 22, 28*f*, 29, 36, 109, 119, 131, 182, 199, 202, 212, 229, 239, 244, 251, 284, 300, 330, 336, 338, 389, 411
  changes 455
  recording 348*f*
  types of 23
  ST-elevation in 119*t*
  tracing 347*f*, 348*f*
Electrocautery 351
Electrolyte disturbances 388
Electromechanical dissociation 320, 326
Electronic article surveillance 350
Electrophysiology procedures 456
Eletrolyte imbalance 379
Ellis van Crevel's syndrome 10
Embolic acute limb ischemia 434
Empiric therapy 228
Encainide 391
Endless loop tachycardia 347
Endocarditis 223, 226, 415
  culture-negative 225
  infective 150, 195, 202, 204, 223, 225*fc*, 228, 229
  subacute infective 224, 224*t*
Endocrine diseases 234
Endothelin receptor antagonists 220, 427, 430
Endothelization 400
Enterococcus faecalis 231
Entricular hypertrophy 308
Epicardial fat 253
Epicardial lead placement,
  indications of 342
Epidural anesthesia 463
Epigenetics 474
Epilepsy 318, 318*t*
Epinephrine 365
Episode, termination of acute 309
Erectile dysfunction 427
Erythrocyte sedimentation rate 137
Esion-related factors 404
Estrogen receptor modulator 465
Ethanol, beneficial effects of 469*b*
Exercise
  heart rate influence 43
  role of 100
  tolerance test 100
  treadmill test 40, 41, 433
    false negative 45
    nondiagnostic 44
Extensive infarction 118*f*
Extracorporeal membrane oxygenation 293
Extracorporeal shock wave lithotripsy 351

F

Fallot's pentad 214
Fallot's tetrad 71
Fallot's tetralogy develop 214
Fallot's triad 214
Familial hypercholesterolemia 474, 475
    pharmacological treatment of 475
Fasting glucose, impaired 438
Fat attenuation
    analysis of 503
    index 503
Fatty acids 512
    saturated 511, 512
Fatty liver 510
Fibrin 373
Fibrinolytic
    administration of 373
    agents 116, 364, 365, 372, 373, 373t
    therapy 373
First heart sound 148, 150
Fistula 210
Flecainide 309, 391, 451
Fluorodeoxyglucose 52
Folley's catheter 292
Fondaparinux 368
Fontan operation 222
Forrester hemodynamic classification 276t
Frusemide 379
Furosemide 445

G

Gallavardin phenomenon 170
Gaseous pollutants 469
Gastrointestinal disease, pre-existing 97
Gemfibrozil 451
Gene
    silencing 477
    therapy 476
Genetic 474
    cardiac diseases 477
    cardiovascular diseases 474, 474b
    diseases 474
    engineering 476
Genomics 474
Geriatric cardiology 478
    necessary 478
Geriatric population 478
Geriatric syndrome 479
Gestational hypertension 447
Giant 'a' wave 15
Gibson's murmur 208
Glomerular filtration rate 378, 453
Glucose tolerance, impaired 438
Glycemic control 443
Glyceryl trinitrate, drug-induced 334
Glycoprotein 365, 406

Glycosides 383
Good stethoscope, characteristics of 17
Graham Steell murmur 176, 177t
Great arteries
    congenitally corrected
        transposition of 446
    transposition of 191, 222
Guanethidine 335
Guide wire 66
Guillain-Barré syndrome 335

H

Haemophilus 225
Hallucination, digitalis-induced 455
Heart 450, 454, 465, 468, 489
    attack 454, 454t
    block 315
    chambers 2f
    muscle, inflammation of 233
    primary tumors of 464
    systemic disease involving 489t
    transplantation 289
Heart disease 438, 442, 444, 461, 474, 478,
        483, 492, 493, 495
    causes of traumatic 472
    hypertensive 259, 264, 265, 268
    mimic 444, 492
    neoplastic 464
    preexisting 445
    pregnancy-induced 445
    prevent 513
    stable ischemic 83
    structural 328
    traumatic 472
    types of 445
Heart failure 8, 201, 259, 272, 276t, 278, 288,
        362, 379, 386, 429, 442, 479, 481,
        482t, 490, 491, 496
    acute 274, 280, 286, 224, 286t
    advanced 280
    care 289
    causes of 279
    chronic 268, 274, 286, 286t
    classification of 278
    cyanosis in 8
    device therapies for 289
    forms of 273
    functional classification for 275
    in infancy, typical features of 201
    interventions for 413
    management 280, 288, 504
    mechanism of 268, 268fc
    nutritional causes of 279
    prevention of 442
    revised staging for 278
    severe 8
    stages of 275, 275t
    therapies, interventions for 288

treatment of 284, 285
with preserved ejection fraction 278, 279, 442, 482
with reduced ejection fraction 274, 278, 279, 288, 482
Heart rate 444
   age-predicted maximum 42
   histogram 38
   maximum 42
Heart-healthy
   diet 500
   oil 511
Hemochromatosis 234
Hemodynamic alterations 207
Hemodynamic changes 160
Hemodynamic classification 275
Hemodynamic consequences 152
Hemoptysis 145, 149
Hemorrhagic complication 302
Hemorrhagic stroke 459
Heparin 187, 301, 364, 369, 424
   before starting 369
   role of 130
   therapeutic level of 368
   unfractionated 368
Hibernating myocardium 62
High-calorie soft drinks 500
High-density lipoprotein 382, 495, 496, 512
   cholesterol 85, 88, 484
   role of 85
High-voltage power lines 350
Hill's sign 176, 177
Holiday heart syndrome 306
Holter monitoring 38, 39, 335
Holter recording 38, 321f
Holt-Oram syndrome 10, 11f
Human immunodeficiency virus 261, 490
Hydralazine 445, 449, 451
Hypercalcemia 380
Hypercholesterolemia 89
Hyperglycemia 380, 439, 440
Hyperhomocysteinemia 451
Hyperinsulinemia 93, 440
   act 88
Hyperkinesia 57
Hypertelorism 10
Hypertension 84, 175, 259, 264, 268, 376, 378, 418, 432, 456, 478, 481, 482, 484, 497, 509
   categories of 260, 260t
   chronic 447
   classification, isolated systolic 264t
   continuum 269
   diagnosis of 262
   drug-induced 265
   essential 265
   isolated systolic 264
   malignant 263
   types of 447

Hyperthyroid 490
Hypertriglyceridemia, treat 382
Hypertrophic cardiomyopathy 7, 226, 233, 235, 238t, 239, 243, 243t, 308, 336, 474
   pharmacologic therapies for 237
Hypertrophic obstructive cardiomyopathy 240, 336, 386, 394
Hyperuricemia 380
Hypocalcemia 312
Hypokinesia 56
Hypotension 291, 332
   postural 332
Hypothyroidism 234
Hypovolemia 237
Hypoxemia, correction of 429
Hypoxia 425
Hysteresis 345

I

Iatrogenic cardiac trauma 472
Idiopathic dilated cardiomyopathy 52t
Idiopathic fibrosis 296
Idioventricular rhythm 296
Iliac artery, left 436f
Implantable cardioverter defibrillator 219, 330, 352
   implantation, limitations of 354
   indications of 354
Implantable loop recorder 38, 40
Incretins 441
Indomethacin 209
Infarction, prevention of 120
Infarct-related artery 410
Infarcts classified 108
Infection 415
   right-sided 224
Infective endocarditis
   acute 224t
   classification of 223b
   classify 223
   clinical hallmark of 224
   peripheral manifestations of 227
   prophylaxis of 230, 230b
   risk factors for 226
   selection of antibiotics for 231b
   treatment of 227, 231
Inhalational anesthetics 462
Inhibited pacing 349
Inodilators 384t
Inotrope 134
   role of 134
Inotropic agents 383
Inoue balloon 413f
Insulin 442
   resistance 440
Interatrial septum 199, 212, 413
Interstitial fibrosis 243

Interventional cardiology 394
Interventional treatments, catheter-based 394
Interventricular septum 36, 239, 240, 429*f*
    components of 200, 200*f*
Intracardiac masses 58
Intracoronary thrombus 129
Intracranial hemorrhage 410, 458
Intravascular ultrasound 59
Intravenous drug abusers 226
Invasive coronary angiography,
    indications of 100
Invasive monitoring
    components of 292
    indications of 133, 291
Ischemia 26, 39, 410, 485
    diagnosis of 25
    episodes 39
Ischemic cardiomyopathy 52, 52*t*, 115
Ischemic chest pain 97
Ischemic heart disease 6, 39, 52, 82, 161, 284, 296, 320, 334, 364, 376, 427, 464, 468, 479, 483, 485, 490
    manifestations of 82
    prevention of 363
    risk stratification for 486
Ischemic mitral regurgitation, stages of 159
Ischemic stroke 459
    reperfusion strategy in 459
Ischemic syndrome, spectrum of 106, 106*fc*
Isosorbide dinitrate 361
Isosorbide-5-mononitrate 361

J

Janeway lesions 227
Jones criteria 139, 141
Jugular pulsation 16*t*
Jugular vein
    external 16
    internal 11, 13*f*
Jugular venous
    pulsation 16
    waves 15*f*
Jugular venous pressure 11, 17, 256, 273, 444
    causes of raised 11
    examination of 12, 13
    normal 424
    waves of 14
Juvenile mitral stenosis 150

K

Kexin type 9 477
Kidney 264
Killip classification 276, 276*t*
Kingella 225
Kissing balloon inflation 409
Kussmaul's sign 17

L

Labetalol 335, 448
Laceration 255
Late systolic peaking 209*f*
L-carnitine 279
Lead polarity 345
Leaflet motion, type of 159
Left anterior
    descending artery 199, 404
    hemiblock 37*f*
Left atrial
    appendage 2*f*
        percutaneous closure of 456
    appendix 306
    enlargement 46, 48, 49*f*, 162, 202
    injection 72
    myxoma 466, 466*f*
Left atrium 196, 197*f*, 199, 202, 212
Left axis deviation 202
Left bundle branch block 26, 27, 34, 35*f*, 36, 36*t*, 282
Left circumflex artery 73*f*
Left heart
    catheters 64, 64*f*
    disease 429
    failure, causes of 274
Left Judkins catheter 65
Left ventricle 1, 2*f*, 48, 49, 202, 212, 222, 239, 355*f*, 404, 429*f*
Left ventricular 24, 114, 119, 162, 178, 197*f*, 199, 239, 243, 275, 276, 279, 336
    dysfunction 394, 502
        diastolic 57, 276
        grading of 56
    ejection fraction 245, 288, 483, 502
    end-diastolic pressure 244, 251
    enlargement 46
    failure 119, 251, 284, 360, 378, 424, 493, 493*t*
        acute 277, 287, 493
        treatment of acute 286
    hypertrophy 26, 28*f*, 36, 212, 239, 268, 311, 336, 419
        common causes of 29
    injections 71
    motion, abnormalities of 57
    outflow tract 236, 239
    systolic function, assessment of 180
    thrombus 58*f*
    volume reduction 289
Lesion
    diffuse 402*f*
    intervention, type C 403
    type A 401*f*
    type B 401, 402*f*
    type C 402*f*
Levocardia 191

Lidocaine 391
Lignocaine 326, 445, 449
   role of 390
Limb ischemia
   acute 433, 434t
   classification, acute 434b
Lipid 443
   abnormalities 497
   profile 381
Lipid-lowering agents 380-382, 382t
Lipoprotein profile 84, 84t
Local coronary vasoconstriction 407
Loeys-Dietz syndrome 474
Low molecular-weight heparin 246, 368, 494
   advantage of 113
Low venous pressure 17
Low-density lipoprotein 85, 382, 432, 496
   cholesterol 85, 511
Lower limb, CT angiography of 436f
Lowering cholesterol, treatment approach for 87
Lung disease 425
Lutembacher's syndrome 193

M

Machine learning 501, 502, 502t, 503, 504
Malar flush 9
Manifold system 67
Marfan's syndrome 10, 175, 474-476
   arachnodactyly in 475f
Marrow procedure 242
Masked hypertension 263
Maternal cardiac risk, predictors of 445, 446b
Mean pressure gradient 154, 173
Mechanical circulatory support devices 293
Mechanical prosthesis 184t
   valve 463
Mechanical valves 184
Medication
   management 504
   perioperative 481
Metabolic cardiac injury 473
Metabolic syndrome 88, 438, 484
   diagnosis of 88t
Metabolism, inborn errors of 474
Metaprolol 266
Metformin 441, 442
Methyldopa 448, 451
Methysergide 255
Metronidazole 371
Mexiletine 391, 451
Microalbuminuria 453
Microvascular dysfunction 284
Milrinone 451
Mini-crush technique 408
MitraClip
   in situ 166f
   system 146, 166, 288

Mitral area 18
Mitral balloon valvuloplasty 144, 157t
Mitral commissurotomy 158t
   closed 157t
Mitral leaflet, anterior 199, 237
Mitral position 185f
Mitral regurgitation 141, 158, 161, 161t, 162, 162t, 164f, 199, 235, 237, 239, 274, 490
   acute 160, 160t
   assessment of severity of 163
   cause of 164
   chronic 160t
   moderate 164f
   severe 163f, 164f
   transcatheter therapies for 166
Mitral stenosis 49f, 58f, 142, 147, 151f, 161, 161t, 162, 162t, 179, 193, 195t, 272
   assessment of 153
   categories of 149
   causes of 147
   drug therapy in 155
   during pregnancy, risk of 446
   features of 149t
   grades of severity of 147, 154t
   interventions for 305
   natural course of 148
   radiologic findings of 151
   severe 150, 154, 154f
   stages of 147
   with atrial fibrillation, treatment of 155
Mitral valve 2f, 137, 199, 237, 239, 253
   disease 142, 194
   prolapse 308, 490
   replacement 144, 156
Mitral valvotomy 156
   closed 156-158
   open 156, 158
Mitral valvular diseases 49, 148
M-mode echo 151, 173, 241f, 466
Moderate-degree endurance exercise 513
Molecular medicine 476
Molecular therapies 476
Monoclonal antibody 465
Monorail balloon 398
Müller's sign 177
Multifocal atrial tachycardia 296, 299
Multifocal ventricular ectopics 40f
Multivessel disease 405, 406
Mural infections 224
Murmur 19, 416
   diagnosis of 20
   early
      diastolic 178, 217
      systolic 178
   ejection systolic 170
   etiologically 19
   intensity of 20

mid-diastolic 148, 194, 202
  quality and configuration of 20
  timing of 20
  two distinct systolic 171
Muscular dystrophy 234
Mustard/Senning operations 222
Myeloproliferative diseases 425
Myocardial damage 234
Myocardial depression 472
Myocardial disease 329
Myocardial failure synonymous 272
Myocardial infarction 7, 24, 26, 36, 55, 58*f*,
      103, 111, 112, 114, 248, 251, 259,
      264, 268, 275, 284, 307, 311, 336,
      373, 392, 404, 405, 418, 419, 468,
      481, 484, 486, 495, 503
  acute 27, 33, 106, 107, 125, 125*t*, 127, 250*t*,
      251, 268, 275, 290, 334, 341, 360, 363,
      419, 419*t*, 423, 423*t*, 454, 480, 486
  anterior wall 114, 114*t*, 117*f*
  cause of 470
  complications of acute 480
  development of 115
  diagnosis of acute 25, 119
  inferior wall 114*t*
  pain of 7*t*
  perioperative 461*b*
  revised cutoffs of 498*t*
  time course of 108*f*
Myocardial ischemia 55
Myocardial mapping 357
Myocardial perfusion 62*f*
  imaging 52, 60
      indications of 61
Myocardial reperfusion 127
Myocardial toxicity, mechanism of 470
Myocardial viability 62
Myocarditis 233, 234
  causes of 233
  etiology of 233*b*
Myocardium 51, 94, 127, 233
  diseases of 233
Myocyte apoptosis 243
Myxedema 9
Myxoma 466
  presentation of 466

N

Nafcillin 231
Narcotic anesthetic 463
Nateglinide 441
Natriuretic peptide, B-type 279, 287
Nausea 388
Neck
  anatomy 13*f*
  vein 14, 16
      examination of 11

Neisseria species 231
Neoplastic diseases 464
Nephropathy, contrast-induced 453
Neurogenic pulmonary edema 455
Neurogenic syncope 333, 334*t*
Nicotine replacement therapy 513
Nicotinic acid 381, 451
Nifedipine, role of 378
Nitrate 103, 359
  preparations 361
  therapy 359
      causes of failure of 360
      tolerance, development of 360
Nitroglycerine 134, 359, 361
Nocturnal angina 95
Noncompliant balloon 398
Noncoronary angioplasty 394
Nonglycosides 383
Nonionizing radiation techniques 45
Nonstatin therapy 87
Non-ST-elevation myocardial
      infarction 109, 378
Nonsteroidal anti-inflammatory drug 302, 371
Non-ST-segment elevation 479
  myocardial infarction 106, 109, 110*f*
Nonvitamin K 303
  oral anticoagulants, position of 303
Noradrenaline 293
Norepinephrine 384
Nuclear cardiology 60
Nutritional deficiency 236

O

Obesity 90, 484
  paradox 511
Obstructive cardiac lesions 334
Occlusive pulmonary vascular disease 422
Omega-3 fatty acids 512
Omeprazole 371
Optical coherence tomography 60
Oral vasodilator, long-term 428
Organophosphorus compound poisoning,
      cardiac manifestations of 471
Orthopnea 4, 5
Orthostatic hypotension 335
Osler nodes 227
Ostium
  primum defect 192, 197, 197*f*
  secundum defect 192, 193
Oximetry method 70
Oxygen 71, 71*t*

P

P wave 297*f*
Pacemaker 337
  battery failure, indications of 351
  dual-chamber 338*f*

function, environmental factors
    influence 350
  generator, components of 337
  inhibited 346*f*
  mediated tachycardia 346
  programmability of 345
  single-chamber 338*f*
  syndrome 346
  types of 338, 338*b*
  unipolar 339
  units
    coded 338
    indications of used 347
Paclitaxel 465
Palliative care 482
Palpitation 6, 145
Paradox, prevention 509
Paradoxical embolism 455
Parasternal area, lower left 18
Parasternal long-axis view 57
Parasternal short-axis view 57
Parenteral anticoagulants 368
Parkinsonism 335
Paroxysmal atrial tachycardia 299
Paroxysmal nocturnal dyspnea 4, 5
Paroxysmal supraventricular tachycardia 392
  types of 297
Partial anomalous pulmonary venous
    connection 194, 199
  drainage 194
Patent ductus arteriosus 48, 70, 207, 208, 212, 226, 415
  closure of 210
Patent foramen ovale 195
Pathological hypertrophy 243, 243*t*
Patient-related factors 404
Penicillin 140
  G 231
Penicillin-resistant streptococci 231
Pentalogy of Fallot 194
Percutaneous balloon
  pericardiotomy 257
  valvuloplasty 412
Percutaneous coronary intervention 59, 103, 104, 109, 122*f*, 395, 404, 450, 456, 462, 487
  current expectations of 400
  indications of 121
  limitations of 404
  types of 126
Percutaneous old balloon angioplasty 396
Percutaneous transluminal coronary
    angioplasty 131, 405
  indications for 405
Percutaneous transseptal myectomy 242
Percutaneous valvuloplasty 456
Perfusion defects, types of 61
Pericardial constriction 255*f*

Pericardial diseases 248
Pericardial effusion
  causes of 465
  classify 249
  diagnosis of 252
  large 252*f*, 253*f*
  quantify 249
  radiologic features of 252
Pericardiocentesis
  complications of 254
  indications of 254
Pericarditis 7, 248, 250, 250*t*
  causes of 248
  classification of 248*b*
Pericardium 248
Perioperative cardiovascular risk 461
Peripartum cardiomyopathy 236
  development of 447
  prognosis of 447
Peripheral arterial disease 432, 435, 480
  classify 433
  clinical significance of 433
  diagnosis of 435, 436
  interventions for 437
  risk factors for 432
  stages of 433*b*
Peripheral vascular diseases 432, 510
Permanent pacemaker 340
  generator 340*f*, 340*t*
  implantation, subclavian puncture for 343*f*
Permanent pacing, indications of 342
Persistent ductus arteriosus 188, 207, 210
  complications of 209
  differential diagnosis of 208
  helping closure of 207
  medical management of 209
  types of 207
Persistent ductus sinus 210*t*
Persistent rupture sinus 210*t*
Petechiae 227
Pharmacoinvasive therapy, utility of 128
Pharmacologic agents 233, 330
Phenylbutazone 371
Phenytoin 391
Phlegmasia
  alba dolens 435
  cerulea dolens 435
Phosphate 279
Phosphodiesterase inhibitors 384, 427, 430
Physiological hypertrophy 243, 243*t*
Physiological pacing 350
Pioglitazone 441
Plasma glucose, fasting 438
Plasminogen activator inhibitor-1 373, 495
Platelets, unique features of 365
Pleural effusion 283
  left-sided 253
Pliable mitral leaflets, signs of 150

Pollution
  indoor 469
  outdoor 469
Polycythemia 428
Polydactyly 11*f*
Polydipsia 438
Polymorphic ventricular tachycardia 471
Polyuria 438
Poor renal perfusion 379
Popliteal artery, right 436*f*
Populations 141
Positive inotropic effect 385
Positron emission tomography 52
Postcapillary pulmonary hypertension 426
Postmyocardial infarction 363
Potency of tablets, loss of 360
Prasugrel 365
Precapillary pulmonary hypertension 426
Preeclampsia 447
Pre-existing mural thrombus,
    propagation of 407
Pregnancy 274, 363, 444
  antihypertensives used in 448
  effect of 445
  physical signs in 444
Presyncope 237
Primary percutaneous coronary intervention
    125, 125*t*, 127, 410, 411
  indications of 412
Primary pulmonary
  arterial hypertension 426
  hypertension 427
Primordial prevention 509
Primum defect 198*t*
Prinzmetal's angina 364
Proarrhythmia 314
Procainamide 391, 451
Propafenone 309
Prophylaxis, secondary 140*b*
Propofol intravenous 463
Propranolol 326, 362, 391
Proprotein convertase subtilisin 477
Prostaglandin 207
  inhibitors 209
Prosthetic valve 184, 448
  diseases 183
  dysfunction 175
  types of 183
Provisional stenting 408
Proximal optimization technique 409
Pseudoinfarction 27
Pseudomonas aeruginosa 231
P-synchronous pacing 348
Pulmonary areas 18
Pulmonary arterial hypertension 202, 425, 426
  echocardiographic features of 426
  sign of 151

Pulmonary arterial pressure 57
Pulmonary artery 2*f*, 48, 70, 71, 196, 212,
    222, 421
  diseases of 422
  enlargement 46
Pulmonary balloon valvuloplasty 144, 213*f*
Pulmonary capillary 48
  hypertension, sign of 151
  pressure 276
  wedge pressure 244, 276
Pulmonary circulation 421
  peculiarities of 421
Pulmonary edema 277, 277*f*, 360
  X-ray of 47
Pulmonary embolism 6, 287, 421, 423, 425,
    425*b*, 490
  classification of 423*b*
  diagnosis of 423
  subsequent development of 424
Pulmonary heart diseases 421
Pulmonary hemosiderosis 50*f*
Pulmonary hypertension 7, 162, 194, 196,
    212, 421, 422, 425, 426, 428
  causes of 426
  common causes of 426
  radiologic features of 47
Pulmonary regurgitation 70, 422
Pulmonary stenosis 19, 71, 194, 212, 213, 217,
    217*f*, 336, 422
  isolated 216*t*, 217
  mild 188
  signs of severe 212
  treatment of 213
Pulmonary valvotomy 214
Pulmonary valvuloplasty 190
Pulmonary vascular disease, severe 199
Pulmonary vasodilators 430
Pulmonary veins 47, 421
Pulmonary veno-occlusive disease 202
Pulmonary venous hypertension,
    sign of 151
Pulse, causes of irregular 296
Pulsed-wave Doppler 164, 174, 181
Pulseless electrical activity 321, 327
Pulsus
  paradoxus 249, 251
    causes of 251
  parvus et tardus 170

Q

Q wave, causes of 27
QT syndrome
  long 91, 296, 312, 328
  short 328
Quincke's pulse 177
Quinidine 391

R

Radiation therapy 465
Radiofrequency ablation 313
Rapid Y descent 15
Rastelli operation 222
Recombinant tissue plasminogen
    activator 109, 454
Re-entrant tachycardia,
    atrioventricular 298, 308
    nodal 297, 297f, 313
Regurgitation, effect of 180
Renal angiography, indications of 79
Renal denervation therapy 394
Renal diseases 450
Renal failure 452
Renal transplant patient 270
Renin-angiotensin
    aldosterone 451
        system 375
    system 267, 287, 288
Reperfusion injuries 374
Respiration, behaviors with 20
Respiratory disorders 422
Respiratory distress 493, 493t
Respiratory tract infection 284
Restenosis 404
Restrictive cardiomyopathy 235, 244, 244t
Retroplacental bleeding 187
Revascularization
    incomplete 407
    procedures, mode of 403
Rheumatic carditis 138t
Rheumatic fever 136, 139, 140b, 141, 147, 150,
        159, 234
    acute 136, 139, 175
    bed rest in 142t
    diagnosis of 138
    diagnostic criteria of 139b
    prevalence of 136
    prophylaxis 140
    secondary prevention of 140
    unique features of 137
Rheumatic heart disease 139, 159, 223, 497
    chronic 136, 142
    prevalence of 136
Rheumatic mitral stenosis 144
Rheumatic valvular disease,
        management of 146, 146b
Rheumatoid arthritis 235, 489
Rhythm
    control of 301
    strips 39
Rib notching 417
Rifampicin 231
Right atrial
    enlargement 46, 212
    injection 71

Right atrium 2f, 71, 192f, 196, 197f, 212, 244,
        256, 338, 355f
    diastolic collapse of 254f
Right axis deviation 199
Right bundle branch block 27, 34, 35f, 36, 36t,
        37, 37f, 37t, 199, 212, 311, 342
Right heart
    catheters 63, 64
    failure 157, 490
        causes of 274, 275
Right ventricle 1, 2f, 48, 49, 71, 73f, 202, 212,
        217, 222, 338, 355f
    diastolic collapse of 254f
    disorder of 273
Right ventricular 114, 119, 196, 197f, 429f
    end-diastolic pressure 244
    enlargement 46
    failure 215
    hypertrophy 2, 30f, 36, 37, 37t, 202, 212
        causes of 31
        diagnosis of 30
    infarction 115, 117t
    injection 71
    outflow tract 189
        obstruction 204
Rivaroxaban 372
Rosiglitazone 441
Roth spot 227
Rule of Halves 269
Rupture sinus of Valsalva aneurysm 210

S

Sarcoidosis 234, 236, 425
Sarcopenic adiposity 510
Secundum atrial septal defect 197f, 198
Secundum defect 198t
Sedentary behavior 484
Seldinger technique 65
Selenium 279
Semiology 150
Septal myotomy-myomectomy 242
Sex hormones 265
Shock 291, 332
Shocking coil 353f
Shunt 70
    anomalies 48, 48t, 211t
        different 211
    classification of 70b
    detected 70
Shy–Drager syndrome 335
Sibutramine 266
Sick sinus syndrome 315, 315f, 342
    development of 350
Silent ischemia 39
Silent killer 263
Silent mitral stenosis 150
Sinoatrial node 73f

Sinus
    bradycardia 349
    of Valsalva aneurysm 210
    rhythm 318*f*, 321*f*, 386
    tachycardia, inappropriate 296
    venosus 193
        defect 192
Situs inversus 191
Situs solitus 191
Skeletal deformity 194
Sleep-disordered breathing 421, 430
    mechanism of 430
Small molecule tyrosine kinase inhibitors 465
Smoking 432, 484
    cessation program 512
Sodium nitroprusside 286
Sodium-glucose cotransporter-2 280
    inhibitors, indications of 442
Sotalol 390, 392
Spinal anesthesia 463
Spinal arteries, anterior 417
Splinter hemorrhage 227
Spontaneous abortion 187
Stable angina 95, 101
    chronic 102, 405, 405*b*
    graded 96
    outline treatment of 102
Staphylococcus 231
Starr-Edwards metallic prosthesis 185*f*
Statins 499
ST-elevation myocardial infarction 364, 411
Stem cell therapy 477
Stenosis accurately, degree of 174
Stent 396, 398
    deployment 396
    implantation of 395
    indications of 399
    platform, advances in 395
Streptococcus viridans 228, 231
Streptokinase 114, 115, 373, 419
Stress
    cardiovascular magnetic resonance 100
    echo 54, 58, 100
    single photon emission computed
        tomography 100
    techniques 330
    test result, abnormal 74
    testing 101
Stroke 259, 430, 454, 454*t*, 478, 480
    acute 266
    cause of 458
    hypertensive developed 268
    infarctive 458
    management 460
    patients 458
    risk 304
Structural heart disease, intervention of 412

ST-segment
    depression 25
    elevation 23*t*
        causes of 23
ST-segment elevation myocardial
        infarction 82, 106, 109, 109*t*,
        120*f*, 127*t*, 411*t*, 412
    atypical features of 124
    reperfusion of 127, 411
Stunned myocardium 62
Submaximal exercise test 42
Sudden cardiac death 83, 172, 178, 237, 239,
        320, 327, 470, 505
    causes of 328, 329
    etiologies of 327
    management of 337
    prevent 330, 363
    risk factors for 329
    survivors of 329
Sudden death 239, 456
    increased risk of 239*b*
    predictors of 239
Sulfamethoxazole 371
Sulfinpyrazone 371
Supraventricular arrhythmias 295
    cardioversion of 325
Supraventricular tachycardia 306, 309, 311,
        311*t*, 324, 356, 378, 392
    ablation 297*f*, 356*f*
    acute 386
Surgery 214, 461
Surgical aortic valve replacement 171, 280
Surgical therapy 331
Sympathomimetic amines 293, 386
Syncope 297, 255, 332, 333, 333*t*, 335, 480
    causes of 334
    episodes of 335
    investigations in 335*t*
Syndrome X 93
Syntax scoring system 78
Syphilitic aortitis 175
Systemic disease 489
Systemic hypertension 470
Systemic inflammation 440
Systemic lupus erythematosus 235, 490
Systemic sclerosis 489
Systemic steroids 265
Systolic anterior motion 237, 241

T

Tachyarrhythmias 295, 309, 332, 333
    mechanism of 295
Tachycardia
    broad complex 310
    detect 353
    duration of 297
    narrow complex 298
    wide complex 32

Takayasu's aortitis 415
Takotsubo cardiomyopathy 490
Takotsubo syndrome 245
    apical ballooning in 246f
Tamoxifen 465
Target organ damage 264
Technetium 61
Temporary pacemaker 63, 340
    generators 340f, 340t
Temporary pacing, indications for 341
Ten volt test 344
Tendon xanthoma 10f
Tenecteplase
    advantages of 372
    disadvantages of 372
Tension pneumothorax 292
Terazosin 335
Tetralogy of Fallot 70, 194, 214, 216t, 217, 217f, 217t, 219, 222, 229, 336
    aortic changes in 216
    complications of 215
    differ 216
    interventions for 219
    physical signs of 215
    radiologic features of 217
Thallium 61
Therapeutic lifestyle changes 511
    prevention of 511b
Thiamine deficiency 236, 279
Thiazides 379
Thienopyridine 365, 405
Three-dimensional echo 54
Thromboembolic phenomena 145, 301
Thromboembolic prevention, risk stratification for 302
Thromboembolism, prevent 301
Thrombolysis 120f, 373
    contraindication for 131
    in stroke, contraindications of 459
Thrombolytic administration, time frame for 131fc
Thrombolytic agents 115, 372
Thrombolytic therapy 120, 121, 125, 125t, 126
    benefit of 120
    contraindications of 121
    reverse 132
Thrombotic cardiovascular disease 365
Thromboxane 365
Thrombus 58, 407
Thump version 324
Thyroid-stimulating hormone 490
Thyrotoxicosis 274
Ticagrelor 365
Tissue-Doppler imaging 54
Tissue-type plasminogen activator 373
Tobacco use 498
Torsades de pointes 312, 313f

Total anomalous pulmonary venous connection 199
Total peripheral resistance 428
Toxic agents 233
Toxins 234, 468
Trans fat, role of 512
Transaortic valve implantation 175
Transcatheter
    aortic valve replacement 171, 280
    device 206
    heart valves 171
    mitral valve
        repair 166
        replacement 166
    therapies 190
Transcutaneous electric nerve stimulation 351
Transesophageal echo 53, 197, 420
Transient Q 27
Transradial approach, complications of 78
Transradial catheterization, advantages of 77
Transthoracic echocardiography 420
Traube's sign 177
Treadmill test 497
Tricuspid area 18
Tricuspid regurgitation 188
    causes of 183
Tricuspid valve 2f, 11, 192f, 490
    disease 183
    replacement 183
Triggered pacing 349
Triglyceride 382
Trimethoprim 371
Troponin 113, 245
Tubercular pericardial effusion 257
Tubercular pericarditis 255f
Turner syndrome 10
T-wave inversions, patterns of 24
Two-dimensional echo 151, 152, 152f
Two-stent strategy 408
Tyrosine kinase inhibitors 465

U

Unstable angina 106, 264, 360, 361
    treatment of 113
Upper lobe diversion 49, 282
Uremia 236
Urinary tract infection 24

V

V waves, prominent 15
Valve, type of 144
Valvotomy, indications of 157
Valvular aortic stenosis, stages of 169
Valvular diseases 6, 179, 474, 478
    clinical presentation of 145b
Valvular dysfunction 167

Valvular heart disease 74, 136, 144, 327, 480
    classification 144b
Valvular lesion 180
Valvular regurgitation 189, 446
Valvular stenosis 394
Vancomycin 230
Variant angina 95
Vascular remodeling 92
Vascular sheath
    and manifold 67f
    use of 66
Vasodilators 430
    clinical uses of 376
    role of 133, 285
Vegetation 225
Veins, diseases of 434
Vena cava
    inferior 2f, 192f, 222, 256
    superior 2f, 71, 192f
Venous graft 104
Venous pressure, bedside
    measurement of 14f
Venous thromboembolism 422, 425, 480
    risk factors 422, 422b
Venous thrombus 435, 435t
Venous waves 15
Ventricular arrhythmias 74, 295
Ventricular asystole 321
Ventricular contraction, premature 114
Ventricular extrasystoles 296
Ventricular fibrillation 114, 311, 312f, 321, 322f, 326, 327, 333, 392
Ventricular inhibited pacing 349f
Ventricular premature complexes, clinical
    significance of 312
Ventricular remodeling 123
Ventricular septal defect 48, 70, 72, 188, 191, 200, 202, 205, 206, 212, 222, 394
    classify 200
    complications of 203
    different degrees of 201
    differential diagnosis of 203
    perimembranous 204f
    treatment for 205
    types of 204
Ventricular septal rupture 291

Ventricular tachycardia 31, 114, 239, 310, 310f, 311, 311t, 320, 321, 322f, 333, 336, 347, 363, 392
Ventricular triggered pacing 349f
Ventriculoarterial discordance 221
Verapamil 309, 341, 392
Vertigo 388
Viral myocarditis 234
Visceral fat deposition,
    clinical importance of 510
Vitamin K antagonist 372
Voice change detection 504
Vomiting 388
Vulnerable myocardium 90
Vulnerable plaque 90

W

Waist circumference 88, 498, 510
Warfarin 301, 302, 305, 364, 369, 371t, 444, 449
    therapy 369, 370
        risk of bleeding during 371
Water bottle appearance 221
Water-hammer pulse 177
Weight loss, unexplained 438
White coat 263
Williams syndrome 9
Wolff-Parkinson-White syndrome 32, 298, 306, 307f, 308, 308f, 309, 357, 392
    prognosis of 308
Wolff-Parkinson-White tachycardias 313
Women's ischemia syndrome evaluation 485

X

Xanthelasma 10, 10f

Y

Yentl syndrome 485
Yoga 513
Young myocardial infarction, VIRGO
    classification for 486t

Z

Zygote 474